CRC SERIES IN NUTRITION AND FOOD

Editor-in-Chief

Miloslav Rechcigl, Jr.

Handbook of Nutritive Value for Processed Food
Volume I: Food for Human Use
Volume II: Animal Feedstuffs

Handbook of Nutritional Requirements in a Functional Context
Volume I: Development and Conditions of Physiologic Stress
Volume II: Hematopoiesis, Metabolic Function, and Resistance to Physical Stress

Handbook of Agricultural Productivity
Volume I: Plant Productivity
Volume II: Animal Productivity

CRC Handbook of Nutritional Requirements in a Functional Context

Volume II
Hematopoiesis, Metabolic Function, and Resistance to Physical Stress

Editor

Miloslav Rechcigl, Jr.

Nutrition Advisor and Chief
Research and Methodology Division
Agency for International Development
U.S. International Development Cooperation Agency
Washington, D.C.

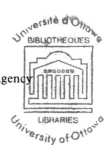

CRC Series in Nutrition and Food
Editor-in-Chief
Miloslav Rechcigl, Jr.

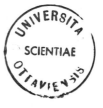

CRC Press, Inc.
Boca Raton, Florida

Library of Congress Cataloging in Publication Data

Main entry under title:

Handbook of nutritional requirements in a functional
context.

(CRC series in nutrition and food)
Bibliography: p.
Includes index.
CONTENTS: v. 1. Development and conditions of
physiological stress.—v. 2. Hematopoiesis, metabolic
function, and resistance to physical stress.
1. Stress (Physiology)—Nutritional aspects—Hand-
books, manuals, etc. I. Rechcigl, Miloslav.
II. Series. [DNLM: 1. Nutrition. QU145 H236]
QP82.2.S8H36   599.01   80-19981
ISBN 0-8493-3956-1 (v. 1.)
ISBN 0-8493-3958-8 (v. 2)

This book represents information obtained from authentic and highly regarded sources. Reprinted material is quoted with permission, and sources are indicated. A wide variety of references are listed. Every
reasonable effort has been made to give reliable data and information, but the author and the publisher
cannot assume responsibility for the validity of all materials or for the consequences of their use.

Direct all inquiries to CRC Press, Inc., 2000 N.W. 24th Street, Boca Raton, Florida 33431.

International Standard Book Number 0-8493-3956-1 (Volume I)
International Standard Book Number 0-8493-3958-8 (Volume II)

Library of Congress Card Number 80-19981
Printed in the United States

PREFACE
CRC SERIES IN NUTRITION AND FOOD

Nutrition means different things to different people, and no other field of endeavor crosses the boundaries of so many different disciplines and abounds with such diverse dimensions. The growth of the field of nutrition, particularly in the last 2 decades, has been phenomenal, the nutritional data being scattered literally in thousands and thousands of not always accessible periodicals and monographs, many of which, furthermore, are not normally identified with nutrition.

To remedy this situation, we have undertaken an ambitious and monumental task of assembling in one publication all the critical data relevant in the field of nutrition.

The *CRC Series in Nutrition and Food* is intended to serve as a ready reference source of current information on experimental and applied human, animal, microbial, and plant nutrition presented in concise tabular, graphical, or narrative form and indexed for ease of use. It is hoped that this projected open-ended multivolume compendium will become for the nutritionist what the *CRC Handbook of Chemistry and Physics* has become for the chemist and physicist.

Apart from supplying specific data, the comprehensive, interdisciplinary, and comparative nature of the *CRC Series in Nutrition and Food* will provide the user with an easy overview of the state of the art, pinpointing the gaps in nutritional knowledge and providing a basis for further research. In addition, the series will enable the researcher to analyze the data in various living systems for commonality or basic differences. On the other hand, an applied scientist or technician will be afforded the opportunity of evaluating a given problem and its solutions from the broadest possible point of view, including the aspects of agronomy, crop science, animal husbandry, aquaculture and fisheries, veterinary medicine, clinical medicine, pathology, parasitology, toxicology, pharmacology, therapeutics, dietetics, food science and technology, physiology, zoology, botany, biochemistry, developmental and cell biology, microbiology, sanitation, pest control, economics, marketing, sociology, anthropology, natural resources, ecology, environmental science, population, law politics, nutritional and food methodology, and others.

To make more facile use of the series, the publication has been organized into separate handbooks of one or more volumes each. In this manner the particular sections of the series can be continuously updated by publishing additional volumes of new data as they become available.

The Editor wishes to thank the numerous contributors many of whom have undertaken their assignment in pioneering spirit, and the Advisory Board members for their continuous counsel and cooperation. Last but not least, he wishes to express his sincere appreciation to the members of the CRC editorial and production staffs, particularly President Bernard J. Starkoff, Earl Starkoff, Sandy Pearlman, Pamela Woodcock, Lisa Levine Eggenberger, John Hunter, and Amy G. Skallerup for their encouragement and support.

We invite comments and criticism regarding format and selection of subject matter, as well as specific suggestions for new data which might be included in subsequent editions. We should also appreciate it if the readers would bring to the attention of the Editor any errors or omissions that might appear in the publication.

Miloslav Rechcigl, Jr.
Editor-in-Chief

PREFACE
HANDBOOK OF NUTRITIONAL REQUIREMENTS
IN A FUNCTIONAL CONTEXT

Nutritional requirements of animal organisms, including those of human beings, vary depending on the physiological state of the organisms. This accounts for vulnerability to malnutrition among certain population groups such as pregnant and nursing women, young infants, children, the aged, and the sick.

Adaptation and resistance to specific climate and environmental stresses is also dependent on the availability of specific nutrients in appropriate amounts. There are also subtle differences in the nutritional requirements for specific physiological processes and body functions as there are differences in the requirements for specific nutrients by different tissues during their development.

The purpose of this Handbook is to bring together all the available information on the nutritional requirements of animal organisms for specific processes and functions. This is believed to be the first systematic treatment of nutrition in a functional context. Apart from furnishing specific nutritional data, this Handbook provides a useful framework for a comparative physiologist or biochemist searching for commonality or differences among various biological systems.

THE EDITOR

Miloslav Rechcigl, Jr. is a Nutrition Advisor and Chief of Research and Methodology Division in the Agency for International Development.

He has a B.S. in Biochemistry (1954), a Master of Nutritional Science degree (1955), and a Ph.D. in nutrition, biochemistry, and physiology (1958), all from Cornell University. He was formerly a Research Biochemist in the National Cancer Institute, National Institutes of Health and subsequently served as Special Assistant for Nutrition and Health in the Health Services and Mental Health Administration, U.S. Department of Health, Education and Welfare.

Dr. Rechcigl is a member of some 30 scientific and professional societies, including being a Fellow of the American Association for the Advancement of Science, Fellow of the Washington Academy of Sciences, Fellow of the American Institute of Chemists, and Fellow of the International College of Applied Nutrition. He holds membership in the Cosmos Club, the Honorary Society of Phi Kappa Pi, and the Society of Sigma Xi, and is recipient of numerous honors, including an honorary membership certificate from the International Social Science Honor Society Delta Tau Kappa. In 1969, he was a delegate to the White House Conference on Food, Nutrition, and Health and in 1975 a delegate to the ARPAC Conference on Research to Meet U.S. and World Food Needs. He served as President of the District of Columbia Institute of Chemists and Councillor of the American Institute of Chemists, and currently is a delegate to the Washington Academy of Sciences and a member of the Program Committee of the American Institute of Nutrition.

His bibliography extends over 100 publications including contributions to books, articles in periodicals, and monographs in the fields of nutrition, biochemistry, physiology, pathology, enzymology, molecular biology, agriculture, and international development. Most recently he authored and edited *Nutrition and the World Food Problem* (S. Karger, Basel, 1979), *World Food Problem: a Selective Bibliography of Reviews* (CRC Press, 1975), and *Man, Food and Nutrition: Strategies and Technological Measures for Alleviating the World Food Problem* (CRC Press, 1973) following his earlier pioneering treatise on *Enzyme Synthesis and Degradation in Mammalian Systems* (S. Karger, Basel, 1971), and that on *Microbodies and Related Particles, Morphology, Biochemistry and Physiology* (Academic Press, New York, 1969). Dr. Rechcigl also has initiated a new series on *Comparative Animal Nutrition* and was Associated Editor of *Nutrition Reports International*.

ADVISORY BOARD MEMBERS

CONTRIBUTORS

A. Aschkenasy, M.D., Sc.D.
Centre National de la Recherche
  Scientifique
Laboratoire d'Hematologie
  Nutritionelle
Paris, France

C. H. Barrows, Sc.D.
Section of Comparative Nutrition
Gerontology Research Center
National Institute on Aging
Baltimore City Hospitals
Baltimore, Maryland

T. K. Basu, B.V.Sc., M.S., Ph.D.
Foods and Nutrition Division
Faculty of Home Economics
The University of Alberta
Edmonton, Canada

U. N. Bhuyan, M.D.
Department of Pathology
All-India Institute of Medical Sciences
New Delhi, India

J. G. Brand, Ph.D.
Monell Chemical Senses Center and
  Department of Biochemistry
School of Dental Medicine
University of Pennsylvania
Philadelphia, Pennsylvania

G. A. Campbell, Ph.D.
Protein Research Laboratory
Veterans Administration Medical
  Center
Bronx, New York

R. K. Chandra, M.D.
Department of Pediatrics
University of Newfoundland
St. John's, Newfoundland

J. W. T. Dickerson, Ph.D.
Division of Nutrition and Food Science
Department of Biochemistry
University of Surrey
Guilford, Surrey, England

C. Eckhert, Ph.D.
School of Public Health
Division of Environmental and
  Nutritional Sciences
University of California
Los Angeles, California

V. R. Edgerton, Ph.D.
Brain Research Institute
Department of Kinesiology
University of California
Los Angeles, California

W. P. Faulk, M.D.
Blond McIndoe Centre for
  Transplantation Biology
East Grinstead, Sussex, England

S. Frankova, D.Sc.
Institute of Psychology
Czechoslovak Academy of Sciences
Prague, Czechoslovakia

G. Goldspink, Ph.D., Sc.D., F.R.M.S.
Department of Zoology
University of Hull
Kingston-upon-Hull, Yorkshire
England

K. Y. Guggenheim, M.D.
Department of Nutrition
Hebrew University-Haddasah Medical
  School
Jerusalem, Israel

E. S. E. Hafez, Ph.D.
Departments of Gynecology,
  Obstetrics, and Physiology
School of Medicine
Wayne State University
Detroit, Michigan

H. Hagedorn, Ph.D.
Department of Entomology
Cornell University
Ithaca, New York

R. E. Hammer, B.Sc.
School of Medicine
Wayne State University
Detroit, Michigan

F. X. Hausberger, M.D., Sc.D.
Department of Anatomical Sciences
Temple University
School of Dentistry
Philadelphia, Pennsylvania

W. J. Hayes, Jr., M.D., Ph.D.
Department of Biochemistry
School of Medicine
Vanderbilt University
Nashville, Tennessee

E. Hietanen, M.D.
Department of Physiology
University of Turku
Turku, Finland

O. Heroux, Ph.D.
Division of Applied Biology
National Research Council
Ottawa, Ontario, Canada

L. S. Hurley, Ph.D.
Department of Nutrition
University of California
Davis, California

D. B. Jelliffe, M.P.H.
School of Public Health
University of California
Los Angeles, California

R. E. Johnson, M.D., D.Phil.
Horn of the Moon Enterprises
Montpelier, Vermont

J. J. Jones, M.D.
3 Esplanade
Liverpool, England

J. Kaltenbach, Ph.D.
Department of Biological Sciences
Mount Holyoke College
South Hadley, Massachusetts

M. Kare, Ph.D.
Monell Chemical Senses Center and
  University of Pennsylvania
Philadelphia, Pennsylvania

H. Karunajeewa, Ph.D.
Department of Agriculture
Animal Research Institute
Werribee, Victoria, Australia

G. T. Keusch, M.D.
Division of Geographic Medicine
Tufts University School of Medicine
New England Medical Center Hospital
Boston, Massachusetts

G. C. Kokkonen, B.A.
Section of Comparative Nutrition
Gerontology Research Center
National Institute on Aging
Baltimore City Hospitals
Baltimore, Maryland

O. Koldovsky, M.D., Ph.D.
Department of Pediatrics
University of Arizona Health Sciences
  Center
Tuscon, Arizona

J. LeMagnen, M.D.
College de France
Paris, France

John T. Maher, Ph.D.
Altitude Research Division
U.S. Army Research Institute of
  Environmental Medicine
Natick, Massachusetts

M. Naim, Ph.D.
Faculty of Agriculture
Hebrew University of Jerusalem
Rehovot, Israel

A. E. Needham, D.Sc.
Department of Zoology
Oxford University
Oxford, England

Y. Ohira, Ph.D.
Brain Research Institute
Department of Kinesiology
University of California
Los Angeles, California

A. Ornoy, M.D.
Department of Anatomy and
  Embryology
Hebrew University-Haddasah Medical
  School
Jerusalem, Israel

J. Quarterman, Ph.D., F.R.S.C.,
  C.Chem.
Nutritional Biochemistry Department
Rowett Research Institute
Bucksburn, Aberdeen, Scotland

R. Rajalakshmi, Ph.D.
Department of Biochemistry
M.S. University of Baroda
Baroda, India

J. A. F. Rook, Ph.D., D.Sc.
Agricultural Research Council
London, England

M. L. Ryder, M.Sc., Ph.D., F.I.Biol.
ARC, Animal Breeding Research
  Organisation
Edinburgh, Scotland

I. M. Sharman, Ph.D., F.R.S.C.
Dunn Nutritional Laboratory
University of Cambridge and Medical
  Research Council
Cambridge, England

W. J. Stadelman, Ph.D.
Department of Animal Sciences
Purdue University
West Lafayette, Indiana

N. C. Stickland, Ph.D.
Department of Veterinary Medicine
University of Edinburgh
Edinburgh, Scotland

G. Stirling, M.D.
Department of Pathology
College of Medicine and Allied Sciences
King Abdulaziz University
Jeddah, Saudi Arabia

A. J. H. Van Es, M.D.
Institute for Livestock Feeding and
  Nutrition Research
Lelystad, The Netherlands

M. Vulterinovna, M.D.
Institute of Clinical Experimental
  Medicine
Prague, Czechoslovakia

I. Wolinsky, Ph.D.
Department of Human Development
  and Consumer Sciences
University of Houston
Houston, Texas

D. H. Woollam, M.D., Sc.D.
Department of Anatomy
University of Cambridge
Cambridge, England

DEDICATION

To my inspiring teachers at Cornell University—Harold H. Williams, John K. Loosli, the late Richard H. Barnes, the late Clive M. McCay, and the late Leonard A. Maynard. And to my supportive and beloved family—Eva, Jack, and Karen.

HANDBOOK OF NUTRITIONAL REQUIREMENTS IN A FUNCTIONAL CONTEXT

Volume I

Development and Conditions of Physiological Stress

Differentiation and Development
Development of Specific Tissues
Conditions of Physiological Stress

Volume II

Hematopoiesis, Metabolic Function and Resistance to Physical Stress

Hematopoiesis
Digestion and Endocrine Functions
Chemical Senses
Metabolism of Foreign Substances
Physical Performance and Behavior
Adaptation and Resistance to Environmental Stress

TABLE OF CONTENTS

Volume II

Hematopoiesis

NUTRITION AND ERYTHROPOIESIS

M. Vulterinová

According to recent findings,[1,2] a balanced diet as regards energy and nutrient content contains all substances needed for normal erythropoiesis. Various nutritional factors such as proteins, amino acids, and iron act as building stones and together with other factors participate in the formation of red blood cells and their maturation. Nutritional factors are utilized not only as material for the formation of red cells but also as a source of energy and as a substantial part of activators of enzyme systems for the repletion and function of cells.

Deficiency of blood-forming substances in the organism results either from absolute deficiency in the diet or relative deficiency when the requirements of the organism are increased on physiological grounds such as growth, pregnancy, and lactation and in pathological conditions. Deficiencies are manifested during injury, infection,[2,3] or during major losses due to impaired nutrient utilization as in the case of diseases of the digestive system associated with malabsorption syndrome.[4-6] Commonly recommended low-protein diets during renal failure are deficient as a source of haematopoietic nutritional factors.[7,8]

The complex of the main nutritional factors which cause changes in erythropoiesis in humans and experimental animals whose diets are deficient in these factors includes, above all: iron, vitamin B_{12}, folic acid, protein (individual amino acids), vitamin C, and vitamin E, and, as regards members of the B complex, includes vitamins B_1, B_2, and B_6. Deficiency of the trace elements Cu, Mo, Mg, and Zn also has an adverse effect. Changes in the peripheral blood count and clinical manifestations are typical in some deficiencies of nutritional factors such as iron, vitamin B_{12}, and folic acid. The participation of other nutritional factors is difficult to evaluate from the blood count alone, even with clear-cut anemia, as the morphology in the peripheral blood stream as well as in the bone marrow overlaps and more sensitive biochemical methods must be used to detect the deficiency.

Erythropoietic disorders (disturbances) affect the nutritional factors and the organism at different times. Yet, the first to be exhausted are the erythropoietic reserves of the nutritional factors; the deficit manifests itself clinically later. It is assumed that nutritional anemia develops only when the deficiency of one or several haematopoietic factors persists for some time.

PREVALENCE OF NUTRITIONAL ANEMIA IN THE POPULATION

Nutritional anemia is defined by a drop of hemoglobin to a below-normal level and a reduced content of one or more essential hematopoietic factors. As nutritional anemias are a worldwide problem, efforts have been made to unify the criteria. A group of WHO experts was established which issued instructions outlining basic methodological procedures in population studies. Based on the assembled data, the expert group elaborated and later modified diagnostic criteria of anemia.[9-12] From all studies, it is obvious that the main criterion remains the hemoglobin level, taking into account age, body weight, sex, pregnancy, etc. The lower borderline of hemoglobin levels in different groups is presented in Table 1.

Based on numerous population surveys, the borderlines of hemoglobin levels changed somewhat in recent years to 14% in men and 12.5% in women. In developing countries, severe anemias (including macrocytic anemias) are encountered and, as population studies show, even in parts of the world with no hunger problem mild anemias

Table 1
CRITERIA FOR THE
DIAGNOSIS OF ANEMIA

Lower borderline of hemoglobin
levels

Children aged 6 months to 6 years	11 g%
Children aged 6 to 14 years	12 g%
Adult males	13 g%
Adult females, nonpregnant	12 g%
Adult females, pregnant	11 g%

Note: Hemoglobin levels are lower than the
figures stated above. The values given
are in g/100 ml.

predominate, caused by deficiency of iron, folic acid, and vitamin B_{12}. Less frequently, this anemia is caused by protein deficiency. Anemia is encountered mainly in women during pregnancy; in different countries, this population ranges from 21 to 80%. Even higher is the incidence of iron deficiency without anemia (defined by the plasma iron level and transferrin saturation), i.e., in 40 to 99%.[10] A combined deficiency of iron and folic acid is frequently found in pregnancy.[12,13] It is known that iron deficiency can mask concomitant morphological abnormalities caused by folic acid or vitamin B_{12} deficiency.[14,15] Iron deficiency is, however, more frequently associated with a drop of the folic acid level.

The mechanism of a reduction of the folic acid level remains obscure. Toskes et al.[16] provided evidence that induced nutritional iron deficiency in rats leads to a decline of folic acid which improves after iron administration.

Less frequently, anemias are observed in children, women in their child-bearing years and during lactation, and in men and women above 65 years of age.[17,18] In all categories, iron deficiency prevails. The second place is held by folate deficiency[19-21] although other nutritional factors such as vitamin B_{12} deficiency[22] and protein deficiency[23,24] also play a part.

IRON DEFICIENCY

Iron is one of the substances known for the longest time to be essential for hematopoiesis. Dietary deficiency of iron and impaired absorption and increased losses of this substance lead to a negative iron balance. The iron content in an adequate diet varies from 15 to 18 mg. The amount absorbed depends on the type of foodstuffs, their combination, and the needs of the organism. Many investigations have provided evidence of higher iron absorption from a diet in which animal proteins predominate (the utilization being 15 to 20%), while from vegetables only 5 to 10% iron is absorbed. Layrisse and Martinez-Torres[25] compared iron absorption in healthy subjects and blood donors from various sources. The results of their numerous investigations are presented in Figure 1.

It may be assumed that a vegetarian diet in some populations and a reduced iron absorption from these sources contribute to the development of anemia and iron deficiency. Factors which block iron absorption include oxalates, phosphates, and phytate, in part, as they bind ionized iron and reduce its solubility.[26-29] This finding could explain the poorer iron absorption from vegetables.

In addition to animal protein, other supporting dietary factors which enhance absorption of ionized iron[30,31] include some proteins in legumes such as black beans,[32]

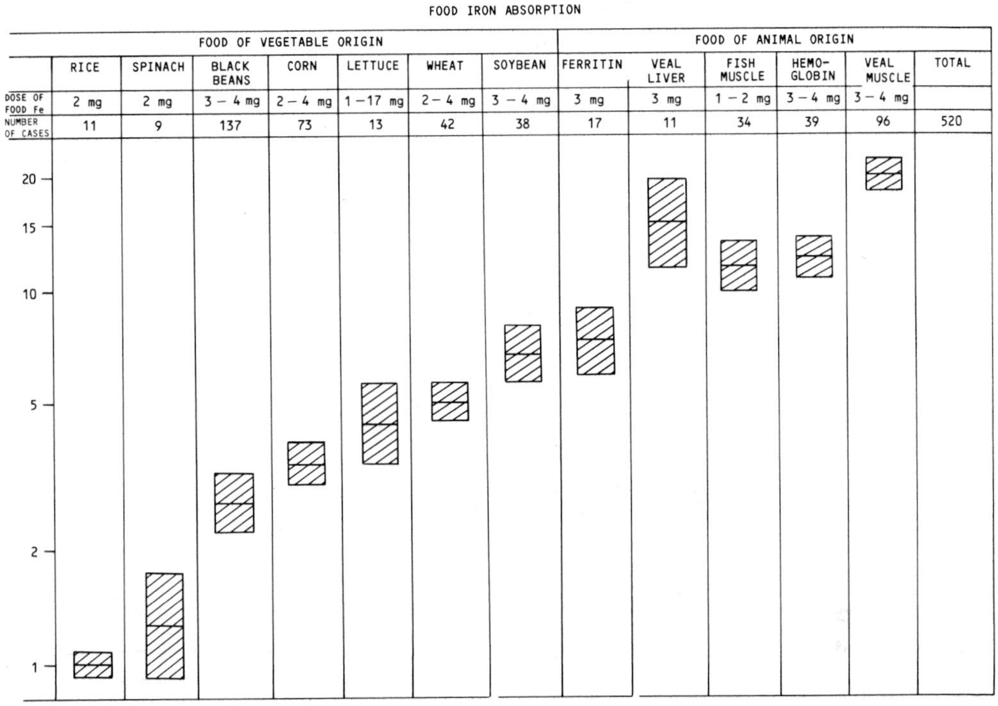

FOOD IRON ABSORPTION

	FOOD OF VEGETABLE ORIGIN							FOOD OF ANIMAL ORIGIN					
	RICE	SPINACH	BLACK BEANS	CORN	LETTUCE	WHEAT	SOYBEAN	FERRITIN	VEAL LIVER	FISH MUSCLE	HEMO-GLOBIN	VEAL MUSCLE	TOTAL
DOSE OF FOOD Fe	2 mg	2 mg	3 — 4 mg	2 — 4 mg	1 —17 mg	2 — 4 mg	3 — 4 mg	3 mg	3 mg	1 — 2 mg	3 — 4 mg	3 — 4 mg	
NUMBER OF CASES	11	9	137	73	13	42	38	17	11	34	39	96	520

FIGURE 1. Iron absorption by adults from a range of foods. The bars represent the mean absorptions and standard errors calculated from the logarithms of the percentage absorptions. Standardized methodology was used for all determinations. (From Layrisse, M. and Martinez-Torres, C., *Progress in Haematology*, Vol. 7, Brown, E. B. and Moore, C. V., Eds., Grune and Stratton, New York, 1971, 137—160. With permission.)

ascorbic acid, and some sugars. A review by Botwell and Finch[33] gives an overall idea of the problem of iron absorption.

Another factor in the control of iron absorption is the role played by iron-storing organs. Many investigations using labeled iron and assessing the absorption by means of a whole-body counter draw attention to the greater absorption in women (22.9%) than in men (16.7%). In chronic blood losses, the absorption may be as high as 54 to 74% of the administered iron.[34-37]

One of the indicators of iron deficiency in the organism is its enhanced absorption. According to Heinrich and Haussmann,[37,38] the prelatent stage is characterized by a reduction of reserves in bone marrow. Provided that absorption from gastrointestinal pathways is not impaired, the organism tries to compensate for iron deficiency by greater absorption. The latent deficiency is manifested later by a decline of the plasma iron level and a rise of the total iron-binding capacity (TIBC) (an indirect indicator of transferrin).

In the subsequent stage there follows a decline of hemoglobin in red cells, a reduction of protoporphyrin in erythrocytes, and a reduced transferrin saturation. Only later do typical changes in the blood count occur such as hypochromasia, microcytosis and clinical maifestations of anemia. Among clinical symptoms, the following predominate: fatigue, headache, vertigo, palpitations, inability to concentrate, anorexia, angular stomititis, painful fissures of the lips, brittle nails, and other organic changes, A more sensitive method which can detect an early deficiency is assessment of stores in marrow, of plasma iron level, and of the total binding capacity (TIBC).

When assessing iron stores in bone marrow, histochemical detection of iron can be used, based on staining of smears with Berlin blue (called Perls reaction). It was introduced into clinical practice by Rath and Finch in 1948.[39] This method, slightly modified, is used even at present by many authors.[36,40-42] When well stained, the preparations can be evaluated according to Weinfeld's scale.[41,43]

From our experience, and according to Hedenberg,[45,46] assessment of iron stores by means of the desferal CIBA test (Desferrioxamine) as a screening test[44] is suited only as an orientation test for the determination of iron deficit.

FOLIC ACID FOLATE DEFICIENCY

Folic acid deficiency is associated with macrocytic anemia in the peripheral blood stream and megaloblastic bone marrow. This morphological appearance resembles vitamin B_{12} deficiency; for the differential diagnosis, further laboratory examinations are needed. A reliable diagnostic method for the early detection of folic acid deficiency is the estimation of serum and red cell levels. For the assessment of folate reserves in tissues, the red cell level reflects reserves better than the amount assessed in serum.[47,48] The primary organ of folate reserves is the liver which, in the case of dietary folate deficiency, is able to meet the needs of the organism for approximately 2 months, and only after that time do deficiency signs develop. Folic acid (pferogeglutamic) is present in food of plant and animal origin. Rich sources of this vitamin are yeast, liver, nuts, spinach, asparagus, and fresh vegetables. The minimum daily requirement of folates (as pteroylglutamic acid) for an adult is 50 to 100 μg (about 80% of this amount is absorbed). The daily requirement may increase as much as ten times under different physiological and pathological conditions (pregnancy, adolescence, hemolytic anemia, infection). A negative folate balance develops if the increased requirements are not met from the diet or when the losses are increased due to impaired absorption.

Folic acid deficiency is encountered in population surveys as well as in clinical studies. Folates are absorbed mainly in the jejunum and to a smaller extent in the ileum. Polyglutamates are broken down by pteroylglutamate hydrolase to monoglutamates, which are absorbed by the mucosal cell.[49] In cells, folates act as coenzymes in various biochemical reactions, characterized by the transfer of simple chemical units which contain one carbon atom. They make possible the process of formylation in purine synthesis and methylation in purimidine synthesis. They are also involved in the metabolism and synthesis of amino acids such as serine, glycine, homocysteine, and glutamic acid and participate in the conversion of formate into 10-formyltetrahydrofolate.

Population surveys show folic acid deficiencies combined with iron and B_{12} deficiencies in pregnant women. Old people eating a very poor diet are also threatened. In clinical practice, deficiencies are found in subjects with an inadequate intake and in subjects with gastrointestinal disorders.

VITAMIN B_{12} DEFICIENCY

Vitamin B_{12} is one of the main nutritional factors needed for hematopoiesis. Primary sources of vitamin B_{12} are animal proteins (especially meat offals), liver, and, to a smaller extent, eggs, milk, cheese, and yeast. In the normal diet, the vitamin B_{12} content varies between 1 to 3 μg (the daily requirement is about 2 μg). In foods the vitamin is bound to protein and is released from that bond by the action of proteolytic enzymes in the stomach. There the released vitamin combines with an intrinsic factor (IF) and forms a complex which is taken to the distal portion of the ileum. There, the released vitamin binds with an intrinsic factor (IF), forming a complex. This complex is then transported into the distal parts of the ileum where it enters the enterocyte by the action of a specific mechanism involving calcium. By using a labeled vitamin B_{12}, it was found that the complex is transported through the membranous enterocyte surface to mitochondria.

Vitamin B_{12} is bound to protein, is probably also bound to fraction alpha and beta, and is linked with transcobalamine I and II.[54-56] Transcobalamine II is transported to stores, in particular the liver, and is mobilized as required. It is maintained that vitamin B_{12} reserves in the liver will (in the absence of IF) last 5 years before they become exhausted, such as the case after total gastrectomy. The causes of vitamin B_{12} deficiency can be divided roughly into three groups: (1) dietary deficiency (2) absence of IF, and (3) increased losses of vitamin B_{12} and bacterial competition in diseases of the small intestine.

The clinical manifestations of vitamin B_{12} deficiency are macrocytic anemia, megaloblastic bone marrow, and other changes, such as a smooth painful tongue, anorexia, diarrhea and a varied neurological symptomatology. Another sign of vitamin B_{12} deficiency is a reduced serum level and a concomitant increase of the folate, LDH, iron, and bilirubin level. An additional early manifestation of vitamin B_{12} deficiency is an increased urinary excretion of methylmalonic acid.

Modern diagnosis of impaired vitamin B_{12} metabolism makes use of various isotope methods. With one of these methods, vitamin B_{12} is labeled with ^{57}Co or ^{59}Co and administered orally after which its serum level cumulation in the liver and excretion in the urine are assessed. In clinical work for the diagnosis of impaired vitamin B_{12} absorption, the classical reliable Schilling test is used.[57]

PROTEIN DEFICIENCY AND ERYTHROPOIESIS

According to Aschkenasy,[60] the pathogenesis of anemia caused by protein deficiency is due to inhibition of erythropoiesis and a reduced life span of red cells. According to Reissman,[58] it seems probable that protein deficiency does not influence the synthesis of plasma proteins directly but does this by reducing erythropoietin formation, i.e., by altered regulation. It is surprising how rapidly erythropoiesis becomes inhibited — after only several days on the deficient diet, proerythroblasts disappear from bone marrow. This mechanism of depressed erythropoiesis plays a part in short-term experiments in particular. The interference with erythropoiesis in chronic protein deficiency leading to protein-energy malnutrition is even more serious.

Chronic protein deficiency interferes with erythropoiesis in several ways:

1. With hemoglobin synthesis where the required amino acids are lacking
2. With the regulation of erythropoiesis as the formation of erythropoietin is declining
3. With the transport of all hemotopoietic factors, in particular iron
4. With the absorption of hemotopoietic factors

Erythropoietin is now considered the main factor in the control of erythropoiesis. When it is deficient, erythrocyte formation in bone marrow is impaired as proper differentiation of the maternal cell does not take place. This applies in particular to precursors of red blood cells; however, during prolonged protein deficiency, inhibition of the red and white blood cell series and even hypoplasia of the bone marrow may develop.[58] Evidence of this is provided by many experimental and clinical observations of protein malnutrition.[59] Some authors found cases of anemia as well as a decline of plasma proteins after 8 weeks on a low-protein diet.[60] In kwashiorkor, anemia is part of the multifactorial deficiency.[61-63]

Protein malnutrition is manifested by a pathological aminogram where amino acids needed for the synthesis of plasma proteins are deficient. The hemoglobin concentration and number of red cells diminishes depending on the reduction of the total blood volume,[64] as was proved in experiments on dogs[65] and rats.[66] There have been several investigations conducted with humans[65,67,68] which drew attention to the proportional weight loss and reduction of total metabolically active body mass in protein-energy malnutrition. At the same time, evidence was presented of the breakdown of the amino acid spectrum which accompanies developing anemia.

Protein deficiency interferes markedly also with the transport of all hematopoietic factors. All vitamins and trace elements are bound to some protein fractions: vitamin B_{12} to alpha and beta globulin, vitamin B_6 mainly to alpha globulin, vitamin C to alpha globulin, and folic acid to all globulins. In this connection, the position of transferrin, the transport protein of iron, is very important. The decline of the transferrin level in protein malnutrition is very significant. This was repeatedly demonstrated in animal experiments and in children with kwashiorkor.[69] During fasting and a diminution of plasma proteins, a reduced transferrin synthesis[70,71] as well as a reduced albumin synthesis was observed. Transferrin is considered a very sensitive indicator of the nutritional status. When a low-protein diet is administered — in experiments with rats or humans — transferrin declines sooner than albumin and hemoglobin.[71-75]

In one experimental investigation, a decline of transferrin as an indicator of induced protein deficiency in rats[76] was observed. The transferrin level rises very rapidly after adequate dietotherapy.[69,76-78] Our investigations also revealed a positive correlation between the transferrin level and the albumin concentration after protein refeeding (Figure 2).

While it has been proved that protein deficiency interferes with iron transport, no agreement has been reached to this point on findings pertaining to plasma levels of iron. In experimental work where the low-protein diet contained adequate amounts of iron, plasma level was often elevated.[79] In other experimental work[80] and in particular clinical work[81-83] low plasma-iron levels are described.

So far, there is no uniform opinion on the question of how protein deficiency affects iron reserves. Some authors found exhausted iron reserves in cases of kwashiorkor.[82-84] On the other hand, in chronically sick patients with hypoalbuminemia[81] and in kwashiorkor,[85,86] the surprising finding of normal or even elevated amounts of stainable iron in bone marrow was reported. Bruschke[87] described enhanced iron deposition in the liver and spleen in chronic starvation. We also found increased iron reserves in reticular cells of the bone marrow and higher levels of sideroblasts in patients with anemia and hypoalbuminemia[88] (Figures 3 and 4).

During protein-energy malnutrition, the absorption of hematopoietic factors is impaired. In degenerative changes of the gastric mucosa, HCl and the intrinsic factor are reduced, thus impairing the binding of vitamin B_{12} with the intrinsic factor. This leads to disorders of vitamin B_{12} absorption. During impaired absorption of vitamin B_{12}, dysmicrobia resulting from the diminished gastric acidity also occurs. At the same time, iron absorption is impaired as ferric ions are precipitated at a pH above 5.[89]

More recent work by Clavin,[30] Sood,[80] and Aschkenasy[60] provides evidence of the marked reduction of iron absorption in protein deficiency. It is not clear, however, whether the reduced absorption is proportional to the inhibition of erythropoiesis. Donatti[90] described a rise of iron absorption in acute fasting after administration of erythropoietin. Reverse conclusions were published by Aschkenasy.[91] In his experiments, injection of erythropoietin enhanced the erythropoietic utilization of absorbed[59] Fe but did not influence the absorption of this isotope. Aschkenasy concludes from this that iron absorption in rats with protein deficiency is not related to the level of erythropoiesis. The mechanism of reduced absorption has not been elucidated to date. In his work on possible intraluminal factors, Lynch[83] emphasizes in particular the effect of achlorhydria. Obviously, a major part is also played by changes of the mucosa

TOTAL IRON BINDING CAPACITY (TIBC)

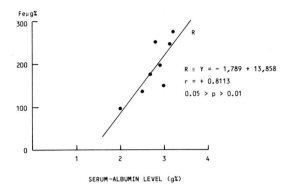

FIGURE 2.   Relationship between TIBC and serum-albumin level in patient in course of protein-realimentation.
(From Vulterinová, M., Vliv karenee bíl kovin na kruet-
vorbu, (Influence de la carence alimentaire en protéines sur
l'hematopoiese en tchéque, Recueil de la Societé pour
l'alimentation Rationnelle, Prague, 85-96, 1969. With permission.)

SIDEROBLASTS

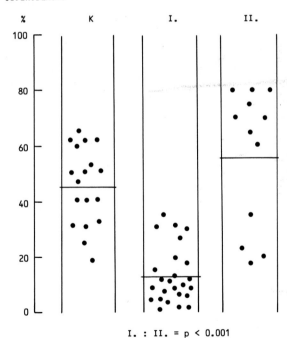

FIGURE 3.   The distribution of iron stored in bone marrow
in three groups. Iron stores established by dyeing of Berlin blue
and evaluated according to Weinfeld. K = control group; I =
patient with anemia; II = patient with anemia and lowered
serum-albumin levels. (From Weinfeld, A., Storage iron in
man, *Acta Med. Scand. Suppl.*, 427, 9—124, 1964. With permission.)

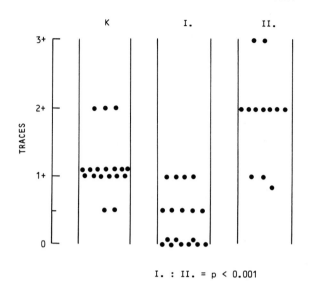

FIGURE 4.　The distribution of iron stored in bone marrow in three groups. Iron stores established by dyeing of Berlin blue and evaluated according to Weinfeld. K = control group; I = patient with anemia; II = patient with anemia and lowered serum albumin levels.

of the small intestine which, as with other organs with a high protein content, suffers from reduced cell proliferation. It is important that iron absorption is reduced during protein deficiency, even in selective iron deficiency, where otherwise, absorption of labeled iron is enhanced[3,35,92] and a combined iron and protein deficiency may easily develop.

The reduced iron absorption in rats with protein-energy deficiency improves after only several days on a hyperprotein diet.[93] Previous work based on feeding rats a low-protein diet with a high iron content drew attention to the expressive deposition of iron in different organs which led to the erroneous interpretation of an enhanced iron absorption.[94,95]

The above mechanisms probably also participate in the development of secondary nutritional anemias which are observed in various diseases, in particular, diseases of the digestive system associated with severe malabsorption syndrome and in patients with chronic renal insufficiency who are on a low-protein diet for prolonged periods.

VITAMIN B₆ DEFICIENCY

Pyridoxine is involved in heme formation; when it is deficient, the amount of porphyrin in red cells declines.[96] Bickers et al.[97] described 20 patients with normocytic hypochromic anemia and Hines[98] described rare instances of macrocytic anemia which improved after pyridoxine treatment. In all these anemias, the plasma and tissue iron level was raised and hemosiderosis may have been present. Incorporation into red cells was retarded. Anemia produced experimentally by a pyridoxine-deficient diet[99] has a similar character. These anemias were investigated experimentally in monkeys, pigs, cats, chicks, and rats. In rats, however, they develop only after 40 to 50 weeks.[60,100,101]

Patients with pyrodoxine-responsive anemia have been studied extensively by Horrigan and Harris[100] and Hines and Harris,[98] whose publications document the fascinating array of biochemical and hematological events seen in these individuals. In many instances, they required other therapeutic measures such as the administration of liver, vitamin B_{12}, folic acid, etc., in addition to vitamin B_6 therapy.

Daily requirements of vitamin B_6 in man are 0.2 to 5 mg depending on age, metabolic status, and protein intake.[99]

THIAMIN DEFICIENCY

Experiments with monkeys provided evidence that thiamin is needed for normal erythropoiesis. Microcytic and macrocytic anemias were described as a consequence of thiamin deficiency.[103]

RIBOFLAVINE DEFICIENCY

Riboflavine participates in the production of erythropoietin through its probable involvement in the maturation of red blood cells.[104] Experimental anemia due to riboflavine deficiency has been described in monkeys and other animals.[105] In addition to anemia, a low concentration of plasmatic protein has been found in all thiamine-deficient animals. In bone marrow, there is a reduction of immature red blood cell elements and megakaryocytes. After riboflavine treatment the above changes tend to normalize. Selective riboflavine-responsive anemias are seldom found in man.[67,104]

VITAMIN C DEFICIENCY

Vitamin C affects hemotopoiesis in several ways. In the gastrointestinal tract, it promotes iron absorption by retarding the formation of poorly absorbed Fe^{+++} complexes and protects bivalent ions against oxidation. This effect is manifested only during oral administration.[105] Vitamin C also plays a part during the transformation of folic acid into its active form, folinic acid, also known as vitamin B_{12}[106] That anemia is associated with scurvy has been confirmed experimentally. Normocytic and normochromic (and in rare instances macrocytic anemia associated with reticulocytosis) raised plasma iron and Fe levels in tissues, caused a reduction of leukocytes in bone marrow, and increased the number of immature cells of the red and white series. It is assumed that the maturation of red cells is impaired, although some authors ascribe these anemias to repeated small blood losses caused by vascular fragility.[107]

VITAMIN E DEFICIENCY

Vitamin E, like vitamin B_{12} and folic acid, is involved in nucleic acid metabolism. It is important as an antioxidant which protects the red cell from hemolysis.[108] In vitamin E deficiency, a reduced life span of red cells was observed.[109] It is known that anemia can be induced experimentally by a diet lacking vitamin E. Anemia is produced in different animal species by different mechanisms. According to Fitch[110] three mechanisms must be considered: anemia caused by blood loss, hemolysis and retarded erythropoiesis. Experimental vitamin E deficiency in chicks led to the development of exudative diathesis with extravasal hemorrhage into tissues. In rodents, anemia during hypovitaminosis E was caused by acute hemolysis when the animals were exposed to stress (oxidant stress). In monkeys and pigs, anemia developed as a result of very slow erythropoiesis; megaloblastic anemia developed which responded very well to the administration of vitamin E, while other nutrients such as iron, vitamin B_{12}, and folic acid did not cause remission. Based on these findings, Majas et al.[111] and others administered, with favorable results, vitamin E to patients with megaloblastic anemia when common therapeutic procedures failed.

Hemolysis proportional to serum tocopherol levels was frequently observed in humans at concentrations below 0.3 mg/100 ml. When vitamin E was administered to volunteers,[112] strengthening of the red cell membrane was proved by erythrograms. The antihemolytic action of vitamin E is also used in clinical work for blood preservation. As regards clinical symptomatology, vitamin E deficiency acts atypically — anemia may be normocytic to macrocytic.[113] Majaj[111] was the first to decribe megaloblastic anemia due to vitamin E deficiency in children with kwahiorkor. In an adequate diet where fats account for 30 to 35% of the caloric volume, the tocopherol content is 10 to 15 mg, which corresponds to the common requirements.

COPPER DEFICIENCY

Copper is a constituent of various enzymes which are involved in the synthesis of protoporphyrin and are essential for erythropoiesis. In animals with dietary copper deficiency, microcytic hypochromic anemia was induced with concomitant iron deficiency. Improvement did not occur after administration of iron but only after addition of copper. Experimental work also provides evidence that copper deficiency in the organism reduces iron absorption and interferes with the iron utilization for hemoglobin. According to the work of Daum and Donner,[116] copper helps to mobilize iron from stores. The mean intake is reported to be 2.5 to 5 mg; however, a positive balance is found already on a dietary intake of 2 mg/day. Under normal conditions, 0.03 mg Cu is retained.[117] In diets with an adequate energy content, a copper content of 2 mg is sufficient. Copper is absorbed in the upper portion of the small intestine and is absorbed more readily in organic complexes than copper sulfate for example. Copper is transported in plasma bound to alphaglobulin (ceruloplasmin). The total amount of ceruloplasmin in blood is 100 mg/100 ml. Copper is roughly equally distributed between plasma and erythrocytes.

Copper levels decline in pregnancy and some diseases although it was not possible to demonstrate anemia caused by copper deficiency alone[116,118]

ZINC DEFICIENCY

The daily dietary zinc intake is 10 to 15 mg. It is not known exactly how much is absorbed. The zinc level in the blood is 700 to 800 μg and 34% of this zinc is bound to globuline. The content in erythrocytes is 1.2 to 1.3 μg and leukocytes contain 3% of the total zinc content of blood. Raised zinc levels were described in untreated pernicious anemia. After treatment with vitamin B_{12}, the levels return to normal. Interference with hematopoiesis was proved experimentally; however, the mechanism of action is not known. After the i.v. administration of labeled zinc, the latter moves very rapidly from plasma into the liver where it is deposited. It also cumulates in the pancreas and then appears in red cells in bone marrow. Experimental investigations detected zinc in dehydrogenase, and it is assumed that it participates in its activity. In humans, zinc deficiency was diagnosed concurrently with iron deficiency, i.e., in hypochromic anemia and also in conjunction with protein-energy malnutrition. Sandstead[114] found zinc deficiency in people with a high phytate diet.[114,115]

COBALT DEFICIENCY

Cobalt is known in its biological function as a constituent of vitamin B_{12}. Vitamin B_{12} contains more than 4% cobalt and is a coenzyme in nucleoprotein synthesis. Cobalt deficiency in animals is manifested as vitamin B_{12} deficiency and the condition is not relieved by administration of cobalt alone, but rather together with vitamin B_{12}.[119]

Cobalt is of interest from a biological and pharmacological standpoint as it stimulates erythropoiesis. It is assumed that during its administration erythropoietin formation increases.[60] Cobalt is also needed for vitamin B_{12} synthesis by bacteria. The dose needed by animals to produce vitamin B_{12} is 0.07 to 0.08 mg Co per day. Its requirement is thus very small and the need is fully met by the dietary intake. Human requirements are not known. The diet contains approximately 5 to 8 μg cobalt. A small proportion is absorbed.

Cobalt deficiency was repeatedly observed in developing countries, along with other nutrient deficiencies. Severe cobalt deficiencies are described in veterinary medicine, in ruminants in particular. In addition to anemia, they also cause severe anorexia and may even be fatal. Some authors report that cobalt reduces iron absorption and exerts a direct influence on iron metabolism.

MOLYBDENUM DEFICIENCY

Trace elements are found in all plant and animal cells. Molybdenum in tissues is bound in molecules of different flavoproteins. In hematopoiesis, it is involved indirectly as xanthine oxidase contains one atom of molybdenum. Xanthine oxidace is important for the mobilization of ferritin iron in the liver, and by this route molybdenum plays a part in iron metabolism. Molybdenum probably, in general, inhibits a copper-containing enzyme.[120,121] So far, we do not know any typical syndrome of molybdenum deficiency in humans or animals. It has been proved, however, that dietary deficiency causes a rise of xanthine-oxidizing activity which returns to normal after supplementation of the diet with a small amount of molybdenum. Iron deficiency anemia also recedes more rapidly after combined iron and molybdenum therapy.[60,122]

REFERENCES

1. **Mašek, J.**, Recommended nutrient allowances in *World Review of Nutrition* Vol. 25, S. Karger, Basel, 1976, 1—107.
2. **Chandra, R. K.**, Nutrition as a critical determinant in susceptibility to infection, in *World Review of Nutrition*, Vol. 25, S. Karger, Basel, 1976, 166—188.
3. **Doberský, P. and Vulterinova, M.**, Poruchy výživy při resekci zaludku, in *Ernährungstörungen nach Magenresektion,* Státni Zdravotnicke Nakladatelstvi, Praha, 1962, 310—312.
4. **Adlersberg, D.**, The malabsorption syndrome in man. Clinical and pathologic aspects. *Am. J. Clin. Nutr.*, 8, 173—178, 1960.
5. **Cook, G. C.**, Malabsorption, *Br. Med. J.*, 1, 613—617, 1967.
6. **Krondl, A., Skala, J., Vulterinová, M., Štastna, R., and Pirk, F.**, *Fat and Malabsorption Syndrome*, Academia, Prague, 1971, 1—209.
7. **Kluthe, R. and Quirin, H.**, *Diätbuch für Nierenkranke,* 2nd ed., Thieme-Verlag, Stuttgart, 1971.
8. **Pechar, J.**, Amino-acids levels and erythropoiesis in uremia and human renal transplantation, 1975, in press.
9. Report of a Study Group on Iron Deficiency Anaemia, *WHO Technical Report Series*, No. 182, World Health Organization, Geneva, 1959.
10. Report of a WHO Scientific Group, Nutritional Anaemias, *WHO Technical Report Series*, No. 405, World Health Organization, Geneva, 1968.
11. Report of a WHO Scientific Group, *WHO Technical Report Series*, No. 503, Nutritional Anaemias, World Health Organization, Geneva, 1972.
12. Report of an IAEA/USAID/WHO Joint Meeting, Control of Nutritional Anaemia with Special Reference to Iron Deficiency, *WHO Technical Report Series*, No. 580, World Health Organization, Geneva, 1975.
13. **Chanarin, I.**, Diagnosis of folate deficiency in pregnancy, *Acta Obstet. Gynecol. Scand.*, 4, 39—42, 1967.

14. 6th Symp. Swedish Nutrition Foundation, Occurrence, Causes and Prevention of Nutritional Anaemias Almquist & Wiksells, Boktryckeri Aktiebolag, Upsala, 1968.
15. **Chanarin, I., Rothman, D., and Berry, V.**, Iron deficiency and its relation to folic-acid status in pregnancy: results of clinical trial, *Br. Med. J.*, 1, 480—485, 1965.
16. **Tokes, P. P., Smith, G. H., Gianella, R. A., and Conrad, M. E.**, Folic acid abnormalities in iron deficiency: The mechanism of decreased serum folate levels, *Am. J. Clin. Nutr.*, 27, 355—372, 1974.
17. **Zamrazilová, E. and Hejda, S.**, Výskyt anémie v naší populaci, (occurrence of anaemia in the present population), *Časopis lékařů českých*, 107, 1496—1500, 1968.
18. **Zamrazilová, E. and Hejda, S.**, Hematologické hodnoty u žen s různými ztrátami železa, (Haematological findings in women with different iron losses), *Československá Gynekologie*, 39, 515—517, 1974.
19. **Levy, S., Hershko, C., Grossowicz, N., Rachmilewitz, M., and Izak, G.**, Prevalence and causes of anaemia in children in Kiryat Shmoneh,Israel, *Am. J. Clin. Nutr.*, 23, 1364—1369, 1970.
20. **Basu, R. N. et al.**, Etiopatogenesis of nutritional anaemia in pregnancy: a therapeutic approach, *Am. J. Clin. Nutr.*, 26, 591—599, 1973.
21. **Colman, N. et al.**, Prevention on folate deficiency in pregnancy by food fortification, *Am. J. Clin. Nutr.*, 27, 339—344, 1974.
22. **Herbert, V.**, Megaloblastic anemia as a problem in world health, *Am. J. Clin. Nutr.*, 9, 1115—1120, 1968.
23. **Viteri, F. E. et al.**, Hematological changes in protein calorie malnutrition, *Vitam. Horm.*, 26, 573—615, 1968.
24. **Finch, C. A.**, Erythropoiesis in protein calorie malnutrition, in *Proc. Sym. Protein Calorie Malnutrition*, Chiang Mai, Thailand, 1973.
25. **Layrisse, M. and Martinez-Torres, C.**, *Progress in Haemiatology*, Vol. 7, Brown, E. B. and Moore, C. V., Eds., Grune and Stratton, New York, 1971, 137—160.
26. **Sharpe, L. M., Peacock, W. C., Cooke, R., and Harris, R. S.**, The effect of phytate and other food factors on iron absorption, *J. Nutr.*, 41, 433—446, 1950.
27. **Hegsted, D. M., Finch, C. A., and Kinney, T. D.**, Influence of diet on iron absorption, *J. Exp. Med.*, 90, 147—156, 1949.
28. **Forth, W. and Rummel, W.**, Abhängigkeit der Eisenresorption von der Eisenbindung durch den Darm, *Med. Pharm.*, 14, 384—390, 1966.
29. **Peters, T., Apt, L., and Ross, J. F.**, Effect of phosphates upon iron absorption studied in normal human subjects and in experimental models using dialysis, *Gastroenterology*, 61, 315—322, 1972.
30. **Klavins, J. N., Kinney, T. D., and Kaufman, N.**, The influence of dietary protein on iron absorption, *Br. J. Exp. Pathol.*, 43, 173—185, 1962.
31. **Brodan, V., Kuhn, E., Brodanová, M., and Válek, J.**, Some factors influencing the course of iron absorption curves, *Rev. Czech. Med.*, 15, 10—23, 1969.
32. **Heinrich, H. C., Bartels, H., Gabbe, E. E., Meineke, B., Nass, W. P., and Whang, D. H.**, Die intestinale Resorption des Nahrungseisens aus dem Hämoglobin der Leber and Muskular bei Menschen mit normalen Eisenreserven and Personen mit prälatentem-latentem Eisenmangel, *Klin. Wachenschr.*, 47. 309—317, 1969.
33. **Bothwell, T. H. and Flinch, C. A.**, *Iron Metabolism*, Little, Brown, Boston, 1962, 92—137.
34. **Heinrich, H. C.**, Die Ganzkörper-Radioaktivitätsmessing in medizinischer Forschung und klinischer Diagnostik, *Therapiewoche*, 51, 2099—2121, 1967.
35. **Heinrich, H. C.**, Pralatende, latende a manifeste Eisenmangelzustande bei Blutspendern, *Muench. Med. Wachenschr.*, 110, 1845—1852, 1968.
36. **Heinrich, H. C., Bartels, H., Heinisch, B., Hausmann, K., and Kuse, R.**, Intestinale ^{59}Fe resorption und pralantender Eisenmangel während der Gravidität des Menschen, *Klin. Wachenschr.*, 46, 199—202, 1968.
37. **Heinrich, H. C., Gabbe, E. E., Kugler, G., Whang, D. H., Hausmann, K., Bartels, H., Kuse, R., and Meinecke, K. H.**, Diagnostischer ^{59}Fe^{2+}-Resorptions-Test und diffus verteiltes Reserveeisen der Knochenmarksmakrophagen bei Magenmucosastrophie und nach Magen-⅔-Resektion bzw. totaler Gastrektomie, *Klin. Wachenschr.*, 49, 825—835, 1971.
38. **Hausmann, K., Kuse, R., Meinicke, B., Bartels, H., and Heinrich, H. C.**, Diagnostische Kriterien der prältenten, latenten und manifesten Eisenmangel, *Klin. Wachenschr.*, 49, 1164—1174, 1971.
39. **Rath, C. E. and Finch, C. A.**, Sternal marrow hemosiderin, *J. Lab. Clin. Med.*, 33, 81—86, 1948.
40. **Hausmann, K., Kuse, R., Sonnenberg, O. W., Bartels, H., and Heinrich, H. C.**, Inter-relations between iron stores, general factors and intestinal iron absorption, *Acta Haematol.*, 42, 193—207, 1969.
41. **Weinfeld, A.**, Storage iron in man, *Acta Med. Scand. Suppl.*, 427, 9—124, 1964.
42. **Pexa, H.**, Depoteisen im Knochemark, *Blut*, 13, 221—231, 1966.
43. **Petrusová, I. and Vulterinová, M.**, Dnešni moznosti stanovení zásob železa, *Ceskoslovenská Gynekologie*, 5, 342—346, 1973.

44. **Wöhler, F.,** Diagnosis of iron storage diseases with desferrioxamine, *Acta Haematol.,* 32, 321—337, 1964.
45. **Hedenberg, L.,** Studies on iron metabolism with desferrioxamine in man, *Scand. J. Haematol.,* 6, 3—86, 1969.
46. **Fielding, J.,** Storage iron and desferrioxamine, *Proc. R. Soc. Med.,* 12, 1218—1221, 1970.
47. **Herbert, V.,** Megaloblastic anaemias: mechanismus and management, *Dis. Mon.,* 2, 1—4, 1965.
48. **Herbert, V.,** Folic acid and vitamin B_{12}, in *Modern Nutrition in Health and Disease,* 5th ed., Goodhart, R. S. and Shils, E. M., Eds., Lea & Febiger, Philadelphia, 1973.
49. **Luhky, A. L., Eagle, F. J., Roth, E., and Cooperman, J. M.,** Relapsing megaloblastic anaemia in an infant due to a specific defect in gastro-intestinal absorption of folic acid, *Am. J. Dis. Child.,* 112, 482—488, 1966.
50. **Rosenberg, I. H. et al.,** Absorption of polyglutamic folate: participation of desconjugating enzymes of the intestinal mucosa. *N. Engl. J. Med.,* 280, 985—988, 1969.
51. **Rothenberg, S. P., da Costa, M., and Rosenberg, Z.,** Radioassay for serum folate, *N. Engl. J. Med.,* 286, 1335, 1972.
52. **Schjönsby, H. and Andersen, K. J.,** The intestinal absorption of vitamin B_{12}, *Scand. J. Gastroenterol.,* 9, 7—11, 1974.
53. **Donaldson, R. M., MacKenzie, I. L., and Trier, J. S.,** Intrinsic factor-mediated attachment of vitamin B_{12} to brash borders and microvillous membranes of hamster intestine, *J. Clin. Invest.,* 46, 1215—1228, 1967.
54. **Olesen, H.,** Serum transcobalamins, *Scand. J. Gastroenterol.,* 9, 13—16, 1974.
55. **Nexö, E. and Gimsing, P.,** Turnover studies with radio-iodine-labelled Transcobalamin I, *Scand. J. Gastroenterol.,* 9, 17—18, 1974.
56. **Gullberg, R.,** In vivo and in vitro release of vitamin B_{12}-binding. Protein characterized by large molecular size, *Scand. J. Gastroenterol.,* 9, 24—26, 1974.
57. **Schilling, R. F.,** The absorption and utilisation of vitamin B_{12}, *Am. J. Clin. Nutr.,* 3, 45—51, 1955.
58. **Reissmann, K. R.,** Protein metabolism and erytropoesis. I. The anemia of protein deprivation, *Blood,* 23, 137—145, 1964.
59. **Dallman, P. R. and Manies, E. C.,** Protein deficiency. Contrasting effects on DNA and RNA metabolism in rat liver, *J. Nutr.,* 103, 1311—1318, 1973.
60. **Aschkenasy, A.,** Nutrition et hématopoièse, in *Protéines,* Vol. 3, Centre National de la Recherche Scientifique, Paris, 1971, 59—71.
61. **Allen, D. M. and Dean, R. F. A.,** The anaemia of Kwashiorkor in Uganda, *Trans. R. Soc. Trop. Med. Hyg.,* 59, 326—341, 1965.
62. **Stekel, A.,** Haematologic studies of severe undernutrition of infancy, *Am. J. Clin. Nutr.,* 3, 320—337, 1969.
63. **Stekel A. and Smith, N. J.,** Haematologic studies of severe undernutrition of infancy, *Am. J. Clin. Nutr.,* 23, 896—904, 1970.
64. **Weech, A. A., Wollstein, M. and Goetsch, E.,** Nutritional edema in dog; development of deficits in erythrocytes, and hemoglobin on diet deficient in protein, *J. Clin. Invest.,* 16, 719—728, 1937.
65. **Metcoff, J., Favour, C. B. and Stare, F. J.,** Plasma protein and hemoglobin in protein-deficient rats; 3— dimensional study, *J. Clin. Invest.,* 24, 82—91, 1945.
66. **Benditt, E. P., Straube, R. L. and Humphreys, E. M.,** The determination of total circulating serum protein and erythrocyte volumes in normal and protein—depleted rats, *Proc. Soc. Exp. Biol. Med.,* 62, 188—192, 1946.
67. **Viteri, F., Alvarado, J., Luthringer, D. and Wood, R. P.,** Hematological changes in calorie malnutrition, *Vitam. Horm.,* 26, 573—615, 1968.
68. **Viteri, F., Béhar, M. and Arroyave, G.,** in *Mammalian Protein Metabolism,* Vol. 2, Munro, H. N. and Allison, J. B., Eds., Academic Press, New York, 1964, 523.
69. **Antia, A. V., McFarlane, H. and Soothill, J. F.,** Serum siderophilin in kwashiorkor, *Arch. Dis. Child.,* 43, 459—462, 1968.
70. **Morgan, E. H.,** Transferrin and transferrin iron, in *Iron in Biochemistry and Medicine,* Jacobs, A. and Worwood, M., Eds., Academic Press, New York, 1974, 29—71.
71. **Morgan, E. H. and Peters, T.,** The biosynthesis of rat serum albumin, *J. Biol. Chem.,* 246, 3500—3507, 1972.
72. **Lahey, M. E., Béhar, M., Viteri, F. and Scrimshaw, N. S.,** Values for copper, iron and iron-binding capacity in the serum in Kwashiorkor. *Pediatrics,* 22, 72.
73. **Adams, E. B., and Scragg, J. N.,** Iron in the anaemia of kwashkiorkor, *Br J. Haematol.,* 11, 676—681, 1965.
74. **El-Schobaki, F. A., El-Hawary, M. F. S., Morcos, S. R., Abdelkhalek, M. K., El-Zawahry, K., and Sakr, R.,** Iron metabolism in Egyptian infants with protein-calorie deficiency, *Br. J. Nutr.,* 28, 81—89, 1972.

75. **McFarlane, H., Ogbeide, M. I., Reddy, S., Adcock, K. J., Adeshina, H., Gurney, J. M., Cooke, A., Taylor, G. O. and Mordie, J. A.**, Biochemical assessment of protein-caloric malnutrition, *Lancet*, 1, 392—395, 1969.

76. **Marečková, O., Skála, I., Pechar, J., Mareček, Z. and Vulterinová, M.**, Časová posloupnost změn biochemických parametrů u experimentálni protein-kalorické malnutrice u krys, (Gradual succession of biochemical parameters in experimental protein caloric malnutrition in rats), *Čs. gastroenterol*, 27, 285—289, 1973.

77. **Vulterinová, M. and Brodan, V.**, Taux du fer plasmatique en physiologie en clinique, *Ann. Hyg. Lang. Fr. Med. Nutr.*, 8, 31—42, 1972.

78. **Vulterinová, M.**, Vliv karence bílkovin na krvetvorbu, (Influence de la carence alimentaire en protéines sur l'hematopoiese en tchéque), Recueil de la Societé pour l'Alimentation Rationnelle, Prague, 85—92, 1969.

79. **Conrad, M. E., Foy, A. L., Williams, M. L., Knospe, W. H.**, Effect of starvation and protein depletion on ferrokinetics and iron absorption, *Am. J. Physiol.*, 213, 557—565, 1967.

80. **Sood, S. K., Deo, M. G., and Ramalingaswami, V.**, Anemia in experimental protein deficiency in the rhesus monkey with special reference to iron metabolism, *Blood*, 26, 421—432, 1965.

81. **Weir, D. R., Dimitrov, N. V., Houser, H. B., Suhrland, L. G., and Myint, T.**, Serum proteins and blood vitamin in anemia of the chronically ill, *J. Chron. Dis.*, 22, 407—419, 1969.

82. **Halsted, Ch. H., Sourial, N., Guindi, S., Kattab, A. K., Capter, J. P., and Patwardhan, V. N.**, Anaemia in kwashiorkor in Cairo, *Am. J. Clin. Nutr.*, 22, 1371—1382, 1969.

83. **Lynch, S. R., Becker, D., Septel, H., Bothwell, T. H., Stevens, K., and Metz, J.**, Iron absorption in kwashiorkor, *Am. J. Clin. Nutr.*, 23, 792—797, 1970.

84. **Pereira, S. M. and Baker, S. J.**, Hematologic studies in Kwashiorkor, *Am. J. Clin. Nutr.*, 18, 413—420, 1966.

85. **Adams, E. B., Scragg, J. N., Naidov, B. T., Liljestrand, S. K. and Cocram, V. I.**, Observation of the aetiology and treatment of anemia in kwashiorkor, *Br. Med. J.*, 3, 451—454, 1967.

86. **Adams, E. B.**, Anaemia associated with kwashiorkor, *Am. J. Clin.*, 22, 1634—1638, 1969.

87. **Brüschke, G.**, Eisenstoffwechsel, Steinkopff, T., Ed., Verlag, Dresden, 1964, 68—80.

88. **Vulterinová, M. et al.**, Změny krvetvorby a poruchy metabolismu železa za některých patologických stavu, (The changes of erythropoiesis and disturbances in iron metabolism in some pathological states), IKEM, Praha, in press.

89. **Cook, J. D., Brown, G. M., Valberg, L. S.**, *J. Clin. Invest.*, 43, 1185—1191, 1964.

90. **Donati, R. M., Chapmean, C. W., Warnecke, M. A., and Gallagher, N. I.**, Iron metabolism in acute starvation, *Proc. Soc. Exp. Biol. Med.*, 117, 50—53, 1964.

91. **Aschkenasy, A.**, Influence de la carence alimentaire en protéines sûr l'absorption digestive et sur la distribution Tissulaire du ^{59}Fe absorbé, chez le rat male. Effect des injections dérythropoietine, *Rev. Fr. Etud. Clin. Biol.*, 11, 1010—1022, 1966.

92. **Turnbull, A.**, Iron Absorption, in *Iron in Biochemistry and Medicine* Jacobs, A. and Worwood, M., Eds., Academic Press, N.Y., 1974, 369—403.

93. **Envonwu, C. O.**, Biochemical and morphological changes in rat submandibular gland in experimental protein calorie malnutrition, *Exp. Mol. Pathol.*, 16, 244—269, 1972.

94. **Gillmann, T., Ganham, P.A.S., and Hathorn, M.**, Experimental nutritional siderosis, *Lancet*, 2, 557—558, 1958.

95. **Sriramacharie, S., Srikantia, S. G., and Gopalan, G.**, Cytosuderosis of liver in protein deficient monkeys, *Indian J. Pathol. Bacteriol.*, 2, 226—236, 1959.

96. **Gepner-Wozniewska, M.**, Metabolismus vitaminu B$_6$ a stav jeho nedostatku u člověka, *Pol. Tyg. Lek.*, 20, 367—570, 1965.

97. **Bickers, J. N., Brown, Ch. I., and Sprague, A. C.**, Pyridoxin responsive anaemia, *Blood*, 19, 304—312, 1962.

98. **Hines, J. D. and Harris, J. W.**, *Am. J. Clin. Nutr.*, 14, 137, 1964.

99. Recommended Daily Allowances, Food and Nutrition Board, National Academy of Sciences, National Research Council, Washington, D.C., 1968.

100. **Horrigan, D. L. and Harris, J. W.**, Pyridoxine-responsive anemias in man, *Vitam. Horm.* 26, 549—568, 1968.

101. **Keyhani, M., Giuliani, D., Giuliani, E. R. and Morse, B. S.**, Erythropoiesis in pyridoxine deficient mice, *Proc. Soc. Exp. Biol. Med.*, 146, 114—119, 1974.

102. **Coursin, D. B.**, Pyridoxine deficiency and erythrocyte function, in *Malnutrition and functions of blood cells*, Proc. Symp. sponsored by the Malnutrition Panels of the United States-Japan Cooperative Medical Science Programm, Kyoto, Japan, 1972, 115—147.

103. **Rogers, L. E., Potter, F. S. and Sidbury, J. B.**, Thiamine-responsive megaloblastic anaemia, *J. Pediat.*, 74, 494—504, 1969.

104. **Lane, M. and Alfrey, C. P.**, The anaemia of human riboflavin deficiency, *Blood*, 25, 432—442, 1965.

105. **Brise, H. and Hallberg, L.**, Effect of ascorbic acid on iron absorption, *Acta Med. Scand.*, Suppl. 376/171, 51, 1962.
106. **Vilter, R. V.**, Vitamin B$_{12}$, folic acid, in *Modern Nutrition in Health and Disease*, Wohl, M. G. and Goodhart, R. S., Eds., Lea & Febiger, Philadelphia, 1964, 421—431.
107. **Goldberg, A.**, The anemia of scurvy, *Q. J. Med.*, 32, 51, 1963.
108. **Green, J.**, Vitamin E and the biological antioxidant theory, *Ann. N.Y. Acad. Sci.*, 203, 29—44, 1972.
109. **Vos, J. and Molennar, J.**, Mitochondrial and mikrosomal membranes from livers of vitamin E deficient ducklings, *Ann. N.Y. Acad. Sci.*, 203, 74—89, 1972.
110. **Fitch, C. D.**, The hematopoietic system in vitamin E-deficient animals, *Ann. N.Y. Acad. Sci.* 203, 172—176, 1973.
111. **Majaj, A. S., Dinning, J. S., Azzan, S. A. and Darby, W. J.**, Vitamin E-responsive degaloblastic anaemia in infants with protein-caloric malnutrition, *Am. J. Clin. Nutr.*, 12, 374—379, 1963.
112. **Hrubá, F., Vulterinová, M., Nováková, V., Placer, Z.**, Reflection of tocopherol saturation in the haemogram of healthy subjects, *Int. J. Vitam. Nutr. Res.*, 41, 521—528, 1971.
113. **Dinning, J. S.**, Vitamin E-responsive anemia in monkeys and man, *Nutr. Rev.* 21, 289—291, 1963.
114. **Sandstead, H. H., Shukry, A. S., Prasad, A. S., Gabr, M. K., El Hifney, A., Mokhtar, N. and Darby, W. J.**, Kwashiorkor in Egypt. I. Clinical and biochemical studies, with special reference to plasma zinc and serum lactic dehydrogenase, *Am. J. Clin. Nutr.*, 17, 15, 1965.
115a. **Sandstead, H. H.**, Zinc nutrition in the U.S.A., *Am. J. Clin. Nutr.*, 26, 1251—1257, 1973.
115b. **Hambridge, K. M.**, Zinc deficiency in children, in *Trace Element Metabolism in Animals*, Vol. 2, Hoekstra, W. G., Suttie, J. W., Ganther, H. E. and Mertz, W., Eds., University Park Press, Baltimore, 1974, 171—183.
116. **Daum, J. and Donner, L.**, K patogenese poruch výmeny železa a medi, *Lékarške Óbzory*, 11, 53, 1962.
117. **Grassmann, E. and Kirchgessner, M.**, On the metabolic availability of absorbed copper and iron, in *Trace Element Metabolism in Animals*, Vol. 2, Hoekstra, W. G., Suttie, J. W., Ganther, H. E., and Mertz, W., Eds., University Park Press, Baltimore, 1974, 523—526.
118. **Gordano, A., Baertl, J. M. and Graham, G. G.**, Copper deficiency in infancy, *Pediatrics*, 34, 324—336, 1964.
119. **MacPherson, A. and Moon, F. E.**, Effects of long-term maintenance of sheep on a low-cobalt diet as assessed by clinical condition and biochemical parameters, in *Trace Element Metabolism in Animals*, Vol. 2, 2nd Int. Symp., University Park Press, Baltimore, 1974, 624—628.
120. **Kovalsky, V. V. and Vorotnitskaya, I. E.**, The role of copper and molybdenum in the regulation of xanthine oxidase and urate oxidase properties, *Dokl. Akad. Nauk. SSSR* 187(6), 1969.
121. **Kovalsky, V. V., Vorotnitskaya, I. E. and Tsoi, G. G.**, Adaptive changes of the milk xanthine oxidase and its isoenzymes during molybdenum and copper action, *Trace Element Metabolism in Animals — 2*, 2nd Int. Symp., University Park Press, Baltimore, 1974, 161—170.

NUTRITION AND LEUKOPOIESIS

A. Aschkenasy

I. INTRODUCTION: SOME DATA ON THE ORIGIN AND PHYSIOLOGY OF LEUKOCYTES

The frequency and gravity of infections in malnourished subjects is well known.[1] This phenomenon is generally ascribed to reduced resistance toward pathogenic agents and their toxins, due mainly to the deficient supply of leukocytes and to the impairment of their functional activities. The latter are themselves controlled by a highly elaborated enzymatic system contained in these cells.[2,3]

The blood concentration of leukocytes is relatively stable (albeit much less in the rat and especially the mouse than in man) because of a dynamic equilibrium between their production on the one hand and their destruction or intestinal elimination on the other. This equilibrium depends to a large extent on the quantitative and qualitative changes of alimentary intake and on the capacity for utilizing the absorbed materials for the development of the leukopoietic tissues, maintenance of normal leukocytic activity, and synthesis of leukocyte-derived immunoglobulins (Ig) and other extracellular factors.

With the possible exception of a fraction of tissular macrophages (although, according to some authors,[4] all of these cells may also derive from bone marrow) and of mast cells, which seem to differentiate *in situ* from histiocytes of the reticuloendothelial system, all leukocytes of adult mammals originate in the bone marrow from unspecialized pluripotential stem cells,[5] yielding both erythroid and leukocytic progeny.

A. Granulocytes

After having differentiated in the bone marrow from the lymphoid stem cell[6] via the stages of myeloblast, promyelocyte, myelocyte, and metamyelocyte, the three categories of granulocytes (neutrophils, eosinophils, and basophils) emigrate into the bloodstream; about half of the leukocytes circulate while another half take part in a marginal pool adherent to endothelial cells.[7] Both of these pools are in rapid equilibrium.

After an intravascular half-life, which in man and in the rat does not exceed a few hours for neutrophils[8,9] and is 8 to 12 hours for eosinophils,[10] the granulocytes penetrate by diapedesis into various tissues in order to participate in nonspecific inflammatory reactions and in immunologic processes.

Granulocytes are also found in the red pulp of the spleen, and especially in the mucosa and submucosa of the alimentary tract, mainly in the small intestine, which is the principal site of elimination of granulocytes in physiological conditions. This concerns neutrophils[11,12] as well as eosinophils, which, in the rat, are about 30-fold more abundant in the intestinal wall than in the blood.[13]

1. Neutrophils

These granulocytes are the first cells to attack the infecting organisms (mainly bacteria, but also some protozoa) in acute inflammatory reactions, while the mononuclear macrophages become predominant only after about 3 days, when the granulocytes are already disintegrating in the infectious foci.

Phagocytosis of bacteria is enhanced by the presence of complement and by the "opsonic" activity of antibodies, which facilitate the attachment of the microbial antigens to the phagocytes.[14] The phagocytic process starts with the entry of the foreign organism into a vesicle formed by interiorization of the cell membrane. Afterwards, the cytoplasmic granules fuse with the phagocytic vacuole and release enzymes in a process called "degranulation," which initiates the digestion of the engulfed organism. The enzymes concerned include hydrolysases, nucleases, β-glucuronidase, lysozyme, and myeloperoxidase in the primary granules, and alkaline phosphatases and lactoferrin in the secondary granules.[15,16]

The attachment of the organism to the phagocyte provokes an increase in glucose metabolism, especially in the oxidation of glucose via the hexose monophosphate (HMP) shunt, leading to the formation of H_2O_2.[17] This product is a strong bactericidal agent in the presence of myeloperoxidase[18,19] and a halide cofactor such as iodine.[20,21]

However, other bactericidal mechanisms are also operative, and involve the intervention of lysozyme in concert with H_2O_2 and lactoferrin, which blocks free iron and thus prevents it from being utilized by the bacteria.[20,21] Finally, the basic granule proteins are also deleterious to the microorganisms.[22-24]

In contrast to the abundant literature on the macrophages, very few data are as yet available concerning the involvement of neutrophils in cell-mediated immunity and antibody production. Recruitment of neutrophils by antigen-activated T lymphocytes has been reported in delayed hypersensitivity,[25] while, on the other hand, microbial antigens, especially Gram-negative bacterial endotoxins, constitute a very strong stimulus for neutropoiesis and mobilization of neutrophils.[26,27]

2. Eosinophils

Increased production of these cells occurs following repeated exposure to protein antigens, as seen in allergic reactions, especially in those produced by parasites.

The hypothesis that eosinophilia is in most cases an immunologic phenomenon is confirmed by the chemotactic attraction exerted on these cells by antigen-antibody complexes[28-30] as well as by the fact that eosinophils preferentially phagocytose IgE-containing immune complexes.[31] Furthermore, it has been shown that eosinophil migration to the site of allergic reactions is induced by specifically sensitized thymus-dependent lymphocytes[32,33] probably acting via a humoral factor, a "lymphokin."[34,35]

In all probability, the allergic reactions induced by soluble dietary proteins and by luminal microflora may be the main cause of the high eosinophil concentration in the intestinal mucosa.

Eosinophils also intervene in the phagocytosis of mast cell granules[36] and in the removal of the excess histamine released from these cells in the *lamina propria* of the stomach during acid secretion.[37,38] This would explain the high number of eosinophils in the gastric glandular mucosa of the rat.[39,40]

3. Basophils

The blood basophils and the closely related tissular mast cells have not yet been studied extensively in connection with the nutritional status of the animal. Yet, like eosinophils, these cells play an important role in allergy. Indeed, they are believed to retain on their surface the immunoglobulin E secreted by B lymphocytes. This basophil-bound Ig permits the binding and neutralization of the allergen in the case of a secondary aggression by the latter.[41] Combination of the allergen and the antibody provokes the release of histamine as well as of other mediators from the basophils.[42,43] The mast cells of the gastric mucosa also play a role in the acid secretion via release of histamine.[38,44]

Another physiological function of blood basophils and mast cells is represented by secretion of heparin from their metachromatic granules. This substance not only plays a role as an anti-coagulant factor but also intervenes in the turnover of lipids after their intestinal absorption (see Section VI.B.2, "Basophils," later in this chapter).[45]

Addendum: Recent Data on the Biochemical Mechanism of Phagocytosis, Bactericidal Activity, and Immunologic Involvement of PMNs

The availability of NADP is known to be a rate limiting factor in hexose monophosphate shunt activity of neutrophils (PMN). NADPH-oxidase in granular leukocytes is required for the formation of both NADP and H_2O_2 and for the subsequent onset of bactericidal activity in PMNs. It has been reported by Shilotri[637] that ascorbic acid-deficient guinea pigs displayed a marked decrease of phagocytosis and of bactericidal activity and that these defects were due to a deficiency of NADPH-oxidase during phagocytosis.[637]

Other interesting recent data concern the involvement of PMNs in inflammatory and immunologic reactions. It has been observed in vitro that (human) PMNs have receptors for and are stimulated by the Fc fragment of immune complexes (IC) and immunoglobulin (Ig) aggregates formed by IgG, IgA, IgD, and by the C_{3b} fractions of complement. Receptors for the Fc fragment of IgM are not present and IgM-IC (or aggregated IgM) interact with the PMN surface via C_{3b} receptors.[638] The PMN-IC interaction results in the phagocytosis of IC with the subsequent release of lysosomal proteolytic enzymes and cationic proteins from PMNs.[638,639] Thus, the interaction of surface receptors with IC may explain the extensive involvement of neutrophils in inflammatory injury of immunologic origin,[640] as well as the presence of large quantities of Ig and C_3 on the PMN surface in autoimmune diseases with circulating IC, e.g., lupus erythematosus, rheumatoid arthritis, and IgM-IgG cryoglobulinemia.[641]

B. Lymphocytes

These cells form the most complex category of leukocytes because of the peculiarities of their evolutive cycle and their many-faceted functions, especially with regard to their intervention in immune responses.[46-53]

1. Duality of Origin and Histological Distribution

A major achievement of recent immunologic investigations was the discovery of the existence of two principal functional types of lymphocytes endowed with distinct immunologic capacities: (1) the T lymphocytes, which are processed by the thymus and initiate the cell-mediated immunity and also certain humoral responses to "thymus-dependent" antigens, and (2) the B lymphocytes, which, at least for the most part, originate directly from the bone marrow in adult mammals.[54,55] However, in birds, a specific lymphoepithelial appendage of the cloaca, the bursa of Fabricius, is the exclusive source of these cells.[46-53]

In actuality, the lymphoid progenitors of the bone marrow in mammals give rise not only to B lymphocytes but also to T lymphocytes. However, whereas one part of these stem cells emigrates directly to the peripheral lymphoid organs, where they become the precursors of B cells (that is, the short production pathway for lymphocytes, involving only two or three intramedullary mitoses[56]), another part (T cell percursors) migrates first to the thymus, where these cells (thymocytes) divide and mature to become T lymphocytes before leaving this organ for the blood vessels. This long production pathway requires about eight intrathymic mitoses.[56,57]

a. Thymus

This organ is formed of two lobes, each of them composed of a large cortex and a much smaller medullary region. The cortex is populated mainly by thymocytes, while the medulla contains a relatively large portion of native cells derived from the reticuloepithelial anlage of the thymus. It is under the inductive, probably humoral, impulsion of the latter cells[58-61] that the cortical thymocytes undergo mitotic division and maturation, and migrate from the periphery to the central area of the thymus. While some of them die locally in the organ, the great majority of thymocytes leave the thymus for the blood and peripheral lymphoid organs after an intrathymic stay not exceeding 48 to 72 hr in the rat and mouse.[62,63] Accordingly, the thymus contains mainly young and immature lymphocytes.[64]

It is not yet clearly established whether thymocytes of the medullary area are derived from a fraction of the cortical cells[65,66] or whether the two cell groups represent different developmental pathways[67] and originate from two types of immigrated stem cells.[68] In addition, there is no consensus as to the filiation between the different types of thymocytes and the peripheral T lymphocytes; although several authors believe that the medullary thymocytes are the sole precursors of the latter cells, a direct emigration of cortical lymphocytes also remains possible.[68] The presence of cells with low or high immunologic capacity among both thymocytes and peripheral T lymphocytes supports this hypothesis.

The thymus reaches its maximum size in the first weeks after birth in the rat and the mouse, and during the total duration of childhood (1 to 15 years) in man.[69] Puberty initiates an irreversible involution which is much more pronounced in man than in laboratory animals. However, even in adult humans, thymic involution is not as complete as was formerly supposed.[69] Besides, the possible development of thymic tumors (thymoma) attests to the persistence of residual tissue that is capable of reactivating.

In addition to the physiological age-dependent changes, two major factors can induce a rapid regression of the thymus: (1) different stresses which act via the successive release into the bloodstream of epinephrine, ACTH, and glucocorticoid hormones, and (2) denutrition and malnutrition. An adrenal-mediated stressing effect may in large part also account for the thymolytic action of nutritional disturbances (see Section II.E, "Hormonal Control of the Leukocyte Changes Induced by Starvation" and Section IV.A. 5.a.iv, "Glucocorticoids," later in this chapter.)

b. Peripheral Lymphoid Organs

The emigration of thymocytes toward these organs starts prior to birth and reaches its maximum during the first week of life in the mouse,[52] which explains why the decrease in T cell population is much more striking after neonatal thymectomy than after removal of the adult thymus.[47]

After having circulated together in the blood vessels, both T and B lymphocytes reach the peripheral lymphoid organs (lymph nodes, spleen, gut-associated lymphoid structures), where they achieve their morphological and functional maturation in distinct histological compartments. This maturation may be in part controlled by humoral factors secreted by the thymus and the bursa equivalent (bone marrow?), respectively.[46,50,70]

The thymus-dependent areas are represented in the lymph nodes by the paracortex, located below and to some extent between the follicles, while the areas populated mainly by B lymphocytes include the outer cortex and the follicles with their germinal centers (the latter appearing only after immunization) as well as the medullary cords containing lymphocytes and plasma cells.[71] The number of both types of cells increases strongly after injection of antigen.

In the spleen, T cells are found essentially in the periarteriolar lymphoid sheet of the white pulp, whereas the B cells occupy the follicles and are also numerous in the red pulp, where they are associated with macrophages and granulocytes. In the mouse, the proportion of T lymphocytes, estimated by using chromosomal markers of histocompatibility antigens, reaches 70 to 80% among the blood lymphocytes and 60 to 80% and 30 to 40% in the lymph nodes and spleen, respectively.[64] These percentages are similar to those found in the mouse with the help of antithymic serum[72] and to the percentages calculated in adult rats by comparing viable lymphocyte levels of thymecto-mized animals to those of intact animals (60 to 80% T cells in the lymph nodes, 30 to 50% in the spleen[73]).

The gut-associated lymphoid structures are represented mainly by lymphoepithelial formations composed of aggregates of follicles (tonsils, Peyer's patches in the wall of the small intestine, and appendix). Throughout the alimentary tract, but particularly at the level of the small intestine, numerous lymphocytes are continuously eliminated into the lumen.[50] It is not yet known to what extent this phenomenon is linked to the principal function of the intestinal lymphocytes, i.e., their intervention in the processing and transport of absorbed soluble proteins, polypeptides, and higher molecular weight lipids.[74] These substances are incorporated into the cells of the lymphoid structures, from which they are transferred to the vascular system, either inside the egressing lymphocytes themselves or in the form of protoplasma droplets shed from these cells.[75]

Furthermore, the lymphoid tissue of the gut plays an important role in the immune responses to the continuous antigen stimulation exerted by the luminal microflora and (or) the alimentary proteins. Indeed, these lymphoid formations produce large quantities of antibodies (mainly IgA), which are synthesized by the numerous plasma cells derived from B lymphocytes present in these structures.[76-78] Good and his co-workers[79-81] have suggested that these formations, along with the tonsils, may act in mammals in a manner analogous to the bursa of Fabricius in birds. This hypothesis (despite being contested because of the capacity of Peyer's patches to react to thymus-dependent antigens even in the absence of the thymus[77,78]) has been strengthened by recent immunologic findings suggesting a complete absence of T cells in these structures.[82]

On the other hand, it has been suggested that the thymic component of the immune activity of Peyer's patches could be represented by the lymphocytes located between the epithelial cells and the basement membrane of the gut wall, since these lymphocytes disappear after neonatal thymectomy.[93]

Because of these differing data, the question of the independence of the gut lymphoid tissue from the thymus is not yet resolved.

2. Life Span of Lymphocytes

The determination of lymphocyte life span by tritiated thymidine incorporation showed the existence of two populations; the largest one is short lived (about 10 days), while the other survives for many weeks or months in rodents[84] and for 4 to 5 years in man.[50]

In the thymus, the great majority of lymphocytes represented by the cortical cells is short lived, while the highest proportion of long-lived lymphocytes is found in the lymph nodes and the thoracic duct lymph; the spleen — and blood — lymphocytes include a large proportion of both cell types.[50] In the case of the thymus, spleen, and lymph nodes, these data are in agreement with those for the mitotic indices, which are five to ten times higher in the thymus than in the lymph nodes or the spleen in the mouse and man[69] and ten times higher in the thymus than in the spleen of the rat[85] (see Table 14 later in this chapter).

Many long-lived T lymphocytes and, to a lesser extent, B lymphocytes recirculate between blood and lymphoid organs. It is from the recirculating pool that antigens induce the recruitment of specific antigen-sensitive lymphocytes into appropriate lymphoid organs.[86]

In the case of the T lymphocytes, the life span also depends on the status of the thymus. Indeed, in the rat, thymectomy even if performed only 25 days after birth is followed by a sharp reduction of the number[73] as well as of the mean viability of the cells in the peripheral lymphoid organs.[87] This may be explained by the arrest of the seeding of new viable T lymphocytes as well as by the exclusion of some protective, probably hormonal, influences of the thymus.

3. Cell Size and Its Correlation with Functional Activity

There are lymphocytes of different size in all lymphoid organs, although the proportion of small lymphocytes (5 to 7 μm nuclear diameter on conventional smears, according to the classification of Bryant[88]) is particularly high (90%) in the thymus.

Medium-sized and large lymphocytes are metabolically more active than small lymphocytes, as indicated by their higher mitochondrial and polyribosomal content,[50,89] their capacity for synthesizing nucleic acids and proteins,[90,91] and their mitotic activity.[69,92]

In actual fact, lymphocyte size, far from being a constant, genetically determined feature, changes with the metabolic activity of the cell. An example of such changes is given by the enlargement of antigen- or mitogen-stimulated lymphocytes during blastic transformation. Indeed, such a transformation is accompanied by important cytological and biochemical changes: development of the Golgi apparatus,[56] increased glucose degradation through the HMP pathway,[93] and strong activation of DNA and RNA synthesis.[90,94] Conversely, the lymphocyte size decreases, either via mitotic division of large and medium-sized lymphocytes, as observed in the thymus[69] and lymph nodes,[50] or without mitoses, following (primarily protein) malnutrition.[95]

4. Sensitivity to Glucocorticoid Hormones

A characteristic feature of the great majority of thymocytes and of an important fraction of peripheral blood and lymphoid tissue lymphocytes is their high sensitivity to glucocorticoids.[96]

The finding that a drop in blood lymphocyte levels, especially of large lymphocytes, observed after a single injection of cortisone does not occur in thymectomized rats[97] indicates the thymic origin of the circulating hormone-sensitive cells. Inside the thymus in the mouse and rat, only some 5% of thymocytes resist a single massive injection of hydrocortisone.[98,99] These resistant cells are located in the medullary area, while the cortex is populated almost exclusively by cortisone-sensitive lymphocytes.[100] Adequate and repeated doses of this hormone are also capable of destroying a part of the medullary thymocytes.[68,101]

The two subpopulations of thymocytes also differ as to their sensitivity to specific antithymic sera which are cytotoxic only for cortical (cortisone-sensitive) lymphocytes,[67,68] the only cells to have full representation of membrane thymus-specific antigens.[64,99] On the other hand, the blastic transformation and mitotic proliferation in response to thymus- and T-cell-specific phytomitogens (phytohemagglutinin, PHA, and concanavalin A (Con A)) are more pronounced in vitro with cortisone-resistant lymphocytes than with cortisone-sensitive lymphocytes, when the results are calculated per cell.[99,102]

Cortisone-sensitive cells also react to PHA, however, and the PHA-induced response of the thymus as a whole must be ascribed much more to the predominant population of cortisone-sensitive, mainly cortical, thymocytes than to the small pool of cortisone-resistant cells of the medulla. This will be shown in comparative experiments on the reactivity of lymphocytes to PHA and cortisone in normally nourished and protein-deprived rats (see Section IV.A.3.d.iv, "Effect of Protein Deprivation on the Lympho-cytic Response to Phytohemagglutinin (PHA)" and Section IV.A.3.d.v, "Compared Action of Protein Deprivation on Cortisone-sensitive and Cortisone-resistant Lympho-cytes" later in this chapter).

PHA responsive peripheral T lymphocytes are also destroyed to a large extent by corticoids in the spleen,[103] as well as in the lymph nodes.[247] The effect is particularly striking in the latter organs since, in the absence of stimulation, there are only very few mitoses, and they are exclusively exhibited by cortisone-resistant cells (see Table 20 later in this chapter).

5. *Immunologic Activity of the Lymphocytes*
a. *Thymus-dependent (T) Lymphocytes*

These cells are the principal agents responsible for cell-mediated immunity. The latter includes cytotoxicity towards allogeneic cells such as viruses and some intracellular bacteria, rejection of foreign tissues, graft-vs.-host reaction (GVHR), and delayed hypersensitivity.[47,50,52,53] Furthermore, T lymphocytes cooperate as "helper cells"[105] in antibody production by B lymphocytes and their plasma cell descendents in response to thymus-dependent antigens, composed exclusively (serum proteins) or partly (heterologous erythrocytes) of protein.

This helper activity is always preceded by differentiation and division of the T lymphocytes.[51] It consists of picking up the antigen, previously processed by macrophages, by means of membranous receptors (of a still unknown nature) and transferring the antigenic determinants to areas occupied by B lymphocytes. This leads to a sufficient concentration of the determinants to trigger antibody production by the latter cells.

It has been suggested that in the terminal phase of T-B interaction the antigen forms a bridge between the T and B receptors, the protein fragment ("carrier") of the antigen being bound to the T cell and the hapten fragment to the B cell.[105] In actual fact, according to more recent findings,[25,86,106,107] the B cells may be stimulated by means of humoral mediators essentially released from antigen-activated T lymphocytes. These factors include T-cell-derived proteolytic enzymes capable of activating components of the complement.

Indeed, the induction of antibody synthesis by B lymphocytes may be conditioned not only by the binding of the antigenic determinants to their specific B cell receptors but also by the T-cell-dependent transfer of activated complement (C'3) to specific receptors on the same lymphocytes.[108] Moreover, not only do T cells induce the production of immunoglobulins by B cells but, conversely, complexes composed of antigen and Ig determinants of these cells are able to activate T lymphocytes. On the other hand, the latter cells secrete a macrophage-activating factor which enhances the degradation of the antigen by phagocytes, thus blocking antibody production (Figure 1).

It has been claimed[98] that only a minor subpopulation of thymocytes (Th 2), identified with the cortisone-resistant lymphocytes of the medulla and considered to be the sole precursor of peripheral T cells, would be immunocompetent, whereas the cortisone-sensitive thymocytes of the cortex (Th 1) are devoid of any immunologic capacity. In reality, resistance to glucocorticoids is exhibited mainly by T cell precursors of the mouse bone marrow, while the response of splenic lymphocytes to sheep red blood cells (SRBC), a thymus-dependent antigen, was found to be cortisone sensitive in the mouse (at least in the early stages of antibody response[104,109]) as well as in the rat.[101]

It has not yet been definitely established whether the helper activity of T lymphocytes and the intervention in cell-mediated immunity such as skin graft rejection and GVHR are performed by distinct subpopulations of these cells[110] or by the same cells, and whether, in the second alternative, there is[111] or is not[112] competition between the humoral and cell-mediated immunologic activity of these cells.

According to Segal et al.,[110] T cells involved in GVHR are resistant to hydrocortisone, while the helper cells are sensitive to the same hormone but become resistant after they have been sensitized to the carrier (protein) fraction of the antigen. On the other hand, there are claims that helper function and delayed hypersensitivity may be carried out by distinct T lymphocytes.[113]

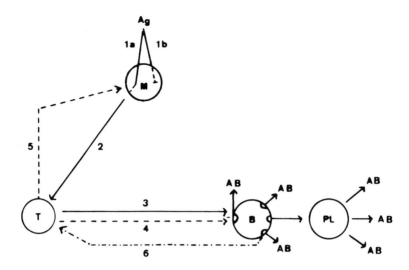

FIGURE 1.   Recent data on the interactions between macrophages (M), T cells, and B cells in the cooperative production of antibodies. Ag: antigen, Pl: plasma cell, AB: antibodies. 1: Antigen is either processed and activated (1a) or completely destroyed (1b) by the macrophage. 2: The M-processed Ag activates the T lymphocytes. 3: The activated T cells intervene in the production of antibodies by B lymphocytes and plasma cells against thymus-dependent antigens. 4: Possible inhibition of AB production by thymus-derived suppressor cells. 5: Inhibition of Ig production can also result from a feedback effect: the release of a macrophage-activating factor by T cells stimulated by IgG-producing complexes (Ag + Ig determinants of B cells). (Drawn mainly from data of Miller.[86])

Even among the cell-mediated reactions themselves, delayed contact hypersensitivity would not depend on the same T lymphocytes, as cytotoxicity[114] and GVHR cells would be more resistant to hydrocortisone than cytotoxic cells.[110]

For some authors[115] there are two subsets of peripheral T cells: One responds strongly to Con A, contains only a few thymic (Θ) antigens, migrates preferentially to the spleen, and is provided with helper, GVHR, and cytotoxic activities, while the other subset is characterized by high responsiveness to PHA, high content of thymic antigens, homing to the lymph nodes, and intervention in the mixed lymphocytic reaction.

On the other hand, if one accepts the hypothesis that the same T lymphocytes are provided with both helper and cell-mediated immunologic functions,[112] the possibility arises that each of these activities corresponds to a distinct stage of cell maturation and (or) to the existence of specific thresholds for the different mitogenic and immunogenic stimulations.[115]

Finally, a category of thymus-derived "suppressor" cells capable of inhibiting antigen-induced lymphocyte proliferation[116] and antibody production[117-119] has been described. Suppressor cells may play a role in a homeostatic control of immune responses.[120]

Thymocytes and T lymphocytes have been divided into several sublines not only on the basis of their immunologic potential but also by virtue of physical separation techniques (cell electrophoresis, velocity sedimentation, BSA density gradient centrifugation).[68,121] However, it was found that identical physical properties may coexist with different immunologic capacities.[68]

b. *Thymus-independent (B) Lymphocytes*

The antigenic determinants that enter into contact with B lymphocytes are captured by specific receptors incorporated in the cell membrane. The receptors of virgin B cells are generally formed of IgM,[122] but the stimulation by antigen induces the secretion of different categories of antibodies: IgM, IgG, IgA, or IgE.

The type of immunoglobulin secreted depends on the structure and dose of the antigen, the route of its introduction, and the time elapsed between immunization and immunologic testing, as well as on the number of antigenic stimulations (the primary response producing mainly IgM, while the secondary response produces increased proportions of IgG).

The functional status of the thymus also plays an important role in the case of thymus-dependent antigens. Indeed, the activity of T lymphocytes controls the equilibrium between the production of IgM and IgG, since it induces the formation of the latter at the expense of the former immunoglobulin. Accordingly, the antibody response elicited by thymus-independent antigens consists mainly of IgM.[86]

Thymus-derived helper cells intervene not only in the production of IgG but also in that of IgE and IgA, the latter being secreted primarily by B lymphocytes of the respiratory and intestinal mucosa.[123]

If the antigen is represented by heterologous erythrocytes, its capture by B lymphocytes can be visualized by the appearance of rosette-forming cells (RFC), which indicate the recognition and binding of the antigen. The same phenomenon can be obtained if lymphocytes from animals immunized to nonerythrocytic antigens are incubated with red cells previously coated with these antigens, regardless of whether the latter were or were not thymus dependent.

The immunologic ("acquired") RFCs also secrete small amounts of specific Ig which diffuse only in the immediate vicinity of the lymphocytes, thus strengthening the antigenic adherence to the membrane.[124,125] However, in man and, to a much smaller extent, in the mouse,[126] formation of rosettes can occur after in vitro contact with SRBC, even in the absence of previous immunization to this antigen. While these "spontaneous" RFCs are either T or B lymphocytes in the mouse,[126] all T cells in man exhibit this phenomenon, and are the only cells capable of doing it, which permits them to be easily counted in the blood.[127] The levels found even in healthy subjects, however, differ considerably according to the techniques used.[128]

The immune response to antigen-containing or antigen-bound erythrocytes is also demonstrated by the appearance of hemolytic plaque-forming cells (PFC) in the presence of complement, these plaques being due to the limited diffusion of hemolytic antibodies around the immunocompetent B cells. At a more advanced stage, the antibodies diffuse into the circulating blood. The principal producers of the serum antibodies are plasma cells, which represent a category of B lymphocytes specialized in an intensive protein synthesis.

In the case of thymus-dependent antigens, the absence or functional inactivation of the thymus can be more or less compensated for by the addition of adjuvants such as Freund's complete adjuvant or BCG, which probably act by replacing or activating the T cells.[129]

Thymus-independent antigens (such as pneumococcal polysaccharides, *Escherichia coli* lipopolysaccharides, synthetic polyamino acids, antigens of *Salmonella H* and *Brucella*,[130] and also dextran sulfate and polyvinylpyrrolidone) stimulate the synthesis of antibodies by B lymphocytes without cooperation of helper cells. This immunologic effect is ascribed to the polymeric structure and slow degradation of the B antigens. Indeed, the repetition of identical antigenic determinants increases the number of stimulated membranous receptors and consequently the triggering action of the determinants.[51]

C. Macrophages

The importance of the cooperation of these cells in humoral as well as cell-mediated immune reactions has been definitely established.[131-133]

Phagocytosis by these cells may result in the complete destruction of the antigen, thus preventing any immunologic reaction, but, in general, the degradation is incomplete, leading instead to increased immunogenicity of the antigen via the release of free antigenic determinants. These determinants are transferred to membrane receptors of T lymphocytes (Figure 1).

Furthermore, macrophages stimulate the proliferation of the antigen-induced T cells[134] and activate the helper cells.[135] They also play a role in the presentation of the antigen to B lymphocytes[136] and trigger the divisions of the latter cells.[137]

Some of these actions may be performed via soluble factors secreted by macrophages in the absence of direct cellular contact.[135,138]

In addition, it has been shown that the immunoactivating effect of macrophages requires the interaction of T lymphocytes sensitized to the appropriate antigen.[139] Indeed, the activated lymphocytes secrete soluble mediators which stimulate the proliferation of macrophages, thus enhancing the bacteriostatic activity of these cells.[86,140] The macrophage-activating factor produced by T cells may be identical to the migration-inhibitory factor (MIF).[141]

The question concering the intervention of macrophages in the processing of thymus-independent antigens is not yet resolved.[133]

D. Some General Considerations on the Nutritional Control of Leukocyte Production and Activity

Almost all nutrients, some of them (vitamins and certain minerals) representing only trace constituents of the diet, are indispensable for proliferation and differentiation of these cells. The need for exogenous material depends on the rate of leukocyte turnover and the number of cells eliminated in the alimentary tract or destroyed either in the hematopoietic organs themselves or during inflammatory and immunologic reactions.

However, the dietary intake intervenes not only as a source of building material for the cellular structures and secreted products but also by inducing adaptive changes in the activity of leukocytic enzymes. In the case of alimentary deficiencies, this may lead to a functional block of these cells, including their immunologic functions.

Furthermore, the nutritional status influences the secretion of different hormones intervening in the turnover of leukocytes. The action of some of them, such as ACTH, TSH, and epinephrine, is mediated by the membrane-bound adenylcyclase system, which is well developed, at least in the lymphocytes, and also depends on nutritional conditions.[142]

It may also be that the diet triggers or impairs the production of specific humoral leukopoietic factors which are not yet well individualized. Such factors have been described in granulopoiesis[27,143-145] and especially in lymphopoiesis, the latter factors being primarily of thymic origin.[146-151]

The following sections will deal with leukocytic alterations provoked by quantitative and (or) qualitative changes of the alimentary intake.

II. STARVATION AND EXCLUSIVE WATER DIET

A. Blood Leukocytes

Only a few, partly conflicting data are available concerning the influence of such diets in both animals and humans (for older references see Jolly[152] and Jackson[153]). More recently, it has been reported that adult rats display a sharp drop in the blood levels of neutrophils and lymphocytes after acute starvation of only 80 to 96 hr with water ad libitum,[154,155] and that leukopenia, especially lymphopenia, increases with the duration of fasting.[156] In our experiments, the lymphocyte levels dropped to 11% of the normal values after 3 days[155] (Table 1).

A striking decrease in the number of blood eosinophils was reported first by Opie[157] in starved guinea pigs. In the rat, moderate, apparently stress-induced, eosinopenia was already noticed after only one night of food removal, apparently because the food is ingested mainly during the night in this species.[158] A much more important and lasting eosinopenia is induced by prolonged aqueous inanition, as has been observed in the dog after 25 to 65 days of such a diet.[159] In this experiment, refeeding was followed by a blood discharge of eosinophils proportional to the level of ingested protein.

In man, prolonged fasting (up to 40 days) was found to provoke leukopenia without a change in the proportion of neutrophils and lymphocytes.[160] However, in obese patients, a diet reduced to water and some vitamins, given for about 44 days, resulted in the exclusive decrease of blood neutrophil levels, which could reach 50% of base line figures after 10 days.[161] A gradually increasing deficiency of folic acid apparently contributed to this effect since the development of neutropenia could be delayed by supplementation with the vitamin.[161] Indeed, in other experiments, serum folate levels were found to decrease significantly after 6 to 8 weeks of fasting.[162]

The fasting neutropenia does not prevent normal responses to intercurrent viral or bacterial infections, which are indeed capable of provoking a nearly twofold increase in leukocyte counts in most instances.[161]

As in laboratory animals, a drop in blood eosinophil levels has been observed in all cases of complete starvation in man.[163]

There are no data available concerning the phagocytic potential of neutrophils, except the report of decreased serum opsonic activity in starved rats.[164]

B. Bone Marrow

In laboratory animals as well as in cachectic humans, earlier authors[152,153] reported a mucoid degeneration of the fat tissue in the bone marrow following prolonged inanition; however, the hematopoietic tissue is also reduced. In starved rabbits, this reduction concerns erythroblasts and lymphocytes to a greater extent than granulocytes, although the latter also display frequent pycnosis of the nuclei.[152] In man, no cellular changes have been observed in the bone marrow after acute starvation.[161]

C. Lymphoid Organs

1. Thymus

The extreme sensitivity of this organ to denutrition in man is not a recent discovery, since, 130 years ago, Simon[165] called the thymus a "barometer of nutrition, and a very delicate one," and Hérard[166] indicated the nutritional factors responsible for the weight changes of the thymus. Hammar[167] was the first to show that in man as well as in the rabbit acute starvation is followed by the almost total disappearance of the lymphocyte

Table 1

EFFECT OF A 3-DAY STARVATION ON THE WEIGHT OF THE LYMPHOID ORGANS, BLOOD LYMPHOCYTE LEVELS, AND VIABILITY OF THE TISSULAR LYMPHOCYTES IN PATHOGEN-FREE MALE SHERMAN RATS

| Diet | Body weight (g) | | Weight of the lymphoid organs and blood lymphocyte levels | | | | | |
| | Initial | Terminal | Thymus (mg) | Lymph nodes (mg) | | Spleen (mg) | Blood lymphocytes/mm³ | |
				Cervical	Mesenteric		First day	Last Day
Balanced diet (18% casein) (6)[a]	210 ± 13[b]	236 ± 10	546.0 ± 43.0 (231.3)[c]	50.7 ± 11.6 (21.5)	33.3 ± 3.9 (14.1)	611.0 ± 32.9 (258.9)	10,430 ± 680	12,240 ± 645
Complete starvation (7)	206 ± 10	141 ± 9	171.8 ± 30.5 (121.8)	18.7 ± 2.3 (13.2)	17.8 ± 1.7 (12.6)	176.5 ± 19.5 (125.2)	10,760 ± 860	1,325 ± 257
Percent difference	—	-40.25	-68.53[g]	-63.12[e]	-46.55[f]	-71.10[g]	—	-89.18[g]
			Percentages of dead (stained)[d] lymphocytes					
Balanced diet	—	—	11.3 ± 1.9	31.2 ± 2.6	31.7 ± 2.6	29.2 ± 2.5	—	—
Complete starvation	—	—	42.0 ± 8.9[f]	43.8 ± 6.0	44.3 ± 5.0[e]	62.1 ± 4.4[g]	—	—

a   Number of rats.
b   Mean ± standard error (SE).
c   Relative weight (per 100 g body weight).
d   Dye (erythrosin) exclusion test: lecture immediately after addition of dye to the cell suspension; for the technique, see Reference 155).
e, f, g   Significantly different from control (balanced diet) values at P levels <0.05, <0.01, and <0.001, respectively.

From Aschkenasy, A., *Arch. Sci. Physiol.*, 25, 275–292,1971. With permission.

population of this organ, starting with the cells of the cortex, while the reticular cells and the Hassall's corpuscles are much more resistant. The same author also remarked on a "paradoxical" appearance of adipose deposits in the thymus of athreptic infants.

Similar changes were reported in starved laboratory animals.[153]

2. Spleen and Lymph Nodes

The reduction of these organs, in particular of the spleen, is as pronounced as that of the thymus, both in man and in laboratory animals (rabbit, guinea pig, and rat) (Table 1).[152,153,155] Prolonged starvation provokes an atrophy of the white pulp in the spleen, while the red pulp displays a high phagocytic activity in relation to the increased intrasplenic destruction of red cells and lymphocytes.[168] The cellular density decreases considerably in both the spleen and the lymph nodes, and the latter organs also lose their follicles after protracted inanition.[152,153]

After only 3 days of starvation in the rat, the splenic and lymph node lymphocytes as well as the thymocytes exhibit a sharp reduction in viability, as measured by a dye exclusion test (Table 1).[155]

3. Gut-associated Lymphoid Structures

Involution of these formations following starvation was reported many years ago in both man and animals.[153] In the guinea pig, the number of thoracic duct lymphocytes originating from the mesenteric lymph nodes and the intestinal wall drops by 25% after 2 days of complete inanition.[169] These findings can be explained by the role played by the intestinal lymphocytes in the transport of absorbed lipids and proteins and in the immunologic responses to the latter nutrients (see Section I.B.1.b, "Peripheral Lymphoid Organs," earlier in this chapter).

Among the intestinal lymphoid organs of birds, the bursa of Fabricius, like the thymus, also undergoes an early involution after starvation with selective atrophy of the cortex.[152] This suggests that the functionally bursa-like lymphoid tissue located in the bone marrow and, possibly, in the intestinal lymphoid structures (see Section I.B.1.b, "Peripheral Lymphoid Organs," earlier in this chapter) might also be deeply injured in prolonged complete inanition, as is the bursa in birds. Therefore, not only thymus-dependent immune responses but also thymus-independent antibody production should be impaired after starvation. However, there are still no data available concerning the immunologic consequences of complete inanition.

D. Neutrophils and Eosinophils in the Gastrointestinal Wall

The number of both cell types, but particularly that of eosinophils, diminishes in the intestinal mucosa and submucosa of starved animals (dog, guinea pig, rabbit, rat), as has already been reported by several early authors.[170-173] An important drop (~50%) of the eosinophil levels also occurs in the gastric mucosa after 3 days of inanition in the rat, but the levels increase again if the starvation is prolonged,[174] suggesting rather a biphasic stress-induced adrenal regulation (stimulation → inactivation).

E. Hormonal Control of the Leukocyte Changes Induced by Starvation

1. Glucocorticoid Hormones

Many arguments play in favor of increased activity of the hypophyso-adrenal axis in acute starvation. Starvation provokes adrenal hypertrophy in the rat[175,176] and guinea pig.[177] With the exception of the terminal stage, where edematous degeneration has been observed in the rat,[178] the hypertrophy of these glands is due to a selective hyperplasia of the fascicular zone[177] and thus may correspond to functional hyperactivity. Indeed, fasting young rats present elevated adrenal and plasma corticoid levels which are directly proportional to the percentage weight loss of the animals.[179]

On the other hand, adrenalectomized mice starved for 96 hr do not present any weight reduction of the thymus[180] nor any significant loss of nitrogen from the total lymphoid organs, while this loss exceeds 30% in intact mice.[181] These findings are in favor of an adrenal control of the starvation-induced lymphoid involution, whereas fasting blood neutropenia may be ascribed to a direct block of the granulocyte maturation in the bone marrow.

2. Androgens

After a 96-hr starvation, the reduction of the lymphoid organs is much less pronounced in intact female mice and in castrated males than in intact male mice.[176] In male rats starved during the same interval, the mobilization of nitrogen from the thymus is entirely prevented by orchidectomy,[176] whereas the degradation of the splenic proteins is not influenced.

3. Thyroid Hormones

Unlike adrenalectomy, removal of thyroid still amplifies the involution of lymphoid tissue in mice starved for 48 hr.[181] This finding, which could be explained by the lymphostimulating capacity of thyroxine,[56,182] demonstrates the persistence of thyroid activity during starvation, apparently providing some protection for the lymphoid organs. Similar observations have been reported in protein-deficient rats.[77]

III. SEMISTARVATION AND BALANCED UNDERNUTRITION

A. Blood and Bone Marrow Leukocytes

Neutropenia in rats[183] and severe lymphopenia in mice[184,185] were reported after protracted undernutrition. On the other hand, when a balanced (18% casein) but quantitatively restrained diet is given to rats pair-fed with animals on a 4% casein diet for 8 weeks, the number of blood leukocytes per cubic millimeter decreases sharply, the drop involving mainly the lymphocytes but in general also the neutrophils (Table 2).[186] A diet lacking only protein reduces the lymphocyte and eosinophil levels, but not those of neutrophils (see Section IV.A.1, "Neutrophils," later in this chapter).

In man, advanced, usually lethal, denutrition, like that which was observed in German concentration camps or in the Warsaw Ghetto, either did not reduce but rather increased the blood leukocytosis[187] or provoked neutropenia and lymphopenia in the absence of infection[188] and eosinopenia with the exception of cases with parasitosis.[189]

In addition, hemodilution accompanying famine edema, resulting from hypoproteinemia and (or) renal or cardiac failure, frequently amplifies the nutritional leukopenia as well as anemia.

Adult volunteers subjected to semistarvation for 24 weeks exhibited a 35% drop of the blood leukocyte levels without apparent changes in the differential count.[190]

Myelograms performed in the Warsaw Ghetto during World War II revealed a paradoxical increase (probably due to a maturation block) in the number of myeloid cells as well as of erythroblasts.[188]

B. Lymphoid Organs

As in complete starvation, the thymus and the spleen are the most injured organs in animal undernutrition,[152,153,186,191] although they are less reduced in balanced undernutrition than in the case of exclusive protein deficiency. Thus, the weight of the thymus was found to be reduced by 50% in rats after 6 weeks of a protein-poor diet (6% casein) given ad libitum in comparison to pair-fed rats receiving a 24% casein diet given during the same interval.[192] Similar results were observed in our laboratory after 8 weeks of a 4% casein diet, as compared to an 18% casein-restricted regimen (Table 2).[186]

Table 2

BLOOD NEUTROPHILS AND LYMPHOCYTES, AND WEIGHTS OF LYMPHOID ORGANS AFTER 8 WEEKS OF A 4% CASEIN DIET, AS COMPARED TO AN 18% CASEIN DIET GIVEN AD LIBITUM OR PAIR-FED IN YOUNG MALE CHARLES RIVER RATS[186]

Diet[a]	Body weight (g)		Blood (per mm³)		Thymus (mg)		Spleen (mg)		Cervical lymph node (mg)	
	Initial	Terminal	Neutrophils	Lymphocytes	Absolute	Relative	Absolute	Relative	Absolute	Relative
18% casein ad libitum (8)[b]	105.4 ±3.0[c]	376.5 ±5.6	2,498 ±1,178	16,963 ±839	790.6 ±70.3	210.6 ±20.2	812.9 ±32.1	216.0 ±8.1	21.8 ±5.8	5.9 ±1.6
18% casein pair-fed (8)	108.4 ±1.3	154.4 ±4.7 (−59.0)[d]	818 ±166 (−67.2)	5,090 ±853 (−70.0)[g]	255.8 ±9.1 (−67.6)[g]	166.8 ±7.8 (−20.8)	317.1 ±32.1 (−61.0)[g]	202.8 ±14.6 (−6.1)	8.2 ±3.3 (−62.4)	5.1 ±1.8 (−13.5)
4% casein (9)	105.9 ±3.1	98.8 ±9.0 (−73.8)	1,949 ±528 (−22.0)	7,444 ±1,165 (−56.1)[g]	129.7 ±32.9 (−83.6)[g]	114.6 ±24.5 (−45.6)[f]	163.1 ±19.0 (−79.9)[g]	164.2 ±11.5 (−21.0)[f]	6.3 ±0.8 (−71.1)[e]	6.4 ±0.5 (+8.5)

a   For the composition, consult References 142 and 232.
b   Number of rats.
c   Mean ± SE.
d   Percent changes with regard to the values of the 18% casein ad libitum group.
e, f, g Significantly different from control values (18% casein ad libitum) at P levels <0.05, <0.01 and <0.001, respectively.

C. Hormonal Control

While, according to Mulinos et al.,[193] undernourished rats would exhibit an involution of adrenals and not a hypertrophy as observed in starved animals,[175] a relative hypertrophy of these glands was reported by others after a calorie-poor diet.[194]

In man, the frequent incidence of some symptoms similar to those of Addison's disease (asthenia, hypotension, pigmentation) in undernourished subjects and, in particular, the reduced urinary excretion of 17-ketosteroids[195,196] suggested an adrenal insufficiency. In actual fact, the latter anomaly concerns genital and not adrenal steroids and is due to a deficiency of glycuroconjugation of these hormones in the liver.

Indeed, the plasma levels of 17-hydroxycorticosteroids, far from being reduced, are frequently above normal in human protein calorie malnutrition (PCM: marasmus), which represents a fairly good equivalent of experimental semistarvation (see Section IV.B.3.c, "Role Played by the Adrenals in the Lymphocytic and Immunologic Anomalies Induced by Protein Malnutrition in Man," later in this chapter).

D. Relationship Between Leukocytic Anomalies and Immunologic Defense Reactions in Animal Undernutrition

Relatively few data are available concerning immunodepression in balanced undernutrition in animals. In recent experiments in our laboratory, young pair-fed rats maintained for 8 weeks on a restricted 18% casein diet exhibited a sharply depressed production of rosette- and plaque-forming cells after immunization to SRBC, while no significant changes in the levels of these immunocytes were observed in rats subjected for the same time to a 4% casein diet ad libitum (Table 3).[186]

Intrauterine growth retardation due to maternal semistarvation in rats was reported to produce a significant impairment of SRBC-antibody formation in the first- (F1) and even in the second- (F2) generation offspring, although the litters had free access to food.[197] These findings are at variance with those of Kenney,[198] who did not observe immune depression in the progeny of protein-deficient rats.

At any case, significant immunologic abnormalities have been observed in the closely related protein-calorie malnutrition (PCM) in man, as will be discussed in Section IV.B.3.b, "Immunologic Activity," later in this chapter.

IV. DEFICIENCIES OF PROTEIN AND AMINO ACIDS

A. Animal Experimentation
1. Neutrophils
a. Effect of Protein Deficiency
i. Quantitative Changes of Neutrophils

Among rats submitted to a protracted protein-free diet, only females were found to develop a moderate neutropenia,[199] while in male rats a drop in the blood neutrophil levels was observed exclusively in cases of associated folic acid deficiency[200,201] and (or) if the microbiological synthesis of this vitamin in the intestine was suppressed by sulfonamides.[202] On the contrary, neutropenia reported in rats receiving a diet with 0.5% lactalbumin[203] might be ascribed to hemodilution with edema exhibited by these animals.

The normal levels of circulating neutrophils in protein-deficient male rats may be explained by the mobilization of reserves of these cells in the bone marrow, the spleen, and the intravascular marginal pool, as well as by their decreased elimination in the intestine because of the quantitative and qualitative impairment of the alimentary intake. In fact, the alterations of neutropoiesis became apparent mainly when the deficient animals were challenged with stress conditions stimulating this activity. Thus, repeated

Table 3

IMMUNOLOGIC CHANGES AFTER 8 WEEKS OF A 4% CASEIN DIET, AS
COMPARED TO AN 18% CASEIN DIET GIVEN AD LIBITUM OR PAIR-FED IN
YOUNG MALE CHARLES RIVER RATS IMMUNIZED TO SHEEP RED BLOOD
CELLS[186]

Diet	Rosette-forming cells per 10^6 viable spleen lymphocytes	Plaque-forming cells per 10^6 viable spleen lymphocytes	Serum antibody titers[a]	
			Hemagglutinins	Hemolysins
18% casein ad libitum (8)[b]	6074 ± 673^c	159 ± 23	3.424 ± 0.097	2.634 ± 0.075
18% casein pair-fed (8)	1377 ± 182^e	54 ± 13^d	3.311 ± 0.114	2.860 ± 0.114
4% casein ad libitum (9)	5373 ± 1230	101 ± 32	$2,876 \pm 0.261$	2.408 ± 0.207

[a]   Values expressed as decimal logarithms of the highest dilution giving agglutination or complete hemolysis.

[b]   Number of rats.

[c]   Mean ± SE.

[d, e]   Statistically different from the 18% casein ad libitum group: $P < 0.01$ and <0.001, respectively.

bleeding, subcutaneous injection of turpentine, or intravenous injection of a peritoneal exudate in the rat[204] as well as intravenous inoculation of *Staphylococcus aureus* in the rabbit[205] are followed by a much lower hyperneutrophilia in the case of a protein-deficient diet than with a balanced one.

On the other hand, although the total influx of neutrophils, induced locally by intraperitoneal (i.p.) injection of glycogen, is much lower in protein-deprived rats[206] and rabbits[207] than in normally nourished controls (which obviously results from the body weight differences between the two groups), the neutrophil levels per milliliter of peritoneal exudate do not differ significantly.[206] Surprisingly, the protein-deprived rats, injected i.p. with glycogen, exhibit an abnormal increase in the number of blood neutrophils per cubic millimeter (Table 4).[206] This may correspond to a "pseudoleukocytosis" induced by mobilization of marginal granulocytes as a consequence of the stressing effect of glycogen via a discharge of epinephrine.[7] Indeed, a similar discrepancy between unchanged or even inhibited local inflammatory accumulation of neutrophils and elevated levels of these cells in the blood has already been observed, even in normal dietary conditions, after injection of epinephrine or cortisone.[26]

It has been reported[206] that stress results in an accelerated mobilization of neutrophils from the bone marrow to peripheral blood in PD rats; this was recently confirmed by Suda et al.[642] These authors noted that after a weak inflammatory stimulus, such as the implantation of cover slips, the percentage of ^{3}H-thymidine-labeled neutrophils in the blood was paradoxically higher 12 and 24 hr later in deficient rats compared to controls. This probably results from the decreased size of the marrow pool in PD animals. However, complete exhaustion of this pool can occur following more severe stress conditions, e.g., repeated bleeding, the injection of turpentine, or certain microbial infections,[204,205] as well as after highly protracted protein deprivation.

Table 4

CHANGES IN THE PERITONEAL AND BLOOD LEVELS OF NEUTROPHILS 5 HR AFTER INTRAPERITONEAL INJECTION OF GLYCOGEN[a] IN NORMALLY NOURISHED AND PROTEIN-DEPRIVED [b] ADULT RATS[c,206]

Diet	Peritoneal neutrophils per ml of harvested liquid	Peritoneal neutrophils per total harvested liquid	Blood neutrophils/mm^3		Percent changes
			Before glycogen injection	After glycogen injection	
18% casein (6)[d]	1,595 ± 236[e]	30,018 ± 5,226	930 ± 160	1,715 ± 182	+84
Protein-free for 2 months (7)	1,027 ± 170	11,255 ± 1,760[g]	1,532 ± 330	4,682 ± 550[h]	+205
18% casein for 2 weeks after 2 months of protein deprivation	1,234 ± 267	12,508 ± 2,692[f]	4,729[i] ± 803[h]	8,561 ± 1,265[h]	+81

a   10 mg glycogen/4 ml physiological saline per 100 g body weight.
b   For the composition of the diets, consult References 142 and 232.
c   Pathogen-free male Sherman rats.
d   Number of rats.
e   Mean ± SE.
f, g, h Statistically different from the 18% casein group: P < 0.05, <0.01 and <0.001, respectively.
i   The high initial count corresponds to the neutrophil discharge induced by protein refeeding.

ii. Functional Changes of Neutrophils

Many studies have been carried out concerning the functional activities of neutrophils in experimental protein deficiency. Thus, blood neutrophils were shown to exhibit reduced phagocytic potency against bacteria (*Salmonella enteritidis*) in protein-deprived rats, but this was observed only in cases of previous immunization to the same microorganism.[208] Therefore, decreased opsonic activity of antigen-antibody complexes would be the real reason for the impaired phagocytosis.

Some other workers also reported reduced phagocytosis in experimental protein malnutrition in rats and mice, with regard to bacteria[209-212] as well as to heterologous red cells.[213] All these experiments, however, were performed not on blood neutrophils but on macrophages of the spleen,[209,212] the peritoneal exudate,[210,213] or the liver.[211]

Differing findings have been published concerning the serum titers of complement. Indeed, the levels were found to be much lower in young rats subjected to a 7% casein diet than in controls nourished with a 27% casein diet,[214] while, according to other authors,[215] adult protein-depleted rats do not display any anomaly in their complement levels.

As to the biochemical parameters of the neutrophilic functions, a striking drop in myeloperoxidase activity was observed in the granulocytes of the intestinal mucosa in protein-deficient rats,[203] but no experimental data are available concerning the same activity in the blood. Nitro-blue-tetrazolium reduction was not depressed in peritoneal neutrophils of protein-deficient rabbits following injection of glycogen.[207]

iii. Neutrophils During Protein Refeeding

In spite of the usual conservation of normal blood neutrophil levels in adult male rats during the course of a protein-free diet, refeeding with a balanced (18% casein) diet given ad libitum rapidly induces a temporary increase in the number of circulating neutrophils.[216-218] This neutrophilia may result not only from an increased supply of leukopoietic protein material but also from a chemotactic attraction and an immunologic stimulation of the neutrophils[219] by the incompletely degraded foreign dietary proteins.

Some experimental data suggest an intervention of the spleen and also of the thymus in this phenomenon. Indeed, neutrophil release is much smaller in rats that have been thymectomized at 25 days of age 1 month before the onset of a protein starvation lasting 2 months (Figure 2),[220] and is also reduced in intact rats that have been injected during the first 10 days of refeeding with highly purified antithymic globulins (see Table 18 later in this chapter).[221]

On the other hand, i.p. injection of glycogen provokes a significantly smaller blood discharge of neutrophils in thymectomized rats than in intact animals if both groups received a recovery diet after prolonged protein deprivation.[206]

Since no neutropenia was reported after thymectomy in rats on a balanced diet,[199] one must conclude that depression of neutropoiesis occurs only when the removal of the adult thymus is completed by a profound involution of the peripheral T cell population. This may provoke the disappearance of a neutrophil-mobilizing T-cell-derived factor similar to the macrophage-activating factor secreted by the same cells.[140] The shortage of such a hypothetical agent may become particularly apparent in the first weeks of protein refeeding after protein starvation because of an increased demand for granulocytes.

Rats deprived of both thymus and spleen display the same changes in neutrophil restoration as do only thymectomized rats, but even splenectomy alone (carried out 1 week before protein deprivation) is sufficent to significantly shorten the neutrophil release induced by the recovery diet (Figure 2).[220] Since, in normally fed rats, removal of the spleen is followed by a blood discharge of neutrophils, the inhibitory effect of the splenectomy on neutrophil restoration after a protein-free diet may be ascribed to the

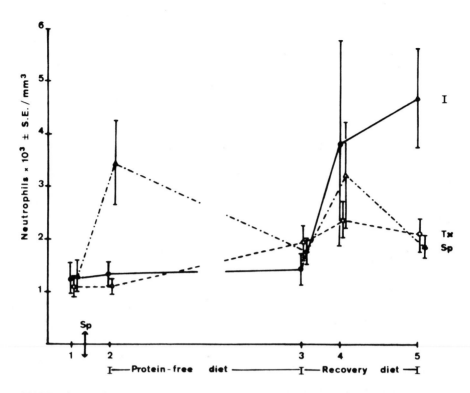

FIGURE 2.   Evolution of blood neutrophil levels (means ± SE) in male Charles River rats during an 85-day period of protein starvation and a 3-week period of a recovery 18% casein diet. Effects of thymectomy (Tx) and splenectomy (Sp) performed at 25 and 48 days of age, 4 weeks and 1 week, respectively, before the onset of protein deprivation. I: intact rats. 1: 1 week before the protein-free diet; 2 and 3: the first and last days of the diet; 4 and 5: the 8th and 22nd days of the recovery diet. ‡: splenectomy. Note the massive release of neutrophils into the blood stream following splenectomy, and the inhibitory effect of both thymectomy and splenectomy on the protein-refeeding-induced discharge of neutrophils. (From Aschkenasy, A., *C.R. Soc. Biol.*, 163, 295–300, 1969. With permission.)

revival of the granulopoietic activity of the spleen (generally limited to the fetal and neonatal periods) under the stress of protein refeeding, so that this organ becomes an important producer of the neoformed neutrophils.

b. Effects of Specific Amino Acid Deprivations

In contrast to a diet completely devoid of amino acids, which is only moderately and inconstantly neutropenic, several, but not all, imbalanced synthetic diets containing an incomplete mixture of amino acids instead of protein lead to a strong impairment of neutropoiesis. This effect was particularly apparent when such incomplete diets were given to rats that had been previously depleted of protein by means of a prolonged protein starvation (Table 5).[217,218] Under such conditions, the most deleterious diets were those lacking lysine, histidine, and, in particular, valine. Indeed, deprivation of the latter amino acid resulted in a virtually complete suppression of neutropoiesis within 10 days. After the same period, the blood neutrophil count increased strongly following a recovery diet with 18% casein ad libitum. The same diet given to rats pair-fed with valine-deprived animals did not augment the blood neutrophilia above the levels of the protein-starvation period, but it did not depress the neutrophil levels as did valine deprivation. Therefore, the neutropenic effect of certain incomplete amino acid diets cannot be ascribed only in the anorexia caused by nearly all imbalanced regimens.

Table 5

COMPARED EFFECTS OF BALANCED DIETS (CASEIN OR COMPLETE AMINO ACID MIXTURE) OR
OF SOME INCOMPLETE AMINO ACID DIETS ON BLOOD NEUTROPHILS AND LYMPHOCYTES OF
RATS WHEN GIVEN DURING A PERIOD OF 10 DAYS AFTER 7 WEEKS OF PROTEIN
DEPRIVATION

Diet following protein deprivation	Neutrophils (per mm^3)			Lymphocytes (per mm^3)		
	1st day	11th day	Mean percent change	1st day	11th day	Mean percent change
18% casein ad libitum (5)[a]	1330 ± 450	3320 ± 920	+149.6	4260 ± 340	6615 ± 320	+55.3
17% complete amino acid mixture[b] (6)	780 ± 85	965 ± 240	+23.7	5200 ± 580	6180 ± 720	+18.8
Without lysine (5)	1300 ± 445	425 ± 65	−67.3[c]	6360 ± 650	6040 ± 680	−5.0
Without sulfur amino acids (6)	1310 ± 255	1560 ± 380	+19.1	9230 ± 470	5270 ± 875	−42.9
Without histidine (5)	1500 ± 420	635 ± 120	−57.7	6660 ± 355	5390 ± 280	−19.2
Without phenolic acids (5)	1170 ± 165	970 ± 85	−17.1	9100 ± 810	5570 ± 835	−38.8
Without tryptophan (6)	905 ± 155	1050 ± 125	+16.0	6540 ± 310	6010 ± 530	−8.1
Without threonine (5)	1080 ± 330	1180 ± 140	+9.2	7540 ± 440	6130 ± 920	−18.7
Without valine (6)	1530 ± 375	205 ± 45	−86.6	9110 ± 850	4750 ± 580	−47.9
18% casein restricted (5)	1000 ± 170	1070 ± 305	+7.0	8190 ± 880	3740 ± 280	−54.3

[a] Number of animals (adult male Charles River rats).
[b] Percentage and composition of the mixture according to Reference 634.
[c] The sharpest drops in leukocyte levels are in boldface type.

Adapted from Aschkenasy, A., *C.R. Soc. Biol.*, 160, 933—937, 1966. With permission.

Contrary to the deprivation of valine, the lack of sulfur amino acids does not provoke neutropenia.[217,218] Nevertheless, i.p. injections of ethionine, a methionine antagonist, given for 40 days, induce chromosomal alterations in bone marrow myelocytes (breaks, gaps, and fragmentation), which can be prevented by simultaneous injections of methionine.[222]

2. Eosinophils

a. Effect of Protein Deficiency

Eosinophils are the first leukocytes to decrease in number in protein-deficient rats; after 3 weeks of a protein-free diet given to adult rats, the eosinophil concentration is 60 to 70% lower in the blood and 50% lower in the gastrointestinal mucosa, while the percentages in the bone marrow are still normal (Table 6).[223] After 2 months of the same diet, these cells disappear almost completely in the blood and bone marrow,[39] whereas the levels of blood neutrophils per cubic millimeter remain unchanged[199] and those of lymphocytes show a drop of about 66% during the same period.[220]

Refeeding with a protein diet (15 or 18% casein) results in a return to normal eosinophil levels, first in the bone marrow and blood (after 5 to 10 days) and somewhat later in the digestive mucosa.[39] This delay may be due to the time necessary for the development of local allergic reactions against alimentary proteins.

b. Effects of Specific Amino Acid Deprivations

No eosinopenia is observed in rats after 3 weeks of a diet lacking only sulfur amino acids or lysine. On the other hand, the levels of blood eosinophils manifest an important drop after deprivation of phenolic amino acids, histidine, arginine, or leucine, and especially after removal of isoleucine or valine. With all these diets, eosinopenia is even more marked than in rats completely devoid of alimentary amino acids (Table 6).[223]

Table 6

BLOOD, BONE MARROW, AND GASTROINTESTINAL EOSINOPHILS[a] IN ADULT MALE PARASITE-FREE WISTAR RATS GIVEN EITHER AN 18% CASEIN DIET OR DIETS CONTAINING 17% OF VARIOUS AMINO ACID MIXTURES FOR 3 WEEKS[b]

Diet	Number of rats	Blood (per mm^3)	Bone marrow (per 10^3 cells)	Gastric mucosa[c]	Ileal villi[c]
18% casein	9	323 ± 60	41.4 ± 8.4	85 ± 5	27 ± 4
Complete mixture of 19 amino acids	10	230 ± 37	32.2 ± 2.9	61 ± 6	30 ± 3
Diet without sulfur amino acids	6	362 ± 70	73.0 ± 10.0	59 ± 7	38 ± 2
Without lysine	6	381 ± 99	69.5 ± 5.6	66 ± 8	28 ± 6
Without tryptophan	6	136 ± 28	30.4 ± 2.9	46 ± 3	17 ± 1
Without phenolic amino acids	10	38 ± 4	18.9 ± 5.1	47 ± 4	12 ± 2
Without histidine	6	69 ± 35	29.0 ± 9.9	41 ± 6	21 ± 2
Without threonine	5	137 ± 36	31.8 ± 8.0	59 ± 7	24 ± 2
Without leucine	5	63 ± 11	39.0 ± 5.8	54 ± 5	27 ± 2
Without isoleucine	4	11 ± 6	12.2 ± 5.9	14 ± 6	8 ± 5
Without valine	5	2 ± 0.4	4.1 ± 1.6	5 ± 4	2 ± 1
Without arginine	5	64 ± 23	25.8 ± 4.3	66 ± 8	17 ± 1
Without amino acids	14	114 ± 19	41.0 ± 6.2	42 ± 1	13 ± 0.5

[a] The counts were performed by the method of Randolph.
[b] Mixtures prepared according to Rose et al.[634]
[c] Per 100 squares of an eyepiece reticle (magnification of 800X).

From Aschkenasy, A., *Rev. Fr. Etud. Clin. Biol.,* 10, 299—307, 1965. With permission.

The lack of valine is by far the most harmful, as it is for neutrophils and lymphocytes, since 3 weeks suffice for the almost complete disappearance of eosinophils in the blood, the digestive tract, and the bone marrow, which contains no more than very few immature precursors of these cells (Table 6).[223]

The harmful effect of imbalanced amino acid diets is still much more pronounced when, instead of being given after a normal diet, they follow a protracted (60 days) complete protein deprivation. In such conditions, eosinopenia due to this deprivation cannot be cured by any recovery diet lacking only one essential amino acid, including methionine or lysine.[217] This contrasts with the absence of eosinopenia after deprivation of these two amino acids if the rats are previously maintained on a balanced diet permitting the accumulation of protein reserves.[223]

c. Physiological Significance of Dietary Eosinopenia

This anomaly may be due principally to the arrest of allergic eosinotactic reactions induced in the digestive mucosa by repeated absorption of soluble proteins. Reduction of the intestinal microflora possibly also intervenes in the depression of local immune eosinophil-concentrating processes. There is also some parallelism between the degree of blood and gut eosinopenia and the extent of thymic involution, as suggested by comparing the effects of different amino acid diets on the two parameters (Table 6 and Table 12, later in this chapter). This could be explained by the hypothesis that T cells intervene in the recruitment of eosinophils for the allergic responses to antigens.[32-35]

The drop in the number of eosinophils in the gastric mucosa of protein- or amino-acid-deprived rats may be of nonimmunologic origin and be related rather to the mucosal aplasia and subsequent arrest of acid secretion, since it has been claimed that these cells absorb excess histamine during gastric secretion.[37,38] However, Teir et al.[174] succeeded in increasing gastric eosinophilia in the absence of any ingestion of protein. This was accomplished not only by injecting pilocarpine, which stimulates gastric secretion, but also after injection of atropine or by performing vagotomy, although the latter two interventions inhibit this secretion.

The dissimilar effects of different amino acid diets on the eosinophils are hardly compatible with an immunologic explanation, since a priori these low-molecular-weight diets should display only a moderate immunogenic potency. Therefore, it appears probable that the eosinopoietic capacity of some amino acids may be due to their direct influence on the mitotic activity of eosinophil precursors and (or) on the functional (enzymatic) activity of adult eosinophils; valine and isoleucine seem to be particularly involved in these processes.

d. Role Played by Glucocorticoid Hormones in Dietary Eosinopenia

Protein deprivation in adult rats provokes an increase in the relative weight of the adrenals, observed after 25 days of diet in some animals, along with, but only at a later stage (~5 weeks), a rise in the corticosterone levels in plasma and (or) adrenals. The latter effects, as well as adrenal hypertrophy, are also observed with diets lacking exclusively certain amino acids (phenolic acids or valine; see Table 27 later in this chapter).[224] The same diets are also particularly harmful for the thymus and the eosinophils. These findings suggest that, at least to a certain extent, dietary eosinopenia may be due to a hypercorticalism provoked by the stressing effect of the imbalanced diets.

In addition, both the eosinophils and the thymus of protein-deficient animals are particularly sensitive to the deleterious action of glucocorticoid hormones. Indeed, the drop in blood eosinophil levels observed 4 hr after i.p. injection of ACTH or cortisone (4 mg and 0.4 mg, respectively, per 100 g body weight) is much more important in protein-deprived rats (-90%) than in normally fed rats of the same age and strain (-50 to 60%).[225] These results may be explained by increased functional activity of the circulating glucocorticoids in protein-deficient animals because of an abnormally high proportion of a free form of these hormones not bound to their carrier protein, as has already been reported in malnourished children.[226]

3. Lymphocytes
a. Effect of Protein Deficiency
i. Lymphoid Organs

All these organs display a considerable decrease in size in protein-deficient rats, but the atrophy of the thymus is the earliest and the most complete manifestation;[227,228] the involution of the spleen is also important.[200,221,228] In the case of the spleen and lymph nodes in general, only the absolute and not the relative weights are reduced (Table 7).[227-229]

Growth of the spleen and thymus has also been found to be delayed in normally fed very young rats if their mothers had be subjected to a 5% protein diet during pregnancy.[198] In actual fact, because of the striking reduction of cellular density per unit weight in protein-deprived rats, the decrease in the populations of all these organs, including the lymph nodes, is still much greater than indicated by the weight changes alone (Table 8).[229] Thus, the reductions in total lymphocyte population found after 2 months of a protein-free diet in adult male rats are 99% for the thymus, 90% for the spleen, and 72% for the cervical lymph nodes.[229]

An important decrease in the number of lymphocytes, with predominant rarefaction of theta-positive lymphocytes, has also been reported in the thymus, spleen, and lymph nodes of mice subjected from weaning to an 8% casein diet for 14 days.[230] The thymic

Table 7

EFFECT OF A PROTEIN-FREE DIET ON THE WEIGHT OF LYMPHOID ORGANS IN PATHOGEN-FREE MALE SHERMAN RATS FOR 2 MONTHS

Diet	Body weight (g)		Thymus (mg)		Spleen (mg)		Cervical lymph node (mg)	
	Initial	Terminal	Absolute	Relative	Absolute	Relative	Absolute	Relative
18% casein (7)[a]	174.7 ± 4.4[b]	454.1 ± 12.1	589.2 ± 63.8	130.1 ± 14.7	802.4 ± 55.2	174.3 ± 10.0	15.6 ± 1.8	3.1 ± 0.3
Protein free (10)	194.3 ± 8.8	112.5 ± 6.1	31.6 ± 3.3	27.9 ± 2.3	159.8 ± 7.6	143.3 ± 5.6	6.1 ± 0.6	5.5 ± 0.4
Percent difference	—	−75.2	−94.6	−78.6	−80.1	−17.8	−60.9	+60.1

a Number of rats.
b Mean ± SE.

From Aschkenasy, A., *Arch. Sci. Physiol.*, 26, 359–366, 1972. With permission.

Table 8

EFFECT OF A PROTEIN-FREE DIET ON THE LYMPHOCYTIC POPULATION IN THE BLOOD AND LYMPHOID ORGANS OF MALE PATHOGEN-FREE SHERMAN RATS[a]

Number of lymphocytes

Diet	Blood (per mm³)	Thymus (×10³)		Spleen (×10³)		Cervical lymph node (×10³)	
		Per mg	Per organ	Per mg	Per organ	Per mg	Per organ
Balanced diet (7)[b]	12,180 ±900	3,680 ±132	2,149,796 ±227,787	970 ±74	779,872 ±69,515	1,021 ±162	16,708 ±4,312
Protein-free diet (2 months) (10)	4,080 ±450	761 ±66	22,665 ±3,961	496 ±28	77,960 ±5,221	733 ±51	4,627 ±710
Decrease (%)	−66.5	−79.3	−98.9	−48.9	−90.0	−28.2	−72.3

a Terminal body weight: 454.1 ± 12.4 g for the controls, 112.5 ± 6.1 g for the protein-deprived rats.
b Number of rats.

From Aschkenasy, A., *Arch. Sci. Physiol.*, 26, 359–366, 1972. With permission.

atrophy was particularly pronounced in the cortex, while the medullary area, containing an important proportion of large reticuloepithelial cells, was relatively preserved.[227,231]

In the spleen and lymph nodes, the rarefaction of cells involves both the thymus-dependent (paracortex) and thymus-independent (follicles and medullary cords) areas.[199,232,233] Also, the erythrosin exclusion test has demonstrated a sharp reduction of viability of the lymphocytes of the thymus, spleen, and mesenteric lymph nodes when protein-deprived rats were compared to weight and age controls (Table 9).[155] In all lymphoid organs, cell viability is completely restored after 2 weeks of protein refeeding.[155]

ii. Lymphocytes of the Digestive Tract

Protracted protein deprivation provokes an almost complete disappearance of Peyer's patches in the rat, but the lymphocytes scattered in the lamina propria of the intestinal villi seem to be as numerous as in normal rats. This impression may be explained by the atrophic retraction of the mucosa. Nevertheless, measurement of the size of lymphocytes of the villi reveals an increased percentage of small lymphocytes at the expense of large lymphocytes and plasma cells. Refeeding with casein restores the normal proportions of these cell types (Table 10).[234]

This finding can be understood in the light of the role played by the gut-lymphoid structures in the immunologic reactions (secretion of antibodies, mainly IgA, by plasma cells) against dietary soluble proteins and also in the synthesis of lipoproteins from absorbed fats and amino acids.[75-78,235] Apparently, both of these activities should be inhibited in the case of protein deprivation.

iii. Blood Lymphocytes

Lymphopenia is constant (Figure 3), although it appears later than eosinopenia.[231,236] There is a simultaneous decrease in the average size of the nucleus and particularly cytoplasm (Table 11), which corresponds to a preponderant rarefaction of large and medium-sized lymphocytes while the number of small lymphocytes is relatively, but not completely, preserved (Figure 4).[237] Indeed, the average drop in the number (per cubic millimeter) of the three morphological types of blood lymphocytes (defined arbitrarily according to their cellular index (CI), the product of two cell diameters measured on blood smears) in male rats after 70 days of protein deprivation was found to be of 91% for the large lymphocytes (CI $> 110 \ \mu m^2$), 67% for the medium-sized lymphocytes, and only 19% for the small lymphocytes (CI $< 80 \ \mu m$ (values calculated from Reference 237).

Refeeding with a balanced diet is followed by a striking increase in the number (Figure 3) as well as in the size (Table 11) of the lymphocytes, the size of the cytoplasm increasing more than that of the nucleus. Accordingly, the proportion of large and medium-sized lymphocytes is augmented at the expense of the small lymphocytes (Figure 4). After 10 days of a recovery diet, the increase in the number of large lymphocytes is lower if this diet contains a mixture of 19 amino acids instead of casein. This is also the case for the weight of the thymus (Figure 5).

If the 18% casein recovery diet is given only in very small amounts (4 to 5 g dry weight per day), the total number of blood lymphocytes drops sharply (Table 5), but the increase in the mean cell size is not prevented while it is by deprivation of only one essential amino acid (see below) (Table 11). Thus, the size increase apparently requires a much smaller supply of complete protein than cellular proliferation.

b. Effects of Selective Deprivation of Certain Essential Amino Acids
i. Lymphoid Organs

As after protein deprivation, the thymus is the organ that suffers the most in the case of a lack of essential amino acids. Thymic atrophy has already been reported in rats

Table 9
VIABILITY OF LYMPHOCYTES IN SOME LYMPHOID TISSUES OF NORMALLY FED AND PROTEIN-DEPRIVED PATHOGEN-FREE MALE ADULT SHERMAN RATS

	Percentages of lymphocytes (± SE) stained with erythrosin[a]			
Group	Thymus	Cervical lymph node	Mesenteric lymph node	Spleen
Controls of the same weight as protein deprived rats (5)[b]	6.2 ±1.2	29.6 ±8.4	34.2 ±7.8	27.0 ±1.2
Controls of the same age (16)	10.3 ±1.6	30.7 ±3.6	28.7 ±2.2	35.2 ±2.5
Rats deprived of proteins since 49 days (12)	28.6 ±5.8	32.6 ±3.5	63.9 ±6.9	53.4 ±2.8
Rats re-fed for 14 days after a protein-free diet (13)	9.8 ±1.4	32.8 ±3.1	34.6 ±3.4	37.5 ±2.0

[a] According to the method of Claesson[635] modified by Aschkenasy.[155] The results of this table have been read immediately after the contact of the cells with erythrosin.
[b] Number of animals.

From Aschkenasy, A., *Arch. Sci. Physiol.*, 25, 275–292, 1971, and *World Rev. Nutr. Diet.*, 21, 151–197, 1975 (S. Karger AG, Basel). With permission.

deprived of phenolic amino acids,[238] threonine,[239] histidine,[240] tryptophan,[241] isoleucine,[242] or valine.[243] In young male rats subjected to diets devoid of various essential or semiessential amino acids for 24 days, the weight reduction of the lymph nodes and (to a lesser extent) the spleen is generally proportional to the drop in body weight. Only the thymus may also exhibit an important decrease in relative weight (per 100 g body weight) (Table 12).[228] The involution of this organ is particularly important in the absence of isoleucine or valine, while relative weight reduction is not significant after deprivation of arginine and is relatively moderate after lack of lysine.

In general, the involution of the thymus parallels the decrease in the number of blood eosinophils and is inversely proportional to the relative weight of the adrenals (compare Tables 6 and 12). Lack of valine, as well as of methionine and cystine, also significantly reduces the proportion of large lymphocytes and plasma cells in the intestinal mucosa (Table 10).[234]

If incomplete amino acid diets are given for 10[244] or 7 days[218] to rats previously subjected to protracted protein starvation, the restoration of the lymphoid organs is either completely or partly inhibited according to both the amino acid omitted from the diet and the organ concerned. In fact, as compared to recovery diets containing either casein or a complete mixture of 19 amino acids, almost all of the incomplete diets depress the relative as well as the absolute weights of the lymphoid organs, particularly of the thymus (Table 13, Figure 5).

ii. Blood Lymphocytes

The lymphopenic effect of methionine deficiency was demonstrated many years ago[245] and confirmed more recently.[234]

Table 10
PERCENTAGES OF LYMPHOCYTES OF DIFFERENT SIZES AND OF PLASMOCYTES AND BASOPHILIC LYMPHOCYTES IN INTESTINAL VILLI IN RATS[a] GIVEN COMPLETE OR INCOMPLETE SEMISYNTHETIC DIETS FOR 3 WEEKS

Diet	Small lymphocytes (%)	Large lymphocytes (%)	Basophilic lymphocytes and plasmocytes (%)	Unclassed lymphocytes (%)
18% casein[b] (6)[c]	73.8 ±4.2[d]	20.5 ±3.5	2.3 ±0.7	3.4 ±1.1
18% complete amino acid mixture[e] (6)	79.6 ±1.8	16.8 ±3.8	1.5 ±0.1	2.1 ±0.7
Without sulfur amino acids[e] (8)	82.0 ±2.5	14.3 ±1.8	0.7 ±0.2	3.0 ±0.7
Without valine[e] (7)	84.1 ±1.5	12.5 ±1.4	0.4 ±0.1	3.0 ±0.7
Without any amino acid (8)	86.8 ±2.8	10.9 ±2.3	0.6 ±0.2	1.7 ±0.6
Recovery with 18% casein for 1 week (7)	78.0 ±2.6	17.7 ±1.9	1.4 ±0.4	2.9 ±0.9

[a] Adult pathogen-free male Sherman rats.
[b] For the composition, consult References 142 and 232.
[c] Number of rats.
[d] Mean ± SE.
[e] The same composition as in Table 5.

From Cao, M. J. and Aschkenasy, A., *C.R. Soc. Biol.,* 164, 277—281, 1970. With permission.

On the other hand, if incomplete amino acid diets are administered after protein deprivation, the lymphopenia provoked by the latter diet not only is not cured but may be aggravated, as is the case with diets devoid of valine or sulfur amino acids.[218,244]

Furthermore, the mean size of the lymphocytes, reduced by protein starvation, does not rise at all after administration of these incomplete diets, and still diminishes after deprivation of valine (Table 11). This results in an almost complete disappearance of large lymphocytes in the blood: ~3 per 100 lymphocytes, whereas these cells still remain at a 11% level after prolonged protein deprivation and rise up to ~50% after 10 days of a complete 18% casein recovery diet.[244]

If the above findings are compared to those reported earlier in this chapter for neutrophils,[217,218] the need for certain amino acids appears to be dissimilar for the production of blood neutrophils and for lymphocytes. Thus, the lack of sulfur amino acids is more deleterious for lymphocytes than for neutrophils, while, on the contrary, deprivation of lysine is more harmful for blood neutrophils than for lymphocytes (Table 5).[218]

The lack of valine or isoleucine, however, is highly deleterious for neutropoiesis and eosinopoiesis, as well as for lymphopoiesis (Tables 5, 6, 12, and 13). Since leukocytes contain enzymes involved in the oxidation and decarboxylation of α-ketonic acids derived from branched-chain amino acids,[246] these cells may be large consumers of valine and isoleucine. This would perhaps explain the sharp depression of leukopoiesis after deprivation of these amino acids.

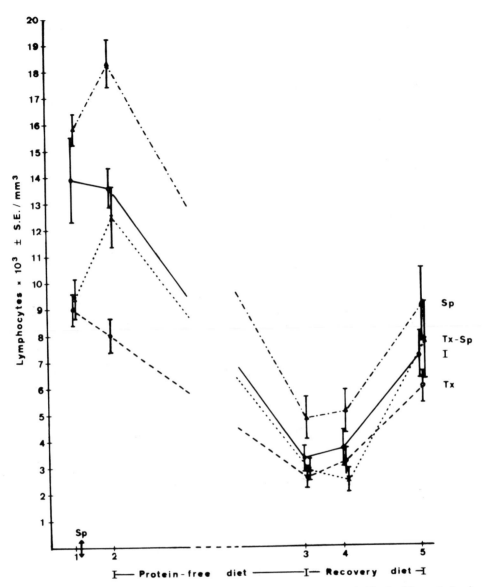

FIGURE 3.   Evolution of blood lymphocyte levels (means ± SE) in male Charles River rats deprived of proteins for 85 days, and restored afterwards with an 18% casein diet for 21 days. Comparison between intact rats (I, •——) and rats thymectomized (Tx, ○— —), splenectomized (Sp, Δ—·—), or deprived of both the thymus and the spleen (Tx-Sp, x...). The same time intervals (1—5) as in Figure 2. ↕: day of splenectomy (1 week before the protein-free diet). Note 1°, the lymphocyte discharge after splenectomy; 2°, the disappearance of the gap between the lymphocyte levels of I and Tx rats after protracted protein starvation. (From Aschkenasy, A., *C.R. Soc. Biol.*, 163, 295—300, 1969. With permission.)

c. *Physiological and Biochemical Nonimmunologic Significance of the Lymphocyte Changes Induced by Protein and Amino-acid Deprivation*

On the basis of previously mentioned data (Section I.B.3, "Cell Size and Its Correlation with Functional Activity") the size decrease induced by the lack of protein may correspond to a functional inactivation of these cells. Indeed, the percentage of mitoses is sharply decreased in the thymus, and also diminishes (albeit to a much lesser extent) in the spleen of protein-deficient rats (Table 14).[85] In nonstimulated lymph nodes, the mitotic activity is very low, even with a balanced diet, which explains the

Table 11
EVOLUTION OF CELLULAR AND NUCLEAR INDICES (μm^2) ± SE OF BLOOD LYMPHOCYTES IN RATS SUBMITTED TO VARIOUS DIETS AFTER A 2-MONTH NITROGEN STARVATION[a]

| | Cellular indices | | Nuclear indices | |
Diet	1st day	11th day	1st day	11th day
18% casein ad libitum	91.0 ± 2.6	116.8 ± 4.3	69.1 ± 1.6	79.1 ± 2.5
Complete mixture of 19 amino acids	84.7 ± 3.0	107.2 ± 3.5	66.1 ± 2.3	74.7 ± 1.6
18% casein, restricted	90.5 ± 1.8	109.1 ± 3.5	66.2 ± 1.0	77.2 ± 1.4
Diet without sulfur amino acids	86.0 ± 3.6	88.2 ± 3.6	66.2 ± 2.8	66.2 ± 1.5
Without lysine	87.2 ± 4.9	90.7 ± 3.0	66.9 ± 2.7	68.6 ± 1.6
Without tryptophan	82.7 ± 4.7	87.4 ± 4.9	63.9 ± 2.8	67.5 ± 3.1
Without phenolic amino acids	83.5 ± 1.6	93.1 ± 2.9	66.6 ± 1.1	68.8 ± 1.6
Without histidine	87.8 ± 2.0	90.6 ± 1.6	67.0 ± 1.7	66.8 ± 1.5
Without threonine	86.3 ± 5.5	89.7 ± 4.1	67.7 ± 4.3	66.8 ± 1.6
Without valine	89.8 ± 4.0	77.1 ± 2.4	69.1 ± 3.1	60.9 ± 1.3
Without amino acid nitrogen[b]	89.4 ± 3.8	85.6 ± 2.5	70.0 ± 3.2	65.0 ± 1.2

[a] Same diets and rats as in Table 5.

[b] In one group, the protein-free diet was prolonged for a supplementary period of 10 days in order to serve as a term of comparison with the other diets.

From Aschkenasy, A., *C.R. Soc. Biol.,* 160, 1787–1792, 1966, and *World Rev. Nutr. Diet.,* 21, 151–197, 1975. With permission.

absence of significant changes after protein deprivation. It is only in the case of previous stimulation with PHA that the antimitotic effect of a protein-free diet can be revealed in these organs (see Table 20 later in this chapter).[85]

Whereas the drop in the mitotic activity in the spleen coincides with an important reduction of DNA synthesis per unit weight, as measured by ^{3}H-thymidine incorporation, the thymus and the lymph nodes surprisingly exhibit an increase in this synthesis despite the sharply decreased (thymus) or unchanged (lymph nodes) mitotic indices (Table 14).[247] This suggests a prolongation or a block of the S and G2 phases of the cell cycle in the latter two organs. Such an anomaly may also occur in the spleen, since the DNA content per cell measured by a biochemical method was found to increase in the spleen as well as in the thymus and lymph nodes of protein-deprived rats (Table 15).[142] This interpretation agrees with the data of Hopper et al.,[248] who found a paradoxical increase in the labeling of intestinal epithelial cells in starved or protein-depleted rats, as well as with similar findings of Deo and Mathur[249] concerning intestinal and bone marrow cells in protein-deprived rats.

It is of interest to mention that a discrepancy between increased DNA levels and mitotic arrest has also been observed in giant metamyelocytes in Addisonian pernicious anemia,[250] which might suggest the existence of a similar disturbance of the cell cycle in deficiencies of protein and cobalamin.

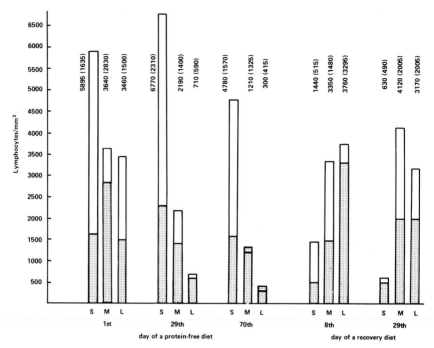

FIGURE 4.   Average levels of small (S), medium (M), and large (L) lymphocytes in intact (the entire columns) or thymectomized (the stippled segments of the columns and values in parentheses) male rats fed protein-free and recovery diets. In the eighth and ninth columns, the cell level in thymectomized rats exceeded those in intact rats. The size of lymphocytes was determined by measurement of cellular and nuclear indices defined as products of two perpendicular diameters. Cells with a cellular index <80 μm^2 were considered small lymphocytes, while those with an index >110 μm^2 were considered large lymphocytes. (From Aschkenasy, A., *Isr. J. Med. Sci.,* 1, 552–562, 1965. With permission.)

On the other hand, the drop in the mitotic indices of lymphocytes is consistent with the finding of an increased turnover of cyclic AMP in these cells, as attested by high adenylcyclase and phosphodiesterase activity in the lymphoid organs as well as by the high levels of this nucleotide in the spleen of protein-deprived rats (Tables 16 and 17).[142] Indeed, an inverse relationship between the mitotic activity and the intracellular turnover of cyclic AMP has been demonstrated.[251]

There are also other indices of functional hypoactivity of lymphocytes in experimental protein malnutrition: The thymocytes of protein-deprived rats exhibit a strong decrease both in the ATPase activity and their potassium content. In the spleen, however, the drop in potassium content occurs at the same time as a moderate increase in ATPase activity. On the other hand, neither blood nor lymph-node lymphocytes present any anomaly of these two biochemical parameters (Figure 6).[252]

Finally, since PHA stimulation of lymphocytes involves increased glucose metabolism through the HMP shunt which parallels the mitotic activity,[253] it is possible that the depression of the PHA response, as observed in vivo after protein deprivation (see below)[254] may correspond to an inactivation of the HMP pathway.

Premitotic Block of the Lymphocyte Cycle in PD Rats

This block was confirmed by the comparative determination of the DNA concentration in ^{3}H-thymidine-labeled lymphocytes on autoradiographs[643] and the liquid scintillation determination of ^{3}H-thymidine incorporation on a per cell basis.[644] It was found that radioactivity per cell was 16 times higher in popliteal lymph nodes (PLN) and 9 times higher in the thymus of PD rats than in the same organs of rats maintained on a control diet of 18% casein (Cs). Mitotic levels, on the other hand, were generally low (~0.6/10^3 cells) in the PLN of both dietary groups and 7 times lower in the thymus of PD rats than in the thymus of Cs controls.[644]

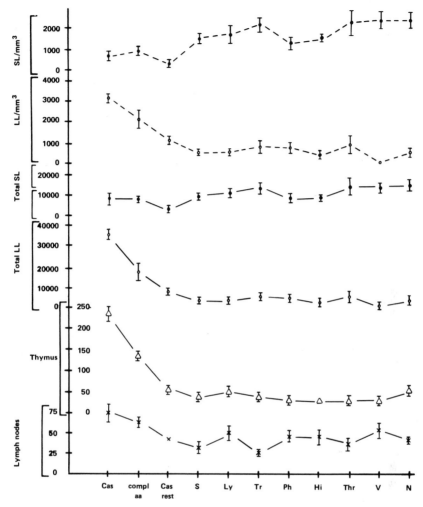

FIGURE 5. Comparison between levels (means ± SE) of small (SL) and large (LL) lymphocytes per cubic millimeter blood and per total blood volume, and weights of thymus and lymph nodes in ten groups of male Sherman rats killed after 10 days of various diets given after prolonged protein starvation. Cas: 18% casein diet ad libitum; compl aa: diet with 17% of a complete mixture of 19 amino acids, prepared according to Rose et al.[634] Cas rest: 18% casein diet quantitatively restricted to amounts of food spontaneously ingested with a diet devoid of valine; S: diet without sulfur amino acids; Ly: without lysine; Tr: without tryptophan; Ph: without phenolic amino acids; Hi: without histidine; Thr: without threonine; V: without valine; N: without any amino acid nitrogen (rats maintained for 10 supplementary days on a protein-free diet). SL: lymphocytes with a cellular index <80 μm^2; LL: cellular index >110 μm^2. (From Aschkenasy, A., *World Rev. Nutr. Diet.*, 21, 151–197, 1975. With permission of S. Karger AG, Basel.)

d. Responsibility of the Involution of the Thymus and the Peripheral T Lymphocytes in Some Cytological Abnormalities Provoked by Lack of Protein

i. Blood Lymphopenia

The blood lymphocyte levels are much higher in intact rats than in lately thymectomized rats, if both are fed a balanced diet. The gap between the two groups is much smaller if the diet is devoid of protein,[95,220,233,255] and it still remains reduced during the first 3 weeks of protein refeeding (Figure 3).[220] These data suggest that the drop in blood lymphocytosis after protein deprivation may be caused to a great extent by the decrease in the number of circulating thymus-derived cells provoked by the involution of this organ.

Large (LL) and medium-sized (ML) blood lymphocytes appear to be influenced to a greater extent by the thymic atrophy than small lymphocytes (SL). Indeed, when rats are maintained on a balanced diet, not only the number of SL but also that of LL and ML is much lower in animals thymectomized 25 days after birth than in the intact littermates,

Table 12

RELATIVE WEIGHTS OF LYMPHOID ORGANS AND ADRENALS (mg/100 g TERMINAL BODY WEIGHT, ±SE) IN YOUNG ADULT MALE WISTAR RATS DEPRIVED FOR 24 DAYS OF VARIOUS AMINO ACIDS OR OF ANY NITROGEN NUTRIENT; COMPARISON WITH CONTROLS GIVEN DIETS WITH 18% CASEIN OR 17% COMPLETE AMINO ACID MIXTURE (TOTAL AMINO ACIDS)

	Diet			Diets deprived of									
	Casein	Total amino acids	Without N	Sulfur amino acids	Lysine	Tryptophan	Phenolic amino acids	Histidine	Threonine	Leucine	Isoleucine	Valine	Arginine
Thymus	130.8 ±5.0	102.7 ±6.8	43.6 ±3.3	46.9 ±1.9	70.4 ±7.8	53.7 ±5.4	35.2 ±5.2	27.6 ±2.2	35.6 ±5.4	38.9 ±3.6	19.9 ±1.0	21.2 ±1.1	85.7 ±14.8
Spleen	164.6 ±4.6	182.0 ±6.3	161.1 ±4.6	170.0 ±3.6	178.5 ±15.7	168.6 ±7.3	149.4 ±8.1	162.2 ±9.1	188.6 ±12.8	173.8 ±6.1	152.3 ±10.1	153.3 ±7.2	183.8 ±11.0
Lymph nodes	22.4 ±2.2	28.5 ±0.7	29.5 ±2.3	35.7 ±4.0	43.8 ±4.4	26.7 ±3.1	30.6 ±1.5	28.6 ±4.6	34.0 ±3.0	27.5 ±2.7	33.4 ±2.7	36.7 ±3.4	24.7 ±0.7
Adrenals	12.2 ±0.7	13.4 ±0.8	17.5 ±0.7	21.1 ±0.4	18.3 ±0.8	16.4 ±1.0	21.4 ±0.8	20.2 ±0.6	20.4 ±0.7	20.9 ±0.8	25.6 ±1.4	21.2 ±0.8	16.6 ±0.7

From Aschkenasy, A., C. R. Soc. Biol., 158, 479–483, 1964. With permission.

Table 13
EFFECTS OF VARIOUS DIETS ON THE LYMPHOID ORGANS WHEN GIVEN FOR 10 DAYS TO RATS PREVIOUSLY DEPRIVED OF PROTEIN DURING 7 WEEKS[a]

Body and lymphoid organ weight	Protein and amino-acid-free diet (5)[b]	18% casein ad libitum (7)	18% casein-restricted diet (5)	Amino acid diets							
				Complete (19 amino acids) (8)	Without sulfur amino acids (6)	Without lysine (5)	Without tryptophan (6)	Without phenolic amino acids (5)	Without histidine (5)	Without threonine (5)	Without valine (6)
Body weight (g) after 2-month protein deprivation	133 ±3	125 ±7	135 ±5	128 ±5	134 ±3	131 ±5	138 ±4	138 ±3	136 ±4	138 ±2	139 ±5
Body weight (g) after 10 days of recovery diets	124 ±4	227 ±13	134 ±3	167 ±5	119 ±2	128 ±5	124 ±4	122 ±3	120 ±4	121 ±2	121 ±4
Thymus (mg)	52.9 ±10.4	237.3 ±22.2	53.8 ±5.8	136.3 ±9.2	36.5 ±4.9	48.7 ±7.5	34.2 ±4.0	28.0 ±3.1	26.1 ±1.6	27.8 ±3.9	27.0 ±1.7
Spleen (mg)	195.7 ±16.8	486.8 ±39.0	225.3 ±6.9	362.8 ±13.7	179.2 ±12.5	219.8 ±16.0	184.6 ±13.2	199.0 ±15.3	278.9 ±23.3	194.2 ±11.0	187.6 ±5.3
Lymph nodes (mg)[c]	33.1 ±1.6	49.0 ±6.0	33.3 ±5.1	43.7 ±3.3	28.1 ±3.5	37.1 ±4.4	25.6 ±1.5	34.5 ±3.2	34.7 ±4.6	30.9 ±3.4	39.0 ±5.0

a The diets and almost all rats are the same as in Table 5.

b Number of rats.

c Total weight of the four largest cervical and two mesenteric lymph nodes.

Adapted from Aschkenasy, A., *Nutrition et Hématopoïèse*, Centre National de la Recherche Scientifique, Paris, 1971, 404, With permission.

Table 14

COMPARED DATA ON DNA SYNTHESIS ACTIVITY PER UNIT WEIGHT AND PROPORTION OF MITOTIC FIGURES AFTER COLCHICINE (PER 10^3 CELLS) IN RATS[a] NOURISHED WITH AN 18% CASEIN DIET OR WITH A DIET DEPRIVED OF PROTEIN FOR 2 MONTHS

Diet[b]	Thymus		Spleen		Popliteal lymph node	
	DNA synthesis[c] per 10 mg (cpm)	Number of metaphases[d] per 10^3	DNA synthesis per 10 mg (cpm)	Number of metaphases per 10^3	DNA synthesis per 10 mg (cpm)	Number of metaphases per 10^3
18% casein diet	147 ± 22[e] (8)[f]	52.3 ± 4.6 (6)	631 ± 152 (8)	5.3 ± 1.0 (6)	60 ± 9 (8)	0.3 ± 0.2 (6)
Protein-free diet	890 ± 184[g] (14)	6.4 ± 1.2[g] (18)	54 ± 17[g] (14)	1.6 ± 0.4[h] (18)	1,309 ± 223[g] (28)	0.2 ± 0.2 (18)

[a] Pathogen-free male adult Sherman rats. The pathogen-free rats used here displayed a very low basic DNA synthetic activity as compared to that found in other experiments.[254]

[b] For the composition of the diet, consult References 142 and 232.

[c] DNA synthesis was measured by ^{3}H-thymidine incorporation with a liquid scintillation counter. The isotope was injected i.p. 1 hr before killing ($1\ \mu Ci\ g^{-1}$). In the protein-deprived group, the counts were performed on pools of two thymuses and spleens and of four lymph nodes (two rats).

[d] The mitoses (metaphases) were counted on Giemsa-stained smears processed by a chromosomal method.[222] The rats were killed 1 hr 30 min after i.p. injection of 0.25 mg/100 g colchicine.

[e] Mean ± SE.

[f] Number of rats.

[g,h] Significant differences ($P < 0.01$ and <0.001, respectively) as compared to the corresponding values found in 18% casein-fed rats.

Table 15

PER CELL CONTENT OF DNA IN THE LYMPHOCYTES OF THE THYMUS, SPLEEN, AND
CERVICAL LYMPH NODES OF ADULT MALE WISTAR RATS MAINTAINED ON A BALANCED OR
PROTEIN-FREE DIET FOR 5 WEEKS

| Diet | DNA (mg) per 10^8 cells of a purified lymphocyte suspension | | |
	Thymus	Spleen	Cervical lymph node
18% casein	0.948 ± 0.018 (6 × 2)[a]	0.992 ± 0.058 (6 × 2)	1.429 ± 0.064 (6 × 8)
Without protein	1.190 ± 0.074[b] (6 × 8)	1.277 ± 0.070[c] (6 × 8)	2.408 ± 0.235[b] (6 × 32)

[a] Number of experiments × number of organs used for each experiment.
[b,c] Significantly different from nondeficient rats, $P < 0.01$ and < 0.05, respectively.

Table 16
COMPARATIVE ACTIVITIES OF ADENYLCYCLASE AND cAMP PHOSPHODIESTERASE (MEANS ± SE) IN THE LYMPHOCYTES OF THE THYMUS, SPLEEN, AND CERVICAL LYMPH NODES OF NORMALLY FED (N) AND PROTEIN-DEPRIVED (PD) RATS[a,142]

| | | | 10^3 counts per minute[b] | | | |
| | | | Adenylcyclase ([³H] cAMP) | | cAMP phosphodiesterase ([³H] 5′AMP) | |
Organ	Group	Weight (g)	Per 10^8 cells	Per mg DNA	Per 10^8 cells	Per mg DNA
Thymus	N (8)[c]	527.8 ± 50.4	8.18 ± 1.04	8.63 ± 1.18	268 ± 28	283 ± 32
	PD (14)	63.3 ± 7.4	53.40 ± 7.89	44.88 ± 6.49	1592 ± 376	1338 ± 330
	Percent change	−88%	+552.8%[d]	+420%[d]	+494%[d]	+373%[d]
Spleen	N (8)	812.5 ± 42.0	33.35 ± 6.25	33.62 ± 6.47	992 ± 120	1000 ± 115
	PD (14)	218.9 ± 8.3	145.86 ± 22.95	114.24 ± 18.18	3708 ± 1012	2904 ± 839
	Percent change	−73%	+337.5%[d]	+233%[d]	+274%[d]	+190%[e]
Cervical	N (8)	20.8 ± 2.9	76.96 ± 11.80	53.86 ± 8.65	1568 ± 199	1097 ± 143
lymph node	PD (14)	5.9 ± 0.4	162.24 ± 29.52	67.38 ± 10.93	2289 ± 432	948 ± 163
	Percent change	−71%	+110.8%[d]	+23%	+46%[e]	0%

[a] Adult pathogen-free male Wistar rats. Terminal body weight 402 ± 10 g for the N rats, 135 ± 2 g for the PD rats. The duration of the diets was 5 weeks.

[b] Quantities of ³H-nucleotides accumulated after incubation of lymphocytes with [2-³H], adenine.

[c] Number of experiments in parentheses. For each experiment, two thymuses, two spleens, and eight cervical lymph nodes for the normal (N) rats, and eight thymuses, eight spleens, and 32 cervical lymph nodes for the protein-deficient (PD) rats were used.

[d, e] Significantly different from N rats (P < 0.01 and < 0.05, respectively).

Table 17
LEVELS (± SE) OF CYCLIC AMP IN THE PURIFIED LYMPHOCYTES OF THE SPLEEN IN NORMALLY FED AND PROTEIN-DEPRIVED RATS[142]

| | Cyclic AMP (μg)[a] | |
Diet[a] (5 weeks)	Per gram DNA[b]	Per 10^8 lymphocytes[b]
Balanced (18% casein)	754 ± 28	0.748 ± 0.091
Protein free	8265 ± 3223	10.553 ± 3.808[c]

[a] For the composition of the diets and the method of dosage used, see Reference 142.

[b] Each value is an average of six experiments. For each experiment, two thymuses, two spleens, and eight cervical lymph nodes for the control rats, and eight thymuses, eight spleens, and 32 cervical lymph nodes for the protein-deprived rats were used.

[c] Significantly different from normally nourished rats (P < 0.01).

the differences being −72% for the SL and −39% for the [LL + ML], respectively, 1 month after thymectomy. On the contrary, after 10 weeks of a lymphopenia-inducing protein-free diet started 55 days after birth, there is no longer a difference in the [LL + ML] levels of intact and thymectomized animals, whereas the gap between SL levels of the two groups remains the same (−67%) as before (−72%) protein starvation (Figure 4).

Although the involution of the thymus may represent an important causal factor of the functional inactivation of blood lymphocytes observed in protein-deficient rats, one must point out that not only intact but also thymectomized rats exhibit a striking loss of [ML + LL] following such a diet (−79% for the former, −60% for the latter animals). On

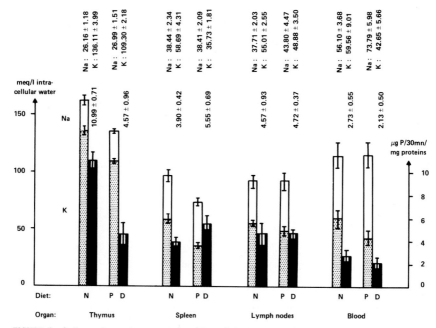

FIGURE 6.   Sodium and potassium contents (meq/l intracellular water) and ATPase activity (μg P/30 min/mg protein) in thymic, splenic, and lymph-node lymphocytes of normal (N) and protein-deprived (PD) pathogen-free male Sherman rats. White segments of columns correspond to Na content, stippled segments to K content, and black columns to ATPase activity. Means ± SE. (From Spach, C. and Aschkenasy, A., *C.R. Soc. Biol.*, 167, 1540–1544, 1973. With permission.)

the other hand, during the first 4 weeks of protein refeeding, an important rise in [ML + LL] levels occurs even in thymectomized rats, although it is much lower in these animals (+130%) than in intact rats (+383%) (Figure 4).[95] Accordingly, dietary blood lymphopenia results not only from thymic atrophy but also from a direct, extrathymic harmful action of the deficient diet on the peripheral, probably both T and B, lymphocytes.

In any case, the preponderant participation of thymus-derived lymphocytes in the restoration of lymphopoiesis during recovery is also attested to by the blocking effect of repeated injections of a purified rabbit anti-rat-thymus serum (Table 18).[221]

ii. Reduced Viability of Tissular Lymphocytes

This anomaly seems to concern mainly the T lymphocytes because an analogous (although less pronounced) phenomenon is observed after late thymectomy in nondeficient rats.[87]

The spleen certainly plays an important role in the fragilization of lymphocytes induced by protein deprivation. Indeed, splenectomy, performed prior to administration of the deficient diet, completely prevents the fragilizing effect of the latter (Table 19).[256] Since the protective influence of splenectomy is lacking in protein-deficient, previously thymectomized rats, the fragilizing effect of the spleen may concern primarily the T lymphocytes rendered less resistant by the atrophy of the thymus, and may be mediated by the phagocytosing activity of splenic macrophages.[168] On the other hand, one can suppose that splenectomy acts by removing the physiological bone marrow block maintained by the spleen, thus permitting the release of newly formed, viable bone-marrow-derived lymphocytes into the blood and to the lymphoid organs.

iii. Dissimilar Effects on Peripheral Lymphoid Organs of Late Thymectomy and of Thymic Atrophy Due to Protein Deprivation

A protein-free diet reduces the quantitative difference between intact and thymecto-

Table 18

PREVENTION OF RESTORATION OF LEUKOPOIESIS (NEUTROPOIESIS AS WELL AS LYMPHOPOIESIS) BY PURIFIED RABBIT ANTI-RAT-THYMUS IMMUNOGLOBULINS (ATHYIG)[a]

Comparison with the Effect of Normal Rabbit Immunoglobulins (NRIg)

Injected product	Neutrophils ± SE per mm³		Lymphocytes ± SE per mm³		Weight (mg) ± SE per 100 g body weight		
	1st day	11th day	1st day	11th day	Thymus	Lymph nodes[b]	Spleen
Physiological saline (6)[c]	1590 ±140	2570 ±570	5355 ±1180	6030 ±1645	139.4 ±20.8	43.7[b] ±6.3	287.5 ±36.0
AThyIg[d] (5)	1545 ±240	960 ±305	4630 ±205	860 ±280	84.0 ±12.0	39.7 ±4.8	232.4 ±15.2
NRIg[d] (5)	1415 ±130	2050 ±350	4785 ±715	4600 ±935	110.2 ±13.4	63.4 ±6.0	312.3 ±19.7

[a] The antiserum was injected into rats from the 1st to the 11th day of an 18% casein diet following an 80-day protein starvation. The rats were male Charles River rats weighing ~250 g before the protein-free diet, ~110 g on the first day of recovery. The weight increase after 10 days of restoration reached +60 ± 9.6% in the controls, while it was sharply reduced in the AthyIg (+25.2 ± 5.4%). The inhibition due to NRIg (+38.6 ± 7.6%) was not significant.

[b] Four cervical and two mesenteric lymph nodes.

[c] Number of rats.

[d] The injected solutions (1 ml/100 g body weight) contained 1 mg protein/ml, and the cytotoxicity titer of AThyIg was 1:128.

From Aschkenasy, A., Bachvaroff, R., and Grabar, P., *C.R. Acad. Sci.*, 267, 1788–1790, 1968. With permission.

mized rats regarding the lymphocyte populations of the spleen and some lymph nodes,[229] as it does with regard to the blood lymphocytes. Nevertheless, the involution of the lymphoid system is more pronounced in protein-deprived thymectomized rats than in intact animals maintained on the same deficient diet, the difference between the two groups being about 50% for the lymph nodes and 30% for the spleen.[229] This finding indicates that in spite of its early involution, the residual thymus retains a certain protective effect on the peripheral T lymphocytes until the most advanced phase of protein malnutrition.

Because of the early arrest of mitotic activity in the thymus, it is improbable that this effect could be due to the continuing emigration of lymphocytes from this organ throughout the development of protein starvation. It is more tempting to consider a persistent secretion of a lymphopoietic hormone. Indeed, the latter seems to be produced by the reticuloepithelial cells of the thymus,[60,61] which, contrary to the great majority of thymocytes, are resistant to prolonged protein deprivation.[227,231] As will be seen later, a protective influence of the thymus could also be shown with regard to some immunologic capacities of protein-deficient animals.

iv. Effect of Protein Deprivation on the Lymphocytic Response to Phytohemagglutinin (PHA)

The involution of the T cell system can also be demonstrated by the sharp reduction of the blastogenic (DNA synthesis)[254] and mitogenic[247] response of popliteal lymph node lymphocytes to PHA when this mitogen is injected into the hind foot pads of rats exhausted by very protracted protein deprivation, as compared to normally nourished

Table 19
PERCENTAGES ±SE OF NONVIABLE LYMPHOCYTES IN VARIOUS LYMPH NODE CELL
SUSPENSIONS FROM INTACT (I), THYMECTOMIZED (Tx), SPLENECTOMIZED (Sp), AND
THYMECTOMIZED-SPLENECTOMIZED (Tx-Sp) RATS,[a] AFTER 1-hr CONTACT WITH
ERYTHROSIN[b]

Effect of a Protein-free Diet, Administered for 8 Weeks

	Popliteal lymph node				Inguinal lymph node				Lumbar lymph node				Cervical lymph node			
Diet	I	Tx	Sp	Tx-Sp	I	Tx	Sp	Tx-Sp	I	Tx	Sp	Tx-Sp	I	Tx	Sp	Tx-Sp
18%	30.9	41.6	33.1	49.5	38.7	46.6	39.6	49.1	36.4	46.3	33.6	54.5	39.7	50.7	31.7	54.4
casein	±3.3	±2.4	±2.7	±5.1	±3.3	±2.5	±2.3	±4.9	±4.6	±3.8	±3.6	±6.2	±4.0	±4.6	±1.6	±7.1
	(9)[c]	(10)	(7)	(8)												
Protein-	56.4	67.7	39.1	51.6	84.4	88.4	47.7	83.7	56.8	63.6	41.3	60.0	60.3	67.9	45.9	54.0
free	±7.0	±6.5	±1.7	±5.9	±6.0	±5.6	±9.7[e]	±6.2	±6.3	±6.8	±2.8[d]	±6.7	±6.6	±5.0	±3.2	±5.9
	(11)	(8)	(9)	(9)												

[a] Pathogen-free Sherman male rats.

[b] The dye-exclusion test was carried out immediately after addition of the dye to the cell suspension in vitro (percentage of dead cells) and 1 hr later (percentage of the totality of fragile cells).[155] This table shows only the values of the second lecture because some changes were more apparent after a 1-hr interval. The protective effect of splenectomy was prevented by the removal of the thymus. The prolonged exposure to the dye explains the high levels of nonviable lymphocytes even in normal, intact rats.

[c] Number of rats.

[d,e] Statistically different from the values of intact (I) rats of the same dietary group; B < 0.05 and < 0.01, respectively.

Adapted from Aschkenasy, A., *C.R. Soc. Biol.*, 167, 1340–1344, 1973. With permission.

controls (Table 20). These data are in agreement with the finding that adult thymectomy also results in a depressed response of mouse spleen cells to thymus-dependent mitogens.[257]

Contrary to the impaired response to PHA observed in rats in vivo, a normal or even increased response has been reported in vitro by Cooper et al.[258] in protein-deficient mice. The experimental diet given by these authors still contained 8% casein, which probably was not low enough to induce a sufficient depletion of PHA-responsive lymphocytes. In addition, the experimental group was compared to a pair-fed control group, the PHA response of which was probably also depressed because of the intake reduction. Finally, it is likely that in vitro, even lymphocytes of protein-deficient animals and humans may be able to assimilate the protein and amino acid constituents of the culture medium, which would make possible their transformation in response to PHA.

v. Comparative Effect of Phytohemagglutinin (PHA) on the Total Lymphocyte Content and Mitotic Activity in Lymph Nodes of PD and Cs Rats

Subplantar PHA injections increased the mitotic frequencies in PLN to a much greater extent in Cs rats (34 times per organ) than in PD rats (12 times). The total PLN lymphocyte population, however, increased more in PD rats (10 times) than in Cs rats (4.5 times).[643] It is possible that PHA increases the membranous resistance of lymphocytes, considerably lowered after protein deprivation,[155] thus decreasing interphase cell mortality. Alternatively, an influx of mitotically inactive T lymphocytes from the thymus into PHA-stimulated lymph nodes should be taken into consideration. Indeed, a decrease of the total cell population of the thymus has been observed after PHA injection in both PD and Cs rats[643] and the loss of thymocytes has also been reported in mice after PHA injection[645] and after immunization.[646]

vi. Compared Action of Protein Deprivation on Cortisone-sensitive and Cortisone-resistant Lymphocytes

The inhibition of PHA responsiveness in vivo in protein deficiency seems to be primarily due to the disappearance of short-lived, cortisone-sensitive lymphocytes.

Table 20
DNA SYNTHESIS[a] AND MITOTIC RESPONSES[a] INDUCED BY PHYTOHEMAGGLUTININ (PHA)[b] IN
POPLITEAL LYMPH NODES OF RATS[a] ON A BALANCED (18% CASEIN) DIET AND ON
A PROLONGED (2-MONTH) PROTEIN-FREE DIET; EFFECT OF A CORTISONE TREATMENT[c]

Cortisone	Nonstimulated	18% casein diet + PHA	Increase (n-fold)	Nonstimulated	Protein-free diet + PHA	Increase (n-fold)
		DNA Synthesis (cpm Per Lymph Node)[d]				
Without cortisone	57 ± 15 (8)[e]	868 ± 146 (8)	15.30^g	566 ± 115 (14)	2121 ± 453 (12)	3.75^f
With cortisone	76 ± 32 (7)	217 ± 60 (6)	2.86^{ns}	39 ± 16 (14)	220 ± 49 (12)	5.68^f
		Mitotic Indices (Per 10^3 Cells)				
Without cortisone	0.33 ± 0.21 (6)	3.83 ± 0.95 (6)	11.61^f	0.20 ± 0.20 (18)	0.83 ± 0.17 (12)	4.15^{ns}
With cortisone	0.33 ± 0.21 (6)	1.33 ± 0.42 (6)	4.03^{ns}	0.17 ± 0.17 (18)	0.17 ± 0.17 (18)	1.00^{ns}

Note: ns = not significant.

[a] Same methods and conditions as in Table 14.
[b] Phytohemagglutinin (Eurobio, Paris, France) was injected by subplantar route into both hind foot pads (1 mg/100 g per foot). The rats were killed on Day 4 after injection.
[c] Cortisone acetate (Roussel, Paris, France) was given subcutaneously (3 mg/100 g/day) from Day 5 before killing to nonstimulated and PHA-stimulated animals.
[d] The counts of cpm were made on pools of two rats in the protein-deprived group.
[e] Number of rats.
[f,g] Statistically significant increase: $P < 0.01$ and < 0.001, respectively.

Indeed, a 5-day treatment with this hormone (3 mg/100 g/day) given to normally nourished rats reduces the rise of DNA synthesis and mitotic activity in popliteal lymph nodes after subplantar injection of PHA to the same extent as does a prolonged protein-free diet (Table 20).[247]

It is interesting to note that in the protein-deprived group, cortisone sharply reduces the ^{3}H-thymidine incorporation into the lymphocytes, not only in the PHA-stimulated rats but also in the nonstimulated animals, thus apparently suppressing the block of the cell cycle due to protein deprivation. The almost complete absence of mitoses, observed at the same time, suggests that the block is only displaced upwards, prior to the S phase of the cell cycle (Table 20).

The mitotic activity of the thymus is also inhibited to a similar degree by protein deprivation and by cortisone in rats that are not stimulated with PHA (Table 21). On the other hand, the deficient diet is deleterious not only for cortisone-sensitive cells of the thymus and of PHA-stimulated lymph nodes (Tables 20 and 21), but also for a fraction of cortisone-resistant cells (T or B lymphocytes) of the spleen (Table 21). Conversely, there are thymic lymphocytes resistant to protein deprivation that can be destroyed by adequate doses of cortisone.

vii. Comparison of the Effects of PHA and Concanavalin A in PD and Cs Rats

Protein deprivation inhibited only PHA mitogenesis, while reactions to Con A were higher in the PLN and only slightly lower in the spleen of PD rats, compared to Cs controls.[647] Paradoxically, PHA reduced the proliferative activity of the thymus in normal rats and did so to a greater extent than in PD rats, while Con A had no effect in either dietary group. By virtue of certain of their peculiarities (high theta-like antigen content and lymph node homing), T cells of the rat selectively affected by protein deprivation resemble PHA-responsive T cells of mice.[648,649] Con A-responsive T cells in both species are low theta and spleen homing. It may be noted that increased Con A responses have been observed in human blood lymphocytes in vitro after subtotal killing of the PHA-reactive cells.[650] The similarity of this observation to the changes seen in PD rats in vivo may be explained by the functional impairment of the thymus in these animals.

Table 21
COMPARATIVE EFFECT OF PROTEIN DEPRIVATION ON CORTISONE-SENSITIVE AND CORTISONE-RESISTANT MITOTIC ACTIVITY IN THE THYMUS AND SPLEEN

Means ± SE

Mitotic indices (per 10^3 cells)[a]

Organ	18% casein diet[a]		Protein-free diet[a]	
	Without cortisone (6)[b]	With cortisone (6)[c]	Without cortisone (18)	With cortisone (18)
Thymus	52.33 ± 4.64	4.00 ± 0.77	6.40 ± 1.20	0
Spleen	5.33 ± 0.99	5.17 ± 0.79	1.60 ± 0.40	3.17 ± 0.54

[a] Same methods and conditions as in Table 14. The animals were adult male pathogen-free Sherman rats.
[b] Number of rats.
[c] The hormonal treatment consisted of five daily subcutaneous injections of cortisone acetate (3 mg/100 g/day).

viii. Cortisone Sensitivities of Cs and PD Lymphocytes

When the DNA synthetic and mitogenic effects of PHA in Cs and PD rats are compared in the presence and absence of cortisone treatment, it appears that the lymphocytes remaining capable of synthesizing DNA after prolonged protein deprivation are cortisone-resistant, as are dividing cells in the spleen. These cells are partially destroyed by the hormone in nondeficient controls.[85,643] Residual non-dividing cells of the atrophic thymus, however, are still more sensitive to cortisone than are normal thymocytes.[85] This is in agreement with earlier data showing the high cortisone sensitivity of the thymus in PD rats which were adrenalectomized.[328] Depressed PHA responses induced by protein deficiency appear to result primarily from the loss of cortisone sensitive T cells and thymocytes. This may be the result of increased glucocorticoid secretion,[224] itself due to a stress effect of the deficient diet. In addition, these hormones are partially protein-bound in the blood to serum albumin and in particular to a specific carrier protein (an α-globulin). Decreased levels of these two proteins during protein malnutrition may thus result in a higher proportion of free corticosteroids and consequently in enhanced lymphocytolysis activity.[651]

ix. Depression of Thymus-Dependent Humoral Immunity After Dietary Leucine Overload

Recent experiments with rats maintained on protein-poor (4%) and leucine-overloaded (7%) diets have confirmed earlier data[186] which showed that immunological reactions to sheep red blood cells (SRBC) were strikingly impaired under these conditions. This impairment included an almost total disappearance of serum Ig hemagglutinins and hemolysins.[652] These anomalies could be prevented by the administration of small quantities of L-isoleucine and L-valine (0.2% each).[652] Leucine-induced immunodepression may thus be ascribed to a secondary deficiency of these two branched-chain amino acids.

x. Immunologic Changes Induced by Synthetic Diets Poor in Certain Amino Acids

It has been reported by Bounous and Konghern[653] that diets containing subnormal concentrations of certain amino acids, particularly phenylalanine and tyrosine, not only did not depress the immunologic responses of mice injected with SRBC, but actually increased the PFC response and serum hemagglutinin titers and also moderately enhanced delayed hypersensitivity to SRBC. The depression of these reactions was observed only when animals were placed on diets severely deficient in several essential amino acids. It has been suggested that certain moderately imbalanced amino acid diets may preferentially inhibit the production or the function of suppressor T cells and that only severe amino acid deficiencies were able to provoke immunodepression.[654-656]

xi. Effect of Protein Deficiency on B Lymphocytes

Recent results have considerably increased our knowledge on the functional changes of B lymphocytes which occur in experimental protein deficiency. Thus as with T lymphocytes, it was found that splenic B lymphocytes separated by nylon wool filtration exhibited anomalies of cyclic nucleotide contents in PD rats. An increased cAMP/cGMP ratio was found in both lymphocyte classes, but this change was due to decreased cGMP levels in T cells and to increased cAMP levels in B cells.[657] The changes in cAMP and cGMP levels in Cs and PD rats were also different in splenic lymphocytes during immunization to SRBC.[658]

Data on the immunologic activity of B lymphocytes differ according to whether the diet used was totally protein deprived (PD) or only protein-poor (4% casein) and greatly amino acid imbalanced (excess leucine). The increased DNA synthesis in PLN of PD rats induced by subplantar LPS injection was much lower than in Cs rats.[254,659] In the spleen, on the other hand, DNA synthesis and mitotic activity were stimulated by LPS to a greater extent in PD rats. The production of circulating antibodies to this B cell-specific antigen was thus not impaired (Table 25).[294] In protein-poor leucine-over-loaded rats, however, antibody production was depressed in vivo not only against SRBC, a thymus-dependent antigen, but was also reduced against LPS, as indicated by low serum agglutinin titers ($\log_{10}$ 1.786 ± 0.257 in leucine-overloaded rats vs. 2.559 ± 0.099 in 4% casein rats without leucine).[652] The complete disappearance of serum immunoglobulins, IgG, reported in SRBC-immunized leucine-overloaded rats,[186] was also observed after LPS immunization.[652] This finding indicates that the latter effect was due to a direct functional deficiency of B lymphocytes, rather than to the arrest of the T cell-controlled switch from IgM to IgG production. In all cases, the anomalies were prevented by administering valine and isoleucine without changing the casein content of the diet.[652]

Totally protein deprived rats exhibited no reduced immunologic responses to LPS 7 days after injection.[294,659] It should be noted that an important percentage of PD rats suddenly died 1 or 2 days after subplantar or intra-peritoneal injection of the endotoxin (54% after 12.5 μg of LPS and 36% after 6.25 μg).[659] Death was due to acute hemorrhagic necrosis of the liver.[659] Neither 18% casein LPS-injected rats nor non-injected PD rats exhibited similar lesions. The pathogenesis of LPS-induced hepatic necrosis is not clear. It may represent an antigen-antibody reaction similar to the Arthus phenomenon. Identical lesions have been reported in rats fed certain protein-poor diets[660,661] and could be prevented by administering sulfur amino acids.[662]

The necrogenic action of LPS could thus result from the selective consumption of certain amino acids (particularly methionine and cystine) or of metabolites involved in the intrahepatic degradation of the endotoxin. This hypothesis is consistent with the finding that the incidence of necrosis was considerably reduced by administering cortisone, since this hormone is known for its catabolic action on the protein stores of several tissues (particularly muscular and lymphoid) but also for its anabolic effect on liver proteins.[663]

The experimental data reported here may also present a clinical interest, since it appears that immunodepression induced by severe quantitative reduction of protein intake or even complete protein removal from the diet almost exclusively involves thymus-dependent responses, while protein deficiency coupled with leucine overload also depresses responses to microbial endotoxins. Human protein malnutrition is often related to the ingestion of subnormal levels of protein combined with an amino acid imbalance, e.g., sorghum particularly rich in leucine. Therefore, the high incidence and severity of certain infections reported under these conditions may be greatly conditioned by a qualitative rather than a quantitative protein deficiency. In addition, the frequency of acute hepatic necrosis in LPS-inoculated PD rats, in contrast to the apparent absence of any hepatotoxicity of similar doses of LPS in normally fed animals,[659] suggests that mortality occurring in infected protein malnourished humans may occasionally result from increased hepatotoxicity of microbial endotoxins, rather than from immunodepression.

xii. Effect of a Protein-free Diet on the Relative Proportions of Splenic T and B Lymphocytes Separated by Nylon-wool Filtration

Recent investigations in our laboratory[259] revealed that after 35 days of a protein-free diet, suspensions of splenic lymphocytes, dissociated by nylon-wool column filtration,[259a] contain the same percentage of nonadherent (mainly T) cells in protein-deprived rats (15.3 ± 1%) and in control rats of the same strain (Sherman) and age (18.9 ± 1.2%); on the contrary, the percentage of adherent, immunofluorescent B lymphocytes is significantly decreased in the deprived rats (26.5 ± 1.0%) as compared to the control levels (38.1 ± 0.7%). The T/B ratio was found to be 0.6 and 0.5, respectively, in the two experimental groups. When interpreting these unexpected results, one must remember that an important fraction of cells of the initial suspension was lost during the filtration process: about 40% for the lymphocytes of a normal spleen, and 60% for the splenic lymphocytes from protein-deprived rats. One cannot exclude the possibility that the major part of the lost cells in the latter animals were B lymphocytes. On the other hand, the absence of a significant decrease in the percentage of splenic T lymphocytes following protein deprivation may suggest that such a diet decreases the functional activity of thymus-dependent cells, rather than their number. Data obtained recently concerning the content of nylon-wool-separated splenic T lymphocytes in cyclic GMP (antagonist of cyclic AMP), as measured by a protein-binding method, have shown a significant drop in the levels of this nucleotide (9.08 ± 0.43 pM in controls; 7.35 ± 0.40 pM per 10^8 cells in protein-deprived rats),[259] lending substance to the hypothesis of inactivation of these cells.

e. Role of the Thymus in the Changes of Blood Lymphocyte Levels After Deprivation of Various Essential Amino Acids

In rats that were subjected either to a balanced diet containing casein or a complete mixture of 19 amino acids after protracted protein deprivation, or to incomplete diets lacking only one essential amino acid, a positive correlation could be established between the levels of circulating large lymphocytes on the one hand and the weight of the thymus on the other. There was no correlation between large lymphocytes and the weight of lymph nodes or between small lymphocytes and the thymus (Figure 5).[260] These findings agree with the hypothesis of an intervention of the thymus in the malnutrition-induced size changes of blood lymphocytes.

f. Influence of Experimental Protein Malnutrition on the Immunologic Activity of Lymphocytes

There is a large body of evidence that the protein-deprivation-induced hypoactivity of lymphocytes also involves many immunologic parameters.

i. Probable Participation of an Immunologic Mechanism in the Lymphopoietic Action of Ingested Protein

Such participation has been shown in experiments in which two groups of adult rats, after having lost the great majority of their lymphocytes by means of an i.p. injection of chlorambucil, were submitted to a protracted protein starvation and afterwards to an 18% casein diet for 10 days. In one of these groups, a 2-week period of the same casein diet was inserted between the chlorambucil injection and the onset of the protein deprivation, permitting comparison of the hematological responses to the recovery diet in casein-sensitized and nonsensitized animals. As judged from the rise of lymphocytes in the blood levels, particularly of large-sized cells, and from the weight increase of the lymphoid organs and reappearance of secondary follicles in the lymph nodes, the restoration of lymphopoiesis was much more pronounced in sensitized than in nonsensitized rats, despite identical body weights at the start of the recovery period. Apparently, those lymphocytes that arose during the period of protein starvation did not memorize any information concerning foreign proteins (Figure 7).[232]

These findings are in keeping with the recent report of exceptionally active proliferation in vitro of blood lymphocytes from children allergic to foods after oral challenge with the allergen.[261] On the other hand, one can hypothesize, as do Wostman et al.,[262] that repeated stimulation by dietary proteins and also by intestinal microorganisms might be essential to the development of immune defenses in order to combat the invasion of exogenous antigenic substances; it is probably also necessary to prevent the proliferation of malignantly transformed host cells.

Nevertheless, it is highly probable that the lymphopoietic action of dietary proteins is primarily a nonimmunologic phenomenon and is mainly due to direct utilization of amino acids as building material for cellular enzymatic and nonenzymatic proteins. Indeed, a diet containing a complete amino-acid mixture instead of casein is not much less lymphopoietic than casein despite its very low immunogeneic potential.[218,244]

ii. Immunodepressive Effects of Protein Deficiency

The main problem consists of determining the respective involvement of T and B lymphocytes.

aa. Involvement of T Lymphocytes

Humoral immunity – The response to heterologous (generally sheep) red blood cells (SRBC), a thymus-dependent antigen, is significantly reduced, as shown by the drop in circulating antibody titers,[208,215,233,255,263-265] the IgG being generally involved more than IgM.[255] The percentage, and especially the total number (per spleen or lymph node), of plaque-forming cells (PFC) is also decreased in rats[255,265-268] as well as in protein-deficient mice (Table 22).[258,269,270]

An inhibitory effect on serum antibody titers and (or) PFC levels in the spleen was observed after incomplete reduction of dietary protein levels in mice (6% casein),[258] as well as after a prolonged protein-free diet in rats (Table 22).[255]

A greater sensitivity of secondary responses was reported in mice subjected to an 8% casein diet for 6 to 7 weeks immediately after weaning, as compared to controls on a 27% casein diet.[271] In the deficient mice, only the titers of IgG were depressed, while in adult rats the respective effect of protein deprivation of IgG and IgM could not be clearly established.[233,255]

The formation of rosette-forming cells (RFC) is impaired much less than that of PFC. The concentration of these cells per 10^3 lymphocytes in adult rats is even higher after 2 months of protein deprivation than on a normal diet (Table 22).[233,255,266] However, the total number of RFC per organ (spleen or lymph nodes) also diminishes during protein starvation,[233,255] although to a lesser extent than the number of PFC.[255] A drop of both the total count and the concentration of RFC was observed only in very young rats at the terminal stage of a protein-free diet.[186,272]

If the immunization to SRBC is carried out via two injections of antigen with Freund's complete adjuvant added, the protein-deprived rats no longer exhibit any drop in the concentration of PFC, and the concentration of RFC is still higher than after a single

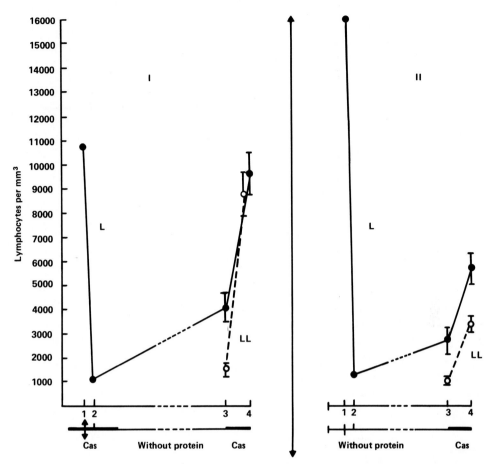

FIGURE 7.   Recovery of blood lymphocytes (means ± SE) after protracted protein starvation in adult male Charles River rats which received an i.p. injection of chlorambucil (12 mg/kg body weight). In Group I, this injection was given 2 weeks before the protein deprivation period, while the rats were still fed an 18% casein diet (Cas). In Group II, chlorambucil was injected after the first week of the protein-free diet. Total lymphocyte (L) count per cubic millimeter of blood: ●—; large lymphocytes (LL, cellular index >110 μm^2): ○ — —; 1: day of first blood cell count just before chlorambucil injection; 2: cell count 4 days after injection; 3 and 4: 1st and 10th days of an 18% casein diet given after the period of protein starvation. This period was more prolonged in Group I (78 days) than in Group II (55 days) in order to obtain a similar body weight (143 ± 3 g and 136 ± 6 g) at the beginning of protein refeeding. (From Aschkenasy, A., *Rev. Fr. Etud. Clin. Biol.*, 13, 792—799, 1968. With permission.)

immunization without adjuvant.[255] The T-cell-stimulating effect of the latter[129] may explain these results.

Indeed, the responsibility of the thymic atrophy and of the subsequent involution of the peripheral T cell system in the decrease of serum antibody levels to SRBC is suggested by several data. First, like a protein-free diet, adult thymectomy is followed by a decrease in the levels of PFC and circulating antibodies in mice[273] as well as in rats.[233,255,266] Second, the levels of serum antibodies, while being much higher in intact rats than in adult thymectomized rats on a balanced diet, become similar in the two groups on a protein-free diet (Table 22).[233,255,265] This suggests a certain resemblance between late thymectomy and dietary thymic atrophy.

However, concerning the total counts (per whole spleen) of PFC and RFC, an important difference is noticed between thymectomized and intact rats, even if both are deprived of protein (Table 22). Apparently, dietary atrophy of the thymus permits the

Table 22
INFLUENCE OF PROTEIN DEPRIVATION AND (OR) LATE THYMECTOMY ON THE IMMUNIZATION TO SHEEP RED BLOOD CELLS[a] IN ADULT MALE PATHOGEN-FREE SHERMAN RATS

Diet[b]	PFC[c] Per 10^6 viable cells	PFC[c] Per spleen	RFC[c] Per 10^3 viable cells	RFC[c] Per spleen	Serum antibody titers[d] Hemagglutinins	Serum antibody titers[d] Hemolysins
(N) I[e] (9)[f]	461 ±63[g]	240,052	3.96 ±0.60	2,062,000	4.214 ±0.078	2.609 ±0.127
(N) Tx[e] (7)	318 ±48	85,976	2.53 ±1.22	689,000	3.483 ±0.111	1.978 ±0.111
(PD) I (7)	111 ±15	7,471	11.54 ±5.92	678,000	3.311 ±0.213	1.677 ±0.145
(PD) Tx (8)	81 ±9	1,626	10.76 ±4.23	216,000	3.349 ±0.133	1.956 ±0.098

[a] The rats were given a single i.p. injection of the antigen without adjuvant, 1 week before killing; 6×10^9 SRBC was injected into control rats (mean body weight ~455 g), and 3×10^9 was injected into protein-deficient rats (body weight ~110 g).

[b] For the composition of the diet, see References 142 and 254. N: balanced diet; PD: protein-deficient diet.

[c] The plaque-forming cells (PFC) were counted by the method of Cunningham and Szenberg, and the number of RFC was determined by the method of Zaalberg. Evaluation of cell viability was made by the dye (erythrosin) exclusion test.

[d] The titers were expressed as $\log_{10}$ values of the highest dilutions giving agglutination or complete hemolysis.

[e] I and Tx: intact and thymectomized rats. The thymus was removed 25 days after birth, 1 month before starting the 2-month experimental diets.

[f] Number of rats.

[g] Mean ± SE.

From Aschkenasy, A., *Life Sci.,* 12(2), 555–562, © 1973; with permission of Pergamon Press Ltd; and from *Ann. Immunol.* (Paris), 124C, 345–362, 1973. With permission.

survival of a much larger number of immunocompetent T lymphocytes than does adult thymectomy performed before and completed by protein starvation. Since the medullary area of the thymus is almost the only one to resist a protracted protein deprivation, one cannot exclude the possibility that the surviving peripheral T cell population in deficient intact rats may be protected by a thymic lymphopoietic and also immunostimulating hormone[148-151] secreted by reticuloepithelial cells of the thymic medulla.

Cell-mediated immunity — This immunity is impaired to a much lesser extent and at a later stage than the production of antibodies.

Indeed, according to Cooper et al.,[269] female mice maintained for three generations on a 4 or 8% casein diet are still able to reject skin allografts even more rapidly than do normal mice. However, Gautam et al.[270] observed a certain tolerance to skin grafts in mice fed a similar 4% casein diet. Also, in our laboratory, a moderately increased duration of the rejection time was remarked when the graft was performed on adult male rats maintained on a protein-free diet for 40 days before the graft and until its complete rejection. The first signs of rejection actually appeared after the same time interval in deficient rats and controls, and an extraimmunologic explanation of the prolonged duration of the rejection process (defective skin nurtiture or vascularization) cannot be discarded.[274]

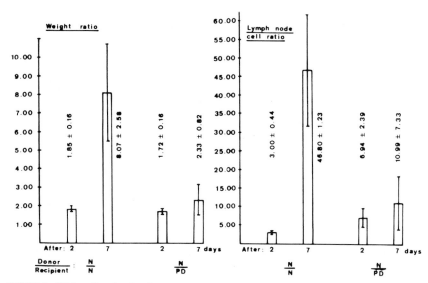

FIGURE 8.   Weight and lymph node cell-content ratios between ipsilateral and contralateral popliteal lymph nodes, 2 and 7 days after subplantar inoculation (into the right foot) of parental spleen lymphocytes: 12×10^6 cells for normally nourished (Sherman $\times$ Wistar) F_1 hybrid male recipients (N); 6×10^6 cells for protein-deprived hybrid recipients (PD). (From Aschkenasy, A., *World Rev. Nutr. Diet.*, 21, 151—197, 1975. With permission of S. Karger AG, Basel.)

On the other hand, increased reactivity was reported in the case of other cell-mediated responses in mice and rats after incomplete protein deprivation. Rats submitted to an 8% casein diet from 3 to 13 weeks of age exhibited a high cytotoxic activity against mastocytoma ascites cells.[275] This has been attributed to the disappearance of a specific serum antibody capable of blocking cellular immunity. Strong GVHR can also be induced in mice by splenic lymphocytes derived from parental donors which have been subjected to an 8% casein diet, and splenomegaly, used as an index of this reaction, is even more important than with donors maintained on a 27% casein diet.[258]

On the contrary, several experiments from our laboratory have shown that protein deprivation (providing that it is complete and protracted) inhibits the GVHR-inducing capacity of donor lymphocytes as well as the cellular defense reactions of the host, depending on whether the deficient diet is given to the donors or to the recipients. Prolonged, complete protein deprivation (2 months, beginning at 10 weeks of age) of the host significantly impairs the evolution of a popliteal lymph node GVHR.[276,277] Indeed, when utilizing the lymph node method, the weight and cellular ratio of ipsilateral/contralateral lymph nodes, as determined 1 week after subplantar inoculation of splenic lymphocytes from normal parental donors, was found to be significantly lower in protein-deprived than in nondeficient, hybrid F_1 recipient rats (Figure 8). This is understandable, since 1 week after inoculation the cellular reaction is mainly of host, not donor, origin.[278]

However, in the spleen-GVHR test,[279] grafted splenic lymphocytes taken from male parental donors deprived of protein for 2 months and recognized by their Y chromosome appear to be incapable of dividing in the spleen of F_1 hybrid female recipients, except in those which themselves have been subjected to a protein-free diet (Table 23).[277,280] Conversely, whichever diet is given to the donors, the proliferation of the grafted lymphocytes is significantly increased in recipients when the latter are subjected to a prolonged protein-free diet (Table 23).[277,280] This finding must be ascribed to the inhibition of host defense reactions, as already shown by the lymph node method (Figure 8).[276,277]

It is useful to point out that only chromosomal techniques have permitted the discovery of the inhibitory effect of protein deprivation on the GVHR-inducing potential

Table 23

MITOSES[a] OF DONOR CELLS IN SPLEEN OF RECIPIENT RATS DURING FIRST WEEK OF A
GRAFT-VS.-HOST REACTION[b]

Effect of Protein Deprivation

Strain and sex		Diet		6 hr		48 hr		7 days	
				Total mitoses ($‰$)	Donor mitoses (%)	Total mitoses ($‰$)	Donor mitoses (%)	Total mitoses ($‰$)	Donor mitoses (%)
Donor	Recipient	Donor	Recipient						
Sherman ♂	(Sherman × Wistar) F$_1$ ♀	Normal	Normal	7.43 ±0.75 (7)[d]	19.93 ±7.05	13.67 ±0.92 (6)	14.51 ±2.08	18.20 ±1.91 (5)	6.93 ±1.99
	♀	Normal	Protein free	1.71 ±0.03 (7)	0	7.50 ±0.99 (6)	11.00 ±4.30	8.67 ±1.98 (6)	17.67 ±3.80
	♀	Protein free	Normal	6.00 ±0.38 (7)	12.23 ±3.73	15.50 ±1.77 (6)	0	19.33 ±2.73 (6)	0.93 ±0.93
	♀	Protein free	Protein free	—	—	7.17 ±0.70	6.36 ±0.94	11.40 ±3.04 (6)	21.00 ±3.67
Sherman ♂ (syngeneic control)	Sherman ♂ (syngeneic control) Uninjected Sherman ♀	Normal	Normal	—	—	9.60 ±0.93 (5) 4.00 ±0.63 (5)	2.00 ±1.23	4.75 ±0.85	

[a] All recipient rats had been injected intraperitoneally with 0.25 mg/100 g of colchicine 1 hr 30 min before killing. The total number of mitoses was established on chromosomal preparations (see Reference 222). The percentages of mitoses of the male donor cells were counted after construction of karyotypes from 100 selected mitotic figures.

[b] The dose of intraperitoneally injected parental splenic lymphocytes (viable cells, unstained by erythrosine) was 120 × 10⁶ or 60 × 10⁶, depending on whether the recipients were fed normally (commercial rat biscuits) or had been fed on a protein-free diet for 2 months.

[c] For the composition of the diet, see References 142 and 254.

[d] Number of rats.

From Aschkenasy, A., *Nature*, 250, 325–327, 1974. With permission.

of the donors. Indeed, the splenic weight index[279] itself is not at all decreased (and even frequently increased) in normal recipients of protein-deprived donor lymphocytes.[277] This agrees with the findings of Cooper et al.[258] in mice grafted with lymphocytes from donors nourished with an 8% casein diet. No more changes were observed in the lymph node weight test in rats in the case of protein-deprived donors.[276]

Thus, taking into account that 1 week after the graft the so-called GVHR is represented mainly by a hyperplasia of host lymphocytes (at least in the splenic and lymph node tests), no valuable conclusions can be drawn as to the real role played by the donor cells without correct identification of the latter.

Inhibition of the host-vs.-graft defenses becomes apparent only at a very late stage of protein starvation, when the thymus and spleen of the recipients are already highly atrophied. Indeed, a significant correlation was found between the strength of GVHR (as indicated by the weight and cell population ratios between stimulated and nonstimulated popliteal lymph nodes in the lymph node test) on the one hand and the weight of the thymus and the spleen on the other (Table 24).[281]

Among other tests of cell-mediated (thymus-dependent) immunity, the lymphocytic response in mixed leukocyte cultures has been found to be impaired in marasmic swine.[282] Also, the inhibition of macrophage migration was reported to be induced in tuberculosis- or BCG-infected protein-deprived mice.[270] On the contrary, contact hypersensitivity to oxazolone, as measured by ear swelling and DNA synthesis in auricular lymph nodes draining the treated skin area, is not at all depressed in rats after 2 months of protein-free diet.[274]

In the light of the above-mentioned findings, it appears that involution of the thymus-dependent lymphoid system induced in rats by protein deprivation may be

Table 24

GRAFT-VS.-HOST REACTION (GVHR) EXPRESSED AS WEIGHT AND CELL RATIOS BETWEEN IPSILATERAL (INOCULATED) AND CONTRALATERAL POPLITEAL LYMPH NODES

Comparison with Weights of Lymphoid Organs in Normally Fed or Protein-deprived Rats

Diet	Thymus (mg)	Ratios iPLN/cPLN		Spleen (mg)	Ratios iPLN/cPLN		Cervical lymph node (mg)	Ratios iPLN/cPLN	
		Weight >3.0	Number of cells >15		Weight >3.0	Number of cells >15		Weight >3.0	Number of cells >15
Balanced	280—470	68.7% (11/16)[a]	68.7% (11/16)[a]	520—660	68.7% (11/16)[a]	68.7% (11/16)[a]	6—19	55.0% (11/20)[a]	60.0% (12/20)[a]
Protein free (4 weeks)	45—120	41.7% (5/12)	50.0% (6/12)	170—220	50.0% (7/14)	57.2% (8/14)	4.1—5.5	40.0% (4/10)	40.0% (4/10)
Protein free (9 weeks)	<45 (2/10)	20.0% (2/10)	20.0%	<155	0 (0/8)	0 (0/8)	<4.0	37.5% (3/8)	37.5% (3/8)

[a] Number of rats with GVHR >3 or >15, respectively, per total number of rats belonging to the different weight groups of each lymphoid organ.

From Aschkenasy, A., *Experientia*, 32, 638—639, 1976. With permission.

conditioned primarily (although not exclusively) by the disappearance of a fraction (subpopulation) of T lymphocytes displaying the following common features: their origin in the thymic cortex;[227,231] their sensitivity to cortisone[247] and to antithymic antibodies;[221] the responsiveness to PHA in vivo;[247,254] the helper activity in humoral responses to thymus-dependent antigens like SRBC;[233,255,266] the intervention in the GVHR (both as initiating donor cells and as cells participating in the host defenses;[276, 277,280,281] and, perhaps to a small extent, in the rejection of skin allografts.[270,274]

On the other hand, the preservation of delayed skin hypersensitivity to oxazolone may be attributed to a distinct long-lived subpopulation which is resistant to protein deprivation[274] as well as to cortisone. It is also possible that the sole differences between the T lymphocytes consist of quantitatively distinct thresholds in the same population for different immunologic stimulants.[115] In such a hypothesis, protein deprivation would simply raise the threshold of the helper activity and of the GVHR inductive and responsive capacities, while not influencing that of other cell-mediated immune reactions. The deficiency of cortisone-sensitive T lymphocytes could be precisely responsible for the elevated threshold of some immune responses.

To a certain degree, this conclusion is at variance with the hypothesis that only cortisone-resistant T cells originating from the thymic medulla are immunocompetent[98,283,284] and responsive to PHA.[102,285] Cortisone sensitivity of PHA-stimulated T cells, however, has already been reported in rat lymph nodes and spleen,[104,247] as well as in the human blood in vitro.[286-288] On the other hand, it has been claimed that optimal immunologic responses to SRBC or in the GVHR cannot be obtained without cooperation of cortisone-resistant and cortisone-sensitive T lymphocytes.[289,290] Therefore, there is no reason to reject the hypothesis that the immunodepression induced by protein deprivation may be due to the disappearance of most of the cortisone-sensitive T cells cooperating with the cortisone-resistant cells in some immunologic reactions.

Finally, a possible intervention of suppressor T lymphocytes in the immunologic anomalies cannot be excluded, since cortisone-resistant thymic and splenic lymphocytes (most of which are also resistant to protein deprivation) have been reported to be a good source of suppressor cell precursors in vitro.[291]

bb. Involvement of B Lymphocytes

These cells are also affected by experimental protein malnutrition, although probably to a lesser extent than T lymphocytes. This malnutrition provokes the regression of not only thymus-dependent (paracortex) but also thymus-independent areas (follicles, medullary cords) of the lymph nodes, as well as the atrophy of splenic follicles inhabited mainly by B lymphocytes.[199,232,233] The marked atrophy of Peyer's patches, a predominantly B-cell-producing organ, also gives evidence for a depressed B cell production and activity.

On the other hand, decreased resistance to pneumococcal antigens, considered thymus independent, has been reported in protein-deficient rabbits and rats.[292]

Finally, as is true of the responses to PHA and SRBC,[254] the blastogenic responses of popliteal lymph nodes after subplantar injection of *E. coli* lipopolysaccharides (LPS) or dextran sulfate (both specific B cell antigens) are also inhibited in protein starvation (Reference 254 and unpublished data). It is true, however, that in the same experiments the reaction of the spleen to LPS was more important with a protein-free diet than with a balanced one. This may be due to the diffusion of the antigen, favored by the involution of the lymph node follicles in the deprived rats.[254]

However, several other findings militate against an important impairment of B cell

Table 25

COMPARED IMMUNE RESPONSES (± SE) 7 DAYS AFTER INTRAPERITONEAL INJECTION OF
MICROBIAL LIPOPOLYSACCHARIDES[a] WITH FREUND'S COMPLETE ADJUVANT ADDED IN
RATS[b] ON AN 18% CASEIN DIET OR ON A PROTEIN-FREE DIET FOR 2 MONTHS[294]

Diet[c]	Terminal body weight (g)	Percentage of viable lymphocytes[d]	Rosette-forming cells[e] per 10^6 viable lympho- cytes	Plaque-forming cells[e] per 10^6 viable lymphocytes	Titers of serum hem- agglutinins[f]	
					Total	IgG
18% casein (11)[g]	317.3	60.7	1642	306	2.462	0.957
	±6.4	±1.2	±329	±125	±0.181	±0.332
Protein	114.0	44.6	2153	139	2.322	0.860
free (10)	±2.2	±2.1	±545	±34	±0.134	±0.325
Difference			NS[h]	NS	NS	NS

[a] Lipopolysaccharides from *Escherichia coli* 055:B5 (Difco, Detroit, Michigan): 10 μg/100 g body weight.
[b] Male Charles River rats.
[c] For the composition of the diets, see References 142 and 254.
[d] The cell viability was evaluated according to the erythrosin exclusion test[155] with lecture immediately after contact with the dye.
[e] Same techniques as in Table 22; see also References 233 and 255. The coupling of LPS to SRBC was performed according to Blackwater et al.[636]
[f] Titers expressed as $\log_{10}$ values. IgG were separated by treatment of the sera with 2-mercaptoethanol.
[g] Number of rats.
[h] Not significant.

activity in protein deficiency. Normal immunologic responses to *Salmonella typhimurium* were observed in rats[208,293] and to *Bacillus abortus* in mice[269] submitted to a protein-free or protein-poor diet.

On the other hand, a protein deprivation lasting 2 months does not significantly influence the humoral response to LPS; the levels of RFC, PFC, and serum antibodies found after i.p. inoculation of this antigen do not differ in protein-deprived and normally fed rats (Table 25).[294]

Concerning the moderate decrease in serum gammaglobulin levels usually observed in rats after protracted protein starvation,[295] it apparently does not involve thymus-independent antibodies, since it has been shown to be controlled by the functional status of the T cell system. Indeed, late thymectomy generally aggravates dietary hypogamma-globulinemia,[296] and thymectomy[297] or injections of antithymic serum[221] impair the restoration of the gammaglobulins during a recovery diet.

g. Immunologic Activity of Lymphocytes in Amino Acid Deficiency or Imbalance

Immunodepression was observed after a dietary excess of phenylalanine[298,299] and after deprivation of tryptophan.[299-301] Diets with limited amounts of phenolic or sulfur amino acids, valine, isoleucine, threonine, or tryptophan were reported to induce a selective depression of tumor growth in mice as well as a reduction of hemagglutinating and blocking antibody responses.[302]

Lysine had no effect on antibody titers when given to rats fed a wheat gluten diet,[215,301] and even decreased 6-day titers when added to a corn diet.[303]

Overload with leucine (7%) in young rats provokes a striking reduction of immunologic responses to SRBC (RFC, PFC, and serum antibodies), but the inhibitory effect is observed only if the diet is itself very poor in protein (4%), while excess leucine is completely innocuous when added to an 18% casein diet (Table 26).[186]

Against expectations, a 4% protein diet not supplemented with extra leucine does not induce significant immunologic depression after 8 weeks of feeding, contrary to what has been observed in rats after complete protein deprivation of the same duration.

It is of parenthetical interest to mention that dietary overload with leucine can result in the development of pellagra (as was reported after feeding with sorgho in certain areas

Table 26

IMMUNOLOGIC DEPRESSION AFTER OVERLOAD WITH LEUCINE IN PROTEIN-DEFICIENT RATS[a]
IMMUNIZED[b] TO SHEEP RED BLOOD CELLS[186]

Diet[c]	Extra leucine (7% of the dry weight of the food)	Body weight (g)		Number of splenic RFC[d] per 10^6 viable lymphocytes	Number of splenic PFC[d] per 10^6 viable lymphocytes	Titers of serum antibodies to SRBC ($\log_{10}$)	
		Initial	Terminal			Hemagglutinins	Hemolysins
18% casein (8)[e]	–	105.4 ±3.0	376.5 ±5.6	6074 ±673	159 ±23	3.424 ±0.097	2.634 ±0.075
18% casein (9)	+	105.3 ±1.6	426.9 ±13.4	8306 ±2250	241 ±60	3.712 ±0.071	2.776 ±0.110
4% casein (9)	–	105.9 ±3.1	98.8 ±9.0	5373 ±1230	101 ±32	2.876 ±0.261	2.408 ±0.207
4% casein (9)	+	107.8 ±3.9	92.4 ±2.8	551 ±184	14 ±3	1.940 ±0.134	1.003 ±0.174
Restricted 18% casein (8)	–	108.4 ±1.3	154.4 ±4.7	1377 ±182	54 ±13	3.311 ±0.114	2.860 ±0.114

[a] Young adult male Charles River rats.
[b] The animals were immunized by single intraperitoneal injection of 2.4 × 10^9 SRBC per 100 g body weight, without adjuvant added. They were killed on Day 8.
[c] The diets were administered for 55 days. The restricted diet was given in amounts ingested by rats on the [4% casein + leucine] diet.
[d] RFC: rosette-forming cells; PFC: plaque-forming cells.
[e] Number of rats.

of India), probably via a disturbing effect of an excess of leucine on the metabolism of tryptophan.[304] The same excess, however, also inhibits the use of valine and isoleucine.[305] Now, lack of these amino acids has been shown to be highly detrimental to the production of lymphocytes[218,234,244] and may probably also depress the immunologic activity of these cells.

Several studies have been devoted to the immunodepressive effect of ethionine, an antagonist of methionine. Such an effect was observed in the case of immunization with synthetic antigenic peptides or SRBC after peroral administration of ethionine in primates and rats,[299,306] as well as after repeated i.p. injections of this antagonist.[307] In the latter experiments, both the production of serum hemagglutinins and hemolysins and that of RFC and PFC were inhibited. Since immunodepression was also noticed after digestive introduction of ethionine,[299,306] this effect could not be ascribed to a hypothetical complete degradation of the antigen by peritoneal macrophages mobilized by this amino acid.

Ethionine also significantly decreases the blastogenic response in vivo to PHA.[308] However, neither rejection of skin allografts nor hypersensitivity to oxazolone is impaired. Thus, as after complete amino acid deprivation, mainly T lymphocytes provided with helper activity and responsive to PHA appear to be inactivated. These cells may represent either a distinct subpopulation or correspond only to a definite stage of immunologic maturation of T cells.

The immunosuppressive effect of ethionine cannot be prevented by injections of ATP or adenosine,[307] which have been tested because of the block of ATP synthesis induced by this amino acid.[309]

Simultaneous administration of methionine together with ethionine actually aggravates the immunologic anomalies.[299,307] Indeed, after immunization with SRBC, almost no RFC are found in the spleen, and the PFC and serum antibody levels fall below the levels observed in rats treated with ethionine alone. These data may be compared to the finding that excess methionine inhibits the production of antibodies in chicks receiving an amino acid diet,[310] as well as in primates[306] and rats[301] fed a soya diet.

Regression of thymus and mesenteric lymph nodes was also observed after methionine overload.[311] When given together with ethionine, however, methionine to a large extent prevents the thymic involution induced by its antagonist,[307] although at the same time amplifying the immunosuppressive effect of the latter. Thus, only immuno-incompetent thymocytes and T lymphocytes seem to be connected with the thymus-protecting action of methionine under these conditions.

We cannot rule out the possibility that the harmful effect of excess methionine may be due to the "antifolate" action of this amino acid, as it was observed in vitro in vitamin-B_{12}-deficient bone marrow cultures in man[312] and the rat.[313] This action involves the block of homocysteine methylation and subsequent accumulation of 5-methyl-THF, which in turn would prevent the folate-dependent methylation of deoxyuridylate to thymidylate, indispensable for DNA synthesis.

4. Macrophages

The phagocytic activity of peritoneal exudate is lower in protein-deprived rats than in normal rats after immunization to *Salmonella typhimurium*.[210] The number of mononuclear macrophages found 5 hr after i.p. injection of glycogen also decreases in rats following a prolonged protein-free diet.[206] However, the defect in macrophages apparently does not play a role in humoral immunodepression due to protein deprivation. Indeed, this effect is not prevented at all in deficient rats when the antigen (SRBC) is injected simultaneously with peritoneal macrophages obtained from isogenic normal rats

3 days after injection of glycogen.[314] On the other hand, deficiency of macrophages may be the principal cause for decrease in natural nonacquired resistance reported in protein-deficient animals.[211]

However, once again, as for several parameters of cell-mediated immune responses, the results reported by Cooper et al.[258,269] in moderately protein-deficient mice indicate rather an enhanced activity of macrophages. Taken together, these conflicting data support the hypothesis that the exhaustion of the functional potential of macrophages, as well as of T and perhaps also of B lymphocytes, observed in advanced stages of protein malnutrition may be preceded by a period of hyperactivity of the same cells, such hyperactivity being the sole anomaly occurring in mice after only partial protein deprivation.

5. Hormonal Control of the Production and Immunologic Activity of Lymphocytes in Experimental Protein Deficiency

a. Hormones and Lymphopoiesis

i. Growth Hormone (GH) and Thymic Hormones

Daily injections of high doses (0.75 mg/day for 14 days) of an active GH preparation (STH, Calbiochem) and (or) of a thymic extract (Comsa)[147] repeated for 2 weeks did not reactivate either lymphopoiesis (blood lymphocyte levels and cell populations of lymphoid organs) or the immunologic responsiveness of rats subjected to protracted protein deprivation.[247] Although these experiments should be completed by utilizing other preparations of thymic hormones, the negative results are consistent with the hypothesis that lack of protein does not injure the production of these factors believed to depend on the reticuloepithelial cells of the thymus.

ii. Thyroid Hormones

The synthesis of thyroxine and triiodothyronine is relatively preserved in protein-deprived diets[315] in spite of the drop in the basal metabolic rate induced by such a diet.[316,317] Moreover, the persistent thyroid activity plays a protective role with respect to leukopoiesis (as well as to erythropoiesis) since thyroidectomy generally aggravates the involution of the thymus and the spleen in protein-deprived rats.[318] Conversely, daily injections of DL-thyroxine reduce the inhibitory effect of a protein-free diet on lymphopoiesis when given during the course of such a diet.[319] They also activate the recovery of lymphopoietic function when given to previously protein-deprived rats restored with a low protein diet (7% casein), the latter permitting by itself only a slow-rate restoration.[236,320]

iii. Androgens

Although the early involution of accessory genital glands indicates a drop in gonadotropic and androgenic secretion after protein deprivation,[227] a residual secretion of these hormones apparently exerts a facilitating effect with regard to the dietary involution of the thymus, since this organ remains much larger in protein-deprived orchidectomized rats than in noncastrated male rats on the same diet.[236,318]

iv. Glucocorticoids

Several findings lead to the conclusion that protein-deficient rats display an increased need for these hormones, the physiological functions of which include, among others, the degradation of various tissular (especially carcass and lymphoid) proteins. This may facilitate the subsequent utilization of the released amino acids for anabolic processes such as the synthesis of many hepatic enzymes, as suggested by the anabolic action of glucocorticoids on the liver.[321,322]

Table 27

EFFECTS OF DIETS DEPRIVED OF PROTEIN OR SOME ESSENTIAL AMINO ACIDS ON ADRENAL
WEIGHTS AND CORTICOSTERONE LEVELS IN PLASMA AND ADRENALS

Diet	Terminal body weight (g)	Relative weight of the adrenals (mg/100 g)	Corticosterone (μg)		
			Per 100 ml of plasma	Per gram of adrenal tissue	In adrenals as a whole per 100 g body weight
Study 1 (25 Days); Wistar Strain					
18% casein (5)[a]	304 ± 4	11.2 ± 0.6	19.8 ± 1.4	36.3 ± 2.2	0.40 ± 0.04
0% protein (7)	132 ± 6	14.6 ± 0.5	23.0 ± 2.6	37.5 ± 4.3	0.53 ± 0.05
Without sulfur amino acids (6)	132 ± 5	16.7 ± 1.4[c]	23.4 ± 3.4	39.5 ± 0.9	0.65 ± 0.08[b]
Without valine (7)	142 ± 4	18.6 ± 0.9[d]	26.6 ± 1.9[b]	36.7 ± 2.8	0.68 ± 0.08[b]
Study 2 (25 Days); Wistar Strain					
18% casein (6)	281 ± 6	14.6 ± 0.6	19.6 ± 2.5	49.4 ± 4.3	0.71 ± 0.06
0% protein (6)	132 ± 2	18.3 ± 0.3[c]	23.3 ± 4.1	40.4 ± 3.0	0.72 ± 0.04
Without isoleucine (5)	119 ± 3	25.3 ± 0.7[d]	22.9 ± 3.7	59.9 ± 8.6	1.51 ± 0.23[c]
Without phenolic amino acids (5)	146 ± 4	19.0 ± 0.9	45.4 ± 3.6[d]	86.2 ± 11.0[b]	1.72 ± 0.36[b]
Study 3 (36 Days); Sherman Strain					
18% casein (7)	315 ± 7	13.9 ± 0.4	10.5 ± 0.5	31.0 ± 1.8	0.42 ± 0.03
0% protein (7)	120 ± 3	19.8 ± 0.5[d]	42.4 ± 5.3[d]	64.9 ± 12.0[b]	1.28 ± 0.24

[a] Number of rats.
[b,c,d] Significantly different from the casein group: P < 0.05, < 0.01, and < 0.001, respectively.

From Aschkenasy, A., Adam, Y., and Joly, P., *Ann. Endocrinol.*, 27, 21–36, 1966. With permission.

Whereas adrenalectomy is tolerated perfectly with a balanced diet, on the condition that the animals are given physiological saline as drinking fluid, adrenalectomized salt-supplemented rats are generally incapable of resisting for more than 2 weeks a diet either completely protein-deprived or containing only 2% casein, unless these animals are provided with accessory adrenal tissue or receive cortisone.[323-325] On the other hand, the existence of spontaneous hypercorticalism in protein-deficient intact animals is suggested not only by a relative hypertrophy of adrenals,[228,231] but also by the usually increased plasma and (or) adrenal levels of corticosterone found after protracted protein starvation in rats[224,272] as well as in primates (Table 27).[326] The negative results reported in mice by Cooper et al.[258,269] can be explained by the presence of 8% casein in their protein-deficient diet, this level certainly being high enough to not provoke an increased need for glucocorticoids, as suggested by the survival of adrenalectomized rats submitted to diets differing in their casein content.[323] In addition, the fact that the lymphoid tissues did not display a disproportionate weight decrease in the experiments of these authors[258,269] also militates against a stressing effect of the 8% casein diet used. Also, Munro[327] observed that after a short period of protein deprivation (11 days), the adrenals, far from being hyperactive, displayed a reduction of their weight as well as of their total phospholipid, protein, and nucleic acid contents. These findings are not at variance with those from my laboratory, which showed that increased corticosterone levels in the plasma were noticed after only 35 days of a protein-free diet in mature rats (Table 27).[224] A progressive increase in the ACTH discharge due to the nutritional stress might be the cause of this adrenal reactivation.

Surprisingly, the anomalies of glucocorticoid secretion are still more pronounced after selective deprivation of certain amino acids (phenolic amino acids, valine, or isoleucine) than with a diet completely devoid of protein and amino acids.[224]

Available evidence suggests that the lymphoid involution provoked by protein deficiency may be conditioned to a large extent by adrenocortical activity. Indeed, adrenalectomized rats that resisted a protein-free diet for more than 3[328] or 5[329] weeks, either because of the presence of accessory adrenal tissue[329] or because of the administration of very low doses of cortisone (100 μg/100 g per day,[328] just enough to permit a survival of at least 3 weeks), exhibited strongly increased blood levels of lymphocytes instead of lymphopenia. These cells apparently originated from the lymph nodes, as judged from the hyperplasia of these organs, whereas the thymus was atrophied to the same extent as in protein-deprived nonadrenalectomized animals.[328]

These findings indicate that high adrenocortical hormonal production and (or) activity, linked to the increased needs of malnourished animals, may be indispensable for the development of blood lymphopenia and the involution of lymph nodes. On the contrary, the atrophy of the thymus occurs as soon as there is the slightest supply of glucocorticoids. The overwhelming predominance of cortison-sensitive cells in the thymus and of cortisone-resistant ones in the lymph nodes (see Section I.B.4, "Sensitivity to Glucocorticoid Hormones," earlier in this chapter) may explain the discrepancy between the above observations.

In addition, the particularly high sensitivity of the protein-deficient thymus to glucocorticoids may be attributed to, as that of eosinophils to the same hormones[225] (see Section IV.A.2.d, "Role Played by Glucocorticoid Hormones in Dietary Eosinopenia," earlier in this chapter), the lack of transcortin, the carrier protein of the latter, and to the subsequent predominance of a free, particularly active form of circulating adrenal corticosteroids.[226]

Thus, the existence of a relative hypercorticalism explains why only lymphocytes, which are the most resistant to cortisone, are able to survive after protracted protein deprivation.

b. Hormones and Immunologic Dysfunction

Growth hormone associated with thyroxine and a thymic extract reportedly activated immunologic reactions of hypophysectomized or hypopituitary animals.[330] However, treatment with GH given alone or together with a thymic extract did not at all enhance the impaired immune responses to SRBC in protein-deprived rats.[247] On the other hand, it may be that the immunologic anomalies of these rats are partly conditioned by the lymphocyte suppressive and immunosuppressive action of endogenous glucorticoids.

Indeed, somewhat similar immunologic alterations (drop in the total number of splenic RFC and PFC, and in the titers of serum antibodies) are observed after prolonged protein deprivation[255,266] and after a 10-day treatment with cortisone (3 mg/day per 100 g body weight).[101] The endogenous glucocorticoids may act not only via their thymolytic effect, as seems to be the case for low doses (1 mg/day) of cortisone, but also directly on the peripheral T lymphocytes.[101]

B. Human Protein Deficiency
1. Neutrophils

No striking changes in the blood levels of leukocytes have been reported in kwashiorkor and marasmus (combined protein-calorie malnutrition — PCM), endemic in some underdeveloped tropical countries.[331,332] The only abnormality frequently observed is the absence of increased neutrophilia during intercurrent severe infections, contrary to what occurs in normally nourished individuals.[1,333] This phenomenon may be due to a faulty mobilization of medullary reserves of granulocytes and also to the decrease of the vascular marginal pool of these cells.

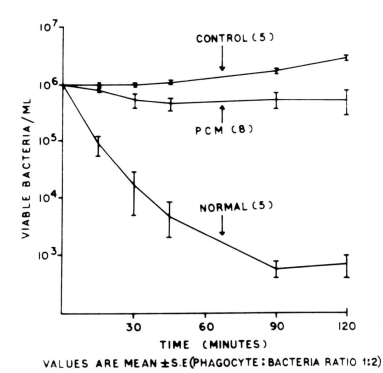

VALUES ARE MEAN ±S.E (PHAGOCYTE : BACTERIA RATIO 1:2)

FIGURE 9. Bactericidal activity of leukocytes isolated from normal children and children with protein-calorie malnutrition. Control: tubes containing bacteria (E. coli) and heat inactivated plasma but no leukocytes. Numbers in parentheses refer to the number of observations. (From Selveraj, R. J. and Bhat, K. S., *Am. J. Clin. Nutr.*, 25, 166—174, 1972. With permission.)

Nevertheless, when interpreting these hematological data, one should also keep in mind that patients with protein malnutrition frequently (especially in case of infection) exhibit edema with hemodilution due to cardiac and renal failure as well as to hypoalbuminemia provoked by both malnutrition and infection. On the other hand, the blood leukocyte levels differ considerably according to the age of the patients and the degree of the malnutrition. Also, some of the reported data have been obtained from subjects already on the way to recovery.

Like the number of neutrophils, the phagocytic potential of these cells and the opsonic activity of the serum are generally within normal limits,[331,334-337] which is in disagreement with some findings reported in protein-deficient animals (see Section IV.A.1.a.ii, "Functional Changes of Neutrophils," earlier in this chapter). However, intracellular killing of bacteria may be reduced in children with kwashiorkor or PCM (Figure 9).[24,332,337,338]

It is interesting to confront these observations with data concerning the biochemical changes associated with phagocytosis. A decrease in glycolysis, as measured by lactate production, was reported in PCM by two groups of authors[332,339,341] but was not confirmed by others.[338] On the other hand, a block of glucose oxidation via the hexose monophosphate shunt, the main biochemical substratum of phagocytosis (see Section I.A.1, "Neutrophils," earlier in this chapter), was demonstrated by the inactivation of two enzymes of this metabolic pathway (glucose 6-phosphate-dehydrogenase and 6-phosphogluconate dehydrogenase) in children with kwashiorkor,[340] as well as by the decreased oxidation of glucose $1\text{-}^{14}C$ to $^{14}CO_2$ by the leukocytes of children with

PCM.[332] In addition, reduced NADPH oxidase activity in leukocytes and the absence of any activation of this enzyme during phagocytosis was reported in PCM.[24,332] As to the unexpected finding of abnormally increased alkaline phosphatase activity,[335] this may be explained by concomitant infection in the examined patients.

Complement levels were found significantly lower in PCM than in normal subjects, particularly in children with kwashiorkor.[342,343] This is another index of impaired phagocytosis because of the important role played by the complement complex in this activity (Section I.A.1). On the other hand, no difference was noted between the results of the nitroblue-tetrazolium test in infants with PCM and in well-nourished children.[344]

2. Eosinophils

Eosinopenia, a characteristic early symptom of experimental protein deprivation, has also been reported in human PCM during World War II (see Section III.A, "Blood and Bone Marrow Leukocytes," earlier in this chapter), but this anomaly is not frequent in malnutrition in tropical regions because of the high incidence of parasitic infestation.

3. Lymphocytes

a. Quantitative and Functional Nonimmunologic Changes; Effect of Phytohemagglutinin

As for eosinophils, there is a striking difference between the data obtained from investigations on semi-starved inmates of concentration camps, in whom lymphopenia was a constant phenomenon,[188] and the findings in infantile kwashiorkor and PCM, where important lymphopenia (<2000 cells per cubic millimeter) was found in only 16 to 20% of cases.[345,346] This may be due to the strong mitotic activity and to the relative resistance of the lymphopoietic system in infants as compared to semi-starved adults, exhausted not only by denutrition but also by hard labor and emotional stress.

As in animals, the thymus is by far the most injured of the lymphoid organs in infantile kwashiorkor.[345,347,348] The spleen, lymph nodes, and tonsils, however, are also involved.[345,346] The histological changes are similar to those found in protein-deprived rats and mice: depletion of the thymic cortex with fibrosis but relatively few changes in the thymic medulla,[153] and diminished cell density in the white pulp of the spleen and in the paracortical areas of the lymph nodes,[345,348] but also reduction of germinal centers,[153] indicating a simultaneous injury of thymus-dependent and independent areas. On the other hand, no changes have been observed concerning the number of intraepithelial lymphocytes of the jejunal mucosa in malnourished children.[349]

Regarding the functional activities of lymphocytes, it may be interesting to note that a reduced migration of these cells to cutaneous lesions in the Rebuck window test was observed in kwashiorkor,[350] yet numerous investigations have concerned the responses to PHA. The majority of the results reported favor a hypoactivity or reduced number of PHA-responsive T cells; thus, impairment of this response in vitro was observed in an important proportion of cases of kwashiorkor and, to a lesser extent, in marasmus.[343,345,346,351-355] However, other authors insist on a large predominance of normal responses in vitro in malnourished children.[343,356,357]

Coovadia et al.[343] pointed to the differing results concerning the transformation of PHA-stimulated lymphocytes when measured by ^{3}H-thymidine uptake (which was below normal in only 29% of the malnourished children) and when assessed by morphological changes (in almost 100% of the patients). In addition, the depressed ^{3}H-thymidine uptake was apparently due to associated folate deficiency, since it could be restored by folic acid therapy, not to protein deprivation.[343] On the other hand, according to Neumann et al.,[355] the percentage of negative reactions to PHA in malnourished children is much higher when the test is performed in vivo (cutaneous delayed hypersensitivity to PHA)

(94%) than with tests in vitro (19%), the latter proportion being even lower than that reported by Coovadia (29%). This finding suggests that positive responses may be ascribed to the protective effect of the protein and amino acid nutrients included in the culture medium. Indeed, incorporation of these nutrients into the lymphocytes should permit a reactivation of the cellular enzymes inhibited by protein depletion.

Since the mitogenic action of PHA on human lymphocytes in vitro can be prevented by glucocorticoid hormones,[286-288] it is reasonable to suppose that, as in protein-deprived rats, mainly the cortisone-sensitive and PHA-responsive fraction of thymocytes and T lymphocytes derived from the thymic cortex may be inhibited in human protein malnutrition.

b. Immunologic Activity

Thymic atrophy was the first phenomenon that suggested a predominant alteration of thymus-dependent lymphocytes in kwashiorkor and marasmus. This hypothesis was strengthened by the frequent incidence of several types of infection involving cellular immunity in subjects with protein malnutrition (tuberculosis, and fungal or viral infections such as measles, rubella, vaccinia, and herpes), as well as by the depression of some specific reactions of this immunity: cutaneous response to tuberculin[346,357-359] and delayed hypersensitivity to 2,4 dinitrochlorobenzene (DNCB)[345,346,357,360-362] or cutaneous reaction to an antigen extract of *Candida albicans*.[346,351,360,361] However, whereas the skin test to *Candida* was found negative only in malnourished children,[346,351,360] not in well-nourished infants with intercurrent infections,[351] a negative tuberculin reaction was also observed during recovery of infections, even in normal infants.[357]

The inhibition of humoral immunity in human protein malnutrition seems to concern mainly the thymus-dependent responses, as is the case in animals. Indeed, the production of antibodies to pneumococcal polysaccharides[355] and TAB vaccine,[363] both B-cell-specific antigens, was found to be normal in the great majority (80%) of cases, while the response to keyhole limpet hemocyanin (KLH), a thymus-dependent protein antigen, was inhibited in 50% of the cases of kwashiorkor.[355] However, depressed responses to TAB vaccine have also been reported in children with PCM.[343] On the other hand, antigens that are supposed to be thymus dependent, such as those of measles and polio viruses, are able to induce strong humoral responses in children with kwashiorkor.[364,365]

The serum levels of all types of immunoglobulins are normal or only moderately reduced in protein-malnourished noninfected subjects.[343,364,366-369] In addition, the Ig levels increase in normal proportions in cases of intercurrent infection.[346,370,371] The reports of high Ig titers in some cases of malnutrition, even in the absence of infection, may be explained by early commencement of dietetic therapy.[365]

The hypothesis of a predominant impairment of T lymphocytes in human protein-calorie malnutrition would be consistent with the frequently observed drop in the number of blood T cells identified by the SRBC rosette test.[362,372] However, other investigators,[373] using the same test, did not find any quantitative changes in T cells, either in marasmus or in kwashiorkor. Similar negative results have been reported in adults acutely malnourished and rendered hypoalbuminemic and lymphopenic by semistarvation diets.[361]

The proportion of B lymphocytes in the peripheral blood, as determined by immunofluorescence in a small number of cases of kwashiorkor, was also found to be of the same order as in normal infants.[343]

Taken together, the above rather conflicting findings suggest the possibility that the depression of responses to T-cell-requiring antigens and T-cell-specific mitogens usually observed may be ascribed (with the eventual exception of very advanced cases of malnutrition) to a functional inactivation of, rather than a percent decrease in, the T cell population.

c. Role Played by the Adrenals in the Lymphocytic and Immunologic Anomalies Induced by Protein Malnutrition in Man

As in protein-deprived rats[224] and primates,[326] the levels of plasma glucocorticoids are generally increased in protein-deficient humans,[226,343,374-377] these levels being higher in PCM than in kwashiorkor.[378]

In addition, the relative increase in the proportion of free cortisol nonconjugated with its serum carrier protein (quantitatively reduced because of the lack of dietary proteins)[226] may lead to a functional activation of the circulating hormone. This strengthens the hypothesis that the hypercorticalism induced by malnutrition may intervene in the involution of the thymus-dependent system.

4. Role Played by Nutritional Deficiencies Other than Lack of Protein on the Leukocytic and Immunologic Consequences of Human Protein or Protein-calorie Malnutrition

Before ending the discussion of proteins and leukopoiesis, it is indispensable to point out the difficulty of separating specific effects of protein and amino acid deprivation from those due to associated deficiencies of other nutrients. Such combined deficiencies are almost constant in protein malnutrition of man. They include the lack of carbohydrates and lipids (as in protein-calorie malnutrition), but also a deficient intake of iron, as well as that of vitamin A and vitamin E, and an inadequate supply of the B complex vitamins, among which the folates are particularly concerned.

All these conditions contribute to the disturbance of the state of balance between production and destruction of leukocytes, and the impairment of their functional activity. This also may adversely influence the immune responses.

Thus, associated iron deficiency may aggravate the inhibitory effect of protein malnutrition on the bactericidal activity of neutrophils,[379] as well as on some cell-mediated mitogenic or immunologic responses (see Section IX.A.1, "Iron Deficiency," later in this chapter). On the other hand, sharp inhibition of some of these responses has been reported in PCM combined with deficiency of folic acid,[343,380] or with those of riboflavin, pyridoxine, and thiamine.[355]

Comparative T and B Lymphocyte Involvement in Malnutrition-Induced Immunodepression

In contrast to the findings of Coovadia et al.,[343] Schopfer and Douglas[664] observed a decrease of the absolute number of complement receptor-bearing B lymphocytes in human protein calorie malnutrition (PCM). As previously reported by other authors (cf. Jackson[153]), they also found decreased cell densities not only in the thymus and in thymus-dependent regions of the lymph nodes and spleen, but also in primarily B lymphocyte inhabited areas of these organs (germinal centers, primary follicles and medullary cords in lymph nodes and red pulp in the spleen). This indicates a parallel decrease of B and T cell populations. These data are consistent with those reported for protein deprived rats.[232,233]

The specificity of the SRBC-rosette test for the identification of human blood T cells has recently been questioned by Kutty et al.[665] It was shown that the physicochemical alteration of the cell membrane, e.g., reduced levels of membrane-associated acetylcholinesterase, was sufficient to inhibit the phenomenon of spontaneous rosette formation. Another error factor is represented by frequently elevated IgE levels, found in the blood of undernourished children as a result of associated parasitic infection.

IgE also inhibits rosette formation in vitro and thus may falsely suggest a decrease of the levels of T lymphocytes.

Mucosal Immunity

In addition to systemic immunity, it has recently been shown that mucosal immunity as well, which depends on the lymphoid formations in the digestive and respiratory systems, is considerably impaired in human PCM. The levels of IgA, the principal immunoglobulin secreted by these formations, were found to be significantly reduced in nasal washings, tears, saliva, and duodenal fluids of malnourished children.[666,667] Chandra[668] also reported that malnourished children immunized with live attenuated poliovirus or measles vaccine had nasopharyngeal washings which contained significantly lower quantities of specific IgA antibody than healthy children; serum antibody levels were comparable in both groups. Impaired mucosal immunity may also favor systemic spread of Gram-negative organisms from the digestive tract and subsequently contribute to explain the frequency and severity of gastrointestinal and respiratory infections in undernourished populations. The attenuated efficiency of the mucosal barrier may also lead to the appearance of allergic and autoimmune reactions, frequently associated with IgA deficiency, as well as to the formation of blood antibodies after the absorption of incompletely digested dietary proteins.[669]

V. LEUKOPOIESIS AND DIETARY CARBOHYDRATES

Fifty to seventy percent of blood glycogen is localized in leukocytes.[381] Whereas the abundance of this compound in granulocytes has been known for a long time,[381-383] the data concerning lymphocytes are contradictory.[56,231]

For leukocytes, glycolysis and oxidative phosphorylation represent the principal source of energy stored in the form of ATP. Alternatively, oxidation of glucose via the hexose-monophosphate shunt leads to the formation of H_2O_2, a potent bactericidal substance. In addition, the same HMP pathway also results in the synthesis of D-ribose, a nucleotide constituent, and also generates the NADPH required for reduction of ribonucleotides to deoxyribonucleotides in the synthesis of DNA.[384]

These biochemical data permit the comprehension of why an inadequate supply of glucose may inhibit phagocytosis[385] as well as cell proliferation. Phagocytosis has also been found to be reduced after overload with glucose, since diabetics display impaired neutrophilic phagocytosis,[386-388] and there is an inverse correlation between the phagocytic capacity and the blood glucose level in diabetic patients.[389]

In normal subjects, ingestion of 100 g glucose, fructose, sucrose, honey, or orange juice all significantly decrease the phagocytic index, whereas the number of neutrophils is not influenced.[390] Ingestion or infusion of glucose, however, is followed by a drop in the blood levels of lymphocytes[391] and eosinophils.[392,393] Since the latter effect also occurs in diabetics,[394] it cannot be ascribed to a stress provoked by discharge of insulin, as has been suggested.[395]

As with phagocytosis, mitotic activity and its biochemical correlate, glucose utilization via the HMP shunt, are sharply decreased in patients with diabetes mellitus. Indeed, incorporation of ^{14}C-thymidine after PHA, as well as the amount of glucose metabolized through the HMP shunt, was found to be much lower in diabetics than in normal subjects.[253]

All these data suggest that disturbed glucose metabolism may impair the destruction and processing of antigens by granulocytes and macrophages on one hand and immunologic reactions of lymphocytes on the other. This would give a metabolic explanation for the frequent incidence of microbial, mycotic, and granulomatous infections as complications of diabetes.

Among the carbohydrates involved in the metabolism of leukocytes, one must also mention heparin, a mucopolysaccharide synthesized by blood basophils and tissular mast cells. It is released during the "degranulation" of these cells.[410]

VI. LEUKOPOIESIS AND DIETARY LIPIDS

A. Effect of Dietary Lipids on Leukocytes

1. Influence on Intraleukocytic Lipids

There are 10 to 20 mg lipids per 10^9 leukocytes in human beings.[396],[397] More abundant in neutrophils than in lymphocytes, they are formed principally of protein-bound phospholipids but also include cholesterol, which exists mainly in a free state contrary to cholesterol in the plasma.[3]

Adult leukocytes are incapable of performing complete synthesis of fatty acids because of the lack of acetyl-CoA-carboxylase, indispensable for the initiating of this synthesis via formation of malonyl-CoA from acetyl-CoA.[398] The cells can utilize, however, fatty acids of the plasma for the biosynthesis of complex lipids.[399]

Changes in the dietary lipids influence the proportions of fatty acids in the lipids of neutrophils. In rats deprived of essential fatty acids, peritoneal neutrophils, mobilized after injection of glycogen, exhibit decreased contents of linoleic and arachidonic acids, whereas the levels of palmitoleic, oleic, and eicosatrienoic acids are increased.[400]

A diet rich in fats stimulates the active transfer of fatty acids from the plasma to the leukocytes, in which they are incorporated mainly into the membrane and the granules.[400]

2. Influence on the Number of Circulating Leukocytes

No anomalies have been reported after dietary lipid deprivation or overload. However, repeated daily intravenous infusions of fat emulsions given to schizophrenic patients for therapeutic purposes have reportedly provoked leukopenia as well as hypochromic anemia, the mechanism of which is as yet not well understood.[401]

B. Intervention of Certain Categories of Leukocytes in the Intestinal Absorption and Transportation of Dietary Lipids

1. Lymphocytes

About 60% of the lipids absorbed in the intestine are drained by the lymphatic vessels; indeed, hypertrophy of lymph nodes was reported a very long time ago in young cats submitted to a fat-rich diet.[402]

According to Shields,[75] lymphocytes of the intestinal mucosa, like those of other lymphoid tissues, secrete cytoplasmic fragments containing lipoproteins which are evacuated afterwards by the lymph. These lipoproteins are believed to be synthesized in the lymphocytes from amino acids and lipids incorporated after their absorption. However, short-chain fatty acids diffuse directly into the portal circulation[403] without first passing through the lymphocytes.

On the other hand, heparin secreted by mast cells of the intestinal mucosa exerts a stimulating action on the production and mobilization of lymphocytes which is antagonistic to that of cortisone.[404-406] This action results in increased entry into the thoracic duct of lymphocytes egressed from the mucosa and mediastinal lymph nodes.[406]

The PHA-induced blastogenic transformation of lymphocytes appears to depend on an equilibrium of the concentrations of unsaturated (UFA) and saturated fatty acids (FA) in the culture medium. Recent studies on human lymphocytes[670] have shown that the blastogenic effect of PHA in a culture medium containing fetal calf serum (FCS) was inhibited by the addition of either saturated or polyunsaturated fatty acids, while the simultaneous addition of both resulted in no inhibition. In contrast to this effect, with human AB serum in the culture medium, fatty acids neither stimulated nor inhibited PHA transformation.

This difference between FCS- and human serum-containing media may be due to the different fatty acid contents in the two media: FCS contains much more saturated fatty acids and much less linoleic acid than human serum and in addition human serum contains more albumin than FCS. The increased levels of this protein may prevent the inhibition of PHA stimulation of lymphocytes by an imbalanced fatty acid concentration in the medium since, according to the authors, a FA/albumin ratio of at least 2:1 is necessary to demonstrate an inhibitory effect of an imbalanced FA concentration.[670]

2. Basophils

Ingestion of a test meal rich in fat is followed by a transitory rise in both the serum lipid levels and in the number of blood basophils,[407,408] with frequent degranulation of these cells.[408,409] Heparin discharged on this occasion[410] activates a lipoprotein-lipase which releases fatty acids from chylomicrons, thus bringing an end to the postprandial hyperlipemia.[403]

Significant correlation between blood basophil and triglyceride levels was reported, whereas there was no connection with serum cholesterol.[411]

VII. LEUKOPOIESIS AND ALCOHOL

A. Animal Experimentation

High doses of ethyl alcohol injected into mice provoke a regression of the thymus, probably via a nonspecific stress effect.[412] On the contrary, no changes in blood leukocyte levels and in the weight of lymphoid organs were observed after 85 days of oral administration to rats of either 12% ethanol or 12% red wine as drinking fluid instead of tap water.[413] The absence of eosinopenia argued against a stressing effect of this diet.

B. Clinical Data

In almost half of the cases, chronic alcohol intoxication induces hypersegmentation of blood neutrophils, as well as macroovalocytosis of red cells. These anomalies are the consequence of a secondary folic acid deficiency, as shown by a decrease in the serum levels of this vitamin in an overwhelming proportion (90%) of alcoholics.[414] On the other hand, intravenous injection of endotoxin is followed in these subjects by a lesser discharge of neutrophils in the blood than in normal controls. In addition, polynucleosis can be replaced by temporary leukopenia in the course of acute infections.[415] The above peculiarities may be explained by the exhaustion of folate reserves after increased consumption of this vitamin in the inflammatory foci.

The finding that the phagocytic activity of leukocytes is not modified after contact with an ethanol solution in vitro[416] is in agreement with the hypothesis that the action of alcohol on neutrophils is only indirect, involving an impairment of folic acid metabolism.

Neutrophils and Macrophages (Recent Data)

The administration of excessively high quantities of ethanol to animals impairs the mobilization of granulocytes and macrophages, as well as leukocyte chemotaxis. No impairment is observed when serum ethanol concentrations are similar to those found in intoxicated humans. It has been found, however, that moderate concentrations of ethanol in humans which produce only mild intoxication reduce the mobilization of neutrophils into the skin and lower serum bactericidal activity against Gram-negative bacteria.[671]

Lymphocytes

Many patients suffering from alcoholic hepatitis exhibit a pronounced decrease in the levels of peripheral blood T lymphocytes[672] and a reduced responsiveness of T cells to PHA.[673,674] This suggests that cell-mediated immunity is impaired. In addition, sera of chronic alcoholics with hepatitis or cirrhosis, have been reported to contain a factor inhibiting PHA or pokeweed mitogen-induced lymphocyte transformation.[671,675-677] The appearance of this serum factor may be due to hepatic dysfunction, rather than to the alcoholic status per se.[671] Furthermore, the lymphocytes of alcohol-treated primates (baboons) were shown to be cytotoxic against autochthonous liver cells even before the appearance of hepatitis or cirrhosis.[678] A hypothesis has been advanced[675] according to which the antigenic stimulation of lymphocytes by a hyalin actin-like protein, accumulated in the liver during alcoholic intoxication, may lead to the secretion of a fibroblast-activating factor by these cells. This factor could be responsible for the conversion of alcoholic hepatitis to cirrhosis.

VIII. DEFICIENCIES OF VITAMINS

A. Vitamins of the B Complex

B vitamins are coenzyme precursors which activate apoenzymes in deficient animals or humans.[417] Since almost all of these enzymes are present in the leukocytes, it is easy to understand why production and activity of these cells is so often impaired in B-vitamin deficiencies. To some extent, the harmful effect of the latter also appears to be mediated by hypophysoadrenal hormonal disturbances.

1. Thiamine

According to early authors,[418,419] human beriberi is frequently accompanied by hyperlymphocytosis and hypertrophy of gastrointestinal lymphoid structures.[420] On the contrary, pigeons deprived of thiamine by a polished rice diet exhibit a drop in the blood lymphocyte levels and an involution of the lymphoid organs, especially of the thymus.[421] The histological alterations of the adrenals (disappearance of fat in the fascicular zone) suggest a stressing effect of the avitaminosis.

Paradoxically, no leukocytic anomalies were observed after protracted administration of a thiamine antagonist (oxythiamine).[422] Furthermore, thiamine-deficient rats do not display any reduction of their immunologic capacities.[423]

An excess of dietary thiamine is well tolerated in rats when they are largely provided with dietary protein. In the case of protein deprivation, however, such an excess amplifies the leukopenia[424] as well as the anemia and hypoalbuminemia of the animals,[425] and also provokes hemorrhagic necrosis of the liver.[426] All of these deleterious effects can be prevented by methionine.[424-426]

These effects may be due to the thiamine-excess-induced imbalance with other B vitamins, especially niacin.[427]

Thiamine pyrophosphate is the coenzyme of transketolase, involved in the hexose monophosphate shunt. The activity of this enzyme has been utilized as a sensitive index of thiamine nutrition. Changes in transketolase activity occurring in response to thiamine deficiency are amplified in leukocytes,[679] since these cells normally contain high levels of thiamine and high enzymatic activities.[679] In addition, a relatively close correlation has been found between the transketolase activities of leukocytes and liver cells.[680]

2. Riboflavin

Dietary lack of this vitamin does not provoke any changes in the leukocyte levels in rats, but those treated with antagonists develop neutrophilic polynucleosis without lymphopenia.[422,428]

On the other hand, malignant lymphoma tissue seems to require more riboflavin than normal tissue, since complete regression of grafted lymphosarcoma has been reported in mice deprived of dietary vitamin B_2 and treated at the same time with an antagonist (isoriboflavin, galactoflavin).[429]

3. Niacin

Despite the participation of this vitamin via the nicotinic enzymes in numerous biochemical processes, and the presence of these enzymes in the leukocytes, there are as yet no reliable data implicating a specific intervention of niacin in leukopoiesis.

Indeed, although leukopenia was reported in niacin deprivation in rabbits[430] and in the "black tongue" in dogs,[431] the protective effect of folic acid[432] suggests rather the responsibility of an associated folate deficiency in this anomaly.

In protein-deprived rats, an excess of dietary nicotinamide increases the blood levels of neutrophils.[424] This may be ascribed to a sparing effect with regard to tissular tryptophan and (or) to folic acid, the intestinal biosynthesis of which seems to be inhibited by protein deprivation (see Section VIII.A.6.a.ii, "Dietary Deprivation and Sulfonamide Leukopenia," below).

4. Pantothenic Acid

Mice deprived of this vitamin for 5 to 6 weeks exhibit blood lymphopenia and involution of the thymus and other lymphoid organs, but lymphopenia is no more apparent at a later stage of avitaminosis.[433] The two opposite effects may be linked successively to an initial stress-induced stimulation of the adrenals (as suggested by their relative hypertrophy) and to a secondary functional exhaustion of these glands. Such biphasic evolution was not observed in rats, perhaps because of the limited duration of the initial stress phase. Indeed, the animals exhibited only signs of adrenal insufficiency such as histochemical alterations of these glands[434] and an absence of lymphopenic and eosinopenic responses to ACTH, epinephrine, or nonspecific stress (swimming in cold water).[435,436]

Adrenal insufficiency in man was also observed following administration of an antagonist of pantothenic acid.[437] The deleterious effect of pantothenic acid deprivation on the adrenals may be attributed to the exhaustion of reserves of coenzyme A, which contains a pantothenate moiety. Its abundance in these glands suggests an intervention of pantothenic acid in the synthesis of corticoids.[436,438,439]

Paradoxically, an excess of pantothenic acid in the diet also inhibits the eosinopenic response in man after swimming.[439] It may be that under these conditions the oxidative reactions participating in the responses to cold stress were enhanced by the increased level of pantothenate in the tissues, thereby reducing the demand for adrenocortical hormones.[439]

The impairment of lymphopoiesis in pantothenic avitaminosis in rats is accompanied by immunologic disturbances. Indeed, a decreased production of antibodies to *Rickettsia*,[440] to heterologous red cells, and to diphtheria toxoid[441] has been reported. On the other hand, splenic lymphocytes from immunized pantothenic-acid-deficient rats are unable to synthesize antibodies in vitro after their passive transfer into normal rats.[442] Reduced formation of antibodies to some microbial antigens (especially tetanus) was also observed in human pantothenic avitaminosis.[443]

Surprisingly, both lymphopenia[444] and immunodepression[445] can be prevented by methionine in pantothenic-acid-deprived rats, although, as related previously (see Section

IV.A.3.g, "Immunologic Activity of Lymphocytes in Amino Acid Deficiency or Imbalance," earlier in this chapter), methionine, when given together with its antagonist, ethionine, aggravates rather than prevents the immunodepression induced by the latter.

5. Pyridoxine

Dietary deprivation of this vitamin is very deleterious to lymphopoiesis in laboratory animals (dogs,[446,447] primates,[448] rats,[446,449,450] and chickens[451]).

Administration of an antagonist, 4-desoxypyridoxine (DOP), induces lymphopenia, even with a nondeficient diet, in normal and leukemic mice[452] and rats.[422,453]

The thymus is always the first target of the lympholytic effect of this avitaminosis,[191,451,454] especially after administration of DOP.[191,454,455] In primates, involution of the spleen and lymph nodes, in addition to atrophy of the thymus,[455] can be observed only by adding an antagonist to a pyridoxine-deprived diet.

Vitamin-B_6-deprived rats exhibit a relative hypertrophy of the adrenals, especially when treated with an antagonist.[191] However, adrenalectomy does not prevent the lympholytic action of the avitaminosis.[456,457]

As in pantothenic acid deficiency, alterations of lymphopoiesis in laboratory animals coexist with a depression of immunologic responses: production of antibodies in rats (against SRBC or influenza virus),[458,459] mice (against *Brucella abortus*),[259] and guinea pigs (against diphtheria toxin),[460] and delayed skin hypersensitivity to tuberculin in guinea pigs inoculated with BCG.[461]

Tolerance of rats to skin homografts is also increased.[462-464] Furthermore, vitamin-B_6-deprived rats were found to have a reduced capacity to respond to foreign lymphoid cells in the mixed lymphocyte reaction, to permit normal lymphocyte transfer reactions, and to incorporate ^{3}H-uridine in vitro into their lymphocytes.[465]

Finally, administration of *dl*-penicillamine, a potent pyridoxine antagonist, to rats fed a diet low in this vitamin completely prevents the development of adjuvant polyarthritis assumed to be an allergic reaction.[466]

Surprisingly, no significant impairment of antibody synthesis has been reported as yet in vitamin-B_6-deficient humans,[467] but there are no recent data available on this subject.

Deprivation of pyridoxine, especially when completed by administration of an antagonist, inhibits the growth of experimental tumors of both lymphoid[453,468] and nonlymphoid origin (sarcoma *180*, Walker carcinoma *256*).[453,469-471] In man, only transitory remissions could be obtained in acute lymphoblastic leukemia after treatment with deoxypyridoxine.[472]

The biochemical mechanisms of the lymphopoietic action of pyridoxine have not yet been fully explained, as is also, to some extent, the case of pyridoxine-responsive anemias.

Among the metabolic activities of this vitamin possibly involved in lymphocytic turnover, one may also consider, in addition to its role in the transamination and conversion of tryptophan to nicotinamide, its probable intervention in the synthesis of C_1 fragments from serine, required for the formation of nucleic acids. This would explain why splenic lymphocytes of vitamin-B_6-deprived rats synthesize less DNA[473] and RNA (especially mRNA) as well as protein, and contain a lower amount of polysomes per unit weight of tissue than do normal rats.[464,474] These findings, however, do not explain why the inhibition does not also concern the production of other leukocytes.

Willis-Carr and St. Pierre[681] recently published new data on the inhibitory effect of vitamin B_6 deficiency on the cell-mediated immunologic activity of T lymphocytes and on their response to mitogens. It was shown that the impaired capacity of T lymphocytes to respond in the mixed lymphocyte reaction (MLR) and to the specific mitogens Con A and PHA, observed in vitamin B_6-deficient rats, resulted from a functional block of thymic epithelial cells. These cells became incapable of converting immature pre-thymic cells to functional T lymphocytes. It was also shown that if splenic, lymph node, and bone marrow lymphoid cells from vitamin B_6-deficient rats were exposed to epithelial cells from a normal thymus, responses underwent a significant increase.

6. Folic Acid
a. Animal Experimentation
i. Antagonists

Deprivation of folates produced by antagonists provokes leukopenia and involution of lymphoid organs (beginning with that of the thymus) in rats and mice[457-477] as well as in swine.[478]

ii. Dietary Deprivation and Sulfonamide Leukopenia

Simple dietary suppression of folates without antagonists is sufficient to induce leukopenia with anemia only in primates,[479] guinea pigs,[480] and chicks,[481] whereas in rats,[192] dogs,[482] and rabbits[483] the biosynthesis of this vitamin by the intestinal microflora to a large extent compensates for the dietary lack of folates. Accordingly, important leukopenia can be obtained in rats only if the biosynthesis is suppressed, either by utilizing germ-free animals[484] or by adding sulfonamides to the deficient diet.[183,485]

Sulfonamide-induced leukopenia is prevented not only by folic acid[485] but also by methionine, provided that the diet is poor in protein (4% casein) and itself lacks this amino acid.[202] On the other hand, the more the diet is deficient in protein, the more the sulfonamides are deleterious to the blood cells as well as to the organism as a whole,[486] which precisely may be linked to the methionine content in the diet.

The protective action of this amino acid could be explained either by the stimulation of the folic-acid-producing microflora or by its sparing effect with regard to this vitamin because of the metabolic relationship between the two factors.

iii. Folate Deficiency as a Consequence of Lack of Protein

A long-lasting protein-deprived diet is in itself sufficient for reducing the body stores of folates. That is the reason why administration of folic acid strongly enhances the weight increase and the recovery of leukopoiesis as well as of erythropoiesis in rats submitted to a protein-poor diet (7% casein) following protracted protein starvation.[216,487] Such an enhancing effect does not occur when the recovery diet contains 15% instead of 7% vitamin-free casein.[216,487]

iv. Immunologic Disturbances

The lymphocyte-stimulating action of folic acid suggests the intervention of this vitamin in immunologic reactions. Indeed, a drop in antibody production has already been observed in folate-deprived rats immunized to either *Rickettsia typhi*[488] or human red cells[489] and to diphtheria toxin,[490] as well as in chicks immunized to *Brucella abortus* or *Salmonella typhosa*.[491]

In some cases, however, folic avitaminosis may exert a stronger depressive effect on the proliferation of viruses or of malignant cells than on the defense reactions against these antigenic cells. This has been reported in mice inoculated with the virus of lymphocytic choriomeningitis or with transplantable lymphoid tumors.[492,493]

The previously reported immunodepressive effect of folic acid deprivation[489] was confirmed by Kuman and Axelrod[682] with the Jerne technique of splenic plaque forming cells (PFC) in folic acid-deprived SRBC-immunized rats. This effect was prevented by the administration of the vitamin shortly before immunization.[682] Similar results were obtained by the same authors with biotin-deficient rats.[682]

v. Intervention of Adrenal Hormones

As in the case of other B-vitamin deficiencies, some responsibility in the leukopenic effect of folic deprivation may be ascribed to an increased, or at least permissive, activity of lympholytic glucocorticoid hormones. Indeed, adrenalectomized mice treated with aminopterin do not exhibit lymphopenia nor lymphoid atrophy, although they do not present hyperlymphocytosis and thymic hypertrophy as do adrenalectomized animals not deprived of folic acid.[477]

b. Clinical Data

i. Leukopenias Accompanying Megaloblastic Anemias

Leukopenia with gigantism of medullary metamyelocytes due to the block of mitoses) and hypersegmentation of blood neutrophils is observed in all megaloblastic anemias, e.g., Addisonian anemia due to a deficiency of vitamin B_{12} provoked by the lack of intrinsic factor, and nutritional and pregnancy anemias induced by an inadequate supply of folates and (or) an increased demand by the fetus.[494,495]

Following voluntary deprivation of folates, hypersegmentation of neutrophils appeared after 7 weeks of such a diet, while excretion of FIGLU (formiminoglutamic acid) after histidine loading did not increase before 13 weeks; blockade of erythroblast maturation occurred only after a still longer interval of time.[496]

The intraleukocytic levels of folates (60 to 123 ng/ml in normal subjects, according to Hoffbrand and Newcombe[497]) are diminished in all megaloblastic anemias accompanied by gigantism of metamyelocytes.[496]

ii. Leukopenias Due to Folic Antagonists

The inhibitory effect of these antagonists (such as aminopterin or methopterin) on leukopoiesis, especially lymphopoiesis, has led to their utilization in the treatment of acute leukemias in children.[498]

iii. Folate Deprivation Resulting from Infection and Inflammatory Polynucleosis

Such a phenomenon was observed in tuberculosis[499] and rheumatoid arthritis.[500] It may be attributed to the high consumption of folates in the inflammatory foci, and to its elevated utilization in the increased metabolism of leukocytes.

iv. Immunologic Anomalies in Folic Acid Deficiency

Depression of delayed skin hypersensitivity to dinitrochlorobenzene (DNCB) and of the lymphocytic response to PHA, both thymus-dependent reactions, was observed in folate-deficient nonobstetric and obstetric patients with megaloblastic anemia and leukopenia (Table 28).[501]

It is highly probable that the resistance to viral, fungal, parasitic, and some bacterial infections, as well as the frequent depression of cell-mediated immunity, observed in protein-calorie malnutrition and kwashiorkor may result not only from a lack of protein but also from an associated folate deficiency. This is particularly the case when the malnutrition is accompanied by megaloblastic anemia, although the latter can be masked by concomitant lack of iron.[502]

c. Biochemical Mechanisms of the Intervention of Folic Acid in the Metabolism of Leukocytes

Among the numerous biochemical reactions requiring folic acid, at least two may be impaired in folate-deficiency leukopenia. The first one is represented by the participation of tetrahydrofolate derivatives in the synthesis of nucleic acids by introducing carbons 8 and 2 into the nucleus of purines, and, in the case of DNA synthesis, by initiating the conversion of deoxyuridylate to thymidylate.[503] Folic acid may also participate in DNA

Table 28

DINITROCHLOROBENZENE (DNCB) AND
PHYTOHEMAGGLUTININ (PHA) TEST RESULTS IN PATIENTS
WITH MEGALOBLASTIC ANEMIA DUE TO FOLIC ACID
DEFICIENCY, AND IN PATIENTS WITH
IRON DEFICIENCY ANEMIA

	Degree of DNCB skin test; number of patients			^{3}H-thymidine uptake (cpm) by lymphocytes before and after PHA stimulation	
Group[a]	O	+	++	Unstimulated[b]	Stimulated[c]
I	11	O	O	507 (219–1, 202)	8,798 ± 3,614
II	6	O	1	480 (176–1, 250)	6,802 ± 2,896
III	5	O	10	326 (130–501)	6,009 ± 3,278
IV	0	2	3	387 (162–672)	23,318 ± 5,474
V	1	4	8	373 (130–719)	26,340 ± 5,681

[a] Group I = nonobstetric, folate deficient; Group II = obstetric, folate deficient; Group III = iron and folate deficient; Group IV = iron deficient; Group V = normal.

[b] Uptake of ^{3}H-thymidine by lymphocytes in presence of saline in nonstimulated cultures.

[c] The cultures were stimulated with 0.1 ml of PHA and were harvested after 48 hr of incubation and 16 hr after addition of tritiated thymidine.

Adapted from Gross, R. L., Reid, J. V. O., Newberne, P. M., Burgess, B., Marston, R., and Hift, W., *Am. J. Clin. Nutr.*, 28, 225–232, 1975. With permission.

metabolism beyond the thymidine-synthetase level. Indeed, leukocytes treated with methotrexate, a folic antagonist, lose the capacity to undergo mitosis in response to PHA, whereas they remain able to synthesize DNA when stimulated by the same mitogen.[504]

The second disturbance, responsible for leukopenia, could be related to the intervention of N^5-methyltetrahydrofolate (N^5-Me THF) as methyl donor in the synthesis of methionine from homocysteine, this reaction requiring a protein-conjugated B_{12}-coenzyme (methylcobalamin). In the absence of this coenzyme, N^5-Me THF cannot be converted to tetrahydrofolate. This prevents the utilization of derivatives of the latter (formyl-, methenyl-, and methylene-tetrahydrofolates) in the folate-mediated synthesis of nucleic acids. In this case, however, the primary causal factor of leukopenia is the lack of cobalamin, not folates, this deficiency acting via the trapping of methyl-TH-folate.

Leukocytes contain enzymes involved in the formation of the above-mentioned folic acid derivatives, which intervene in nucleotide synthesis. N^5-Methyl-THF, the methyl donor in methionine formation, is also present in the leukocytes.[505]

A decrease in the intralymphocytic levels of $N^{5,10}$-methylene-THF was demonstrated in human primary (nutritional) and secondary (Addisonian anemia) folate deficiencies by testing the ^{14}C-formate incorporation into serine, the reaction being mediated by this folic derivative (see Section VIII.A.7.c, "Biochemical Background of the Action of Vitamin B_{12} on the Leukocytes," below).[506,508]

As could be anticipated, the need of leukocytes (granulocytes as well as lymphocytes) for folates parallels the intensity of nucleic acid synthesis. This is the reason why PHA-stimulated lymphocytes take up folates more avidly than do nonactivated resting cells.[509] On the other hand, the folic enzyme activities[505] as well as the folate contents[497,510] are higher in the immature cells of acute and chronic leukemias than in adult leukocytes.

6-Mercaptopurine, an antimitotic agent utilized in the treatment of myeloid leukemias, directly inhibits two folic enzymes: N^{10}-formyl-THA-synthetase and methylene-THF-dehydrogenase.[511]

7. Vitamin B_{12} (Cobalamin)
a. Animal Experimentation

It is almost impossible to provoke significant hematological, particularly leukocytic, changes in monogastric mammals deprived of cobalamin without associated folate deficiency. Thus, in pigs, marked neutropenia was observed only after combined deprivation of both vitamins, but this anomaly responded to folic acid alone, not to vitamin B_{12}.[512] Similar observations were reported in guinea pigs.[482] Deprivation of cobalamin alone was also devoid of any hematological effect in germ-free rats.[513] Only rats born from B_{12}-deprived mothers exhibited a moderate anemia and leukopenia (mainly neutropenia) with a rapid rise of leukocytic levels after administration of vitamin B_{12}.[514,515]

In ruminants, vitamin B_{12} deficiency with severe and lethal anemia and aplasia of the bone marrow develops if the animals are subjected to a cobalt-deficient diet (see Section IX.D, "Cobalt," later in this chapter).[482,516]

In the absence of direct examples of experimental leukopenia induced by lack of cobalamin in monogastric mammals, it may be interesting to mention some indirect arguments in favor of the lymphopoietic potential of this vitamin.

A protective effect of vitamin B_{12} with regard to the thymus was observed in rats exhibiting a thymic regression either of dietary origin (prolonged protein and vitamin B_{12} deprivation followed by an incomplete recovery diet containing 7% casein)[517] or provoked by administration of a thyroid extract[518] or cortisone.[519] In the first case, exogenous cobalamin apparently accelerated the restoration of the thymus by increasing the stores of the vitamin exhausted by protein deprivation and by the subsequent block of its intestinal synthesis. Furthermore, the renewal of the B_{12}-controlled methionine synthesis compensated for the deficiency of this amino acid supplied in suboptimal amounts in the 7% protein diet.[517]

In the other two cases, the exogenous vitamin was useful because of the high consumption of this factor in experimental hyperthyroidism or because of its increased excretion due to hypercorticalism.[520]

Despite the role played by vitamin B_{12} in the synthesis of nucleic acids, its intervention in immunologic responses has not yet been demonstrated either in animals or in man.[521]

b. Clinical Data
i. Vitamin Content in Blood Leukocytes; Transcobalamins

The intracellular levels are very high (480 ng/ml),[522] which is due to the capture of the vitamin by these cells, mainly neutrophils.

Indeed, leukocytes produce a B_{12}-binding protein, transcobalamin I (TC 1), similar to the serum TC I, itself of granulocyte origin.[523,524] Two other TC (II and III) exist both in the plasma and neutrophils;[525,526] like TC I, TC III is produced exclusively by granulocytes,[527] while TC II is synthesized probably not only in leukocytes[526,528] but also in the liver.[529] The secretion of large amounts of TC I by immature and adult granulocytes[523,530] explains the high serum levels of cobalamin found in patients with myeloid leukemia.[531,532]

ii. Vitamin B_{12} and Leukopoiesis

Leukopenia, which accompanies Addisonian pernicious anemia, concerns mainly the neutrophils, and, like leukopenia of primary folic deficiency, is characterized by a gigantism of metamyelocytes and nuclear hypersegmentation of adult neutrophils. The latter anomaly represents the leukocytic counterpart of the nuclear fragmentation (karyorrexis) observed in acidophilic megaloblasts.[533] These anomalies rapidly disappear after administration of folic acid as well as of vitamin B_{12}, and are apparently due to an inadequate utilization of folic acid because of the lack of vitamin B_{12} (see below).

It may be mentioned that there is not only decreased production but also increased destruction of neutrophils in pernicious anemia, as shown by the high serum levels of muramidase (lysozyme),[534] a lysosomic enzyme released during the lysis of granulocytes.[535] Quantitative cytochemical and autoradiographic investigations showed that a high proportion of giant metamyelocytes are in the G2 phase of the cell cycle, which probably indicates a slower rate of DNA synthesis and premitotic arrest.[250] These findings are similar to the results concerning the lymphocytes of protein-deprived rats.[142] The giant metamyelocytes may be effete cells dying within the bone marrow by phagocytosis or autolysis.[250] The circulating hypersegmented neutrophils have diploid DNA contents, and, consequently, are not produced by maturation of giant metamyelocytes without cell division.[250]

Patients with Addisonian pernicious anemia also exhibit reduced lymphocyte response to PHA in vitro. On the other hand, vitamin B_{12} as well as folic acid are able to reactivate this response in folate-deficient patients.[501] It is very probable that the inadequate DNA synthesis in vitamin B_{12} deficiency is due to a secondary blockade in folate metabolism.

c. Biochemical Background of the Action of Vitamin B_{12} on the Leukocytes

In mammals, the intervention of this vitamin has been demonstrated definitively in two enzymatic reactions: methylation of homocysteine to methionine (via the protein-bound methyl-B_{12}-coenzyme) and isomerization of L-methylmalonyl coenzyme A (CoA) to succinyl CoA (via the deoxyadenosyl-B_{12} coenzyme [dAB_{12}]).[536,537]

Methionine is incorporated into protein, while methylmalonyl CoA and its immediate precursor, propionyl CoA, are important intermediates in the catabolism of several amino acids and fatty acids. Both reactions are depressed in vitamin-B_{12}-deficient humans, as evidenced by increased excretion of homocystine, methylmalonate, and propionate in the urine.[537]

Impaired methylmalonyl CoA-mutase activity has also been demonstrated in vitro in leukocytes of B_{12}-deficient patients.[508,538] An increase in enzyme activity was noticed after the addition of dAB_{12}, required as cofactor.[538] However, in patients, no correlation was apparent between the leukocytic enzyme levels on the one hand and the excretion of urinary methylmalonate and hematological alterations on the other. Therefore, it seems that this enzyme is not directly concerned with the hematopoietic function.

In addition, leukocytes of vitamin-B_{12}-deficient miniature pigs display a markedly reduced capacity to oxidize $3\text{-}^{14}C$ propionate to $^{14}CO_2$, even before the appearance of megaloblastic anemia and methylmalonicaciduria. Prolonged incubation of the leukocytes in vitro with dAB_{12}, cyanocobalamin, or hydroxocobalamin partly corrects this metabolic block.[537]

The blockade of homocysteine transmethylation in the absence of cobalamin prevents the synthesis of methionine, and consequently provokes the trapping of N^5-methyl-THF. This leads to reduced concentrations of methionine[539,540] and increased levels of N^5-methyl-THF[541] in the serum of patients with Addisonian anemia. The trapping of methylfolate in turn provokes the arrest of the synthesis of folate derivatives indispensable for the synthesis of RNA ($N^{5,10}$-methenyl- and N^{10}-formyl-THF) and for the methylation of deoxyuridylate to thymidylate ($N^{5,10}$-methylene-THF). The latter folic compound also intervenes in the incorporation of formate into serine, explaining

Table 29

LEUKOCYTE METABOLISM OF PROPIONATE, SUCCINATE, AND SERINE IN VITAMIN-B_{12}- OR FOLIC-ACID-DEFICIENT PATIENTS

Patients	Propionate oxidation[a] (n mole $^{14}CO_2$/3 hr/10^8 leukocytes)		Succinate oxidation (n mole $^{14}CO_2$/3 hr/10^8 leukocytes)		Serine formation from formate[b] (n mole ^{14}C-serine/ 4 hr/10^9 leukocytes)	
	Mean ± SD	Range	Mean ± SD	Range	Mean ± SD	Range
Addisonian megaloblastic anemia	2.8 ± 2.3[d] (19)[c]	0.2—6.8	28.6 ± 13.5 (9)	12.6—60.8	—	—
Addisonian deficiency without anemia	4.3 ± 2.4[d] (12)	1.1—7.9	63.1 ± 31.7 (6)	28.2—105	4.7 ± 1.6[d] (10)	3.3—7.6
Folate deficiency with low B_{12}	5.0 ± 1.3[e] (6)	3.4—5.7	30.0 ± 14.3 (3)	16.2—44.9	5.9 ± 2.2[d] (6)	2.4—9.4
Control subjects	14.4 ± 7.3 (19)	7.6—32.8	29.5 ± 13.1 (19)	14.0—58.0	10.1 ± 3.3 (34)	6.2—12.8

[a] The in vitro leukocyte oxidation of propionate was measured as an index of the activity of deoxyadenosylcobalamin, a coenzyme for methylmalonyl CoA-mutase in the pathway of propionate conversion to succinate. Lack of this enzyme would retard oxidation of propionate but not of succinate.

[b] Serine biosynthesis was measured as an index of methylcobalamin function. Cobalamin deficiency impairs methyltransferase, and thus blocks tetrahydrofolate regeneration from methylfolate and subsequently ^{14}C-formate conversion to ^{14}C-serine via folate intermediates.

[c] Number of determinations.

[d,e] Statistically different from control values at the levels of $P < 0.001$ and < 0.01, respectively.

From Robertson, J. S., Hsia, Y. E., and Scully, K. J., *J. Lab. Clin. Med.*, 87, 89–97, 1976. With permission.

Table 30

ASCORBIC ACID LEVELS IN THE BLOOD PLASMA (PAA) AND IN LEUKOCYTES (LAA) OF ELDERLY SUBJECTS (OVER 75 YEARS)

Effect of Smoking and Fruit Consumption

	Fruit score 0—3			Fruit score 4—7		
	Male smokers	Male nonsmokers	Women	Male smokers	Male nonsmokers	Women
Number	40	39	154	9	21	102
Mean PAA (mg/100 ml)	0.16	0.20	0.24	0.27	0.37	0.45
Mean LAA (μg/10^8 cells)	14.1	14.8	19.8	20.00	20.8	23.1

From Burr, M. L., Elwood, P. C., Hole, D. J., Hurley, R. J., and Hughes, R. C., *Am. J. Clin. Nutr.*, 27, 147–151, 1974. With permission.

why this reaction is impaired in lymphocytes from patients with Addisonian anemia as well as in those of folic-acid-deficient subjects (Table 29).[507,508]

B. Ascorbic Acid

No changes in blood leukocyte levels have been reported in scorbutic guinea pigs.[542] However, the hyperleukocytosis induced by peritoneal irritation is much lower in these animals than in nondeficient controls,[543,544] and the phagocytic activity of the peritoneal exudate is also deeply affected.[544]

In man, phagocytosis of *Micrococcus candidus* by neutrophils decreases in the same measure as does the ascorbic acid intake.[545] On the other hand, in man, this vitamin strongly activates intraleukocytic glucose oxidation via the hexose-monophosphate shunt, which in the neutrophils represents an important biochemical parameter of phagocytosis.[546]

All these data may explain the high levels of ascorbic acid in leukocytes (granulocytes as well as lymphocytes).[547] These levels exceed by far those found in erythrocytes and in the plasma.[548]

According to Lloyd and Sinclair,[549] the concentrations of the vitamin in a healthy man and woman range between 15 and 32 mg/100 g of leukocytes, as opposed to 0.30 to 1.60 mg/100 ml of serum or red cells. Brook and Grimshaw[550] found 24.6 ± 1.3 $\mu g/10^8$ leukocytes in males and 30.7 ± 1.4 μg in females. Indeed, the levels are lower in leukocytes of men than in those of women, as they are lower in cigarette smokers than in nonsmokers,[550,551] and lower in elderly people than in young persons (Table 30).[552]

Dietary factors seem to play a predominant role in the age differences since in elderly subjects significant correlation was found between the leukocyte and plasma ascorbic acid levels on the one hand and the intake of green vegetables and, especially, fresh fruit on the other (Table 30).[552]

During dietary deprivation of vitamin C, the levels of the latter remain normal for a much longer time in leukocytes (103 days) than in the plasma (41 days), but it is only after 134 days that follicular hyperkeratosis, considered to be the first clinical symptom of human scurvy, appears.[553]

The concentration of ascorbic acid in leukocytes seems to be correlated with the ratio of dehydroascorbic acid/reduced ascorbic acid in the plasma.[549]

A direct relationship between the phagocytic activity of peritoneal neutrophils and the ascorbic acid content of these cells has been found in the guinea pig.[544]

One may also mention the existence of metabolic interactions between ascorbic acid and folic acid, since the former intervenes as hydrogen donor in the conversion of pteroyl-glutamic acid to THFA;[554] hence, impairment of this conversion in human scurvy[555] may in turn contribute to depress the functional activities of leukocytes.

The intervention of ascorbic acid in antibody production is still a matter of dispute. Indeed, reduced production of diphtheria antitoxin was reported in scorbutic guinea pigs by some authors,[556,557] but it was not confirmed by others.[521] Deprivation of vitamin C has also been claimed to decrease resistance to infection,[558] but this could also be a consequence of impaired phagocytosis.

Several contradictory data have recently been published concerning the participation of this vitamin in the metabolic events controlling the phagocytic and microbicidal activities of neutrophils.

Incubation of normal human neutrophils with ascorbic acid resulted in increased chemotaxis,[683,684] but this effect was not found in neutrophils isolated from patients with Felty's syndrome or with splenic lupus erythematosus. Both diseases are characterized by leukopenia and the frequent association of infections.[685] It was suggested that ascorbic acid may promote the oxidative denaturation of bacterial constituents thus potentiating bacterial killing.[686]

Ascorbic acid is also assumed to preserve cell integrity by inactivating free radicals and oxidants which are produced during phagocytosis. Nonetheless, only very high ascorbic acid doses (2 g/day) given to healthy adult male volunteers for 2 weeks could reduce intracellular killing of bacteria in leukocytes, while doses of 200 mg/day were ineffective.[688] This effect of massive doses may be due to the inhibition of NADPH-oxidase by dehydroascorbic acid. It has also been reported that during phagocytosis, leukocytes of vitamin C-deficient guinea pigs exhibited a reduced secretion of lysosomal acid phosphatase, which plays an important role in the intracellular digestion of phagocytosed bacteria.[637,688]

Some of the above results are in disagreement with negative experimental observations of McCall et al.,[689] recently confirmed by Stankova et al.,[690] who found no effect of ascorbic acid deficiency on the production of hydrogen peroxide and the killing of *Staphylococcus aureus*.

Ascorbic acid also affects intraleukocyte levels of cyclic nucleotides. Activation of phagocytosis by the vitamin[545,546] has been shown to coincide with an increase of cyclic AMP levels in normal leukocytes.[683–685] However, the levels of leukocyte cAMP have also been found to be greatly elevated in a patient with the Chediak-Higashi syndrome, characterized by an increased susceptibility to pyrogenic infection and the existence of anomalous lysosome-like giant granules in these white cells.[691] Boxer et al. suggest that high cAMP concentrations could inhibit the assembly of microtubules and thus impair bactericidal activity. The leukocyte cAMP levels in this patient were reduced after incubating cells with ascorbic acid and vitamin therapy led to a significant increase of the chemotactic and bactericidal activities of the patient's leukocytes.[691]

Among the other participations of ascorbic acid in white blood cell functional activity, we may mention the enhanced T lymphocyte blastogenesis in the lymphocytes of humans,[692] monkeys,[693] and mice[694] after the oral administration of the vitamin. On the other hand, decreased delayed hypersensitivity to tuberculin has been observed in scorbutic guinea pigs.[695,696] Ascorbic acid thus participates in T cell-controlled humoral as well as in cell-mediated immunity, although the major hematological role of this vitamin seems to be the enhancement of chemotaxis and of hexose monophosphate shunt activity in PMN.[697]

C. Fat-soluble Vitamins

The bacteriocytic activity in the rat and mouse has been found to decrease after inoculation of *Salmonella* if the animals were deficient in vitamin A.[559,560] On the other hand, recent data suggest the intervention of this vitamin as an immune adjuvant,[561-564] enhancing humoral and cell-mediated immunity in mice through the activation of T lymphocytes.

Deprivation of vitamin E in primates induces not only hemolytic anemia but also hyperneutrophilia.[565] No leukocytic anomalies have as yet been reported in human avitaminosis E.[566]

It is of interest to mention that the plasma levels of vitamins A and E are depressed in kwashiorkor and PCM.[567,568] This may be due to the fall of the concentration of their respective carrier proteins; these are all lipoproteins of the plasma for vitamin E, and the retinol-binding protein for vitamin A.[417] In addition, vitamin A deficiency alone results in a lowering of serum albumin levels in the rat.[569] Therefore, a possible contribution of lack of vitamin A to the leukocytic and immunologic disturbances induced by protein malnutrition cannot be excluded.

Vitamin A has been reported to enhance the humoral and cell-mediated immunities of mice via the activation of T lymphocytes.[561-564] It is interesting to note that the vitamin A derivative retinoic acid (RA) has recently been found to stimulate the induction of cell-mediated cytotoxicity to allogenic tumor cells in mice when administered at low doses both in vivo and in vitro. RA does not, however, stimulate lymphocyte proliferation in response to Con A and PHA or in mixed lymphocyte culture and does not affect the delayed hypersensitivity reaction of the humoral response to erythrocytes.[698] It thus appears that RA is a specific adjuvant for the induction of cytotoxic T cells (T killer cells), responsible for the anti-tumor activity of RA.[698]

IX. MINERAL NUTRIENTS

A. Iron

1. Iron Deficiency

In man, iron-deficiency anemia may be accompanied by leukopenia[5] with hyper-segmentation of neutrophils[570] and appearance of giant metamyelocytes in the bone marrow.[571] These abnormalities have been ascribed to concomitant folate deficiency, as suggested by frequently reduced folate levels in the serum of iron-deprived patients and rats,[571,572] as well as by increased excretion of FIGLU after histidine loading in man[570] and rats.[573] The folic deficiency may be due not simply to an inadequate intake of the vitamin but to a disturbance of folic acid metabolism provoked by inactivation of some iron-containing or iron-dependent enzymes. Indeed, the hematological as well as biochemical symptoms of folate deprivation reported in iron deficiency can be cured by iron alone.[570]

Thus, the block of the conversion of histidine to glutamic acid, responsible for the urinary excretion of FIGLU, must be ascribed to the lack of formiminotransferase, which is activated by iron.[573] Incidently, hypersegmentation of neutrophils has been observed in inborn defects of this enzyme.[574]

On the other hand, the depressed activity of certain leukocytic enzymes involved in the oxidative reactions and the intracellular killing of bacteria (cytochromeoxidase[575] and myeloperoxidase[576,577]), as reported in iron deficiency, may be attributed to the presence of iron in these enzymes. Also, neutrophils of the guinea pig and man contain an iron-binding protein similar to the lactoferrin of milk.[578] This protein is endowed with bactericidal activity,[20,579] probably because it sequesters iron, preventing bacteria from utilizing this metal for their growth. Accordingly, microbial proliferation may be enhanced in case of lactoferrin deficiency.

Ferritin, an iron-containing protein, is also in the leukocytes. Among these cells, the circulating macrophages (monocytes) contain much higher levels (seven to eight times) of this protein than do granulocytes and lymphocytes.[580] This is related to the large amount of iron released in the macrophages following phagocytosis of senescent erythrocytes, as well as to the abundance of iron-containing enzymes in these cells, involved in the biochemical processes of bactericidal activity.

For all these reasons, the iron-deficiency-induced morphological anomalies of leukocytes are frequently accompanied by functional inactivation of these cells. Thus, the bactericidal capacity of neutrophils[336,346] and also significant impairment of the nitroblue tetrazolium test have been reported in human iron deficiency, although phagocytosis and opsonic activity were found to be normal.[346]

As to the immunologic responses of lymphocytes, according to the tests used, cell-mediated immunity is either depressed (lymphocyte responses to purified protein derivative [PPD] and to *Candida* antigen)[581] or not impaired (hypersensitivity to DNCB).[501] Responses to PHA were also found to be normal in children and young adults with severe iron-deficiency anemia.[501,582]

Several recent publications support the idea that iron deficiency leads to decreased immune responses. High mortality rates, already reported in iron-deprived rats after infection with *Salmonella typhimurium*,[571,699] were also reported in rats infected with *Streptococcus pneumoniae*, where susceptibility to the microorganism was considerably higher than in non-deprived rats.[700]

As shown in a recent critical review,[701] data concerning humans are much more difficult to interpret because of the variability and the frequent ignorance of the exact nutritional status of the patients and the possible incidence of associated occult infections or parasitic infestations. Cell-mediated immunity was nevertheless found to be defective in humans with iron deficiency.[581,582,701-705]

The responses of lymphocytes to mitogens and antigens were reduced,[702-704] as was the number of blood T cells determined by the standard assay with unsensitized SRBC.[702-705] In addition, the macrophage migration inhibitory factor, the only lymphokine studied, decreased in iron-deficient patients and became normal after repletion.[703]

In contrast to cell-mediated immunity, humoral immunologic reactions in iron-deficient humans were always found to be normal: neither serum titers of IgG, IgA, and IgM nor those of IgA in saliva were found to be decreased.[704,705]

2. Iron Overload

Excess administration of iron may be at least as harmful to the antimicrobial defense reactions of the leukocytes as is iron deprivation, when this excess is given by oral or, especially, parenteral route to malnourished persons such as children and adults with kwashiorkor. Indeed, such subjects present a reduced iron-binding capacity of serum transferrin due to the low levels of this protein, thereby facilitating microbial proliferation. This may bear some responsibility in the high incidence of systemic infections in malnourished infants treated with injections of iron dextran.[583]

Similar conditions are realized endemically in some geographical areas (e.g., in the Bantus of South Africa) where protein malnutrition frequently coexists with both alcoholic cirrhosis and dietary excess of iron.[584] In addition, since transferrin is at least partly synthesized by lymphocytes,[585] the dietary decrease of this synthesis may contribute to depress the immunologic activity of these cells.

B. Copper

Relatively little is known about the effects of copper deficiency on leukocytes, except for the frequency of neutropenia in copper-deprived pigs[586] as well as in marasmic infants nourished with modified cow's milk, adequate with respect to intake of vitamins and iron but poor in copper.[587] Even in cases with severe neutropenia, however, normal neutrophilic responses to infection have been observed.[587] The biochemical background of this hematological anomaly is as yet unknown, but one may point out that copper participates in the activity of some leukocytic enzymes, especially cytochromeoxidase, which contains identical proportions of iron and copper, the latter changing its valence according to the oxidized or reduced state of the enzyme.[384]

C. Zinc

There are 880 μg of zinc per 100 ml of blood, 75% being present in adult erythrocytes and only 3% in leukocytes.[588] The concentration of zinc, however, is 25 times higher in the latter cells (about 0.01 μg/10^6 leukocytes) in man[589] than in the former.[516] The highest levels are found in blood eosinophils and basophils,[589] and, in particular, in tissular basophils (mast cells), which contain 40 times more zinc than the blood leukocytes.[590] Plasma cells are completely devoid of this mineral.[591]

About 80% of the total granulocytic zinc is probably incorporated in an enzymatic zinc-protein complex, and only some 10% exists in alkaline phosphatase, one of the leukocytic zinc-containing enzymes.[591] Nevertheless, decreased activity of this enzyme was reported in leukocytes of zinc-deficient humans and rabbits.[592]

In light of all these data, adequate intake of zinc should be indispensable for normal activity of leukocytes. Therefore, one cannot exclude some relationship between these findings on one hand and blood lymphopenia and atrophy of the spleen[593,594] exhibited by zinc-deprived animals (rats, piglets) on the other. Nevertheless, a corticoid-mediated stress effect is much more likely because of the adrenal hypertrophy observed in deficient pigs.[594] In addition, leukocytes of zinc-deficient rats do not contain lesser amounts of this metal than normal rats.[595]

However, participation of zinc at some stage of leukopoiesis remains certain. Indeed, this metal intervenes in the synthesis of nucleic acids[596,597] as well as in that of proteins,[598] and its essentiality for the PHA-induced transformation of human blood lymphocytes has also been affirmed.[599]

Interesting data have recently been published concerning the participation of zinc in the functional activity of neutrophils and lymphocytes. Chvapil et al.[706] studied the effects of zinc on oxygen consumption, ingestion of yeast particles, and killing of *Escherichia coli* by canine blood neutrophils in vitro. It was found that low quantities of zinc stimulated the functioning of neutrophils, but that higher quantities were associated with a reduced oxidizing metabolism of phagocytosing neutrophils and decreased bactericidal activity. This inhibitory effect was observed only in the presence of magnesium. These results obtained in vitro are consistent with earlier observations showing a decrease of serum zinc levels in patients suffering from extensive burns, in whom phagocytosis was very active,[707] or in those with various infectious processes.[708] The latter authors (Wannemacher et al.) suggested the existence of an endogenous leukocytic mediator-like factor which would induce a depression of the levels of zinc and of other nutrients during infection. Metcoff[709] demonstrated an inverse correlation between zinc levels and the activities of several leukocyte enzymes (pyruvate kinase, adenylate kinase, glucose-6-phosphate dehydrogenase), adenine nucleotide levels and protein synthesis by leukocytes derived from mother blood and cord blood of their offspring.

In spite of the particularly high zinc concentration in bone marrow basophils and tissue mast cells,[590] it was found that adult rats on a zinc-deprived diet (1 ppm vs. 50 ppm in control diets) exhibited a significant increase in the basophil content of both bone marrow and other tissue basophils (mast cells).[710] According to the author, this paradoxical phenomenon may indicate an increased turnover rate of these cells, caused by the depletion of zinc reserves in the tissues.

Zinc also undoubtedly intervenes in the metabolism of lymphocytes and their thymus-dependent immunologic activity.[711] Zinc deficiency has indeed been shown to impair PHA-induced DNA synthesis in lymphocytes[711] and also depresses the production of anti-SRBC antibodies by mice.[712] Thus, in mice maintained on a zinc-deprived diet for 9 weeks prior to immunization with SRBC, the number of spleen PFC was only 10% that of control mice.[712] The titers of serum immunoglobulins IgM and IgG also decreased, even when results were compared to those of restricted pair-fed animals, and not only to the reactions of controls fed ad libitum.[713] Reconstitution of deficient mice with thymocytes prior to immunization restored immunocyte production to a large extent. Zinc deprivation did not, however, affect B cell-specific responses to a hapten-carrier antigen.[712] Cell-mediated immunity function has also been found to be impaired by a dietary zinc deficiency in mice,[714] which confirms the specific zinc dependence of thymus-controlled immunologic reactions.

D. Cobalt

Being a specific constituent of vitamin B_{12}, cobalt is naturally indispensable for leukopoiesis as well as for erythropoiesis. However, in monogastric mammals, the amounts of cobalt necessary for metabolic functions are very low. Indeed, 0.04 μg of cobalt permits the synthesis of 1 μg of vitamin B_{12}, generally considered to be an amount almost sufficient to fulfill the daily requirement of man.[516]

It is only in ruminants (sheep and cattle) that lack of cobalt induces profound pathological changes, including severe anemia, because of a particularly high need for vitamin B_{12} in these animals. Indeed, this vitamin is necessary for the tissular oxidation of organic acids (propionic, acetic, and butyric) formed by the fermentative breakdown of cellulose in the rumen. This oxidation constitutes the main source of metabolic energy in ruminants.[600]

Among the major symptoms of cobalt deficiency in these animals is anemia with aplasia of the bone marrow, demonstrating the involvement of this mineral in overall hematopoiesis.

In normal monogastric mammals, administration of large amounts of cobalt induces polycythemia[516,600] without hyperleukocytosis. This may be due to the fact that the anomaly is apparently caused to a major extent by overproduction of erythropoietin devoid of leukopoietic potential.[601]

Surprisingly, cobalt was reported to increase the resistance of mice to pneumococcal and staphylococcal infections, if this resistance was depressed after excessive administration of manganese.[602] No recent data are available regarding a possible immunologic effect of cobalt.

E. Sodium and Potassium

Deprivation as well as overload of these nutrients disturbs the leukocytic equilibrium.

1. Dietary Deprivation

Protracted lack of sodium has been reported to induce blood eosinopenia in women.[603]

Deprivation of potassium in young rats provokes an arrest of growth and severe visceral lesions, including involution of the lymphoid follicles of the spleen and digestive tract.[604] Thymus and lymph nodes were not examined in this study.

The importance of tissular alteration due to the lack of potassium may be related to the intervention of this electrolyte in the synthesis of protein, as has been demonstrated in microorganisms.[605] On the other hand, secondary lack of potassium is a usual consequence of prolonged protein deprivation because of its release from the catabolized tissues. This is why the addition of potassium to a recovery diet administered to protein-deprived rats considerably enhances the weight restoration of these animals.[606] The enhancing effect of excess potassium is particularly striking if the protein-deprived rats are restored with a diet containing only 7% casein and, in addition, are treated with small doses (1 mg/day) of ACTH. Then potassium not only prevents any mortality in the treated rats but also amplifies the restoration of blood leukocyte levels.[236,322]

2. Overload

a. Parenteral Administration

Slow intravenous infusion of a hypertonic solution of NaCl provokes an important hyperneutrophilia in dogs.[607] A transitory rise in neutrophil levels was observed even after injection of physiological saline in man[608] as well as in the rabbit.[609] This reaction seems to be due to a splenic discharge provoked by the stress of the injection, since it is suppressed by splenectomy.[607]

Concerning eosinophils, intraperitoneal injection of physiological saline is sufficient for inducing in the rat a 30% drop in the blood levels of these cells after 4 hr. This stress effect is prevented by adrenalectomy.[610] On the other hand, eosinopenia provoked by injection of hypertonic NaCl solution (0.05 g/0.5 ml) is as important (40 to 50%) in adrenalectomized as in intact rats.[610]

Intraperitoneal hypertonic KCl solution (0.05 g/0.5 ml) induces eosinopenia only in intact rats, not in adrenalectomized animals given physiological saline as drinking fluid. Death occurs frequently in the latter animals, however, apparently because of the lack of protection exerted by cortical hormones against the potassium excess.[610] Therefore, it may be that potassium released from tissues injured by stressing agents[611] plays a role in stress eosinopenia by enhancing the stimulation of the hypophysoadrenocortical axis.

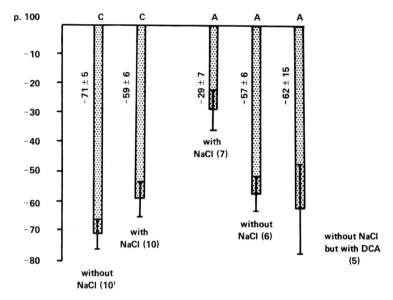

FIGURE 10. Reduction of the eosinopenic response (percentage changes ± SE) to cortisone (1 mg) by administration of physiological saline as drinking water to adrenalectomized (A) rats, as compared to the effect in intact control (C) rats. The preparation of adrenalectomized rats by subcutaneous injections of deoxy-corticosterone (DCA: 1 mg/day for 5 days) is devoid of the protective effect of NaCl. Numbers of rats are in parentheses. (From Aschkenasy, A., *Ann. N.Y. Acad. Sci., 77*, 574–588, 1959. With permission.)

b. Oral Administration

Replacement of drinking water by a 1% NaCl solution increases both the regression of the thymus and eosinopenia in protein-deprived rats.[231],[612] This phenomenon may be ascribed to the stimulation of the adrenals, since hypertrophy of these glands has been reported after overload with salt.[613],[614] However, this effect of physiological saline was observed only in male rats, not in females.[612]

On the other hand, in adrenalectomized normally nourished rats, the drop in blood eosinophil levels 4 hr after intraperitoneal injection of cortisone (1 mg) was found to be much smaller (−29 ± 7%) if the animals received 1% saline as drinking fluid than if they were given tap water (−71 ± 5%) (Figure 10).[610] The protective effect of NaCl against the eosinopenic effect of cortisone was not observed in intact rats, probably because the latter animals were capable of controlling blood electrolyte levels by adjusting the functional activity of their adrenals. Surprisingly, deoxycorticosterone acetate injected in adrenalectomized rats did not manifest the same effect as ingestion of saline water.[610]

F. Magnesium
1. Role Played in Phagocytosis

Depletion of bivalent cations (Ca^{++} and Mg^{++}) by resins or EDTA prevents the neutrophils from phagocytosing bacteria as well as from aggregating and adhering to glass. Magnesium per se is able to restore these capacities,[615],[616] but addition of calcium may be needed for optimal adherence.[615]

Magnesium and zinc are important for the maintenance of leukocyte alkaline phosphatase activity.[592],[617] In actual fact, this enzyme is heterogeneic, being formed of two metallo-isoenzymes, one containing zinc and the other magnesium.[618] Therefore, the intervention of magnesium in phagocytosis may be related to its participation in the activity of this enzyme.

2. Dietary Deprivation

Lack of magnesium provokes important leukocytic alterations in the rat, mainly concerning the granulocytic cell lines; after no more than 10 days of deprivation, there is a striking increase in the number of eosinophils.[619,620] This increase coincides with hyperemic and pruriginous reactions, and with the rise of plasma and urinary histamine levels.[621] Eosinophilia decreases at a later stage, although remaining above normal. In the same animals, degranulation of mast cells occurs in the peritoneal cavity and other tissues.[622] A decrease in the number of these cells and release of histamine from the basophilic granules are also observed.[623]

After 6 to 12 months of a magnesium lack, rats exhibit important blood neutrophilia with myeloid hyperplasia of the bone marrow.[624,625] The lymphocytes are also concerned since lymphosarcomatous tumors[622,626] and malignant thymoma with leukemoid metastases[625] have been reported in rats subjected to a protracted magnesium deficiency. These experimental data are at variance with the observations reporting increases in plasma and erythrocyte magnesium levels in chronic lymphoid leukemia and lymphosarcoma.[627]

In magnesium-deprived rats, histological examination has discovered perivascular lesions of an allergic type disseminated in various tissues: necrosis with accumulation of neutrophils, eosinophils, and, at a later stage, of macrophages.[628]

One may mention in relation to these findings that asthmatic patients display reduced plasma levels of magnesium[629] as well as increased levels of eosinophils in the blood and the bronchi.

G. Calcium

Phagocytosis, as well as the mobility of leukocytes, is activated in vitro by calcium,[630] while its deletion exerts an inhibitory effect.[615] For some investigators,[615,631] the adhesion of neutrophils to glass may also necessitate the presence of calcium in addition to that of magnesium.

Furthermore, calcium intervenes in the induction of mitoses, as was shown for thymic lymphocytes as well as for the cells of inflammatory foci.[632,633]

Calcium and Magnesium

A recent report[715] on children in Cameroon with a double deficiency of these electrolytes showed that there was a significant reduction in the serum concentrations of complement components C_3, C_4 and (C_3 proactivator) and that there was a significant correlation between calcium and C_3 and between magnesium and C_3PA. These correlations may be explained by the hypothesis that calcium is required for the conventional pathway of the complement systems, while magnesium is essential for the alternate pathway of these systems.[715] These findings are important because protein calorie malnutrition and kwashiokor are frequently accompanied by mineral deficiencies due to intestinal malabsorption and diarrhea. The decreased serum levels of C_3 reported in cases of this type of malnutrition[342,343] may be at least partially due to an associated lack of calcium and magnesium.

Comparative experiments were performed with mice fed either a magnesium-deficient diet (4 mg Mg/100 g) or a control diet (40 mg/100 g).[716] Following immunization with SRBC, the immune response was determined by the levels of PFC and RFC in the spleen. While a quantitative limitation of the control diet paradoxically enhanced the PFC response without affecting RFC levels, the magnesium-deficient diet produced a drastic reduction of the primary and secondary humoral immune responses, as indicated by the decreased concentrations of both PFC and RFC. Magnesium thus appears to be indispensable for the helper activity of T cells.

Lithium

In contrast to the negative conclusions of Stein et al.,[717] some new data suggest that lithium stimulates granulopoiesis. First, it has been reported that the total body granulocyte pool, as determined by the unsaturated vitamin B_{12} binding capacity in vivo and granulocyte colony proliferation in vitro, increased in patients given lithium as treatment for manic-depressive psychosis.[718] Lithium was also found to enhance the production of colony stimulating activity (CSA) by mouse lung in vitro.[719] Gupta et al.[720] reported increased levels of CSA in vivo in the urine and serum of patients with Felty's syndrome. Finally, Rossof and Feher[721] observed that the addition of lithium resulted in an increased production of canine marrow colony forming units (CFU) in the agar culture system. These data obtained in vitro remain to be confirmed more directly before the granulopoietic action of lithium becomes unequivocal.

SUMMARY

The alterations of leukopoiesis in different states of denutrition and malnutrition have been reviewed after the presentation of some recent data on the production and physiological functions of the white cells, with special consideration of the immunologic activity of lymphocytes.

The nutrients intervene primarily as building materials for the structures of the nucleus and cytoplasm of leukocytes. The leukopoietic responses induced by some nutrients (proteins) are, however, also partly of immunologic nature.

On the other hand, the harmfulness of several nutritional deficiences is more or less conditioned by the stressing effect of these diets acting via the release of glucocorticoid hormones selectively harmful to lymphocytes and eosinophils.

A hormonal mechanism seems to play a major role in lymphocytic alterations of acute starvation. Hypercorticalism also intervenes in the effects of certain avitaminoses (pyridoxine, pantothenic acid, folic acid) as well as in protracted protein deficiency, involving the involution of the lymphoid system and probably also the partial depression of immunologic responses.

In almost all experimental nutritional deficiences except acute starvation and balanced undernutrition, eosinophils and lymphocytes are injured much more than neutrophils. Thus, in protein-starved rats, eosinopenia and lymphopenia contrast with very few quantitative changes in the blood neutrophils when there is no edema with hemodilution nor associated deficiencies of other nutrients. Lymphopenia is accompanied in these animals by a significant decrease in the size of the circulating lymphocytes.

Among the lymphoid organs, the thymus is the first to be injured, while the lymph nodes are the last. The involution of the thymus mainly concerns the cortisone-sensitive thymocytes of the cortex, while the lymphocytes and reticuloepithelial cells of the thymic medulla are relatively resistant. In the spleen and the lymph nodes, the thymus-independent zones seem to be damaged to almost the same extent as the thymus-dependent areas.

From comparative experiments carried out on intact and thymectomized rats subjected to protein starvation, one may conclude that, to a large extent, the drop in the number and size of blood lymphocytes is conditioned by the early involution of the thymus.

The functional inactivation of the lymphoid system is attested to by several findings: a decrease in the intracellular content of potassium; almost complete disappearance of mitoses, particularly apparent in the thymus, with a premitotic blockade of the cell cycle, as suggested by the paradoxical increase in DNA synthesis and (or) levels per unit weight in the lymphoid organs; and inhibition of the blastogenic and mitogenic lymphocyte response to phytohemagglutinin in vivo.

The finding of an increased turnover of cyclic AMP in protein-deficient lymphocytes is in accord with the arrest of cell divisions.

The alterations of leukopoiesis are still more pronounced in the case of exclusive lack of certain essential amino acids than after complete amino acid deprivation. However, the extent of the damage depends on the nature of the amino acid lacking and the leukocyte line concerned. Lack of valine and, to a lesser degree, isoleucine is the most harmful for all leukocyte types studied. Indeed, neutrophils and eosinophils disappear almost completely from the blood, bone marrow, and intestinal mucosa, and only a few small lymphocytes remain alive after deprivation of valine.

In all prolonged nutritional deficiencies producing involution of the lymphoid organs (incomplete starvation, and deficiencies of pyridoxine, panthotenic acid, folic acid, or proteins) the immune responses have been found to be disturbed. This is also the case after administration of ethionine, antagonist of methionine. An excess of certain dietary amino acids (leucine or methionine) also depresses immunologic reactions.

The thymus-controlled immunologic system seems to be the most involved, as indicated by the predominant inhibition of the thymus-dependent humoral responses and of some (but not all) cell-mediated reactions.

Experimental protein deprivation selectively provokes the disappearance of a functional subpopulation of T lymphocytes characterized by their responsiveness to phytohemagglutinin, and their sensitivity to the lympholytic action of antithymic serum and cortisone.

Although, considered on a per-cell basis, these T lymphocytes are less immunocompetent than cortisone-resistant T cells derived from the thymic medulla, the cooperation of the two cell types may be necessary for enhancing certain thymus-dependent responses; hence, these responses are depressed in protein malnutrition.

Production of antibodies to thymus-independent antigens is, according to most authors, not inhibited in protein-deficient animals.

In human protein malnutrition, the immunologic alterations are more difficult to analyze than in animals, because of the frequent association of various infections on the one hand and additional nutritional deficiencies on the other.

Iron deprivation frequently induces leukopenia as well as a moderate impairment of cell-mediated immunity. An iron overload is at least as harmful as deficiency with regard to antimicrobial defenses, mainly because of the decreased antibacterial activity of lactoferrin in the leukocytes.

Leukocytic abnormalities have also been reported in deficiences of copper, potassium, and, especially, magnesium.

REFERENCES

1. Scrimshaw, N. S., Taylor, C. E., and Gordon, J. E., Interactions of nutrition and infection, *WHO Monogr. Ser.*, 57, 148, 1969.
2. Cline, M. J., *Physiol. Rev.*, 45, 674–720, 1965.
3. Beck, W. S., *Ser. Haematol.*, 1, 69–93, 1968.
4. Volkman, A. and Gowans, J. L., *Br. J. Exp. Pathol.*, 46, 50–61, 1965.
5. Wintrobe, M. M., *Clinical Hematology*, 6th ed., Lea and Febiger, Philadelphia, 1967.
6. Ackerman, G. A., *Ann. N.Y. Acad. Sci.*, 113, 537–565, 1964.
7. Cartwright, G. E., Athens, J. W., and Wintrobe, M. M., *Blood*, 24, 780–803, 1964.
8. Craddock, C. G., Jr., Perry, S., Ventzke, L. E., and Lawrence, J. S., *Blood*, 15, 840–855, 1960.
9. Craddock, C. G., Jr., *Prog. Hematol.*, 3, 92–104, 1962.
10. Foot, E. C., *Br. J. Haematol.*, 11, 439–445, 1965.
11. Ambrus, C. M. and Ambrus, J. L., *Ann. N.Y. Acad. Sci.*, 77, 445–486, 1959.
12. Teir, H., Rytömaa, T., and Cederberg, A., *Acta Pathol. Microbiol. Scand.*, 58, 401–413, 1963.
13. Rytömaa, T., *Acta Pathol. Scand. Suppl.*, 140, 1960.
14. Johnston, R. B., Jr., Klemperer, M. R., Alper, C. A., and Rosen, F. S., *J. Exp. Med.*, 129, 1275–1290, 1969.

15. Spicer, S. S. and Hardin, J. H., *Lab. Invest.,* 20, 488, 1969 (cited by Keusch[23]).
16. Lehrer, R. I., Hamfin, J., and Cline, M. J., *Nature,* 223, 78–79, 1969.
17. Selvaraj, R. J. and Sbarra, A. J., *Nature,* 211, 1272–1276, 1966.
18. Rechcigl, M. and Evans, H. W., *Nature,* 199, 1001–1002, 1963.
19. Cagan, R. H. and Karnovsky, M. L., *Nature,* 204, 255–257, 1964.
20. Klebanoff, S. J., *J. Exp. Med.,* 126, 1063–1078, 1967.
21. Klebanoff, S. J., *Semin. Hematol.,* 12, 117–142, 1975.
22. Zeya, H. I. and Spitznagel, J. K., *J. Bacteriol.,* 91, 755, 1966 (cited by Sbarra et al.[24]).
23. Keusch, G. T., in *Malnutrition and Functions of Blood Cells,* Shimazono, N. and Arakawa, T., Eds., National Institute of Nutrition, Tokyo, 1973, 97–111.
24. Sbarra, A. J., Selvaraj, R. J., Paul, B. B., Strauss, R. R., Jacobs, A. A., and Mitchell, G. W., Jr., *Am. J. Clin. Nutr.,* 27, 629–637, 1974.
25. Miller, J. F. A. P., *J. Allergy Clin. Immunol.,* 55, 1–9, 1975.
26. Fruhman, G. J., *Ann. N.Y. Acad. Sci.,* 113, 968–1002, 1964.
27. Bierman, H. R. and Hood, J. E., *Br. J. Haematol.,* 22, 145–153, 1972.
28. Sabesin, S. M., *Proc. Soc. Exp. Biol. Med.,* 112, 667–670, 1963.
29. Litt, M., *Ann. N.Y. Acad. Sci.,* 116, 964–983, 1964.
30. Kay, A. B. and Austen, K. F., *Clin. Exp. Immunol.,* 11, 37–42, 1972.
31. Ishikawa, T., Wicher, K., and Arbesman, C. E., *Fed. Proc. Fed. Am. Soc. Exp. Biol.,* 31, 744, 1972.
32. Basten, A. and Beeson, P. B., *J. Exp. Med.,* 131, 1288–1305, 1970.
33. McGarry, M. P., Speirs, R. S., Jenkins, V. K., and Trentin, J. J., *J. Exp. Med.,* 134, 801–814, 1971.
34. Colley, D. G., *J. Immunol.,* 110, 1419–1423, 1973.
35. Greene, B. M. and Colley, D. G., *J. Immunol.,* 113, 910–917, 1974.
36. Welsh, R. A. and Geer, J. C., *Am. J. Pathol.,* 35, 103–108, 1959.
37. Räsänen, T., *Acta Pathol. Microbiol. Scand.,* 62, 170–176, 1964.
38. Barzilaï, A., Delaney, J. P., Ritchie, W., and Wangensteen, O. H., *Isr. J. Med. Sci.,* 2, 781–784, 1966.
39. Aschkenasy, A. and Jobard, P., *Nouv. Rev. Fr. Hematol.,* 1, 202–212, 1961.
40. Aschkenasy, A., *C.R. Soc. Biol.,* 158, 278–280, 1964.
41. Ishizaka, T., Tomioka, H., and Ishizaka, K., *J. Immunol.,* 106, 705–710, 1971.
42. Greaves, M. W. and Burdis, B. D., *Int. Arch. Allergy Appl. Immunol.,* 34, 313–323, 1968.
43. Keller, R., *Int. Arch. Allergy Appl. Immunol.,* 34, 139–144, 1968.
44. Räsänen, T., *Acta Pathol. Microbiol. Scand. Suppl.,* 56, 126, 1958.
45. Haikonen, M., Räsänen, T., and Taskinen, C., *Acta Physiol. Scand.,* 74, 368–371, 1968.
46. Good, R. A., Gabrielsen, A. E., Cooper, M. D., and Peterson, R. D. A., *Ann. N.Y. Acad. Sci.,* 129, 130–154, 1966.
47. Miller, J. F. A. P. and Osoba, D., *Physiol. Rev.,* 47, 437–520, 1967.
48. Roitt, I. M., Greaves, M. F., Torrigiani, G., Brostoff, J., and Playfair, J. H. L., *Lancet,* ii, 367–371, 1969.
49. Claman, H. N. and Chaperon, E. A., *Transplant. Rev.,* 1, 92–113, 1969.
50. WHO Scientific Group, Factors regulating the immune response, *WHO Tech. Rep. Ser.,* No. 448, 1970.
51. Miller, J. F. A. P., Basten, A., Sprent, J., and Cheers, C., *Cell. Immunol.,* 2, 469–495, 1971.
52. Raff, M. C., *Nature,* 242, 19–23, 1973.
53. Culliton, B. J., *Science,* 180, 45–47, 89, 1973.
54. Unanue, E. R., Grey, H. M., Rabellino, E., Campbell, P., and Schmidtke, J., *J. Exp. Med.,* 133, 1188–1198, 1971.
55. Osmond, D. G. and Nossal, G. J. V., *Cell. Immunol.,* 13, 117–131, 132–145, 1974.
56. Yoffey, J. M. and Courtice, F. C., *Lymphatics, Lymph and the Lymphomyeloid Complex,* Academic Press, London, 1970, 469, 620–640.
57. Leblond, C. P. and Sainte-Marie, G., in *Haemopoiesis: Cell Production and its Regulation,* Ciba Foundation Symposium, Wolstenholme, G. E. W. and O'Connor, M., Eds., J. & A. Churchill, London, 1960, 152–172.
58. Owen, J. J. F. and Ritter, M. A., *J. Exp. Med.,* 129, 431–442, 1969.
59. Wekerle, H., Cohen, I. R., and Feldman, H. W., *Eur. J. Immunol.,* 3, 745–748, 1973.
60. Waksal, S. D., Cohen, I. R., and Waksal, H. W., *Ann. N.Y. Acad. Sci.,* 249, 492–498, 1975.
61. Scheid, M. P., Goldstein, G., and Boyse, E. A., *Science,* 190, 1211–1213, 1975.
62. Craddock, C. G., Nakai, G. S., Fukata, H., and Vanslager, L.M., *J. Exp. Med.,* 120, 389–412, 1964.

63. Joel, D. D., Chanana, A. D., and Cronkite, E. P., *Ser. Haematol.,* 7, 464–481, 1974.
64. Waksman, B. H. and Colley, D. C., *Cell Interactions and Receptor Antibodies in Immun Responses,* Mäkelä, O., Cross, A., and Kosunen, T. U., Eds., Academic Press, New York, 1971, 53–70.
65. Weissman, I. L., *J. Exp. Med.,* 137, 504–510, 1973.
66. Fathman, C. G., Small, M., Herzenberg, L. A., and Weissman, I. L., *Cell. Immunol.,* 15, 109–128, 1975.
67. Shortman, K. and Jackson, H., *Cell. Immunol.,* 12, 230–246, 1974.
68. Droege, W. and Zucker, R., *Transplant. Rev.,* 25, 3–25, 1975.
69. Metcalf, D., *The Thymus,* Springer-Verlag, Berlin, 1966, 2–3, 8–9, 54–61.
70. Osoba, D. and Miller, J. F. A. P., *Nature,* 199, 653–654, 1967.
71. Parrott, D. M. V., De Sousa M. A. B., and East, J., *J. Exp. Med.,* 123, 191–203, 1966.
72. Raff, M. C., in *Cell Interactions and Receptor Antibodies in Immune Responses,* Mäkelä, O., Cross, A., and Kosunen, T. U., Eds., Academic Press, London, 1971, 83–90.
73. Aschkenasy, A., *J. Physiol.* (Paris), 64, 293–302, 1972.
74. Walker, W. A., Isselbacher, K. J., and Bloch, K. J., *Am. J. Clin. Nutr.,* 27, 1434–1440, 1974.
75. Shields, J. W., *Am. J. Gastroenterol.,* 50, 30–36, 1968.
76. Crabbé, P. A., Bazin, H., Eyssen, H., and Heremans, J. F., *Int. Arch. Allergy Appl. Immunol.,* 34, 362–375, 1968.
77. Cooper, G. N. and Turner, K., *Aust. J. Exp. Biol. Med. Sci.,* 45, 363–378, 1967.
78. Cooper, G. N., Thonard, J. C., Crosby, R. L., and Dalbow, M. H., *Aust. J. Exp. Biol. Med. Sci.,* 46, 407–414, 1968.
79. Cooper, M. D., Peterson, R. D. A., South, M. A., and Good, R. A., *J. Exp. Med.,* 123, 75–102, 1966.
80. Fichtelius, K. E., Finstad, L., and Good, R. A., *Lab. Invest.,* 19, 339–351, 1968.
81. Perey, D. Y. E., Cooper, M. D., and Good, R. A., *Science,* 161, 265–266, 1968.
82. Veldkamp, J., Van Der Gaag, R., and Willers, J. M. N., *Immunology,* 25, 761–771, 1973.
83. Fichtelius, K. E., Yunis, E. J., and Good, R. A., *Proc. Soc. Exp. Biol. Med.,* 128, 185–188, 1968.
84. Claësson, M. H., *Scand. J. Haematol.,* 15, 256–260, 1975.
85. Aschkenasy, A., *Life Sci.,* 21, 253–260, 1977.
86. Miller, J. F. A. P., *Ann. Immunol.* (Paris), 125C, 213–229, 1974.
87. Aschkenasy, A., *C. R. Soc. Biol.,* 165, 1820–1825, 1971.
88. Bryant, B. J., *Eur. J. Immunol.,* 2, 38–45, 1972.
89. Fichtelius, K. F. and Larsson, S. E., *Acta Anat.,* 32, 114–125, 1958.
90. Rieke, W. O., Everett, N. B., and Caffrey, R. W., *Acta Haematol.,* 30, 103–110, 1963.
91. Rieke, W. O. and Schwarz, M. R., *Blood,* 23, 502–516, 1964.
92. Potmesil, M. and Goldfeder, A., *Exp. Cell Res.,* 77, 31–40, 1973.
93. MacHaffie, R. A. and Wang, C. H., *Blood,* 29, 640–646, 1967.
94. Valentine, F. T., in *Cell-Mediated Immunity,* Revillard, J. R., Ed., Karger, Basel, 1971, 6–42.
95. Aschkenasy, A., *Isr. J. Med. Sci.,* 1, 552–562, 1965.
96. Dougherty, T. F., Berliner, M. L., Schneebeli, G. L., and Berliner, D. L., *Ann. N.Y. Acad. Sci.,* 113, 825–843, 1964.
97. Aschkenasy, A., *C.R. Soc. Biol.,* 164, 951–956, 1970.
98. Blomgren, H. and Andersson, B., *Cell. Immunol.,* 1, 545–560, 1971.
99. Stobo, J. D. and Paul, W. E., *Cell. Immunol.,* 4, 367–380, 1972.
100. Ishidate, M. and Metcalf, D., *Aust. J. Exp. Biol. Med. Sci.,* 41, 637–649, 1963.
101. Aschkenasy, A., *Acta Haematol.,* 56, 212–220, 1976.
102. Blomgren, H. and Svedmyr, E., *Cell. Immunol.,* 2, 285–299, 1971.
103. Aschkenasy, A., unpublished data.
104. Claman, H. N., Levine, M. A., and Cohen, J. J., in *Cell Interactions and Receptor Antibodies in Immune Responses,* Mäkelä, O., Cross, A., and Kosunen, T. U., Eds., Academic Press, London, 1971, 333–344.
105. Mitchison, N. A., *Eur. J. Immunol.,* 1, 18–27, 1971.
106. Yu, H. and Gordon, J., *Nature New Biol.,* 244, 20–21, 1973.
107. Valentine, F. T., *Ann. N.Y. Acad. Sci.,* 221, 317–323, 1974.
108. Dukor, P. and Hartmann, K. U., *Cell. Immunol.,* 7, 349–356, 1973.
109. Vann, D. C., *Cell. Immunol.,* 11, 11–18, 1974.
110. Segal, S., Cohen, I. R., and Feldman, M., *Science,* 175, 1126–1128, 1972.
111. Gordon, J. and Yu, H., *Nature New Biol.,* 244, 21–22, 1973.
112. Kettman, J. and Dutton, R. W., *Fed. Proc. Fed. Am. Soc. Exp. Biol.,* 31, 3254, 1972 (abstr.).

113. Elliott, B. E. and Haskill, J. S., *Nature,* 252, 607–608, 1974.
114. Dennert, G. and Hatlen, L. E., *Nature,* 257, 486–488, 1975.
115. Dyminski, J. W. and Smith, R. T., *Ser. Haematol.,* 7, 524–547, 1974.
116. Folch, H. and Waksman, B. H., *Cell. Immunol.,* 9, 12–24, 25–31, 1973.
117. Armstrong, W. D., Diener, E., and Shellam, G. R., *J. Exp. Med.,* 129, 393–410, 1969.
118. Gershon, R. K., Cohen, P., Hencin, R., and Liebhaber, S. A., *J. Immunol.,* 108, 586–590, 1972.
119. Taussig, M. J., *Nature,* 248, 236–238, 1974.
120. Baker, P. J., *Transplant. Rev.,* 26, 3–20, 1975.
121. Wioland, M., Sabolovic, D., and Burg, C., *Nature New Biol.,* 237, 274–276, 1972.
122. Marchalonis, J. J., *Science,* 190, 20–29, 1975.
123. Van Muiswinkel, W. B. and Van Soest, P. L., *Immunology,* 28, 287–291, 1975.
124. Biozzi, G., Stiffel, C., and Mouton, C., in *Immunity, Cancer and Chemotherapy,* Mihich, E., Ed., Academic Press, London, 1967, 103.
125. Moav, N. and Harris, T. N., *J. Immunol.,* 105, 1501–1511, 1970.
126. Bach, J. F. and Dardenne, M., *Cell. Immunol.,* 3, 1–10, 1972.
127. Wybran, J., Carr, M. C., and Fudenberg, H. H., *J. Clin. Invest.,* 51, 2537–2543, 1972.
128. Steel, C. M., Evans, J., and Smith, M. A., *Br. J. Haematol.,* 28, 245–251, 1974.
129. Allison, A. C. and Davies, A. J. S., *Nature,* 233, 330–332, 1971.
130. Mosser, G., Good, R. A., and Cooper, M. D., *Int. Arch. Allergy Appl. Immunol.,* 39, 62–81, 1970.
131. Nossal, G. J. V. and Ada, G. L., *Antigens, Lymphoid Cells, and the Immune Response,* Academic Press, New York, 1971.
132. Unanue, E. R., *Adv. Immunol.,* 15, 95–165, 1972.
133. Unanue, E. R. and Calderon, J., *Fed. Proc. Fed. Am. Soc. Exp. Biol.,* 34, 1737–1742, 1975.
134. Rosenthal, A. S. and Shevach, E. M., *J. Exp. Med.,* 138, 1194–1212, 1973.
135. Erb, P. and Feldmann, M., *Cell. Immunol.,* 19, 356–367, 1975.
136. Pierce, C. W., Kapp, J. A., Wood, D. D., and Benacerraf, B., *J. Immunol.,* 112, 1181–1189, 1974.
137. Schrader, J. W., *J. Exp. Med.,* 138, 1466–1480, 1973.
138. Calkins, C. E. and Golub, E. S., *Cell. Immunol.,* 5, 579–586, 1972.
139. Mackaness, G. B., *J. Exp. Med.,* 129, 973, 1969.
140. Hadden, J. W., Sadlik, J. R., and Hadden, E. M., *Nature,* 257, 483–485, 1975.
141. David, J. R., *Fed. Proc. Fed. Am. Soc. Exp. Biol.,* 34, 1730–1736, 1975.
142. Srivastava, U., Spach, C., and Aschkenasy, A., *J. Nutr.,* 105, 924–938, 1975
143. Bierman, H. R., *Ann. N.Y. Acad. Sci.,* 113, 753–765, 1964.
144. Gordon, A. S., Handler, E. S., Siegel, C. D., Dornfest, B. S., and Lo Bue, J., *Ann. N.Y. Acad. Sci.,* 113, 766–789, 1964.
145. Metcalf, D., *Exp. Hematol.,* 2, 157–173, 1974.
146. Metcalf, D., *Ann. N.Y. Acad. Sci.,* 73, 113–119, 1958.
147. Comsa, J., *Am. J. Med. Sci.,* 250, 79–85, 1965.
148. Goldstein, A. L., Guha, A., Zatz, M. M., Hardy, M. A., and White, A., *Proc. Natl. Acad. Sci. U.S.A.,* 69, 1800–1803, 1972.
149. Trainin, N. and Small, M., *J. Exp. Med.,* 132, 885–897, 1970.
150. Bach, J. F., Dardenne, M., Pleau, J. M., and Bach, M. A., *Ann. N.Y. Acad. Sci.,* 249, 186–210, 1975.
151. Goldstein, G., *Ann. N.Y. Acad. Sci.,* 249, 177–183, 1975.
152. Jolly, J., *Traité Technique d'Hématologie,* Vol. 2., A. Maloine, Paris, 1923, 678–680, 789.
153. Jackson, C. M., *The Effects of Inanition and Malnutrition upon Growth and Structure,* P. Blakiston's and Son, Philadelphia, 1925, 125–126, 136–137, 238–299.
154. Schulz, J. and Muller, H., *Nature,* 196, 178, 1962.
155. Aschkenasy, A., *Arch. Sci. Physiol.,* 25, 275–292, 1971.
156. Archambeau, J. O., Stryckmanns, P., and Brenneis, H., *Radiat. Res.,* 36, 396, 1968.
157. Opie, E., *Am. J. Med. Sci.,* 127, 217–239, 1904.
158. Dury, A., *Am. J. Physiol.,* 163, 96–103, 1950.
159. Wilhelmj, C. M., Milani, D. P., Meyers, V. W., Gunderson, D. E., Shuput, D., Racher, E. M., and McCarthy, H. H., *J. Lab. Clin. Med.,* 43, 888–896, 1954.
160. Shapiro, Y. L., *Patol. Fiziol. Eksp. Ter.,* 7, 447, 1963 (cited in Drenick and Alvarez[161]).
161. Drenick, E. J. and Alvarez, L. C., *Am. J. Clin. Nutr.,* 24, 859–863, 1971.
162. Harper, S. M., Drenick, E. J., and Swenseid, M. E., *Am. J. Clin. Nutr.,* 23, 4–7, 1970.
163. Gastaldi, F. and Fedeli, S., *Arch. Sci. Med.,* 97, 3, 1954.
164. Saba, T. M. and DiLuzio, N. R., *Proc. Soc. Exp. Biol. Med.,* 128, 869–875, 1968.

165. Simon, J., *A Physiological Essay on the Thymus Gland,* Renshaw, London, 1845 (cited in Jackson[153]).
166. Hérard, H. V., Du Spasme de la Glotte, thesis, Paris, No. 3, 1847 (cited by Jackson[153] from Hammar[167]).
167. Hammar, J. A., *Arch. Anat. Physiol. Anat. Abt.,* suppl. bd., pp. 91–182, 1906.
168. Feder, D. and Gordon, A. S., *Anat. Rec.,* 103, 536, 1949 (abstr.).
169. Reinhardt, W. A. and Yoffey, J. M., *Am. J. Physiol.,* 187, 493–500, 1956.
170. Heidenhain, R. and Pflügers, A., *Arch. Ges. Physiol.,* 1888, Suppl. 43, 1–103, 1948 (cited by Jackson[153]).
171. Erdely, A., *Z. Biol.,* 46, 119–152, 1905 (cited by Jackson[153]).
172. Simon, L. G., *C.R. Soc. Biol.,* 59, 648–650, 1905.
173. Biggart, J. H., *J. Pathol. Bacteriol.,* 35, 799–816, 1932.
174. Teir, H., Wegelius, U., Sundell, B., Päivärinne, I., and Kunsi, T., *Acta Med. Scand.,* 152, 275–283, 1955.
175. Mulinos, M. G. and Pomerantz, L., *Am. J. Physiol.,* 132, 368–374, 1941.
176. Szego, C. M. and White, A., *Endocrinology,* 48, 576–590, 1951.
177. D'Angelo, S. A., Gordon, A. S., and Charipper, H. A., *Proc. Soc. Exp. Biol. Med.,* 68, 527–529, 1948.
178. Cameron, A. T. and Carmichael, J., *Can. J. Res.,* 24 E, 37–48, 1946.
179. Slater, G. G., *Endocrinology,* 70, 18–23, 1962.
180. Selye, H., *Br. J. Exp. Pathol.,* 17, 234–248, 1936.
181. White, A. and Dougherty, T. F., *Endocrinology,* 41, 230–242, 1947.
182. Aschkenasy, A., *Sem. Hôp. Pathol. Biol.,* 34, 683–697, 1958.
183. Kornberg, A., Daft, F. S., and Sebrell, W. H., *Arch. Biochem.,* 8, 431–437, 1945.
184. Woodruff, J. F., *J. Infect. Dis.,* 121, 164–181, 1970.
185. Woodruff, J. F. and Woodruff, J. J., *Proc. Natl. Acad. Sci. U.S.A.,* 68, 2108–2111, 1971.
186. Chevalier, P. and Aschkenasy, A., *Am. J. Clin. Nutr.,* 30, 1645-1654, 1977.
187. Waitz, R. and Wellers, G., *Sang,* 19, 340–348, 1948.
188. Szejnman, M., in *Maladie de Famine,* Apfelbaum, E. et al., Eds., American Joint Distribution Committee, Warsaw, 1946, 227–258.
189. Braude-Heller, A., Rotbalsam, J., and Elbinger, R., in *Maladie de Famine,* Apfelbaum, E. et al., Eds., American Joint Distribution Committee, Warsaw, 1946, 173–187.
190. Keys, A., Brožek, J., Henschel, A., Mickelsen, O., and Taylor, H. L., in *The Biology of Human Nutrition,* University of Minnesota Press, Minneapolis, 1950, chap. 14.
191. Grégoire, C., *Arch. Int. Pharmacodyn.,* 78, 313–335, 1949.
192. Reinhardt, W. O., *Ann. N. Y. Acad. Sci.,* 113, 844–866, 1964.
193. Mulinos, M. G., Pomerantz, L., and Lojkin, M. E., *Endocrinology,* 31, 276–281, 1942.
194. Da Costa, E. and Clayton, K., *Fed. Proc. Fed. Am. Soc. Exp. Biol.,* 9, 356, 1950.
195. Miller, E. O., Mickelsen, O., and Keys, A., *Proc. Soc. Exp. Biol. Med.,* 67, 288–292, 1948.
196. Huseby, R. A., Reed, F. C., III, and Smith, T. E., *J. Appl. Physiol.,* 14, 31–36, 1959.
197. Chandra, R. K., *Science,* 190, 289–290, 1975.
198. Kenney, M. A., *J. Nutr.,* 98, 202–208, 1969.
199. Aschkenasy, A., *Rev. Fr. Etud. Clin. Biol.,* 10, 709–723, 1965.
200. Aschkenasy, A., *Sang,* 17, 34–61, 1946.
201. Kornberg, A., *J. Biol. Chem.,* 164, 203–212, 1946.
202. Aschkenasy, A., Polonovski, C., and Rolland, G. J., *J. Physiol.* (Paris), 41, 469–489, 1949.
203. Nelson, D. P. and Newberne, P. M., *Nutr. Rep. Int.,* 8, 283–300, 1973.
204. Asirvadham, M., *J. Infect. Dis.,* 83, 87–100, 1948.
205. Bhuyan, U. N. and Ramalingaswami, V., *Am. J. Pathol.,* 69, 359–367, 1972.
206. Aschkenasy, A., *C. R. Soc. Biol.,* 166, 287–291, 502–507, 1972.
207. Bhuyan, U. N., Mohapatra, L. N., and Ramalingaswami, V., *Indian J. Med. Res.,* 62, 42–52, 1974.
208. Delmonte, L., Eyquem, A., and Aschkenasy, A., *Ann. Inst. Pasteur* (Paris), 102, 420–436, 1962.
209. Mills, C. A. and Cottingham, E., *J. Immunol.,* 47, 503–504, 1943.
210. Guggenheim, K. and Buechler, E., *J. Immunol.,* 58, 133–137, 1948.
211. Steffee, C. H., *J. Infect. Dis.,* 86, 12–26, 1950.
212. La Via, M. F., Barker, P. A., and Wissler, R. W., *J. Lab. Clin. Med.,* 48, 237–254, 1956.
213. Hook, R. R., Jr., Hutcheson, D. P., and Woodward, K., *Nutr. Rep. Int.,* 9, 191–196, 1974.
214. Trnka, Z., *Folia Biol.* (Prague), 2, 306, 1956 (cited by Kenney et al.[215]).
215. Kenney, M. A., Arnrich, L., Mar, E., and Roderuck, C. E., *J. Nutr.,* 85, 213–220, 1965.
216. Aschkenasy, A. and Aschkenasy-Lelu, P., *Arch. Sci. Physiol.,* 1, 225–255, 1947.

217. Aschkenasy, A., *C. R. Soc. Biol.,* 160, 933–937, 1966.
218. Aschkenasy, A., *Arch. Sci. Physiol.,* 25, 415–430, 1971.
219. Keller, H. U. and Sorkin, E., *Immunology,* 9, 441–447, 1965.
220. Aschkenasy, A., *C. R. Soc. Biol.,* 163, 295–300, 1969.
221. Aschkenasy, A., Bachvaroff, R., and Grabar, P., *C. R. Acad. Sci.,* 267, 1788–1790, 1968.
222. Aschkenasy, A. and André, F., *C. R. Soc. Biol.,* 166, 1241–1245, 1972.
223. Aschkenasy, A., *Rev. Fr. Etud. Clin. Biol.,* 10, 299–307, 1965.
224. Aschkenasy, A., Adam, Y., and Joly, P., *Ann. Endocrinol.,* 27, 21–36, 1966.
225. Aschkenasy, A., *Nouv. Rev. Fr. Hematol.,* 1, 213–218, 1961.
226. Schonland, M. M., Shanley, B. C., Loening, W. E. K., Parent, A. M., and Coovadia, H. M., *Lancet,* ii, 435–436, 1972.
227. Aschkenasy, A., *Ann. Endocrinol.* (Paris), 14, 353–365, 1953.
228. Aschkenasy, A., *C. R. Soc. Biol.,* 158, 479–483, 1964.
229. Aschkenasy, A., *Arch. Sci. Physiol.,* 26, 359–366, 1972.
230. Jose, D. G., Stutman, O., and Good, R. A., *Nature,* 241, 57–58, 1973.
231. Aschkenasy, A., *Nutrition et Hematopoièse,* Centre National de la Recherche Scientifique, Paris, 1971.
232. Aschkenasy, A., *Rev. Fr. Etud. Clin. Biol.,* 13, 792–799, 1968.
233. Aschkenasy, A., *Immunology,* 24, 617–633, 1973.
234. Cao, M. J. and Aschkenasy, A., *C. R. Soc. Biol.,* 164, 277–281, 1970.
235. Jacobs, F. A. and Largis, E. E., *Proc. Soc. Exp. Biol. Med.,* 130, 692–696, 1969.
236. Aschkenasy, A., *Am. J. Clin. Nutr.,* 5, 14–25, 1957.
237. Aschkenasy, A., *Isr. J. Med. Sci.,* 1, 552–562, 1965.
238. Maun, M. E., Cahill, W. M., and Davis, R. M., *Arch. Pathol.,* 39, 294–300, 1945.
239. Scott, E. B. and Schwartz, C., *Proc. Soc. Exp. Biol. Med.,* 84, 271-276, 1953.
240. Maun, M. E., Cahill, W. M. and Davis, R. M., *Arch. Pathol.,* 41, 25–31, 1946.
241. Scott, E. B., *Am. J. Pathol.,* 31, 1111–1129, 1955.
242. Scott, E. B., *Proc. Soc. Exp. Biol. Med.,* 92, 134–140, 1956.
243. Scott, E. B., *J. Exp. Molec. Pathol.,* 3, 610-621, 1964.
244. Aschkenasy, A., *C. R. Soc. Biol.,* 160, 1787–1792, 1966.
245. Dinning, J. S., Payne, L. D., and Day, P. L., *Arch. Biochem.,* 27, 467–469, 1950.
246. Goedde, H. W., Langenbeck, U., and Brackertz, D., *Humangenetik,* 6, 189–190, 1968.
247. Aschkenasy, A., *Proc. 10th Int. Congr. Nutr., Kyoto,* 1976, 132-133.
248. Hopper, A. F., Wannemacher, R. W., Jr., and McGovern, P. A., *Proc. Soc. Exp. Biol. Med.,* 128, 695–698, 1968.
249. Deo, M. G. and Mathur, M., *26th Int. Congr. Physiol. Sci., New Delhi,* Vol. 10, All-India Institute of Medical Science, New Delhi, 1974, 110–111 (abstr.).
250. Wickramasinghe, S. N. and Pratt, J. R., *Acta Haematol.,* 44, 37–46, 1970.
251. Sheppard, J. R., *Nature New Biol.,* 236, 14–16, 1972.
252. Spach, C. and Aschkenasy, A., *C. R. Soc. Biol.,* 167, 1540–1544, 1973.
253. Brody, J. I. and Merlie, K., *Br. J. Haematol.,* 19, 193–201, 1970.
254. Aschkenasy, A., *Nature,* 254, 63–65, 1975.
255. Aschkenasy, A., *Life Sci.,* 12(2), 555–562, 1973; *Ann. Immunol.* (Paris), 124C, 345–362, 1973.
256. Aschkenasy, A., *C. R. Soc. Biol.,* 167, 1340–1344, 1973.
257. Jacobs, D. M. and Byrd, W., *Nature,* 255, 153–155, 1975.
258. Cooper, W. C., Good, R. A., and Mariani, T., *Am. J. Clin. Nutr.,* 27, 647–664, 1974.
259. Spach, C. and Aschkenasy, A., *J. Physiol.* (Paris), in press.
259a. Pincus, J. H., Lincoln, P., and Reisfeld, R. A., *Transplantation,* 18, 544–548, 1974.
260. Aschkenasy, A., *World Rev. Nutr. Diet.,* 21, 151–197, 1975.
261. May, C. D. and Alberto, R., *Int. Arch. Allergy Appl. Immunol.,* 43, 525–535, 1972.
262. Wostmann, B. S., Pleasants, J. R., and Bealmear, P., *Fed. Proc. Fed. Am. Soc. Exp. Biol.,* 30, 1779–1784, 1971.
263. Cannon, P. R., Chase, W. E., and Wissler, R. W., *J. Immunol.,* 47, 133–147, 1943.
264. Benditt, E. P., Wissler, R. W., Woolridge, R. L., Rowley, D. A., and Steffee, C. H., *Proc. Soc. Exp. Biol. Med.,* 70, 240–243, 1949.
265. Aschkenasy, A., *C. R. Acad. Sci. Ser. D,* 273, 2384–2387, 1971.
266. Kenney, M. A., Roderuck, C. E., Arnrich, L., and Piedad, F., *J. Nutr.,* 95, 173–178, 1968.
267. Mathur, M., Ramalingaswami, V., and Deo, M. G., *J. Nutr.,* 102, 841–846, 1972.
268. McFarlane, H. and Hamid, J., *Clin. Exp. Immunol.,* 13, 153–164, 1973.
269. Cooper, W. C., Mariani, T., and Good, R. A., *Fed. Proc. Fed. Am. Soc. Exp. Biol.,* 29, 364, 1970 (abstr.).

270. Gautam, S. C., Aikat, B. K., and Sehgal, S., *Indian J. Med. Res.,* 61, 78–85, 1973.
271. Malave, I. and Layrisse, M., *Cell. Immunol.,* 21, 397–343, 1976.
272. Hamid, J., Sayeed, A., and McFarlane, H., *Br. J. Exp. Pathol.,* 55, 94–100, 1974.
273. Raff, M. C. and Cantor, H., *Progr. Immunol.,* 1, 83–93, 1971.
274. Aschkenasy, A., *J. Physiol.* (Paris), 71, 259A, 1975 (abstr.).
275. Jose, D. G. and Good, R. A., *Nature,* 231, 323–325, 1971.
276. Aschkenasy, A., *C. R. Soc. Biol.,* 167, 430–434, 1973.
277. Aschkenasy, A., *Ann. Immunol.* (Paris), 125C, 803–820, 1974.
278. Elkins, W. L., *Progr. Allergy,* 15, 78–187, 1971.
279. Simonsen, M., *Progr. Allergy,* 6, 349–467, 1962.
280. Aschkenasy, A., *Nature,* 250, 325–327, 1974.
281. Aschkenasy, A., *Experientia,* 32, 638–639, 1976.
282. Lopez, V., Davis, S. D., and Smith, N. J., *Pediatr. Res.,* 6, 779–788, 1972.
283. Cohen, J. J., Fischbach, M., and Claman, H. N., *J. Immunol.,* 105, 1146–1150, 1970.
284. Cohen, J. J. and Claman, H. N., *J. Exp. Med.,* 133, 1026–1034, 1971.
285. Jacobson, H. and Blomgren, H., *Cell. Immunol.,* 4, 93–105, 1972.
286. Nowell, P. G., *Cancer Res.,* 21, 1518–1521, 1961.
287. Ono, T., Terayama, H., Takaku, F., and Nakao, K., *Biochim. Biophys. Acta,* 161, 361–367, 1968.
288. Heilman, D. H., Gambrill, M. P., and Leichner, J. P., *Clin. Exp. Immunol.,* 15, 203–212, 1973.
289. Tigelaar, R. E. and Asofsky, R., *J. Immunol.,* 110, 567–574, 1973.
290. Cohen, P. and Gershon, R. K., *Ann. N.Y. Acad. Sci.,* 249, 451–461, 1975.
291. Kontiainen, S. and Feldmann, M., *European Immunology Meeting, Amsterdam,* Oxonian Press, Oxford, Engl., 1975 (abstr.).
292. Wissler, R. W., *J. Infect. Dis.,* 80, 250–263, 264–277, 1947.
293. Metcoff, J., Darling, D. B., Scanlon, M. H., and Stare, F. J., *J. Lab. Clin. Med.,* 33, 47–66, 1948.
294. Aschkenasy, A., *J. Nutr.,* 108, 1527–1539, 1978.
295. Aschkenasy, A. and Courcon, J., *C. R. Soc. Biol.,* 161, 74–78, 1967.
296. Aschkenasy, A., *C. R. Soc. Biol.,* 161, 1280–1283, 1967.
297. Aschkenasy, A., *C. R. Soc. Biol.,* 163, 44–48, 1969.
298. Ryan, W. L., *JAMA,* 191, 295–296, 1965.
299. Gershoff, S. N., Gill, T. J., III, Simonian, S. J., and Steinberg, A. I., *J. Nutr.,* 95, 184–190, 1968.
300. Axelrod, A. E. and Pruzansky, J., *Vitam. Horm.* (N.Y.), 13, 1–27, 1955.
301. Kenney, M. A., Magee, J. L., and Piedad-Pascual, F., *J. Nutr.,* 100, 1063–1072, 1970.
302. Jose, D. G. and Good, R. A., *J. Exp. Med.,* 137, 1–9, 1973.
303. Smith, M. M. and Kenney, M. A., *J. Am. Diet. Assoc.,* 54, 500, 1969 (cited by Kenney et al.[301]).
304. Belavady, B., Srikantia, S. G., and Gopalan, C., *Biochem. J.,* 87, 652–655, 1963.
305. Benton, D. A., Harper, A. E., Spivey, H. E., and Elvehjem, C. A., *Arch. Biochem. Biophys.,* 60, 147–155, 1956.
306. Gill, T. J., III and Gershoff, S. N., *J. Immunol.,* 99, 883–893, 1967.
307. Aschkenasy, A., *Ann. Nutr. Aliment.* 29, 137–150, 1975.
308. Aschkenasy, A., *Eur. Afr. Div. 3rd Meet. Int. Soc. Haematol., London,* Kent Paper Co., London, 1975 (abstr.).
309. Farber, E., *Fed. Proc. Fed. Am. Soc. Exp. Biol.,* 32, 1534–1539, 1973.
310. Bhargava, K. K., Hanson, R. P., and Sunde, M. L., *J. Nutr.,* 100, 241–248, 1970.
311. Klavins, J. V., Kinnay, T. D., and Kaufman, N., *J. Nutr.,* 79, 101–104, 1963.
312. Waxman, S., Metz, J., and Herbert, V., *J. Clin. Invest.,* 48, 284–289, 1969.
313. Cheng, F. W., Shane, B., and Stokstad, E. L. R., *Br. J. Haematol.,* 31, 323–336, 1975.
314. Aschkenasy, A., *C. R. Soc. Biol.,* 167, 200–206, 1973.
315. Aschkenasy, A., Nataf, B., Piette, C., and Sfez, M., *Ann. Endocrinol.* (Paris), 23, 311–332, 1962.
316. Aschkenasy, A., *J. Physiol.* (Paris), 52, 9–10, 1960.
317. Aschkenasy, A., *C. R. Soc. Biol.,* 157, 1950–1954, 1963.
318. Aschkenasy, A. and Pariente, P., *Acta Haematol.,* 9, 29–46, 1953.
319. Aschkenasy, A., *Sang,* 25, 15–30, 1954.
320. Aschkenasy, A. and Dray, F., *Sang,* 25, 461–489, 1954.
321. Aschkenasy, A. and Blanpin, O., *Ann. Endocrinol.* (Paris), 16, 789–793, 1955.
322. Aschkenasy, A., *C. R. Soc. Biol.,* 149, 495–499, 1955.
323. Aschkenasy, A., *Ann. Endocrinol.* (Paris), 16, 199–224, 1955.

324. Leathem, J. H., *Arch. Int. Pharmacodyn. Ther.,* 110, 103–113, 1957.
325. Aschkenasy, A., *C. R. Soc. Biol.,* 154, 1783–1787, 1960.
326. Enwonwu, C. O., Stambaugh, R. V., and Jacobson, K. L., *Am. J. Clin. Nutr.,* 26, 1287–1302, 1973.
327. Munro, H. N., in *Mammalian Protein Metabolism,* Vol. 1, Munro, H. N. and Allison, J. B., Eds., Academic Press, New York, 1964, 381–481.
328. Aschkenasy, A., *C. R. Soc. Biol.,* 158, 708–711, 1964.
329. Aschkenasy, A., *Rev. Belge Pathol. Med. Exp.,* 24, 365–376, 1955.
330. Pierpaoli, W., Baroni, C., Fabris, N., and Sorkin, E., *Immunology,* 16, 217–230, 1969.
331. Balch, H. H. and Spencer, M. T., *J. Clin. Invest.,* 33, 1321–1328, 1954.
332. Selvaraj, R. J. and Bhat, K. S., *Am. J. Clin. Nutr.,* 25, 166–174, 1972.
333. Trowell, H. C., Davies, J. N. P., and Dean, R. F. A., *Kwashiorkor,* E. Arnold, London, 1954.
334. Bieler, M. M., Ecker, E. E., and Spies, T. D., *J. Lab. Clin. Med.,* 32, 130, 1947 (cited by Balch and Spencer[331]).
335. Tepada, C., Argueta, V., Sanchez, M., and Albertazzi, C., *J. Pediatr.,* 64, 753, 1964 (cited by Faulk et al.[365]).
336. Arbeter, A., Echeverri, L., Franco, D., Munson, D., Velez, H., and Vitale, J. J., *Fed. Proc. Fed. Am. Soc. Exp. Biol.,* 30, 1421–1428, 1971.
337. Seth, V. and Chandra, R. K., *Arch. Dis. Child.,* 47, 282–284, 1972 (cited by Faulk et al.[365]).
338. Douglas, S. D. and Schopfer, K., *Clin. Exp. Immunol.,* 17, 121–128, 1974.
339. Yoshida, T., Metcoff, J., and Frank, S., *Am. J. Clin. Nutr.,* 21, 162–166, 1968.
340. Whitehead, R. G., in *Calorie Deficiencies and Protein Deficiencies,* McCance, R. A. and Widdowson, E. M., Eds., J. & A. Churchill, London, 1968, 109–117.
341. Yoshida, T., Metcoff, J., Frank, S., and Delapena, C., *Nature,* 214, 525–526, 1967.
342. Sirisinha, S., Suskind, R., Edelman, R., Charupatana, C., and Olson, R. E., *Lancet,* i, 1016–1020, 1973.
343. Coovadia, H. M., Parent, M. A., Loening, W. E. K., et al., *Am. J. Clin. Nutr.,* 27, 665–669, 1974.
344. Wolfsdorf, J. and Nolan, R., *S. Afr. Med. J.,* 48, 528–530, 1974.
345. Smythe, P. M., Schonland, M., Brereton-Stiles, G. G., Coovadia, H. M., Grace, H. J., Loening, W. E. K., Mafoyane, A., Parent, M. A., and Vos, G. H., *Lancet,* ii, 939–944, 1971.
346. Chandra, R. K., *J. Pediatr.,* 81, 1194–2000, 1972.
347. Vint, F. W., *East Afr. Med. J.,* 13, 332–340, 1937.
348. Watts, T., *J. Trop. Pediatr.,* 15, 155, 1969 (cited by Schlesinger and Stekel[357]).
349. Schwartz, F. C. M., Chitiyo, M. E., and Wolfsdorf, J., *S. Afr. Med. J.,* 48, 2128, 1974.
350. Freyre, S. A., Chabes, S., and Chabes, A., *J. Pediatr.,* 82, 523–526, 1973.
351. Geefhuysen, J., Rosen, E. V., Katz, J., Ipp, T., and Metz, J., *Br. Med. J.,* 4, 527–529, 1971.
352. Grace, H. J. and Armstrong, D., *S. Afr. Med. J.,* 46, 402–403, 1972.
353. Sellemeyer, E., Bhettay, E., Truswell, A. S., Meyers, O. L., and Hansen, J. D. L., *Arch. Dis. Child.,* 47, 429, 1972 (cited by Munson et al.[371]).
354. Law, D. K., Dudrick, S. J., and Abdon, N. I., *Ann. Intern. Med.,* 79, 545–550, 1973.
355. Neumann, C. G., Lawlor, G. J., Jr., Stiehm, E. R., Swendseid, M. E., Newton, C., Herbert, J., Ammann, A. J., and Jacob, M., *Am. J. Clin. Nutr.,* 28, 89–104, 1975.
356. Jose, D. G., Welch, J. S., and Doherty, R. L., *Aust. Paediatr. J.,* 6, 192, 1970 (cited by Munson et al.[371]).
357. Schlesinger, L. and Stekel, A., *Am. J. Clin. Nutr.,* 27, 615–620, 1974.
358. Harland, P. S. E. G., *Lancet,* ii, 719–721, 1965.
359. Lloyd, A. V. C., *Br. Med. J.,* 3, 529–531, 1968.
360. Edelman, R., Suskind, R., and Olson, R. E., *Lancet,* i, 506–508, 1973.
361. Bistrian, B. R., Blackburn, G. L., Scrimshaw, N. S., and Flatt, J. P., *Am. J. Clin. Nutr.,* 28, 1148–1155, 1975.
362. Bang, B. G., Mahalanabis, D., Mukherjee, K. L., and Bang, F. B., *Proc. Soc. Exp. Biol. Med.,* 149, 199–202, 1975.
363. Pretorius, P. J. and De Villiers, L. S., *Am. J. Clin. Nutr.,* 10, 379–383, 1962.
364. Rosen, E. U., Geefhuysen, J., and Ipp, T., *S. Afr. Med. J.,* 980–982, 1971.
365. Faulk, W. P., Demaeyer, E. M., and Davies, A. J. S., *Am. J. Clin. Nutr.,* 27, 638–646, 1974.
366. Najjar, S. S., Stephan, M., and Asfour, R. Y., *Arch. Dis. Child.,* 44, 120, 1969 (cited by Munson et al.[371]).
367. McFarlane, H., Reddy, K., Adcock, K. J., Adeshina, H., Cooke, A. R., and Akene, J., *Br. Med. J.,* 4, 268–270, 1970.
368. Alvarado, J. and Luthringer, D. G., *Clin Pediatr.,* 10, 174, 1971 (cited by Munson et al.[371]).
369. Samuel, A. M., Patel, B. D., and Mankodi, N., *Indian J. Med. Res.,* 60, 1278–1283, 1972.

370. Cohen, S. and Hansen, J. D., *Clin. Sci.*, 23, 351–359, 1962.
371. Munson, D., Franco, D., Arbeter, A., Velez, H., and Vitale, J. J., *Am. J. Clin. Nutr.*, 27, 625–628, 1974.
372. Ferguson, A. C., Lawlor, G. J., Neumann, C. C., and Stiehm, E. R., *Clin. Res,*, 22, 227A, 1974 (abstr.).
373. Rabson, A. R., Geefhuyzen, J., Rosen, E. U., and Joffe, M., *Br. Med. J.*, 1, 40, 1975.
374. Alleyne, G. A. O. and Young, V. H., *Clin. Sci.*, 33, 189–200, 1967.
375. Rao, K. S. J., Srikantia, S. G., and Gopalan, C., *Arch. Dis. Child.*, 43, 365–367, 1968.
376. Lunn, P. G., Whitehead, R. C., Hay, R. W., and Barker, B. A., *Br. J. Nutr.*, 29, 399–422, 1973.
377. Regala-Castillo, K., Pascasio, F. M., and Bantista, F. A., *Asian J. Med.*, 10, 85–88, 1974.
378. Suskind, R., Amatayakul, K., Lietzmann, C., and Olson, R. E., in *Endocrine Aspects of Malnutrition*, Gardner, L. J. and Amscher, P., Eds., Kroc Foundation, Santa Ynez, Calif., 1973, 99.
379. Higashi, O., Sato, Y., Takamatsu, H., and Oyama, M., *Tohoku J. Exp. Med.*, 93, 105–113, 1967.
380. Burgess, B. J., *S. Afr. Med. J.*, 48, 1870–1872, 1974.
381. Olsson, J., Dahlguist, A., and Norden, A., *Acta Med. Scand.*, 174, 123–127, 1963.
382. Wachstein, M., *Blood*, 4, 54–59, 1949.
383. Valentine, W. N., Follette, J. H., and Lawrence, J. S., *J. Clin. Invest.*, 32, 251–257, 1953.
384. White, A., Handler, P., and Smith, E. L., *Principles of Biochemistry*, 3rd ed., McGraw-Hill, New York, 1964, 351–352.
385. Cohn, Z. A. and Morse, S. I., *J. Exp. Med.*, 111, 667–687, 1960.
386. Da Costa, J. C. and Beardsley, E., *Am. J. Med. Sci.*, 136, 361, 1908 (cited by Sanchez et al.[390]).
387. Richardson, R., *Am. J. Med. Sci.*, 204, 29–35, 1942.
388. Bybee, J. D. and Rogers, D. E., *J. Lab. Clin. Med.*, 64, 1–13, 1964.
389. Kijak, E., Foust, G., and Steinman, R. R., *J. Soc. Calif. Dental Assoc.*, 32, 349, 1964 (cited by Sanchez et al.[390]).
390. Sanchez, A., Reeser, J. L., Lau, H. S., Yahiku, P. Y., Willard, R. E., McMillan, P. J., Cho, S. Y., Magie, A. R., and Register, U. D., *Am. J. Clin. Nutr.*, 26, 1180–1184, 1973.
391. Freeman, H. and Elmadjian, F., *J. Clin. Endocrinol.*, 6, 668–674, 1946.
392. Jordan, P. H., Last, J. H., Pitesky, I., and Bond, E., *Proc. Soc. Exp. Biol. Med.*, 73, 243–246, 1950.
393. Hungerland, H. and Raming, P., *Klin. Wochenschr.*, 29, 582–583, 1951.
394. Schrade, W., *Klin. Wochenschr.*, 31, 656–662, 1953.
395. Abelin, I. and Pfister, H., *Klin. Wochenschr.*, 28, 790, 1950.
396. Gottfried, E. L., *J. Lipid Res.*, 8, 321–327, 1967.
397. Schwandt, P., Birk, J., and Ehrhart, H., *Klin. Wochenschr.*, 46, 687–689, 1968.
398. Majerus, P. W. and Lastra, R., *J. Clin. Invest.*, 46, 1596–1602, 1967.
399. Elsbach, P., *Biochim. Biophys. Acta*, 84, 8–17, 1964.
400. Yu, B. P., Kummerow, F. A., and Nishida, T., *J. Nutr.*, 89, 435–440, 1966.
401. Kaley, J. S., Meng, H. C., and Bingham, C., *Am. J. Clin. Nutr.*, 7, 652–656, 1959.
402. Lefholz, R., *Am. J. Anat.*, 32, 1–35, 1923.
403. Sinclair, H. M., in *Nutrition: A Comprehensive Treatise*, Vol. 1, Beaton, G. H. and McHenry, E. W., Eds., Academic Press, New York, 1964, 41–114.
404. Godlowski, Z. Z., *Br. Med. J.*, 1, 854–855, 1951.
405. Hamilton, L. H., *Endocrinology*, 61, 392–397, 1957.
406. Jansen, C. R., Cronkite, E. P., Mather, G. C., Nielsen, N. O., Rai, K., Adamik, E. R., and Sipe, C. R., *Blood*, 20, 443–451, 1962.
407. Zollner, H., *Folia Haematol.* (Leipzig), 90, 394–400, 1968.
408. Lennert, K. and Parwaresch, M. R., *Schweiz. Med. Wochenschr.*, 100, 1410–1415, 1970.
409. Shelley, W. B. and Juhlin, L., *Am. J. Med. Sci.*, 242, 211–222, 1961.
410. Engelberg, H., *Proc. Soc. Exp. Biol. Med.*, 97, 304–308, 1958.
411. Grabener, E., *Med. Klin.* (Munich), 70, 510–515, 1975.
412. Santisteban, G. A., *Q. J. Stud. Alcohol*, 22, 1–13, 1961.
413. Aschkenasy, A., Spach, C., and Aschkenasy-Lelu, P., *Ann. Nutr. Aliment.*, 23, 195–214, 1969.
414. Herbert, V., Zalusky, R., and Davidson, C. S., *Ann. Intern. Med.*, 58, 977–988, 1963.
415. McFarland, W. and Libre, E. P., *Ann. Intern. Med.*, 59, 865–877, 1963.
416. Stokes, P. E. and Lasley, B. J., *J. Clin. Invest.*, 43, 1302, 1964 (abstr.).
417. Olson, R. E., *Am. J. Clin. Nutr.*, 28, 626–637, 1975.
418. Takasu, K., *Mitt. Med. Ges. Tokyo*, 17, 395–404, 1903 (cited by Jackson[153]).
419. Nagayo, M., *JAMA*, 81, 1435–1437, 1923.

420. Tasawa, R., *Z. Exp. Pathol. Ther.*, 17, 27–46, 1915.
421. Deane, H. W. and Shaw, J. H., *J. Nutr.*, 34, 1–20, 1947.
422. Doctor, V. M., *Blood*, 14, 1244–1249, 1959.
423. Carter, B. B. and Axelrod, A. E., *Proc. Soc. Exp. Biol. Med.*, 67, 416–417, 1948.
424. Aschkenasy, A., *Ann. Biol. Clin.*, 5, 262–272, 1947.
425. Aschkenasy, A., Boissier, J., and Rolland, G. J., *Bull. Soc. Chim. Biol.*, 31, 1019–1028, 1949.
426. Aschkenasy, A. and Mignot, J., *C.R. Soc. Biol.*, 140, 208–210, 1946; 141, 19–20, 1947.
427. Malaguzzi Valeri, C., *Klin. Wochenschr.*, 22, 391–392, 1943.
428. Musser, E. A. and Heinle, R. W., *Blood*, 13, 464–474, 1958.
429. Stoerk, H. C. and Emerson, G. A., *Proc. Soc. Exp. Biol. Med.*, 70, 703–704, 1949.
430. Goldsmith, G. A., in *Nutrition: A Comprehensive Treatise*, Vol. 2, Beaton, G. H. and McHenry, E. W., Eds., Academic Press, New York, 1964, 109–206.
431. Handler, P., *Int. Z. Vitaminforsch.*, 19, 393–451, 1948.
432. Krehl, W. A. and Elvehjem, C. A., *J. Biol. Chem.*, 158, 173–179, 1945.
433. Melampy, R. M., Cheng, D. W., and Northrop, L. C., *Proc. Soc. Exp. Biol. Med.*, 76, 24–27, 1957.
434. Deane, H. W. and McKiblin, J. M., *Endocrinology*, 38, 385–400, 1946.
435: Dumm, M. E., Ovando, P., Roth, P., and Ralli, E. P., *Proc. Soc. Exp. Biol. Med.*, 71, 368–371, 1949.
436. Winters, R. W., Schultz, R. B., and Krehl, W. A., *Endocrinology*, 50, 377–384, 1952.
437. Bean, W. B. and Hodges, R. E., *Proc. Soc. Exp. Biol. Med.*, 86, 693–698, 1954.
438. Cowgill, G. R., Winters, R. W., Schultz, R. B., and Krehl, W. A., *Int. Z. Vitaminforsch.*, 23, 275–298, 1952.
439. Ralli, E. P. and Dumm, M. E., *Vitam. Horm.* (N.Y.), 11, 133–158, 1953.
440. Wertman, K. and Sarandria, J. L., *Proc. Soc. Exp. Biol. Med.*, 76, 388–390, 1951.
441. Axelrod, A. E., Carter, B. B., McCoy, R. H., and Geisinger, R., *Proc. Soc. Exp. Biol. Med.*, 66, 137–140, 1947.
442. Stavitsky, A., Pruzansky, J., and Axelrod, A. E., unpublished, 1954 (cited by Axelrod, A. E. and Pruzansky, J.[490]).
443. Hodges, R. E., Bean, W. B., Ohlson, M. A., and Bleiler, R. E., *Am. J. Clin. Nutr.*, 11, 85–93, 1962.
444. Dinning, J. S., Neatrour, R., and Day, P. L., *J. Nutr.*, 53, 557–562, 1954.
445. Ludovici, P. P., Axelrod, A. E., and Carter, B. B., *Proc. Soc. Exp. Biol. Med.*, 76, 670–672, 1951.
446. Morgan, A. F., Groody, M., and Axelrod, A. E., *Am. J. Physiol.*, 146, 723–738, 1946.
447. Hawkins, W. W. and Evans, M. K., *Am. J. Physiol.*, 170, 160–167, 1952.
448. McCall, K. B., Waismann, H. A., Elvehjem, C. A., and Jones, E. S., *J. Nutr.*, 31, 685–697, 1946.
449. Carpenter, K. J. and Kodicek, E., *Br. J. Nutr.*, 2, IX, 1948.
450. Butler, L. C. and Morgan, A. F., *Proc. Soc. Exp. Biol. Med.*, 85, 441–444, 1954.
451. Asmar, J. A., Daghir, N. J., and Azar, H. A., *J. Nutr.*, 95, 153–159, 1968.
452. Weir, D. R., Heinle, R. W., and Welch, A. D., *Proc. Soc. Exp. Biol. Med.*, 72, 457–461, 1949.
453. Rosen, F., Mihich, E., and Nichol, C. A., *Vitam. Horm.* (N.Y.), 22, 609–641, 1964.
454. Stoerk, H. C. and Zucker, T. F., *Proc. Soc. Exp. Biol. Med.*, 56, 151–153, 1944.
455. Mushett, C. W., Stebbins, R. B., and Barton, M. N., *Trans. N.Y. Acad. Sci.*, 9, 291–296, 1947.
456. Stoerk, H. C., *Ann. N.Y. Acad. Sci.*, 52, 1302–1317, 1950.
457. Mueller, J. F., Weir, D. R., and Heinle, R. W., *Proc. Soc. Exp. Biol. Med.*, 77, 312–315, 1951.
458. Stoerk, H. C. and Eisen, H. N., *Proc. Soc. Exp. Biol. Med.*, 62, 88–89, 1946.
459. Axelrod, A. E. and Hopper, S., *J. Nutr.*, 72, 325–330, 1960.
460. Axelrod, A. E., Hopper, S., and Long, D. A., *J. Nutr.*, 74, 58–64, 1961.
461. Axelrod, A. E., Trakatellis, A. C., Block, H., and Stinebring, W. R., *J. Nutr.*, 79, 161–167, 1963.
462. Stoerk, H. C., Eisen, H. N., and John, H. M., *J. Exp. Med.*, 85, 365–371, 1947.
463. Axelrod, A. E., Fisher, B., Fisher, E., Lee, Y. C. P., and Walsh, P., *Science*, 127, 1388–1389, 1958.
464. Axelrod, A. E. and Trakatellis, A. C., *Vitam. Horm.* (N.Y.), 22, 591–607, 1964.
465. Robson, L. C. and Schwartz, M. R., *Cell. Immunol.*, 16, 135–144, 1975.
466. Baumgartner, R., Obenaus, H., and Stoerk, H. E., *Proc. Soc. Exp. Biol. Med.*, 146, 241–244, 1974.
467. Wayne, L., Will, J. J., Friedman, B. I., Becker, L. S., and Vilter, R. W., *Arch. Intern. Med.*, 101, 143–155, 1958.
468. Stoerk, H. C., *J. Biol. Chem.*, 171, 437–438, 1947.
469. Bischoff, F., Ingraham, L. P., and Ruff, J. J., *Arch. Pathol.*, 35, 713–716, 1943.

470. Kline, B. E., Rusch, H. P., Baumann, C. A., and Lavik, P. S., *Cancer Res.,* 3, 825–829, 1943.
471. Skipper, H. E., Thomson, J. R., and Schabel, F. M., Jr., *Cancer Chemother. Rep.,* 29, 63–76, 1963 (cited by Rosen et al.[453]).
472. Weir, D. R. and Morningstar, W. A., *Blood,* 9, 173–182, 1954.
473. Trakatellis, A. C., Axelrod, A. E., Montjar, M., and Lamy, F., *Nature,* 202, 154–157, 1964.
474. Montjar, M., Axelrod, A. E., and Trakatellis, A. C., *J. Nutr.,* 85, 45–51, 1965.
475. Franklin, A. L., Stokstad, E. L. R., Belt, M., and Jukes, T. H., *J. Biol. Chem.,* 169, 427–435, 1947.
476. Philips, F. S. and Thiersch, J. B., *J. Pharmacol. Exp. Ther.,* 95, 302–311, 1949.
477. Dougherty, J. H. and Dougherty, T. F., *J. Lab. Clin. Med.,* 35, 271–279, 1950.
478. Cartwright, G. E., Tatting, B., Ashenbrueker, H., and Wintrobe, M. M., *Blood,* 4, 301–323, 1949.
479. Langston, W. C., Darby, W. J., Shukers, C. F., and Day, P. L., *J. Exp. Med.,* 68, 923–940, 1938.
480. Slungaerd, R. K. and Higgins, G. M., *Blood,* 11, 123–142, 1956.
481. Hogan, A. G. and Parrott, E. M., *J. Biol. Chem.,* 132, 507–517, 1940.
482. Stokstad, E. L. R., *Vitam. Horm.* (N.Y.), 26, 443–463, 1968.
483. Simpson, R. E., Schweigert, B. S., and Pearson, P. B., *Proc. Soc. Exp. Biol. Med.,* 70, 611–612, 1949.
484. Daft, F. S., McDaniel, E. G., Herman, L. G., Romine, M. K., and Hegner, J. R., *Fed. Proc. Fed. Am. Soc. Exp. Biol.,* 22, 129–133, 1963.
485. Daft, F. S. and Sebrell, W. H., *Vitam. Horm.* (N.Y.), 3, 49–72, 1945.
486. Shehata, O. and Johnson, B. C., *Proc. Soc. Exp. Biol. Med.,* 67, 332–335, 1948.
487. Aschkenasy, A., Aschkenasy-Lelu, P., and Rolland, G. J., *Bull. Soc. Chim. Biol.,* 31, 1451–1465, 1949.
488. Wertman, K., Crisley, F. D., and Sarandria, J. L., *Proc. Soc. Exp. Biol. Med.,* 80, 404–406, 1952.
489. Ludovici, P. P. and Axelrod, A. E., *Proc. Soc. Exp. Biol. Med.,* 77, 526–530, 1951.
490. Axelrod, A. and Pruzansky, J., *Vitam. Horm.* (N.Y.), 13, 1–27, 1955.
491. Little, P. A., Oleson, J. J., and Roesch, P. K., *J. Immunol.,* 65, 491–498, 1950.
492. Haas, V. H., Stewart, S. E., and Briggs, G. M., *Virology,* 3, 15–21, 1957.
493. Briggs, G. M., *Am. J. Clin. Nutr.,* 7, 390–396, 1959.
494. Herbert, V., *The Megaloblastic Anemias,* Grune & Stratton, New York, 1959.
495. Varadi, S., Abbott, D., and Elwis, A., *J. Clin. Pathol.,* 19, 33–36, 1966.
496. Herbert, V., *Trans. Assoc. Am. Physicians,* 75, 307, 1962.
497. Hoffbrand, A. V. and Newcombe, B. A., *Br. J. Haematol.,* 13, 954–966, 1967.
498. Farber, S., *Blood,* 4, 160–167, 1949.
499. Roberts, P. D., Hoffbrand, A. V., and Mollin, D. L., *Br. Med. J.,* 2, 198–202, 1966.
500. Gough, K. R., McCarthy, C., Read, A. E., Mollin, D. L., and Waters, A. H., *Br. Med. J.,* 1, 212–217, 1964.
501. Gross, R. L., Reid, J. V. O., Newberne, P. M., Burgess, B., Marston, R., and Hift, W., *Am. J. Clin. Nutr.,* 28, 225–232, 1975.
502. Van der Weyden, M., Rother, M., and Firkin, B., *Br. J. Haematol.,* 22, 299–307, 1972.
503. Stokstad, E. L. R. and Koch, J., *Physiol. Rev.,* 47, 83–116, 1967.
504. Rozenszajn, L. A. and Radnay, J., *Blood,* 43, 401–409, 1974.
505. Grignani, F., Martelli, M., Tonato, M., and Colonna, A., *Acta Haematol.,* 34, 72–87, 1965.
506. Ellegaard, J. and Esmann, V., *Scand. J. Clin. Lab. Invest.,* 31, 9–19, 1973.
507. Ellegaard, J. and Esmann, V., *Br. J. Haematol.,* 24, 571–577, 1973.
508. Robertson, J. S., Hsia, Y. E., and Scully, K. J., *J. Lab. Clin. Med.,* 87, 89–97, 1976.
509. Das, K. C. and Hoffbrand, A. V., *Br. J. Haematol.,* 19, 203–221, 1969.
510. Swendseid, M. E., Bethell, F. H., and Bird, O. D., *Cancer Res.,* 11, 864–867, 1951.
511. Wilmanns, W., *Dtsch. Med. Wochenschr.,* 88, 900–907, 1963.
512. Cartwright, G. E., Tatting, B., Kurth, D., and Wintrobe, M. M., *Blood,* 7, 992–1004, 1952.
513. Valencia, R. and Sacquet, E., *Ann. Nutr. Aliment.,* 22, 71–76, 1968.
514. Borson, H. J., Singman, D., Lepkovsky, S., Dimick, M. K., Gase, V., and Perry, R., *Am. J. Physiol.,* 162, 714–720, 1950.
515. Newberne, P. M. and O'Dell, B. L., *Proc. Soc. Exp. Biol. Med.,* 100, 335–337, 1959.
516. Underwood, E. J., *Trace Elements in Human and Animal Nutrition,* 2nd ed., Academic Press, New York, 1962, 164.
517. Aschkenasy, A. and Pariente, Ph., *Rev. Hematol.,* 6, 166–183, 1951.
518. Pentz, E. I., Graham, C. E., Ryan, D. E., and Klein, D., *Endocrinology,* 47, 30–35, 1950.
519. Meites, J., *Metab. Clin. Exp.,* 1, 58–67, 1952.

520. Meites, J., Feng, Y. S. L., and Wilwerth, A. M., *Am. J. Clin. Nutr.,* 5, 381–392, 1957.
521. Axelrod, A. E., *Am. J. Clin. Nutr.,* 24, 265–271, 1971.
522. Thomas, J. W. and Anderson, B. B., *Br. J. Haematol.,* 2, 41–43, 1956.
523. Meyer, L. M., Cronkite, E. P., Miller, I. F., Mulzac, C. W., and Jones, I., *Blood,* 19, 229–235, 1962.
524. Simons, K. and Weber, T., *Biochim. Biophys. Acta,* 117, 201–208, 1966.
525. Bloomfield, F. J. and Scott, J. M., *Br. J. Haematol.,* 22, 33–42, 1972.
526. Zittoun, J., Marquet, J., and Zittoun, R., *Br. J. Haematol.,* 31, 299–310, 1975.
527. Carmel, R., *Br. J. Haematol.,* 22, 53–62, 1972.
528. Carmel, R. and Coltman, C. A., Jr., *Blood,* 37, 31–39, 1971.
529. Retief, F. P., Vandenplas, L., and Visser, H., *Br. J. Haematol.,* 16, 231–240, 1969.
530. Miller, A. and Sullivan, J. F., *J. Lab. Clin. Med.,* 53, 607–616, 1959.
531. Mollin, D. L. and Ross, G. I. M., *Br. J. Haematol.,* 1, 155–172, 1955.
532. Rachmilewitz, M., Izak, G., Hochman, A., Aronovitch, J., and Grossowicz, N., *Blood,* 12, 804–813, 1957.
533. Aschkenasy, A., *Sang,* 18, 389–401, 1947.
534. Perillie, P. E., Kaplan, S. S., and Finch, S. C., *N.E. J. Med.,* 277, 10–12, 1967.
535. Fink, M. E. and Finch, S. C., *Clin. Res.,* 14, 316, 1966.
536. Silber, R. and Moldow, C. F., *Am. J. Med.,* 48, 549–554, 1970.
537. Seashore, M. R., Hsia, V. E., Scully, K., Durant, J. L., and Rosenberg, L. E., *Am. J. Clin. Nutr.,* 26, 873–875, 1973.
538. Contreras, E. and Giorgio, A. J., *Am. J. Clin. Nutr.,* 25, 695–702, 1972.
539. Karlin, R., Creyssel, R., Creyssel, H., and Croizat, P., *Nouv. Rev. Fr. Hematol.,* 5, 721–727, 1965.
540. Parry, T. E., *Br. J. Haematol.,* 16, 221–229, 1969.
541. Herbert, V., Larrabee, A. B., and Buchanan, J. M., *J. Clin. Invest.,* 41, 1134–1138, 1962.
542. Piliero, S. J. and Gordon, A. S., *Acta Haematol.,* 11, 114–128, 1954.
543. Perla, D. and Marmorsten, J., *Arch. Pathol.,* 23, 543–683, 1937.
544. Nungester, W. J. and Ames, A. M., *J. Infect. Dis.,* 83, 50–54, 1948.
545. Mills, C. A., *Blood,* 4, 150–159, 1949.
546. Cooper, M. R., McCall, C. E., and De Chatelet, L. R., *Infect. Immun.,* 3, 851–853, 1971.
547. Mohanram, M. and Srikantia, S. G., *Clin. Sci.,* 32, 215–222, 1967.
548. Stephens, D. J. and Hewley, E. E., *J. Biol. Chem.,* 115, 653–658, 1936.
549. Lloyd, B. B. and Sinclair, H. B., in *Biochemistry and Physiology of Nutrition,* Vol. 1, Bourne, G. H. and Kidder, G. W., Eds., Academic Press, New York 1953, 369–471.
550. Brook, M. and Grimshaw, J. J., *Am. J. Clin. Nutr.,* 21, 1254–1258, 1968.
551. Calder, J. H., Curtis, R. C., and Fore, H., *Lancet,* i, 556, 1963.
552. Burr, M. L., Elwood, P. C., Hole, D. J., Hurley, R. J., and Hughes, R. C., *Am. J. Clin. Nutr.,* 27, 147–151, 1974.
553. Crandon, J. H., Lund, C. C., and Dill, D. B., *N.E. J. Med.,* 223, 353–369, 1940.
554. Nichol, C. A. and Welch, A. D., *Proc. Soc. Exp. Biol. Med.,* 74, 52–55, 1950.
555. Gabuzda, G. J., Jr., Phillips, G. B., Schilling, R. F., and Davidson, C. S., *J. Clin. Invest.,* 31, 756–761, 1952.
556. Hartley, P., *Proc. R. Soc. Med.,* 36, 147–148, 1942.
557. Long, D. A., *Br. J. Exp. Pathol.,* 31, 183–188, 1950.
558. Natvig, H., *Nutr. Abst. Rev.,* 12, 198–199, 1942.
559. Lassen, H. C. A., *J. Hyg.,* 30, 300, 1930 (cited by Scrimshaw et al.[1]).
560. Lassen, H. C. A., *Experimental Studies in the Course of Paratyphoid Infections in Avitaminotic Rats with Special Reference to Vitamin A Deficiencies,* Levin and Munksgaard, Copenhagen, 1931, 247 (cited by Scrimshaw et al.[1]).
561. Dresser, D. W., *Nature,* 217, 527–529, 1968.
562. Florsheim, G. L. and Bollag, W., *Transplantation,* 15, 564–567, 1972 (cited by Felix et al.[564]).
563. Meltzer, M. S. and Cohen, B. E., *J. Natl. Cancer Inst.,* 53, 585, 1974 (cited by Felix et al.[564]).
564. Felix, E. L., Loyd, B., and Cohen, M. H., *Science,* 189, 886–888, 1975.
565. Dinning, J. S. and Day, P. L., *J. Exp. Med.,* 105, 395–402, 1957.
566. Darby, W. J., *Vitam. Horm.* (N.Y.), 26, 685–699, 1968.
567. Arroyave, G., *Am. J. Clin. Nutr.,* 22, 1119–1128, 1969.
568. Olson, J. A., *Vitam. Horm.* (N.Y.), 26, 1–63, 1968.
569. Vakil, U. K., Roels, O. A., and Trout, M., *Br. J. Nutr.,* 18, 217, 1964 (cited by Arroyave[567]).
570. Chanarin, I., Bennett, M. C., and Berry, V., *J. Clin. Pathol.,* 15, 269–273, 1962.
571. Roberts, P. D., St. John, D. J. B., Sinha, R., Stewart, J. S., Baird, I. M., Coghill, N. F., and Morgan, J. O., *Br. J. Haematol.,* 20, 165–176, 1971.

572. Toskes, P. P., Smith, G. W., Bensinger, T. A., Giannella, R. A., and Conrad, M. E., *Am. J. Clin. Nutr.,* 27, 355–361, 1974.
573. Vitale, J. J., Restrepo, A., Velez, H., Risker, J. B., and Hellerstein, E., *J. Nutr.,* 88, 315–322, 1966.
574. Arakawa, T., Ohara, K., Tahahashi, Y., et al., *Ann. Paediatr.,* 205, 1–11, 1965.
575. Beutler, E., *Ser. Haematol.,* 6, 41–55, 1965.
576. Higashi, O. and Sato, Y., *Tohoku J. Exp. Med.,* 93, 105–113, 1967.
577. Baggs, R. B. and Miller, S. A., *J. Nutr.,* 103, 1554–1560, 1973.
578. Masson, P. L., Heremans, J. F., and Schonne, E., *J. Exp. Med.,* 130, 643–656, 1969.
579. Reiter, B., Brock, J. H., and Steel, E. D., *Immunology,* 28, 83–95, 1975.
580. Summers, M., Worwood, M., and Jacobs, A., *Br. J. Haematol.,* 28, 19–26, 1974.
581. Joynson, D. H. M., Walker, D. M., Jacobs, A., and Dolky, A. E., *Lancet,* ii, 1058–1059, 1972.
582. Kulapongs, P., Vithayasai, V., Suskind, R., and Olson, R. E., *Lancet,* ii, 689–691, 1974.
583. Weinberg, E. D., *Science,* 184, 952–956, 1974.
584. MacDonald, R. A., *Am. J. Clin. Nutr.,* 23, 592–603, 1970.
585. Soltys, H. D. and Brody, J. I., *J. Lab. Clin. Med.,* 75, 250–257, 1970.
586. Wintrobe, M. M., Cartwright, G. E., and Gubler, C. J., *J. Nutr.,* 50, 395–419, 1953.
587. Cordano, A., Placko, R. P., and Graham, G. G., *Blood,* 28, 280–283, 1966.
588. Vallee, B. L., *Physiol. Rev.,* 39, 443–490, 1959.
589. Dennes, E., Tupper, R., and Wormall, A., *Biochem. J.,* 82, 466–476, 1962.
590. Angyal, A. M. and Archer, G. T., *Aust. J. Exp. Biol. Med. Sci.,* 46, 119–121, 1968.
591. Szmigielski, S. and Litwin, J., *Blood,* 25, 56–62, 1965.
592. Trubowitz, S., Feldman, D., Benante, C., and Kirman, D., *Proc. Soc. Exp. Biol. Med.,* 95, 35–38, 1957.
593. Macapinlac, P. M., Pearson, W. N., and Darby, W. J., in *Zinc Metabolism,* Prasad, A. S., Ed., Charles C Thomas, Springfield, Ill., 1966, 142.
594. Miller, E. R., Luecke, R. W., Ullrey, D. E., Baltzer, B. V., Bradley, B. L., and Hoefer, J. A., *J. Nutr.,* 95, 278–286, 1968.
595. Dreosti, I. E., Tao, S., and Hurley, L. S., *Proc. Soc. Exp. Biol. Med.,* 128, 169–174, 1968.
596. Sandstead, H. H. and Rinaldi, R. A., *J. Cell Physiol.,* 73, 81–83, 1969.
597. Terhune, M. W. and Sandstead, H. H., *Science,* 177, 68–69, 1972.
598. Hsu, J. M., Anthony, W. L., and Buchanan, P. J., *J. Nutr.,* 99, 425–432, 1969.
599. Alford, R. H., *J. Immunol.,* 104, 698–703, 1970.
600. Hawkins, W. W., in *Nutrition: A Comprehensive Treatise,* Vol. 1, Beaton, G. H. and McHenry, E. W., Eds., Academic Press, New York, 1964, 309–372.
601. Fisher, J. W. and Langston, J. W., *Ann. N.Y. Acad. Sci.,* 149, 75–87, 1968.
602. Hitchings, G. H., Falco, E. A., and Sherwood, M., *Fed. Proc. Fed. Am. Soc. Exp. Biol.,* 8, 207, 1949.
603. Thomas, C. B., *Ann. Intern. Med.,* 39, 289–306, 1953.
604. Kornberg, A. and Endicott, K. M., *Am. J. Physiol.,* 145, 291–298, 1946.
605. Lubin, M., *Fed. Proc. Fed. Am. Soc. Exp. Biol.,* 23, 994–1001, 1964.
606. Cannon, P. R., Frazier, L. E., and Hughes, R. H., *Metab. Clin. Exp.,* 1, 49–57, 1952.
607. Tullis, J. L., *J. Clin. Invest.,* 26, 1098–1108, 1947.
608. Bluemel, C. S. and Lewis, R., *Am. J. Physiol.,* 67, 464–466, 1924.
609. Beard, L. A. and Beard, J. W., *Am. J. Physiol.,* 85, 169–177, 1928.
610. Aschkenasy, A., *Ann. N.Y. Acad. Sci.,* 77, 574–588, 1959.
611. Selye, H., *Annual Report on Stress,* Acta, Montreal, 1951, 107–108.
612. Aschkenasy, A., *Sang,* 28, 400–446, 1957.
613. Schettler, G., *Klin. Wochenschr.,* 30, 229, 1952.
614. Leschi, J., *C.R. Acad. Sci.,* 239, 720–721, 1954.
615. Allison, F., Jr., Lancaster, B. A., and Crosthwaite, J. L., *Am. J. Pathol.,* 43, 775–795, 1963.
616. Bryant, R. E., *Proc. Soc. Exp. Biol. Med.,* 130, 975–977, 1969.
617. Valentine, W. N., Tanaka, K. R., and Fredricks, R. E., *J. Lab. Clin. Med.,* 55, 303–310, 1960.
618. Rosner, F. and Lee, S. L., *J. Lab. Clin. Med.,* 79, 228–239, 1972.
619. Kruse, H. D., Orent, E. V., and McCollum, E. V., *J. Biol. Chem.,* 96, 519–539, 1932.
620. Hungerford, G. F. and Karson, E. F., *Blood,* 16, 1642–1650, 1960.
621. Bois, P., Gascon, A., and Beaulnes, A., *Nature,* 197, 501–502, 1963.
622. Bois, P., *Br. J. Exp. Pathol.,* 44, 151–155, 1963.
623. Bois, P., *Nature,* 204, 1316, 1964.
624. Battifora, H., McCreary, P., Laing, G. H., and Hass, G. M., *Presbyterian-St. Luke's Hosp. Med. Bull.,* 5, 2–11, 1966 (cited in *Leuk. Abstr.,* 14, 67, 1966).

625. McCreary, P. A., Battifora, H. A., Hahneman, B. M., Laing, C. H., and Hass, G. M., *J. Lab. Clin. Med.,* 72, 991, 1968 (abstr.).
626. Jasmin, G., *Rev. Can. Biol.,* 22, 383–389, 1963.
627. Rosner, F. and Gorfien, P. C., *J. Lab. Clin. Med.,* 72, 213–219, 1968.
628. Lowenhaupt, E., Schulman, M. P., and Greenberg, D. M., *Arch. Pathol.,* 49, 427–433, 1950.
629. Haury, V. G., *J. Lab. Clin. Med.,* 27, 1361–1375, 1942.
630. Delaunay, A., *Ann. Inst. Pasteur* (Paris), 70, 372–375, 1944.
631. Rabinowitz, Y., *Blood,* 23, 811–828, 1964.
632. Perris, A. D. and Whitfield, J. F., *Nature,* 214, 302, 1967; 216, 1350, 1967.
633. Perris, A. D. and Whitfield, J. F., *Proc. Soc. Exp. Biol. Med.,* 130, 1198–1201, 1969.
634. Rose, W. C., Osterling, M. J., and Womack, M., *J. Biol. Chem.,* 176, 753–762, 1948.
635. Claesson, M. H., *Scand. J. Haematol.,* 6, 87–92, 1969.
636. Blackwater, M. J., Levert, L. A., and Hijmans, W., *Immunology,* 28, 847–854, 1975.
637. Shilotri, P. G., *J. Nutr.,* 107, 1513–1516, 1977.
638. Henson, P., *J. Exp. Med.,* 134, 114s–135s, 1971.
639. Camussi, G., Mencia-Huerta, J. M., and Benveniste, J., *Immunology,* 33, 523–534, 1977.
640. Weissman, G. and Dukor, P., *Adv. Immunol.,* 12, 283–322, 1970.
641. Camussi, G., Tetta, C., and Cappio, F. C., *Int. Arch. Allergy Appl. Immun.,* 58, 135–139, 1979.
642. Suda, A. K., Mathur, M., Deo, K., and Deo, M. C., *Blood,* 48, 865–875, 1976.
643. Aschkenasy, A., *Ann. Nutr. Alim.,* 32, 15–40, 1978.
644. Aschkenasy, A., *Nutr. Rep. Internat.,* 18, 177–185, 1978.
645. Bryant, B. J., Hess, M. W., and Cottier, H., *Immunology,* 28, 115–120, 1975.
646. Modabber, F., *Contemp. Topics Immunobiol.,* 2, 207, 1973.
647. Aschkenasy, A., *Ann. Nutr. Alim.,* (Paris), 33, 259–270, 1979.
648. Greaves, M. and Janossy, G., *Transpl. Rev.,* 11, 87–130, 1972.
649. Stobo, J. D. and Paul, E. W., *J. Immunol.,* 110, 362–375, 1973.
650. Rawson, A. J. and Huang, T. C., *Cell. Immunol.,* 17, 310–314, 1975.
651. Baldijao, C., Atinmo, T., Pond, W. G., and Barnes, R. H., *J. Nutr.,* 106, 952–957, 1976.
652. Aschkenasy, A., *J. Nutr.,* 109, 1214–1222, 1979.
653. Bounous, G. and Kongshavn, P. A. L., *Immunology,* 35, 257–266, 1978.
654. Gershon, R. K., *Contemp. Topics Immunology,* 3, 1, 1974.
655. Price, P. and Bell, R. G., *Immunology,* 31, 953–960, 1976.
656. Price, P. and Turner, K. J., *Clin. Exp. Immunol.,* 35, 25, 1979.
657. Spach, C. and Aschkenasy, A., *J. Nutr.,* 107, 1729–1736, 1977.
658. Spach, C. and Aschkenasy, A., *J. Nutr.,* 109, 1265–1273, 1979.
659. Aschkenasy, A., *J. Nutr.,* 108, 1527–1539, 1978.
660. Himsworth, H. P. and Glynn, L. E., *Clin. Science,* 5, 93–123, 1944.
661. Aschkenasy, A. and Mignot, J., *C. R. Soc. Biol. (Paris),* 140, 206–208, 1946.
662. Himsworth, H. P. and Glynn, L. E., *Clin. Science,* 5, 133–137, 1979.
663. Silber, R. H. and Porter, C. C., *Endocrinology,* 52, 518–525, 1953.
664. Schopfer, K. and Douglas, D. S., *Clin. Immunol. Immunopath.,* 5, 21–29, 1976.
665. Kutty, K. M., Chandra, R. K., and Chandra, S., *Experientia,* 32, 289–291, 1976.
666. Sirinha, S., Suskind, R., Edelman, R., Asvapaka, C., and Olson, R. E., *Pediatrics,* 55, 166–170, 1975.
667. Reddy, V., Raghuramulu, N., and Bhaskaram, C., *Arch. Dis. Child.,* 51, 871–874, 1976.
668. Chandra, R. K., *Brit. Med. J.,* 2, 583–585, 1975.
669. Chandra, R. K., *Arch. Dis. Child.,* 50, 532–534, 1975.
670. Tonkin. C. H. and Brostoff, J., *Int. Arch. All. Appl. Immunol.,* 57, 171–176, 1978.
671. Johnson, W. D. Jr., *Ann. N.Y. Acad. Sci.,* 252, 343–347, 1975.
672. Bernstein, I. M., Webster, K. H., Williams, R. C. Jr., and Strickland, R. G., *Lancet,* ii, 488–490, 1974.
673. Tisman, G. and Herbert, V., *J. Clin. Invest.,* 52, 1410–1414, 1973.
674. Leevy, C. M., Chen Th., and Zetterman, R., *Ann. N. Y. Acad. Sci.,* 252, 106–115, 1975.
675. Hsu, C. C. S. and Leevy, C. M., *Clin. Exp. Immunol.,* 8, 749–760, 1971.
676. Newberry, W. M., Shorey, J. W., Sanford, J. P., and Combes, B., *Cell. Immunol.,* 6, 87–97, 1973.
677. Young, C. P., Van der Weyden, M. B., Rose, I. S., and Dudley, F. J., *Experientia,* 35, 268–269, 1979.
678. Paronetto, F. and Lieber, Ch. S., *Proc. Soc. Exp. Biol. Med.,* 153, 495–497, 1976.
679. Cheng, Ch. H., Koch, M., and Shank, R. E., *J. Nutr.,* 106, 1678–1685, 1976.

680. Markkanen, T. and Paltola, O., *Acta Haematol.,* 44, 78–84, 1970.
681. Willis-Carr, J. I. and St. Pierre, R. L., *J. Immunol.,* 120, 1153–1159, 1978.
682. Kumar, M. and Axelrod, A. E., *Proc. Soc. Exp. Biol. Med.,* 157, 421–429, 1978.
683. Goetzl, E. J., Wasserman, S. I., Gigli, I., and Austen, K. F., *J. Clin. Invest.,* 53, 813–818, 1974.
684. Sandler, J. A., Gallin, J. I., and Vaughan, M., *J. Cell Biol.,* 67, 480–484, 1975.
685. Goetzl, E. J., *Ann. Rheumatic Dis.,* 35, 510, 1976.
686. Fudenberg, H. H., Stites, D. P., Caldwell, J. L., and Wells, J. V., *Basic and Clinical Immunology,* Lange Medical Publications, Los Altos, Cal., 1976.
687. Baehner, R. L., Boxer, L. A., Allen, J. M., and Davis, J., *Blood,* 50, 327–335, 1977.
688. Shilotri, P. C., and Bhat, K. S., *Am. J. Clin. Nutr.,* 30, 1077–1081, 1977.
689. McCall, C. E., De Chatelet, L. R., Cooper, M. R., and Ashburn, P., *J. Infect. Dis.,* 124, 194–198, 1971.
690. Stankova, L., Gerhardt, N. B., Nagel, N., and Bigley, R. H., *Infect. Immun.,* 12, 252–256, 1975.
691. Boxer, L. A., Watanabe, A. M., Rister, M., Besch, H. P. Jr., Allen, J., and Baehner, R. L., *N. Engl. J. Med.,* 295, 1041–1045, 1976.
692. Yonemoto, R. H., Cretien, P. B., and Fehniger, T. F., *Am. Soc. Clin. Oncol.,* Abstracts 17, 288, 1976.
693. Hsu, C. K., *Fed Proc.,* 36, 1177, 1977.
694. Siegel, B. V. and Morton, J. I., *Experientia,* 33, 393–395, 1977.
695. Mueller, P. S. and Kies, M. W., *Nature (London),* 195, 813, 1962.
696. Zweiman, B., Schonwetter, F. W., and Hildreth, F. A., *J. Immunol.,* 96, 296–300, 1966.
697. Leibovitz, B. and Siegel, B. V., *Int. J. Vit. Nutr. Res.,* 48, 159–164, 1978.
698. Dennert, G. and Lotan, R., *Eur. J. Immunol.,* 8, 23–29, 1978.
699. Baggs, R. B., and Miller, S. A., *J. Infect. Dis.,* 130, 409–411, 1974.
700. Chu, S. W., Welch, K. J., Murray, E. S., and Hegsted, D. M., *Nutr. Rep. Intern.,* 14, 605–609, 1976.
701. Strauss, R. G., *Am. J. Clin. Nutr.,* 31, 660–666, 1978.
702. Bhaskaram, C. and Reddy, V., *Brit. Med. J.,* 3, 522, 1975.
703. Macdougall, L. G., Anderson, R., McNab, G. M., and Katz, J., *J. Pediatr.,* 86, 833, 1975.
704. Chandra, R. K., *J. Pediatr.,* 86, 899, 1975.
705. Srikantia, S. G., Prasad, J. S., Bhaskaram, C., and Krishnamachari, K. A. V. R., *Lancet,* 1, 1307, 1976.
706. Chvapil, M., Stankova, L., Zukoski, C. IV, and Zukoski, C. III, *J. Lab. Clin. Med.,* 89, 135–146, 1977.
707. Lennard, E. S., Bjornson, A. B., Petering, H., and Alexander, J., *J. Surg. Res.,* 16, 286–298, 1974.
708. Wannemacher, R., Pekarek, R. S., Klainer, A. S., Bartelloni, P., Dupont, H., Hornick, R., and Beisel, W., *Infect. Immun.,* 11, 873–875, 1975.
709. Metcoff, J., in *Malnutrition and the Immune Responses,* Suskind, R. M., Ed., Raven Press, New York, 1977, 285–292.
710. Bélanger, L. F., *J. Nutr.,* 108, 1315–1321, 1978.
711. Chesters, J. K., *Biochem. J.,* 130, 133–139, 1972.
712. Fraker, P. J., Haas, S. M., and Luecke, R. W., *J. Nutr.,* 107; 1889–1895, 1977.
713. Luecke, R. W., Simonel, C. E., and Fraker, P. J., *J. Nutr.,* 108, 881–887, 1978.
714. Fernandes, G., Nair, M., Onoc, K., *Proc. Natl. Acad. Sci.,* 76, 457–461, 1979.
715. Chevalier, Ph., Cornu, A., Delpeuch, F., and Joseph, A., *C. R. Acad. Sci., Paris,* 288, Ser. D, 267–270, 1979.
716. Guenounou, M., Armier, J., and Gaudin-Harding, F., *Intern. J. Vit. Nutr. Res.,* 48, 290–295, 1978.
717. Stein, R. S., Hanson, G., Koethe, S., *Blood,* 50 suppl. 1, 161, 1977.
718. Tismar, G., Herbert, V., and Rosenblatt, S., *Brit. J. Haematol.,* 24, 767–771, 1973.
719. Harker, W. G., Rothstein, G., Clarkson, D., *Blood,* 49, 263–267, 1977.
720. Gupta, R. C., Robinson, W. A., and Kurnick, J. E., *Am. J. Med.,* 61, 29–32, 1976.
721. Rossof, A. H., and Feher, K. M., *N. Engl. J. Med.,* 298, 280–281, 1978.

EFFECT OF NUTRITIONAL FACTORS ON MACROPHAGE PRODUCTION AND FUNCTION*

Gerald T. Keusch

INTRODUCTION

The macrophage was described originally as a large phagocytic cell which played a primary role in the removal of cellular debris due to injury or inflammation.[1] The greater complexity of the cell system of which the tissue macrophage is a component, and of the various roles played by these cells in inflammation and in immune responses, has only recently begun to be appreciated. We are at an even more primitive level of understanding when one asks, in addition, what is the impact of nutritional factors on macrophage production and function? This section will review current concepts of the macrophage and describe what is known of the affect of nutritional deprivation of the host on macrophage function and, then, pose a number of questions for future investigation.

THE NORMAL MACROPHAGE

Macrophage Production

The macrophage is the end result of differentiation of a primitive cell arising in the bone marrow.[2] At an early stage the precursor cell may be identified as a monoblast, a small, round cell without pseudopods, but possessing surface receptors for immunoglobulin and complement, and enzymatic activity including esterase, peroxidase, and lysozyme.[3,4] With further development, monocytes are released into the blood stream as functional, though not fully mature, cells.[5] Within several days of entrance into the blood stream, however, monocytes become tissue associated where they complete their development into more specialized macrophages.[6-8] This maturational process can be directly observed during in vitro culture of peripheral blood monocytes.[9,10] Increased turnover of macrophages is therefore reflected by peripheral blood monocytosis due to increased production and/or release of marrow precursors.[11] This is often noted in specific infections, e.g., tuberculosis, as well as in malignancy, connective tissue diseases, and vasculitis and various granulomatous diseases in which macrophages play an important role.[12]

In the rat, striking monocytosis can be produced by injection of incomplete Freund's adjuvant, colloidal carbon, or bovine serum albumin directly into cervical lymph nodes.[13] Serum from these animals is capable of causing monocytosis in normal animals, indicating the presence of a humoral factor involved in monocyte proliferation. This has been called "monocytogenic hormone". The same or similar factor inducing monocytosis, or FIM, is found during induced peritoneal exudates in mice and results in peripheral monocytosis when injected intravenously.[14,15] The time course of FIM production in the exudate mirrors the peripheral monocyte count.[16] FIM is a thermolabile protein, 18,000 to 24,000 daltons mol wt, unrelated to complement or clotting factors, apparently produced and released by activated macrophages, and without chemotactic or colony stimulating activity by in vitro bone marrow colony assay.[16,17]

Cultured mouse fibroblasts appear to produce a different factor which stimulates DNA synthesis in mouse peritoneal macrophages, and is called "macrophage growth

---

* The literature review for this paper covered the period through April 1978. The paper was submitted in June 1978.

factor'' (MGF).[18,19] MGF is a glycoprotein of molecular weight approximately 60,000 daltons, which migrates electrophoretically as an α-globulin, and is co-purified with, and may be identical to the granulocyte "colony stimulating factor" of mouse L cell cultures.[20,21]

Once mature, macrophages do not appear to de-differentiate or proliferate, and they have a prolonged life span ranging from months to years.[22] During differentiation, macrophages enlarge and show an increase in their content of enzyme containing granules.[9]

Macrophage Activation

The changes described above are even more prominent during the process of activation of macrophages by infection or immunologic engagement.[23] Activation is usually triggered by soluble mediator molecules, called lymphokines, released from sensitized lymphocytes.[24] Activated macrophages show an increase in ruffling of their plasma membrane, increase in content of lysosomal enzymes, hypertrophy of the Golgi zone, stimulation of oxidative metabolism, and in some instances, increased IgG receptor activity of the cell surface.[23] At the same time, these cells can be shown to possess an enhanced capacity for adhering to and spreading out on charged surfaces such as glass (perhaps representative of in vivo phenomena),[25] and they are more efficient at phagocytosis and intracellular killing of microorganisms.[26,27] Although the release of the activation mediators from lymphocytes is antigen specific, that is it occurs only during contact of a previously sensitized lymphocyte with the specific antigen, the activated macrophage is nonspecific in its ability to ingest and kill microorganisms, including totally unrelated species.[26,27]

Macrophage Metabolism in Phagocytosis

Within seconds of exposure to bacteria, there is a dramatic change in oxygen uptake and glucose metabolism by macrophages.[23,28] Increased oxygen consumption and oxidation of glucose through the hexose monophosphate shunt pathway is accompanied by an increase in hydrogen peroxide release and superoxide production.[29] Although similar metabolic changes occurring in phagocytizing polymorphonuclear leukocytes are clearly related to their bactericidal capacity,[30] there is no such correlation for macrophages.[31] These cells lose the peroxidase enzyme involved in the halide-peroxide-myeloperoxidase bactericidal reaction and apparently possess other bactericidal mechanisms of importance.[31,32]

Macrophages produce and secrete a number of proteins which may play a key role in host defense mechanisms. These proteins include an endogenous pyrogen, the second and fourth components of complement, interferon, lysozyme, transferrin, colony stimulating factor and plasminogen activator.[23,33-36]

Macrophage Surface Membrane Receptors in the Immune Response

Monocytes and macrophages have surface receptors for both the Fc portion of IgG_1 and IgG_3,[39] and for C_{3b}.[40] Binding to IgG has been further localized to a specific decapeptide of the CH_3 domain of the Fc fragment. These receptors turn over during phagocytosis[41] and are the recognition site on the cell membrane for microorganisms coated with IgG or C_{3b} opsonins.[42]

Mononuclear phagocytes respond with directed motion to certain stimuli, a process termed "chemotaxis".[43] Chemotactic factors present in inflammatory lesions are the underlying mechanism whereby cells are attracted to the site. These factors include soluble fragments of complement derived from C_3 and C_5, kallikrein, and lymphokines produced by lymphocytes.[23,43,44] The process is complex and must be under some sort of regulating or feedback control, for both humoral and cellular suppressors (inactivators) of chemotaxis have been described.[45] The actual movement appears to be due to alterations of microfilaments involving a sol-gel transformation of an actinomyosin like contractile protein.[46] Several cytoplasmic constituents are important as well, including calcium, GMP, GTP, and cyclic AMP.

Macrophage Functions in the Immune Response

Not only are macrophages functionally suited to recognize and ingest particulate antigen, but they are also so situated in the body in lymph nodes, liver, and spleen to maximally interact with antigen. Concentration of antigen within macrophages can be directly demonstrated by injection of radiolabeled antigen, particularly when of large size, polymerized, aggregated, or particulate.[48,49] Intracellular antigen is then metabolized, probably within intracellular vesicles, and extensive degradation may take place.[49] Some antigens are modified by the macrophage by attachment of a small molecular weight RNA of approximately 4S, a process known as "processing".[50] In a sense, this RNA appears to function as an adjuvant in that it results in a marked increase in the immunogenicity of certain antigens, especially T-cell antigens. The actual mechanism and importance of this processing in vivo, however, remain unclear.

Not only may intracellular macrophage antigen processing be important, but additionally antigen may be present on the cell membrane in a fashion capable of stimulating an immune response.[51] The specific configuration and the concentration required for membrane-attached antigen to trigger lymphocytes is not known. Membrane-bound antigen is much less immunogenic in the presence of soluble antigen,[52] indicating the importance of the way in which antigen is presented to lymphoid cells.

MALNUTRITION AND THE MACROPHAGE

Macrophage Mobilization

Granuloma formation, the normal host response to infection with *Mycobacterium tuberculosis* requires mobilization of monocytes into the infected area and subsequent *in situ* transformation into epithelioid cells. The latter process occurs concomitantly with macrophage activation and enhanced microbicidal capacity.[54] In a series of classic experiments years ago, Lurie[55] demonstrated that immunity to tuberculosis was directly related to the rapidity of mobilization of the monocyte/macrophage and the subsequent formation of definable granulomata. Because of these relationships among mononuclear cell mobilization, granuloma formation, and clinical resistance to tubercle bacilli, animal models employing the BCG strain as a probe have explored the impact of malnutrition upon macrophage function. Virtually nothing is known about marrow production under conditions of deprivation; however, some studies have been performed which assess macrophage mobilization. For example, Bhuyan and Ramalingaswami[56,57] have shown that low protein diets in the guinea pig and rabbit (2% and 0% casein, respectively) impair granuloma formation in these animals. In the guinea pig, low-protein diets result in marked impairment of local nodule formation in the skin in response to intradermal challenge with BCG. Whereas macrophages are abundant in controls within 1 to 2 weeks, 3 to 4 weeks are required before a clear response is seen in the protein deficient animals. Even then it is significantly suppressed compared to the normal diet animals. While numerous bacilli are found extracellularly early in infection, even after 4 to 5 weeks, when the intracellular population is dramatically reduced in the controls, many discrete organisms remain in the malnourished animals. Similar findings are present in draining lymph nodes, in which macrophages are rare and inconspicuous for the first few weeks. Progressive accumulation of macrophages is seen thereafter, but they tend to remain discrete or, at best, to develop into focal immature or mature epithelioid cells without either granuloma formation or caseation necrosis. Tuberculin skin sensitivity either does not develop at all, or is markedly impaired, in the protein-deficient animals.[56]

In the rabbit experiment, animals were immunized with 0.2 mg BCG at the end of 8 weeks of control (20% casein) or experimental (0% casein) diet. They were challenged with intravenous BCG, 5.0 mg/kg, 4 weeks later and observed for an additional 4 weeks. The response to immunization in the protein-deficient animal was impaired, with poor development of the primary complex, ill-formed granulomas, and minimal-to-no tuberculin skin sensitivity. Not unexpectedly, the accelerated granuloma response to BCG challenge in sensitized animals was severely blunted in the deficient rabbits, particularly in the lung, spleen, and bone marrow. There was greater preservation of the granuloma response in the liver of the malnourished rabbits, with considerable giant cell formation as well, perhaps a consequence of the large number of tissue macrophages normally resident in liver and, therefore, a diminished dependence upon migration of blood monocytes into the lesion. It is nevertheless clear from this study that the normal response to BCG reinfection, that is, faster mobilization and activation of macrophages in the cell mediated immune response, does not take place in the protein deficient animal.

Another relevant experiment has been performed using mice injected with *Schistosoma mansoni* into the pulmonary microvasculature.[58] In this model, the normal response is formation of granulomas around the eggs resulting from a typical cell mediated immune response. It is this inflammatory reaction which is, in fact, responsible for clinical illness due to *S. mansoni*.[59] Mice fed on 4, 8, 12, or 20% (control) protein diets, or restricted in caloric intake to 50 or 75% of control, were challenged 4 weeks later with *Schistosoma* eggs. Early granuloma formation (16 days) in the deprived mice was significantly depressed, particularly in animals given the most deficient diet. However with time, increasing reactions were seen, approaching control by 32 days. The principal effect, then, was to delay mobilization of macrophages necessary to produce a granuloma.[58]

Extensive experience with cutaneous cell mediated immune responses in humans, in which a critical effector role is played by macrophages migrating to the site, documents severe depression of macrophage mobilization into the local inflammatory response during protein-calorie malnutrition.[60] Direct observation of macrophage mobilization in response to abrasion of the skin confirms that these cells not only are delayed in entering the resulting exudates in malnourished hosts, but also never reach the same cell number achieved in exudates in healthy individuals.[61,62] Confirmatory data have been obtained employing protein deficient rats.[63]

These results, however striking, do not pinpoint a macrophage specific defect. Chemotactic responses of macrophages depend on humoral as well as cellular factors, defects in either potentially being capable of diminishing cell migration.[64] T-cells are known to play a central and critical role in development of antigen specific cell mediated immune responses,[65] such as the granulomas of tuberculosis or schistosomiasis. The studies described do not distinguish between primary and secondary impairment of macrophage function. It may not be the fault of the macrophage in the malnourished host that the inflammatory response is impaired. For example, a study of experimental protein calorie malnutrition in the rat showed that macrophages from severely deficient animals were not impaired in their in vitro chemotactic responsiveness to a chemotactic stimulus induced in normal rat serum.[66] However, both in vivo generation of chemotactic factors and the number of mononuclear cells entering an irritative peritoneal exudate produced with 1% glycogen were depressed in the deficient, compared to control, animals. Previous observations of impaired in vivo macrophage mobilization into rat skin and casein peritoneal exudate during protein deprivation[63] can thus be explained as a humoral defect, without presupposing a cellular lesion.

Monocyte/Macrophage Phagocytosis

Like movement toward chemotactic stimuli, phagocytosis is also a cooperative process involving the cells and humoral factors termed "opsonins". The humoral factors of importance for opsonization of bacteria are derived from immunoglobulin G and complement, principally from C_{3b}. These proteins, deposited on the surface of the microorganism, are then recognized by receptors on the membrane of the macrophage for the Fc fragment of immunoglobulin or C_{3b}. This promotes close contact between organism and cell and triggers the phagocytic response.[67] Studies of phagocytosis by either fixed or wandering mononuclear phagocytes under conditions of nutritional stress show distinctive and divergent results. Deo, Bhan, and Ramalingaswami[68] demonstrated, by histologic examination of liver, impaired Kupfer cell phagocytosis of colloidal carbon by protein-starved Rhesus monkeys, without correction of the defect by preopsonization of the particles in normal pooled monkey serum. Carbon clearance from serum was also significantly decreased in these animals, as might be predicted from the pathology data. These findings suggest that cellular, and not humoral, phagocytic defects might be present in the animals. Similar depressed carbon clearance rates of unopsonized carbon were found in protein-deficient rats[68] and mice,[69] and also in malnourished Rhesus monkeys challenged with P^{32} labeled *E. coli*.[70]

Although many studies prior to these failed to yield consistent data, more recent and more refined protocols employing colloidal polyvinyl pyrrolidone (PVP), which is cleared by fixed mononuclear cells,[71] show that in protein deprived mice clearance is indeed slow.[72] Coovadia and Soothill[72,74] have used I^{125} PVP of greater than 120,000 mol wt to measure mononuclear phagocyte clearance functions because this particle is exponentially cleared from plasma by tissue macrophages, principally in liver. PVP clearance can be blocked by prior carbon administration and it is stimulated by estrogens.[71] Under basal conditions, it is a relatively stable and reproducibly measurable parameter in normal animals.[73] In their studies, Coovadia and Soothill[72] fed four inbred strains of mice diets containing 4 to 27% protein or diets specifically depleted in phenylalanine and tryptophan. Alterations in PVP clearance could be detected as early as 3 days after instituting a deficient diet and the defect was repaired as quickly when a normal diet was resumed. Two disappearance rates for I^{125} PVP can be calculated from such data, termed K and α, the absolute clearance rate and the clearance corrected for the weight of the liver and spleen. These rates reflect overall phagocytic capacity in the animal and, if one assumes a uniform number of mononuclear cells per gram of tissue, probably the function of individual cells respectively.[73] Protein malnutrition resulted in consistent decreases in K, associated with simultaneous increases in the α function.[72] If loss of hepatocytes and Kupfer cells proceeds in parallel, then decreased K and increased α clearance rates can be explained simply by a diminished number of functioning phagocytic units, without concomitant alteration in the function of individual units. The same mechanism would be consistent with the data of Deo and colleagues[68] and could also explain the inability of preopsonization to alter clearance in their study if each remaining Kupfer cell was already functioning at maximum capacity. Cooper and colleagues[75] created a chronic marginal protein insufficiency model in mice and tested the ability of glass-adherent peritoneal macrophages to phagocytize Fe^{59}-labeled *Listeria monocytogenes*. Phagocytosis was not only unimpaired, but actually increased by about 60% in the protein-deficient cells compared to control.

Experiments with circulating monocytes and peritoneal macrophages support the concept that protein calorie malnutrition does not affect the phagocytic function of mononuclear phagocytes. Keusch and colleagues[76] studied glycogen-induced rat peritoneal macrophages in vitro during the course of development of a fatal protein-calorie malnutrition. Surface receptors for IgG present on these cells were not quantitatively altered during a 4-week period of observation on a 0.5% casein diet. In the presence of normal rat serum, phagocytosis of latex particles, *S. aureus, E. coli,* and *Salmonella enteritidis* ser Enteritidis and Typhimurium all remained perfectly normal when equal numbers of control or deficient cells were compared in vitro.[66,76] However, significant impairment in phagocytosis was found when macrophages from well-nourished animals were incubated in serum from the malnourished rats.[66] Consistent with these findings, using rat macrophages, Douglas and Schopfer[77] showed normal phagocytosis by peripheral blood monocytes from children with acute kwashiorkor, employing IgG-coated sheep erythrocytes or latex spherules as the challenge particle.

Macrophage Function and Antibody Affinity

Soothill and colleagues[73] have recently shown interstrain differences for carbon clearance from serum in a number of inbred mouse strains, presumably reflecting a genetic influence on fixed macrophage function. When the α clearance function was correlated with the affinity of antibody produced against a highly purified unadjuvantized human serum transferrin, there was a significant direct relationship. Mononuclear cell blockade with a large intraperitoneal dose of carbon just prior to immunization of a high clearance/high affinity antibody mouse strain (Ajax) increased the percentage of antibody nonresponse and decreased the relative affinity of the antibody in the responders, suggesting that macrophage function is important in the quality of the immune response. In a subsequent paper Soothill et al.[69] have shown that moderate protein restriction in Ajax mice also decreases carbon clearance, K, corrected clearance, α, and relative affinity of antitransferrin antibody. On the basis of these data, the suggestion is made that macrophage function per se is altered by the induced malnutrition. However, a primary defect seems less likely than a secondary defect in view of the information reviewed in the previous section. PVP clearance, which is generally considered to be the most accurate test of resting macrophage function, indicates that protein restriction increases, not decreases, α clearance.[72] This puts into question the accuracy of the carbon studies. Other effects of protein-calorie deprivation, such as synthesis of opsonic factors by liver, may be involved instead.

Macrophage Metabolism

Data on the impact of malnutrition upon monocyte/macrophage metabolism are extremely limited. Perhaps the most comprehensive recent study is that by Keusch and colleagues[66] in which oxygen consumption and oxidation of $1\text{-}^{14}\text{C}$-glucose were studied in resting and phagocytizing peritoneal macrophages serially during development of a severe, fatal, protein-calorie malnutrition. Oxygen consumption per resting cell was unchanged during a 4-week period of protein restriction. However, the phagocytosis associated burst in oxygen uptake was progressively and markedly blunted in the malnourished cells. Glucose oxidation showed a tendency to diminish in resting malnourished cells, particularly after 2 weeks on the diet, but this did not reach statistical significance. Phagocytosis associated glucose oxidation, however, diminished by 30% during the first week on the diet, and by 60% in the third and fourth weeks. The ratio of phagocytizing to resting activity decreased from 4.8 in the controls to 2.9 in the deprived animals. Values were restored to normal within a week of refeeding a normal diet.

Alveolar macrophages differ metabolically from other mononuclear phagocytes, living as they do in a tissue with a high oxygen tension of 70 to 110mm Hg. Aerobic oxidative processes are thus important and constitute the major source of cellular ATP, in contrast to other macrophages and monocytes.[28] Oxidative metabolism is also increased during phagocytosis by alveolar macrophages; however, it does not lead to production of superoxide radicals, as is the case with other types of macrophages, particularly when activated, and polymorphonuclear leukocytes.[78,79] Watson and colleagues[80] have recently shown that the activity of superoxide dismutase in alveolar macrophages, the enzyme which catalyzes the dismutation of superoxide to peroxide, functioning to protect the cell from the highly reactive superoxide ion, is increased during chronic moderate malnutrition. The authors propose that such a marginal malnutrition may cause macrophage activation, presumably mediated through T-lymphocytes. The effect of more severe malnutrition upon superoxide dismutase was not studied nor was superoxide production itself reported.

Macrophage Bactericidal Activity

Macrophages are the key effector killer cells for a group of pathogens, including *Mycobacterium tuberculosis, Salmonella typhi,* and *Brucella abortus* in humans, *Listeria monocytogenes* and *Salmonella enteritidis* in mice, and *Salmonella typhimurium* in rats. Intracellular bacterial activity has been studied during experimental severe protein-calorie malnutrition in rats, employing *Staphylococcus aureus, Escherichia coli,* and *Salmonella enteritidis* and *typhimurium* as probes.[66] The malnutrition had no effect on the killing function of the cells when normal rat serum was used as opsonin. However, there was a significant decrease in opsonic activity of malnourished-rat serum, which markedly reduced macrophage phagocytosis and, secondarily, intracellular killing.

Deo et al.[68] have previously reported that it takes two and a half times as long to clear the blood of viable *Escherichia coli* in malnourished Rhesus monkeys as it does in normals, possibly due to opsonin deficiency, a decrease in the absolute number of tissue macrophages, and perhaps a defect in the T-cell mediated activation mechanism, although the last mentioned would probably not be a factor in such a short-term experiment.

QUESTIONS FOR FUTURE RESEARCH

It is disappointing to realize, when one attempts to review the literature on an important question, that the state of the art is, to put it mildly, primitive. Such is the case, however, when the subject is nutritional influences on macrophage function. Not only have there been few relevant studies, but also those performed have not usually isolated the macrophage for study from the large number of potentially confounding variables present in vivo. For the mononuclear phagocytes are part of a larger functional system, or perhaps more correctly stated as functional systems, in which both humoral factors and cellular factors (certainly including immunoglobulin, complement, and both T- and B-lymphocytes) play essential roles. Which is (are) the rate-limiting component(s) for granuloma formation, activation of macrophage intracellular bactericidal mechanisms, secretion of macrophage products, immune surveillance, antigen processing, antibody formation, or cytotoxicity functions?

Those data currently available suggest that the monocyte and macrophage retain considerable functional activity during protein-calorie malnutrition. However, only a few functions have been carefully studied and even in these investigations, clear metabolic alterations were detectable. Therefore, it is important to investigate the broader range of macrophage activities, both in vitro and in vivo, a considerable task given the versatility of the individual cells and the mononuclear phagocyte system in general. What is normal in vitro may be quite abnormal in vivo if a limiting accessory factor is deficient. In this case, it might be possible to replace the deficient component and immediately restore the desired macrophage function. While this approach can be considered for humoral factors, it is really not feasible to consider lymphocyte transfusions because of the well-known graft-vs.-host immune reactions. However, lymphocyte-macrophage interactions are themselves mediated by soluble factors secreted by the lymphoid cells which could conceivably be produced and administered to the malnourished host. In addition, there are a number of nonspecific macrophage activators, such as the antihelminthic drug levamisole and double-stranded polyinosinic acid-polycytidylic acid copolymers,[81,82] which could be administered to malnourished subjects in order to bypass the poorly functioning usual activation mechanism. These possibilities are not ready for implementation; however, they are at least amenable to investigation now. Such studies could provide considerable guidance for future therapeutic interventions, either to amplify deficient function or to modulate specific functions in certain disease states, such as auto-immunity or diseases in which pathology results from the immune response to an exogenous agent.

It is also apparent that whereas some information is available on the effects of protein-calorie malnutrition on the macrophage, virtually nothing is known of specific nutrient deficiencies, or excesses, including vitamin A, vitamin C, folic acid, iron, zinc, or other trace metals. At the same time, there may be a synergy between several deficiencies, or excesses, mild in themselves, but with major effects when present together. Studies along these lines also present an opportunity for the double-edged therapeutic sword, to relieve or create specific functional deficits in order to combat a disease.

It is evident from the foregoing discussion that a major research effort is being proposed in almost casual terms. All things cannot be done at once, and the frankly impossible takes even longer. However, the number at risk in industrialized nations, partly due to food fadism and excessive food intake in a growing sector of the population, alters the priorities somewhat. When one adds to this the dictum that we are in many ways what we eat, the imperatives become stronger yet. The role of good nutrition in growth, development, and maintenance of the normal individual and the impact of malnutrition, of whatever sort, upon these various biological parameters is as fundamental a question as one might ask.

REFERENCES

1. Metchnikoff, E., *Lectures on the Comparative Pathology of Inflammation,* Dove Publications, New York, 1891 (reprinted 1968).
2. vanFurth, R. and Cohn, Z. A., The origin and kinetics of mononuclear phagocytes, *J. Exp. Med.,* 128, 415, 1968.
3. Cline, M. J. and Sumner, M. A., Bone marrow macrophage precursors. I. Some functional characteristics of the early cells of the mouse macrophage series, *Blood,* 40, 62, 1972.
4. Goul, J. L., Schotta, C., van Furth, R., Identification and characterization of the monoblast in mononuclear phagocyte colonies grown *in vitro, J. Exp. Med.,* 142, 1180, 1975.
5. Whitelaw, D. M., Bell, M. F., and Batho, H. F., Monocyte kinetics: observations after pulse labeling, *J. Cell. Physiol.,* 72, 65, 1968.
6. Roser, B., The distribution of intravenously injected peritoneal macrophages in the mouse, *Aust. J. Exp. Biol. Med. Sci.,* 43, 553, 1965.
7. Whitelaw, D. M., The intravascular life span of monocytes, *Blood,* 28, 455, 1966.
8. Ebert, R. H. and Florey, H. W., The extravascular development of the monocyte observed *in vivo, Br. J. Exp. Pathol.,* 20, 342, 1939.
9. Nichols, B. A., Bainton, D. F., and Farquhar, M. G., Differentiation of monocytes. Origin, nature and fate of their azurophil granules, *J. Cell Biol.,* 50, 498, 1971.
10. Sutton, J. S. and Weiss, L., Transformation of monocytes in tissue culture into macrophages, epithelioid cells, and multinucleated giant cells. An electron microscope study, *J. Cell Biol.,* 28, 303, 1966.
11. Whitelaw, D. M. and Batho, N. F., The distribution of monocytes in the rat, *Cell Tissue Kinet.,* 5, 215, 1972.

12. **Maldonado, J. E. and Hanlon, D. G.,** Monocytosis: a current appraisal, *Mayo Clin. Proc.,* 40, 248, 1965.
13. **Willoughby, D. A., Coote, E., and Spector, W. G.,** A monocytogenic humoral factor released after lymph node stimulation, *Immunology,* 12, 165, 1967.
14. **Dannenberg, A. M., Jr.,** Macrophages in inflammation and infection, *N. Engl. J. Med.,* 293, 489, 1975.
15. **vanWaarde, D. E., Hulsing-Hesselink, E., and vanFurth, R.,** A serum factor inducing monocytosis during an acute inflammatory reaction caused by newborn calf serum, *Cell Tissue Kinet.,* 9, 51, 1976.
16. **vanWaarde, D. E., Hulsing-Hesselink, E., Sandkuyl, L. A., and vanFurth, R.,** Humoral reputation of monocytopoiesis during the early phase of an inflammatory reaction caused by particulate substances, *Blood,* 50, 141, 1977.
17. **vanWaarde, D. E., Hudsing-Hesselink, E., and vanFurth, R.,** Properties of a factor increasing monocytopoiesis (FIM) occurring in serum during the early phase of an inflammatory reaction, *Blood,* 50, 727, 1977.
18. **Manel, J. and Defendi, V.,** Regulation of DNA synthesis in mouse macrophages. I. Sources, action and purification of the macrophage growth factor (MGF), *Exp. Cell Res.,* 65, 33, 1971.
19. **Manel, J. and Defendi, V.,** Regulation of DNA synthesis in mouse macrophages. II. Studies on the mechanism of action of the macrophage growth factor, *Exp. Cell Res.,* 65, 377, 1971.
20. **Cifone, M., Mocarelli, P., and Defendi, V.,** *In vitro* production of a macrophage growth factor, *Exp. Cell Res.,* 96, 96, 1975.
21. **Stanley, E. R., Cifone, M., Heard, P. M., and Defendi, V.,** Factors regulating macrophage production and growth: identity of colony-stimulating factor and macrophage growth factor, *J. Exp. Med.,* 143, 631, 1976.
22. **vanFurth, R.,** The origin and turnover of promonocytes, monocytes and macrophages in normal mice, in *Mononuclear Phagocytes,* vanFurth, R., Ed., Blackwell Scientific Publications, Oxford, 1970, chap. 10.
23. **Kay, N. E. and Douglas, S. D.,** Mononuclear phagocyte. Development, structure, function and involvement in immune response, *N.Y. State J. Med.,* 77, 327, 1977.
24. **David, J. R.,** Macrophage activaton by lymphocyte mediators, *Fed. Proc.,* 34, 1730, 1975.
25. **Rabinovitch, M., and deStefano, M. J.,** Macrophage spreading *in vitro.* I. Inducers of spreading, *Exp. Cell Res.,* 77, 323, 1973.
26. **Mackaness, G. B.,** The monocyte in cellular immunity, *Semin. Hematol.,* 7, 172, 1970.
27. **Simon, H. B. and Sheagren, J. N.,** Enhancement of macrophage bactericidal capacity by antigenically stimulated immune lymphocytes, *Cell. Immunol.,* 4, 163, 1972.
28. **Karnovsky, M. L., Simmons, S., Glass, E. A., Shafer, A. W., and D'Arcy Hart, P.,** Metabolism of macrophages, in *Mononuclear Phagocytes,* vanFurth, R., Ed., Blackwell Scientific Publications, Oxford, 1970, chap. 7.
29. **Nelson, R. D., Mills, E. L., Simmons, R. L., and Quie, P. G.,** Chemiluminescence response of phagocytizing human monocytes, *Infect. Immun.,* 14, 129, 1976.
30. **Johnston, R. B., Jr., Keele, B. B., Jr., Misra, H. P., Lehmeyer, J. E., Webb, L. S., Baehner, R. L., and Rajagopalan, K. V.,** The role of superoxide anion generation in phagocytic bactericidal activity. Studies with normal and chronic granulomatous disease leukocytes, *J. Clin. Invest.,* 55, 1357, 1975.
31. **deChatelet, L. R., Wang, P., and McCall, C. E.,** Bactericidal mechanisms of macrophages, in *Microbiology 1975,* Schlessinger, D., Ed., American Society of Microbiology, Washington, D.C., 1975, 215.
32. **Adler, L. M., Gee, J. B. L., and Root, R. K.,** H_2O_2 formation and utilization by human monocytes, *Clin. Res.,* 26, 522A, 1978.
33. **Bodel, P.,** Studies on the mechanism of endogenous pyrogen production. III. Human blood monocytes, *J. Exp. Med.,* 140, 954, 1974.
34. **Colten, H. R. and Frank, M. M.,** Biosynthesis of the second (C_2) and fourth (C_4) components of complement *in vitro* by tissues isolated from guinea pigs with genetically determined C_4 deficiency, *Immunology,* 22, 991, 1972.
35. **Glasgow, L. A.,** Leukocytes and interferon in the host response to viral infections. I. Mouse leukocytes and leukocyte produced interferon in vaccinia virus infection *in vitro, J. Exp. Med.,* 121, 1001, 1965.
36. **Gordon, S., Todd, J., and Cohn, Z.,** *In vitro* synthesis and secretion of lysozyme by mononuclear phagocytes, *J. Exp. Med.,* 139, 1228, 1974.
37. **Chervenick, P. A. and LoBuglio, A. F.,** Human blood monocytes: stimulators of granulocyte and mononuclear colony formation *in Vitro, Science,* 178, 164, 1972.
38. **Gordon, S., Unkeless, J. C., and Cohn, Z. A.,** Induction of macrophage plasminogen activator by endotoxin stimulation and phagocytosis, *J. Exp. Med.,* 140, 995, 1974.

39. **Huber, H., Douglas, S. D., Nusbacher, J., Kochwa, S., and Rosenfield, R. E.,** IgG subclass specificity of human monocyte receptor sites, *Nature (London),* 229, 419, 1971.

40. **Lay, W. H. and Nussenzweig, V.,** Receptors for complement on leukocytes, *J. Exp. Med.,* 128, 991, 1968.

41. **Schmidt, M. E. and Douglas, S. D.,** Disappearance and recovery of human monocyte IgG receptor activity after phagocytosis, *J. Immunol.,* 109, 914, 1972.

42. **Griffin, F. M., Bianco, C., and Silverstein, S. C.,** Characterization of the macrophage receptor for complement and demonstration of its functional independence from the receptor for the Fc portion of immunoglobulin G., *J. Exp. Med.,* 141, 1269, 1975.

43. **Ward, P. A.,** Leukotactic responses, *J. Reticuloendothel. Soc.,* 19, 247, 1976.

44. **Snyderman, R. and Mergenhagen, S. E.,** Chemotaxis of macrophages, in *Immunobiology of the Macrophage,* Nelson, D. S., Ed., Academic Press, New York, 1976, 323.

45. **Snyderman, R. and Pike, M. C.,** An inhibitor of macrophage chemotaxis produced by neoplasms, *Science,* 192, 370, 1976.

46. **Hartwig, J. H. and Stossel, T. P.,** Isolation and properties of actin, myosin, and a new actin-binding protein in rabbit alveolar macrophages, *J. Biol. Chem.,* 250, 5696, 1975.

47. **Seyberth, H. W., Schmidt-Gayk, H., Jacobs, K. H., and Hackenthal, E.,** Cyclic adenosine monophosphate in phagocytizing granulocytes and alveolar macrophages, *J. Cell. Biol.,* 57, 567, 1973.

48. **Nossal, G. J., Abbot, A., and Mitchell, J.,** Antigens in immunity. XIV. Electron microscopic radioautographic studies of antigen capture in the lymph node medulla, *J. Exp. Med.,* 127, 263, 1968.

49. **Ehrenreich, B. A. and Cohn, Z. A.,** The uptake and digestion of iodinated human serum albumin by macrophages *in vitro, J. Exp. Med.,* 126, 941, 1967.

50. **White, S. L. and Johnson, A. G.,** Studies on the cellular site of action of macrophage RNA-antigen complexes, *Cell Immunol.,* 21, 56, 1976.

51. **Unanue, E. R.,** The immune response of mice to keyhole limpet hemocyanin bound to macrophages, *J. Immunol.,* 102, 893, 1969.

52. **Unanue, E. R. and Calderon, J.,** Evaluation of the role of macrophages in immune induction, *Fed. Proc.,* 34, 1737, 1975.

53. **Shima, K., Dannenberg, A. M., Jr., Ando, M., Chandrasekhar, S., Seluzicki, J., and Fabrikant, J. I.,** Macrophage accumulation, division, maturation, and digestive and microbial capacities in tuberculous lesions. I. Studies involving their incorporation of tritiated thymidine and their content of lysosomal enzymes and bacilli, *Am. J. Pathol.,* 67, 159, 1972.

54. **Dannenberg, A. M., Jr., Ando, M., and Shima, K.,** Macrophage accumulation, division, maturation, and digestive and microbicidal capacities in tuberculous lesions. III. The turnover of macrophages and its relation to cellular immunity in primary BCG lesions and those of reinfection, *J. Immunol.,* 109, 1109, 1972.

55. **Lurie, M. B.,** Resistance to tuberculosis: Experimental Studies in Native and Acquired Defense Mechanisms, Harvard University Press, Cambridge, 1964.

56. **Bhuyan, U. N. and Ramalingaswami, V.,** Immune responses of the protein deficient guinea pig to BCG vaccination, *Am. J. Pathol.,* 72, 489, 1973.

57. **Bhuyan, U. N. and Ramalingaswami, V.,** Systemic macrophage mobilization and granulomatous response to BCG in the protein deficient rabbit, *Am. J. Pathol.,* 76, 313, 1974.

58. **Akpon, C. A. and Warren, K. S.,** The inhibition of granuloma formation around *Schistosoma mansoni* eggs, *Am. J. Pathol.,* 79, 435, 1975.

59. **Warren, K. S.,** The immunopathology of schistosomiasis: a multidisciplinary approach, *Trans. R. Soc. Trop. Med. Hyg.,* 66, 417, 1972.

60. **Edelman, R.,** Cell-mediated immune response in protein-calorie malnutrition — a review, in *Malnutrition and the Immune Response,* Suskind, R., Ed., Raven Press, New York, 1977, 47.

61. **Freyre, E. A., Chabes, A., Poemape, O., and Chabes, A.,** Abnormal rebuck skin window in kwashiorkor, *J. Pediatr.,* 82, 523, 1973.

62. **Kulapongs, P., Edelman, R., Suskind, R., and Olson, R. E.,** Defective local leukocyte mobilization in children with kwashiorkor, *Am. J. Clin. Nutr.,* 30, 367, 1977.

63. **Gray, I.,** Effect of protein nutrition on leukocyte mobilization, *Proc. Soc. Exp. Biol. Med.,* 116, 414, 1964.

64. **Sorkin, E., Borel, J. F. Stetcher, V. J.,** Chemotaxis of mononuclear and polymorphonuclear phagocytes, in *Mononuclear Phagocytes,* vanFurth, R., Ed., Blackwell Scientific Publications, Oxford, 1970, chap. 25.

65. **Mackaness, G. B.,** Cellular immunity, in *Mononuclear Phagocytes,* vanFurth, R., Ed., Blackwell Scientific Publications, Oxford, 1970, chap. 28.

66. **Keusch, G. T., Douglas, S. D., Hammer, G., and Braden, K.,** Macrophage antibacterial functions in experimental protein-calorie malnutrition. II. Cellular and humoral factors for chemotaxis, phagocytosis, and intracellular bactericidal activity, *J. Infect. Dis.,* in press, 1978.

67. **Stossel, T. P.,** The mechanism of phagocytosis, *J. Reticuloendothel. Soc.,* 19, 237, 1976.

68. Deo, M. G., Bhan, I., and Ramalingaswami, V., Influence of dietary protein on phagocytic activity of the reticuloendothelial cells, *J. Pathol.*, 109, 215, 1973.
69. Passwell, J. H., Steward, M. W., and Soothill, J. F., The effects of protein malnutrition on macrophage function and the amount and affinity of antibody response, *Clin. Exp. Immunol.*, 17, 491, 1974.
70. Ratnakar, K. S., Mathur, M., Ramalingaswami, V., and Deo, M. G., Phagocytic function of reticuloendothelial system in protein deficiency — a study in Rhesus monkeys using ^{32}P-labeled *E. coli*, *J. Nutr.*, 102, 1233, 1972.
71. Morgan, A. G. and Soothill, J. F., Measurement of the clearance function of macrophages with ^{125}I-labeled polyvinyl pyrrolidone, *Clin. Exp. Immunol.*, 20, 489, 1975.
72. Coovadia, H. M. and Soothill, J. F., The effect of protein restricted diets on the clearance of ^{125}I-labeled polyvinyl pyrrolidone in mice, *Clin. Exp. Immunol.*, 23, 373, 1976.
73. Passwell, J. H., Steward, M. W., and Soothill, J. F., Inter-mouse strain difference in macrophage function and its relationship to antibody responses, *Clin. Exp. Immunol.*, 17, 159, 1974.
74. Coovadia, H. M. and Soothill, J. F., The effect of amino acid restricted diets on the clearance of ^{125}I-labeled polyvinyl pyrrolidone in mice, *Clin. Exp. Immunol.*, 23, 562, 1976.
75. Cooper, W. C., Good, R. A., and Mariani, T., Effects of protein insufficiency on immune responsiveness, *Am. J. Clin. Nutr.*, 27, 647, 1974.
76. Keusch, G. T., Douglas, S. D., Braden, K., and Geller, S., Macrophage antibacterial functions in experimental protein-calorie malnutrition. I. Description of the model, morphologic observations, and macrophage surface IgG receptors, *J. Infect. Dis.*, in press, 1978.
77. Douglas, S. D. and Schopfer, K., Phagocyte function in protein-calorie malnutrition, *Clin. Exp. Immunol.*, 17, 121, 1974.
78. Gee, J. B. L., Vassallo, C. L., Bell, P., Kaskin, J., Basford, R. E., and Field, J. B., Catalase-dependent peroxidative metabolism in the alveolar macrophage during phagocytosis, *J. Clin. Invest.*, 49, 1280, 1970.
79. Drath, D. B. and Karnovsky, M. L., Superoxide production by phagocytic leukocytes, *J. Exp. Med.*, 141, 257, 1975.
80. Watson, R. R., Rister, M., and Baehner, R. L., Superoxide dismutase activity in polymorphonuclear leukocytes and alveolar macrophages of protein malnourished rats and guinea pigs, *J. Nutr.*, 106, 1801, 1976.
81. Schmidt, M. E. and Douglas, S. D., Effects of levamisole on human monocyte function and immunoprotein receptors, *Clin. Immunol. Immunopathol.*, 6, 299, 1976.
82. Schmidt, M. E. and Douglas, S. D., Effects of synthetic single- and multi-stranded polynucleotides on human monocyte IgG receptor activity *in vitro*, *Proc. Soc. Exp. Biol. Med.*, 151, 376, 1976.

Digestion and Endocrine Function

NUTRITION AND THE DEVELOPMENT OF DIGESTION AND ABSORPTION

O. Koldovsky

Table 1
INCIDENCE OF "LACTOSE NONDIGESTORS" IN DIFFERENT POPULATIONS AND DIFFERENT AGE GROUPS

Population (number of subjects)	Lactose test load (in water)	Criteria used for evaluation of lactose absorption	Remarks	Ref.	Symbol
Chinese, Malays and Indians living in Singapore (98)	50 g; in children below 25 kg — 2 g/kg body weight	Lactose malabsorption was diagnosed if maximal rise of blood glucose was less than 20 mg% after lactose and higher than 20 mg% after glucose load	Hospitalized for nongastrointestinal disease; glucose test also (½ dose)	22	▲
Baganda (72)	2 g/kg	Highest blood glucose values recorded	Glucose + galactose load given to those with blood glucose increase less than 20 mg%; subjects hospitalized for nongastrointestinal diseases or children from a home for healthy babies	23	▽
Baltimore: Negro (20) Baltimore: White (20)	50 g/m² body surface	Lactose-induced symptoms of abdominal discomfort	Healthy children from a comprehensive care pediatric clinic (all received welfare care)	24	◇ whites ◆ blacks
Student families from Asia, Africa, and Latin America residing in USA (34)	50 g in adults; 30 g in children	Rise in blood glucose less than 25 mg%	All adults with less than 25 mg% increase had symptoms; only 2 out of 4 "intolerant" children had symptoms	25	•
Thai[a] Thai orphanages (parents with leprosy & tuberculosis) (172)	2 g/kg	Rise of blood glucose by 20 mg% and more considered as "tolerance"	Sucrose and glucose tolerance also studied; data for American and Thai adults included	26	◐ ◑
Nigeria-Yoruba (90)	2 g/kg, maximum	Only the highest increase of blood glucose was recorded	Healthy subjects; also sucrose tolerance; unweaned and weaned	27	*
Nigeria-Yoruba (89)	2 g/kg, in children under 25 kg, and 1 g/kg in children over 25 kg of body weight	Same data as Reference 27	In weaned children also glucose-galactose test	28	⊠

Table 1 (continued)
INCIDENCE OF "LACTOSE NONDIGESTORS" IN DIFFERENT POPULATIONS AND DIFFERENT AGE GROUPS

Population (number of subjects)	Lactose test load (in water)	Criteria used for evaluation of lactose absorption	Remarks	Ref.	Symbol
Peru-Mestizo population (90)	50 g/m²	(a) Maximal increase of blood sugar below 26 mg% (b) Also presence of symptoms	Children originally admitted for marasmus or kwashiorkor and their siblings	29	△
Hyderabad-India (27)	2 g/kg	Same criteria as in Reference 29	Healthy adults	30	▨
Finnish village (129 children, 158 adults)	1 g/kg (maximum 50 g)	Values above 25 mg% increase judged normal; between 20—24 mg repeated with double dose; above 20 mg% judged normal	Volunteers from a random sample	31	⊢O⊣
Mexican-American children (MA) (282) and Anglo-American children (AA) (51) of Northern European descent	2 g/kg	(a) Lower sucrase than 25% judged as malabsorption of lactose (b) Presence of gastrointestinal symptoms recorded	Both parents of Mexican-Americans had Spanish surnames	32	×(MA) ⊗(AA)
Japanese children	3.5 g/kg (maximum 50 g)	Lactose malapsorption was diagnosed if maximal rise of blood glucose was less than 20 mg%	% of lactose nondigestors: under 1 year — 0% 1—2.9 years — 33% 3—7.9 years — 46% 8—adults — 100%	32a	

Compiled by O. Koldovsky

a Similar results in Flatz et al.[33] (75 adults, 37 children). Addition of ⊥ to symbols denotes use of the presence of abdominal symptoms to characterize a subject as a "lactose nondigester". Î = Persons with normal lactose tolerance test (LTT) judged according to changes of blood glucose level. △ = both with normal and abnormal LTT but without abnormal symptoms.

Table 2
LACTASE ACTIVITY IN INFANT AND CHILD DUODENAL AND JEJUNAL MUCOSA[66,67]

Activity given in μmoles/min/g protein, except where noted.[a]

Age groups						
Below 1 year	1—3 years	3—5 years	5—7 years	Adult	Notes	Ref.
				44 (22)	Biopsy, near ligamentum	56
				2(12)[b]	Treitzi V.A. hospital patients	
	4.3(6)[c]				Biopsy, race not specified	57[d]
45(8)	38(5)	100(2)		40(8)	Biopsy of lower duodenum; race not specified; children: patients with no gastrointestinal disorders; adults: volunteers	58
10.5(4)[c]					Autopsy, jejunum, newborn Bagandas; 6—38 hrs after death	59
	6.8(38)			5(75)	Thai	60
				42(23)	American adults living in Thailand (biopsy of jejunum)	
35(3)	36(5)	64(1)	35(1)		Biopsy, lower duodenum; race not specified; previous history of diarrhea (function or psychological)	61
	22(6)	18(5)	14(4)		Biopsy, jejunum; Chinese, Malays and Indians living in Singapore	62
28(6)				16.6(8)	Surgery or autopsy, race not given	63
				2.7(6)[b]		
	54(9)	15(6)		7.8(12)	Jejunal biopsy; Hyderabad, India	64

Compiled by O. Koldovsky.

[a]   Number in parentheses indicates number of cases.
[b]   Data for lactase "deficit" groups.
[c]   Per gram wet weight.
[d]   Data of Townely et al.[57] should probably be multiplied by 10; data of Cook[65] should probably be multiplied by 20.

Table 3

JEJUNAL α-GLUCOSIDASES IN CHILDREN AND ADULTS

μmol/min/mg protein (unless noted)

Country	Maltase	Sucrase	Isomaltase	Trehalase	No. of cases	Age	Remarks	Ref.
Uganda	40[a]	15[a]	4[a]	10[a]	4	Newborn	Baganda tribe; autopsy 1—38 hr after death	68
Zambia	332	83	100	26	26	17—59	Zambians admitted for nongastrointestinal complaints; jejunal biopsy	69
U.S.A.	266	87	97	—	22	Adult	No organic G.I. disease; no race given	70
Switzerland	567	166	151	—	17	Adult	Jejunal biopsy specimen taken near ligomentum Treitzi; patients without G.I. symptoms	71
Australia	305[b]	80[b]	86[b]	25[b]	8	Less than 1 year	Biopsy of duodeum	72
	228	108	93	24	4	Between 1—2 years		
Thailand	210	50	—	—	38	Thai children 1 month — 6 yr	Jejunal biopsy in healthy subjects	73
	280	80	—	—	73	Thai adults		
	380	105	—	—	23	American adults in Thailand		
U.S.A.	193	32	—	—	6	Less than 1 yr	Autopsy within 2—8 hr after death and surgery; race and exact location of biopsy not given	74
India	249	88	—	—	9	7 months—3 yr	Jejunal biopsy: apparently healthy subjects	75
	335	115	—	—	6	3 years—7 yr		
	323	97	—	—	12	Adults		
U.S.A.	21[c]	6[c]	6[c]	—	6	1—3 years old	Race and biopsy location not given	76

U.S.A.	234	67	—	170	14—80 years old	145 Whites, 22 Negroes, 3 American Indians; no location of biopsy given	77

Compiled by O. Koldovsky.

Note: Additional data on full-term and premature newborns can be found in Apollonia et al.[79] and on 0 to 15-year-old Australian aborigines in Elliot et al.[80]

a   To convert per protein, multiply by approximately 10 (See Antonowicz et al.[78]).
b   Duodenal specimens.
c   To convert per protein multiply by approximately 20 (see Cook[68]).

Table 4

BILE SALT CONCENTRATION IN DUODENAL JUICE (also see Figure 11)

Gestation age	Age	Conditions	No. of cases	Mean (mEg/l)	Ref.
—	Adults	Postprandial	12	7.50±1.31[a]	16
—	Adults	Postprandial, maximal values	6	20.6±5.36[a]	16
		Postprandial, minimal values	6	2.83±0.40[a]	
		Fasting, minimal values	6	6.66±0.84[a]	
—	Adults	Fasting, minimal values	19	8.1(2.8—20)	169
40	3—15 days	Before feeding	8	2.08±0.61[a]	170
		During feeding (breast milk)	8	1.02±0.14[a]	
35	14 days	2 hr after last feeding	9	3.8±0.9[a]	171
(fed breast milk)	14 days	During first hour after meal	9	1.87±0.21[a]	
37	14 days	2 hr after last feeding	9	8.8±2.05[a]	
(fed milk)	14 days	During first hour after meal	9	2.63±0.59[a]	
Very low birth	12 days	Postprandial	10	1.39±0.39[a]	172
weight	57 days		10	3.62±0.55[a]	
Low birth weight	a) 10—19 days		12	2.0±1.3[a]	173
	b) 20—34 days		7	5.8±2.7[a]	
	group a) after 2—3 weeks		4	Threefold rise as compared to group a)	
Control subjects	21—240 days		8	6.8±2.7[a]	

Compiled by O. Koldovsky.

[a] S.E.M.

Table 5

COMPARISON OF THE BILIARY LIPID COMPOSITION OF CHILDREN WITH BILE OF ADULTS

	Cholesterol (moles %)	Bile acids (moles %)	Phospholipids (moles %)	Ref.
Gallbladder bile of adults	6.0	73.5	20.4	174
	7.6	71.9	20.5	175
Duodenal bile of adults	7.1	72.5	20.4	176
	8.9	—	—	177
Duodenal bile of children	5.0	80.3	14.7	178

Table 6

LEVELS OF GASTRIN, GLUCAGON AND SECRETIN IN VENOUS PLASMA OF INFANTS[209,210]

	Gastrin		Glucagon		
	Oxytocin[a]	No oxytocin[a]	C terminal (pancreat.)	N-terminal	Secretin
Maternal plasma (at birth)	52±14.7[b]	29.5±6.9	57±8	62±5	12.5±3.6
Cord plasma	59±15	89.0±20.9	432±54[a]	227±26[a]	
Cord plasma (combined from 2 groups)	64±12.5		336±42	17±12	92.8±23.9
4-day-old infants	151±15.8		891±239	1318±264	299±58

[a]   Use of oxytocin during delivery; otherwise both groups were combined.
[b]   Mean ± S.E.M. (groups were formed by 11, 19 or 22 subjects).

From Koldovsky, O., *Physiology of the Perinatal Period,* Stave, U., Ed., Plenum Publishing, New York, 1978. With permission.

Table 7

NITROGEN ABSORPTION IN PREMATURE INFANTS AS STUDIED IN
VARIOUS INSTITUTIONS

Diet	Age (weeks)	Nitrogen Intake (g/ kg/day)	Absorption (% of intake)	Number of infants studied	Notes	Ref.
Breast milk	3—8	0.35—0.40	81.6	5		211
Cow milk	2—8	0.43—1.44	89.6	6	a) % of absorption independent of intake	212
Breast milk					b) No age dependency between 2 and 8 weeks	
Casein (whole)	2—6	0.67—1.34	90			213
Casein hydrolysate			91			
Breast milk		0.46	0.82			214
"Humanized" Cow milk	2—9	0.47	81			
		0.75	83	12		
Cow milk		0.78	90			215
		0.72	90			
		0.20	91			
Formulas with casein Hydrolysate	1—5	Approx. 0.8—1.0	96.5	25		216
			95.6			
			95.6		Absorption was higher on formulas containing medium-chain triglycerides than long-chain triglycerides	
			91.3			

Compiled by O. Koldovsky.

Table 8
NITROGEN ABSORPTION IN FULL-TERM INFANTS AS STUDIED IN VARIOUS INSTITUTIONS

Diet	Intake (g/kg/day)	Absorption (% of intake)							Ref.
		>15 days	>30 days	>60 days	>90 days	>100 days	>150 days	Older	
Breast milk	0.26—0.35			84.5(4)					217
Not specified	0.25—0.50						87(1)	85.82(2)	218
Pasteurized breast milk	0.20—0.45	84(3)	85(5)	85(11)	84(9)	87(13)	83(8)	83(12)	219
Fresh breast milk	0.18—0.37		81.86(2)	81(6)	79(4)	86(6)	81(1)	84(4)	220
Fresh breast milk	0.28—0.43			79.82	85(7)	89.90(2)			
Cow milk	0.37—0.55	86.82(2)	81(3)	82(4)	79(5)	84(5)	83(9)	84(9)	221
Cow milk	0.20—0.41		87(4)	87(10)	90(10)	87(13)	87(12)	84(6)	222
Cow milk	71—88	—	—	89(6)	90(5)	90(7)	90(6)		223
a) Evaporated	0.0	—	—		84(4)	88(4)	91(4)		
b) OLAC	0.82—96	—							
c) Whole	0.92—1.08		83(4)	88(6)	85(7)	90(4)			224
Breast milk	0.33—0.44	83(10)[a]		82—87(3)					
Cow milk (S26)	0.40—0.51	85(10)[a]		86—92(5)					
Cow milk (SMA)	0.43—0.51	86(10)[a]		81—84(3)					225
Breast milk	0.45	82(10)[b]							
Cow milk	0.83	89(10)[b]							
Cow milk diet a)	1.86	88(19)[a]							226
b)	1.31	84(12)[a]							
c)	1.16	77(12)[a]							
d)	1.20	77(11)[a]							

Compiled by O. Koldovsky.

Note: Figures for absorption rounded upwards. Number in parentheses denotes number of cases.

a   Infants 5 to 7 years of age.
b   Infants 2 weeks old.

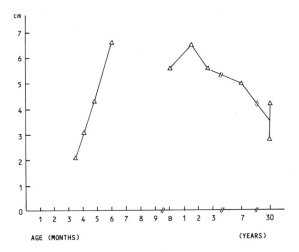

FIGURE 1. Length of the small intestine of human fetuses, children and adults. Ordinate: length of small intestine in cm per cm of length of the body (C-H length). Abscissa: age in months and years, respectively, B = birth. Data for fetuses recalculated from Lindberg[1] for newborn and older from Beneke.[2] (From Koldovsky, O., *Development of the Functions of the Small Intestine in Mammals and Man,* S. Karger, Basel, 1969. With permission.)

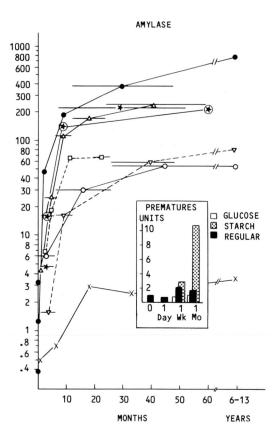

FIGURE 2. Amylase activity in duodenal fluid of infants of different ages. Symbols: X — Klumpp and Neale,[4] △ — Anderson,[9] □ — Auricchio et al.,[8] O — Delachaume-Salem and Sarles,[6] ☆ — Farber et al.,[10] ∇ — Gibbs,[5] ● — Zoppi et al.[3] and Hadorn et al.,[7] and * — Ingomar and Terslev.[11] Ordinate: open symbols denote concentration, full symbols denote output per 50 min/kg of body weight (logarithmic scale). Abscissa: age in months. Insert: Changes in output of amylase (per 50 min/kg of body weight) in prematures on different diets during the first months of life. Black columns indicate infants fed regular diet; white columns, diet with glucose; dotted columns, diet with starch.[3] Horizontal lines denote the age range of studied group (not given if smaller than size of the symbol). All samples were collected from fasted subjects, Klumpp and Neale[4] reported values both from fasted subjects and after test meal. Gibbs[5] used stimulation by secretin (the data without secretin gave similar pattern); Zoppi,[3] Delachaume-Salem,[6] and Hadorn et al.[7] used pancrozymin secretin; Auricchio et al.[8] used pancrozymin secretin; Auricchio et al.,[8] used test meal stimulation. Vazquez[12] reported no change in amylase activity during the first 3 weeks of life in full term infants. Véghelyi[13] did not find different activity in children 11 months to 2 years old as compared to those 8 to 11 years old. (From Koldovsky, O., *Physiology of the Perinatal Period,* Stave, U., Ed., Plenum Publishing, New York, 1978. With permission.)

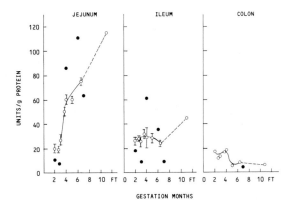

FIGURE 3. Comparison of development of sucrase in jejunum, ileum and colon of human fetuses and newborn. Abscissa: age in postconceptional weeks, FT = one full term born exencephalus. Ordinate: μmol of sucrose split per minute and gram of protein. Open circles: total of 44 fetuses studied, short vertical lines: 2 S.E.M. (Jirsova et al.)[14] Full circles: total of 6 fetuses studied (Sheehy and Anderson).[15] (From Koldovsky, O., *Physiology of the Perinatal Period*, Stave, U., Ed., Plenum Publishing, New York, 1978. With permission.)

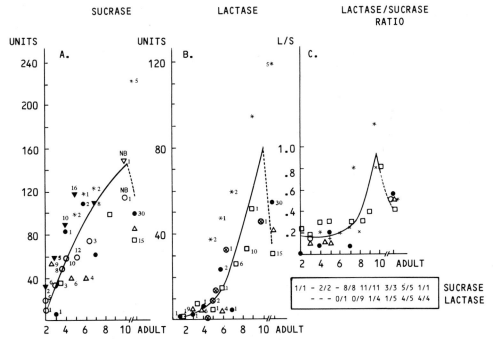

FIGURE 4. Sucrase and lactase activity in small intestine of human fetuses. Figures A and B: Data for sucrase and lactase (mean values from individual papers) are expressed as μmoles/min/g protein (□*△O) or in arbitrary units per gram wet weight (⊗ ∇). Small figures at symbols denote number of fetuses studied. Figure C: Ratio of lactase/sucrase as calculated from corresponding data. Table at the bottom compiled from data of Ibrahim and Hoppe-Seylers[21b] and Ibrahim et al.[21c] The age corresponds to that in the figure above; the denominator = number of fetuses tested, the numerator = number of fetuses with a positive test for the disaccharidase. Symbols and References: □ — Auricchio et al.,[16] △ — Dahlquist and Lindberg,[17] * — Eggermont,[18] ∇ — Fomina,[19] ⊗ — Heilskov,[20] O — Jirsova et al.,[21] ● — Sheehy and Anderson.[21a] (From Koldovsky, O., *Physiology of the Perinatal Period,* Stave, U., Ed., Plenum Publishing, New York, 1978. With permission.)

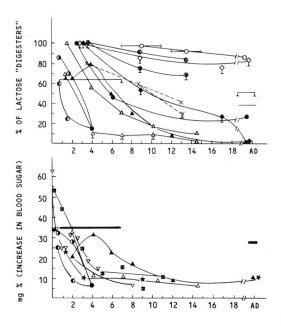

FIGURE 5.   Incidence of "lactose nondigestors" in different populations and different age groups. Addition of ⊥ to symbols denotes use of the presence of abdominal symptoms to characterize a subject as a "lactose nondigestor". △ = persons with normal lactose tolerance test (LTT) judged according to changes of blood glucose levels; △ = both with normal and abnormal symptoms. See Table 1 for detailed explanation of symbols. (From Koldovsky, O., *Physiology of the Perinatal Period*, Plenum Publishing, New York, 1978. With permission.)

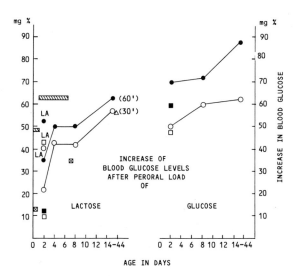

FIGURE 6. Rise of blood glucose levels after peroral load of lactose and glucose in infants during first 6 weeks of life. Open symbols: Values 30′ after sugar load; full symbols 60′ values. Triangles and circles — values from premature infants; squares — from full term infants; LA — values in children who received lactose perorally. Data of Boellner et al.[34] (O, □, ●, ■), Jarret and Holman[35] (△, ▲,) Cook[36] (■), and Anyon and Clarkson[37] (□, full term). A postnatal, lactose-connected rise in blood sugar was found to be highly significant.[1] The data of Cook,[36] due to the large scatter, did not significantly differ between the two age groups. Infants were fasted 4 hr[34,35] or 6 hr[36] before being fed with lactose (1.75 g/kg body weight; Cook used 2 g/kg body weight). Boellner et al.[34] studied 49 infants of undisclosed race; Cook's subjects were Bagandas; Jarrett and Holman studied 16 U.S. Negroes and 4 U.S. Caucasians. Blood glucose was determined using the glucose-oxidase method[34,36,37] and the "true glucose" technique.[35] (From Koldovsky, O., *Physiology of the Perinatal Period*, Stave, U., Ed., Plenum Publishing, New York, 1978. With permission.)

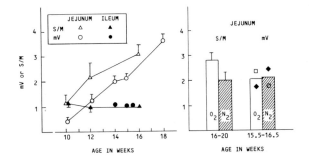

FIGURE 7.   Development of active glucose transport in human fetuses. Left part: prenatal development of glucose transport as studied in vitro (technique of everted sacs) in oxygen atmosphere. Abscissa — age in postconceptional weeks. Ordinate — S/M = ratio of concentration of glucose in serosal fluid to glucose in mucosal fluid at the end of 60 min. incubation period (triangles); mV = the potential difference of glucose transfer (circles). Open symbols denote jejunum; full symbols denote ileum. Short vertical lines denote S.E.M. Right part: Comparison of transport in oxygen (open) and nitrogen (full) atmosphere. Age of the fetuses given under the columns. Short vertical curves denote S.E.M.; small rectangles in the right part of the figure denote individual values.[38,39] (From Koldovsky, O., *Physiology of the Perinatal Period,* Stave U., Ed., Plenum Publishing, New York, 1978. With permission.)

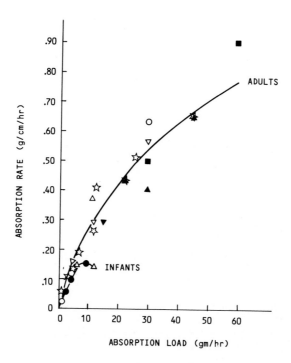

FIGURE 8.   Rate of glucose absorption from the perfused jejunum in infants and adults. Symbols: Infants: 2 to 4 months old, △ — Ref. 40; 7 to 21 months old, ● — Ref. 41; 3 weeks to 6 months old, ○ — Ref. 41 (compiled by Yunoszai[52]). Adults: ■ — Ref. 44, ▼ — Ref. 45, ○ — Ref. 46, * — Ref. 47, ▽ — Ref. 48, ☼— Ref. 49, △ — Ref. 50, ▲ — Ref. 12. (Compiled by Fordtran and Ingelfinger.[43]) The concentration of glucose solution applied to infants varied between 0.15 to 16% and 0.12 to 10% to adults. (From Koldovsky, O., *Physiology of the Perinatal Period,* Stave, U., Ed., Plenum Publishing, New York, 1978. With permission.)

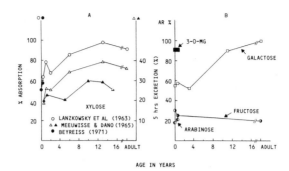

FIGURE 9.   Postnatal changes in absorption of monosaccharides in children. A: Absorption of xylose. Left ordinate: % absorption of xylose (O — Ref. 53, ● — Ref. 54), right ordinate: 5 hr excretion in % (△ — Ref. 53, ▲ — Ref. 55). B: Absorption of galactose, fructose, arabinose, and 3-O-methylglucose. Ordinate AR% s.a.p.o. / s.a.i.v. × 100 (s.a. denotes surface area under curve depicting the changes of given sugar levels in blood after peroral load (p.o.) and after i.v. application of an identical dose between 0 and 120 min.[54]). (From Koldovsky, O., *Physiology of the Perinatal Period*, Stave, U., Ed., Plenum Publishing, New York, 1978. With permission.)

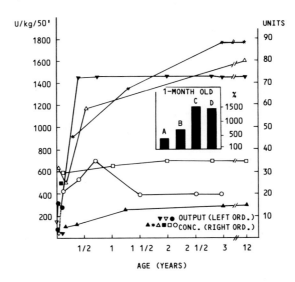

FIGURE 10.   Lipase activity in the duodenal juice of infants and children. Right ordinate: Data of (O,[81] △,[82] and
□[83] — full term; ■ — prematures) are given as concentration of lipase in units (short vertical lines in data of Anderson[81] denote S.E.M.: data of Droese[83] are multiplied by
five.) Left ordinate: Lipase activity as units secreted per 50
min/kg (∇[84] — full term; ● — prematures; ∇ — not defined; ▼[85] and *[86] — 3 age groups according to body weight:
4 to 8 kg, 8 to 12 kg, above 12 kg; ▲[87] — values after test
meals, similar to fasting values). Insert: Effect of different
diets in lipase activity in prematures 1 month old. Data expressed as a percent of values found in these infants at
birth. Diet A was a high-fat diet with glucose; diets B, C,
and D were low-fat diets; diet B contained starch.[84] Vas-
quez[88] reported a significant (80%) increase during the first
3 weeks of life. Veghelyi[89] did not see substantial developmental differences in multiple determinations on 47 children from 1 to 11 years of age. Samples were obtained: (a)
without stimulation,[81,82] (b) after magnesium sulphate stimulation,[83] (c) after pancreozymin-secretin stimulation,[84-86]
and (d) after test meal.[87] (From Koldovsky, O., *Physiology
of the Perinatal Period,* Stave, U., Ed., Plenum Publishing,
New York, 1978. With permission.)

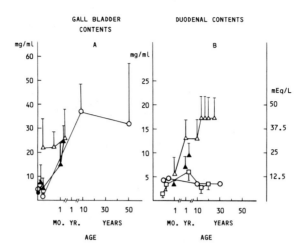

FIGURE 11.   A. Bile acid concentration in gall bladder bile in infants and adults (postmortem samples). (O — full-term; ● — prematures),[90] (△ — full-term; ▲ — prematures),[91] vertical lines denote one SD. B. Bile acid concentration in duodenal contents (see also Table 4) (From Koldovsky, O., *Physiology of the Perinatal Period,* Plenum Publishing, New York, 1976. With permission.) □ (in mEq/l) — samples obtained after 6 to 8 hr fasting[92] O(in mEq/ l) — after about 6 hr fasting,[93] △ — full term,[91] ▲ — prematures; mg/ml samples obtained after choleretic stimulation (magnesium sulphate); vertical lines denote one SD.

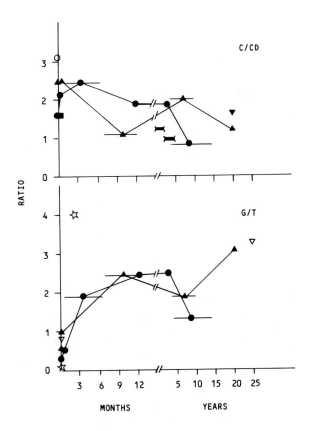

FIGURE 12. Postnatal changes in composition of bile acids in duodenal juice. Data from: ▲ — Ref. 94, 95; ● — Ref. 96; ▼ — Ref. 97; ■ — Ref. 98; ○ — Ref. 99; * — Ref. 100; ▽ — Ref. 101; ▣ — Ref. 102. Upper part: ratio of cholic to chenodeoxycholic acids. Lower part: ratio of glycine to taurine conjugates. Horizontal lines denote age range. (From Koldovsky, O., *Physiology of the Perinatal Period,* Stave, U., Ed., Plenum Publishing, New York, 1978. With permission.)

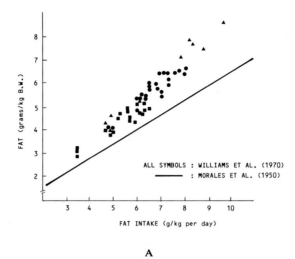

A

FIGURE 13.   Fat retention in infants and children fed different doses of fat. A) Fat intake and retention expressed per kilogram of body weight. Full symbols represent 55 full-term infants,[103] 1 week of age, fed four adapted formulas or breast milk. Regression line[104] in 24 determinations on eight 3-week-old prematures fed skimmed milk and butter fat. (From Koldovsky, O., *Physiology of the Perinatal Period,* Stave, U., Ed., Plenum Publishing, New York, 1976. With permission.) B) Regression line #1 retention of fat in infants, 3 to 9-week old.[105] Regression line #2 represents children with mild diarrhea, 24 determinations, type of fat not given.[106] Regression line #3 represents data calculated from seven cases by Holt et al.[106] (**Compiled by O. Koldovsky.**) C) Fecal fat excretion plotted against fat intake on three diets: ● — breast milk, ○ — SMA/S26, and ▽ — O.M.I.® Fullterm infants, 1 week old.[107] According to the authors, correlation between the fecal fat and fat intake had an exponential form. (**Compiled by O. Koldovsky.**) D) Retention of fat in coeliac children; each child was studied at different levels of fat intake. Each symbol denotes a different subject: ○ — 20-month-old; ● — 8-month-old; ■ — 7½-year-old; and 4 other patients,[108] ▼, ▲, △, ▽.[105] (From Koldovsky, O., *Physiology of the Perinatal Period,* Stave, U., Ed., Plenum Publishing, New York, 1978. With permission.)

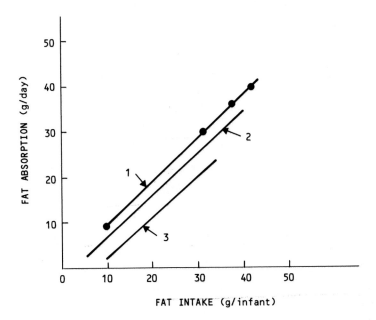

FIGURE 13B

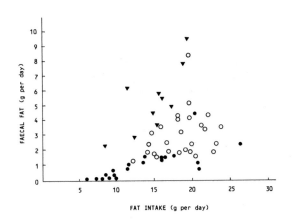

FIGURE 13C

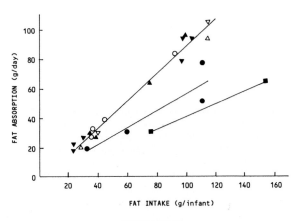

FIGURE 13D

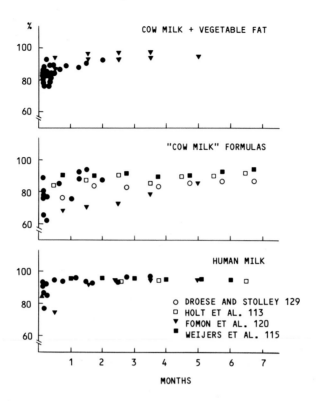

FIGURE 14.   Fat absorption in full-term infants (expressed as percent of intake).[109-128] (From Koldovsky, O., *Physiology of the Perinatal Period,* Stave, U., Ed., Plenum Publishing, New York, 1978. With permission.)

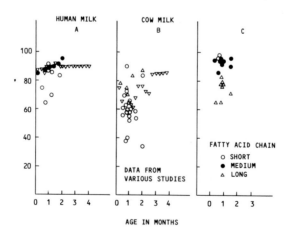

FIGURE 15.   Absorption of human (A) and cow milk (B) fat and comparison of retention of triglycerides of various fatty acids chain length (C) in prematures (expressed as % of fat intake). Symbols and References: 15A. — ▽,[129,130] ●,[135] ○;[131-134,136] 15B. — ▽,[130] △,[139] ●,[135] ○;[131-135,137,138,140-148] 15C. — Ref. 143,145-148. (From Koldovsky, O., *Physiology of the Perinatal Period,* Stave, U., Ed., Plenum Publishing, New York, 1978. With permission.)

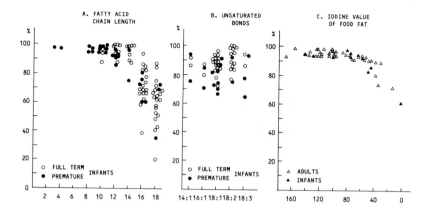

FIGURE 16. Absorption of various fats classified according to, A., fatty acid chain length, B., unsaturated bonds, and, C., iodine value (expressed as percent of fat intake).[149-163]

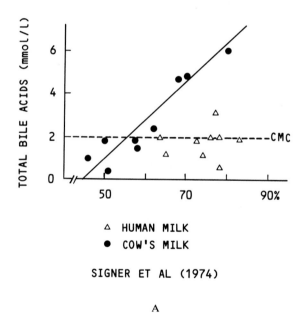

SIGNER ET AL (1974)

A

FIGURE 17. Relationship between fat absorption and bile acids concentration in infants. A) Abscissa: fat absorption in % of fat intake; △ = human milk fat; ● cow's milk fat. Infants 11 to 14 days of age from gestations lasting 35 to 37 weeks, respectively. (CMC — critical micellar concentration).[164] B) Ordinate: Percent of infants with fat absorption higher than 80% (open part of the column) or lower than 80% (black parts).[165,166] (From Koldovsky, O., *Physiology of the Perinatal State,* Stave, U., Ed., Plenum Publishing, New York, 1978. With permission.)

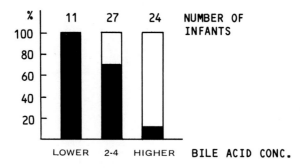

LAVY ET AL (1971) & LAVY (1974)

FIGURE 17B

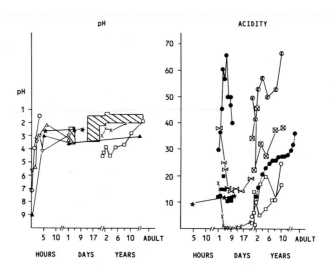

FIGURE 18A AND B.   Postnatal changes in gastric pH and acidity in infants. pH Determination: ∇, 32 full-term infants — fasting;[179] △, 53 full-term infants — fasting;[180] *, 25 full-term — newborn: fasting, older infants: 1 hour after meal;[181] ▲, 14 prematures — before feeding, feeding tube remained *in situ*;[182] ○, 12 full-term — feeding, feeding tube remained *in situ*;[183] □, 74 full-term — fasting;[184] ×, 40 children — fasting;[185] ▨ , Compilation of older data, after histamin stimulation.[186] Free and total acidity: ■ free, ● total (fasting values of 58 prematures followed on consecutive days);[187] * buffer value;[181] □ free, ⊠ total acidity (fasting), ○ free, ● total acidity (after test meal);[184] (10) free, ⋈ total acidity (50 full-term, fasting);[188] (11) ●--●--●free acid (following a test meal [boys], values in girls [not shown] do not increase after 9 years).[189] (From Koldovsky, O., *Physiology of the Perinatal Period,* Stave, U., Ed., New York, 1978, B. Compiled by O. Koldovsky.)

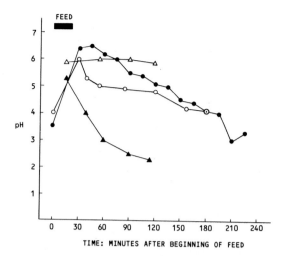

FIGURE 19.   The effect of feeding on pH values of the stomach contents of infants of different age. Data: O — 10 premature babies, 13 days old;[190] ● — 25 full-term newborn infants;[192] △ — infants, 1 to 2 months old;[192] ▲ — children, 3—13 years old.[192] (From Koldovsky, O., *Physiology of the Perinatal Period,* Stave, U., Ed., Plenum Press, New York, 1976. With permission.)

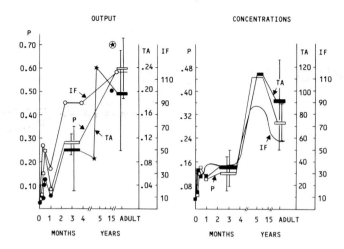

FIGURE 20.   Postnatal development of secretion of pepsin (P), titr-
able acid (TA), and intrinsic factor (IF) in infants.[193] Further TA data
taken from references 194 (●) 195 (★), and 196 (✪), assuming mean
adult weight = 70 kg). Ordinates: P — A: ng/hr/kg, B: mg/mℓ; TA
— A: mEq/hr/kg, B: mEq/ℓ; IF — A: ng B_{12}/hr/kg, B: ng B_{12}/mℓ.
(A) Output per kilogram of body weight and hour. Horizintal length
of rectangles denotes the extent of the age group. Short vertical lines
denote the range of values (used only in 2- to 3-month-old and adult
groups). (B) Concentration per kilogram of body weight and hour.
(From Koldovsky, O., *Physiology of the Perinatal Period,* Stave, U.,
Ed., Plenum Press, New York, 1976. With permission.)

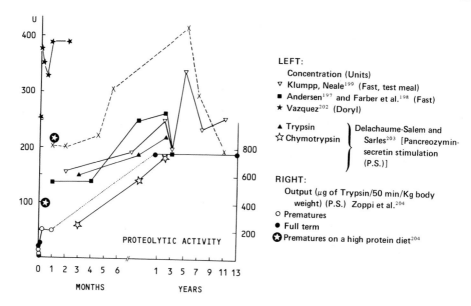

LEFT:

Concentration (Units)
▽ Klumpp, Neale[199] (Fast, test meal)
■ Andersen[197] and Farber et al.[198] (Fast)
★ Vazquez[202] (Doryl)

▲ Trypsin ⎫ Delachaume-Salem and
☆ Chymotrypsin ⎬ Sarles[203] [Pancreozymin-
⎭ secretin stimulation (P.S.)]

RIGHT:

Output (µg of Trypsin/50 min/Kg body weight) (P.S.) Zoppi et al.[204]
○ Prematures
● Full term
✪ Prematures on a high protein diet[204]

FIGURE 21. Postnatal changes in proteolytic activity in the duodenal juice. In recent years the definition of trypsin activity as opposed to other protease activities has been qualified. (The reader is advised to check original papers for a detailed description of method and substrates.) Earlier studies determined changes of viscosity of gelatine;[197-199] later, casein[200] and hemoglobin[201] were used as substrates. Whereas the data of Anderson[197] do not show any statistically significant differences between age groups (even with the considerable number of subjects studied — 54), the data of Zoppi et al.[204] show both a significant postnatal increase and a significant effect of the high protein diet in the early postnatal period. Previous data from the same laboratory[205] in a smaller group of children did not show statistical difference between various age groups (0 to 1/2, 1/2 to 1, 1 to 5, and 5 to 13 years old).

In addition to these data, mean trypsin values (fasting and after test meal) in 42 children 1 to 6 years of age (mean: 2 1/2 years) were published. Mean concentration and output of trypsin per body weight were reported to be 50% higher in six infants 1 to 11 months of age (mean: 7 months) than in six children (2 to 11 years; mean: 5 1/2 years).[201] An extensive study[200] found no difference in trypsin activity in children 1 to 2 years old as compared to 8 to 11 years old; the values in the intermediate age group were similar, but with an unexplained 30% lower activity in 2- to 3-yearold children. No postnatal change was found in α-chymotrypsin and carboxypeptidase activity in 27 infants and children from 6 weeks to 13 years.[205] Results of the same group[204] with trypsin, where previous reports also indicate no postnatal changes, suggest that these findings should be judged as preliminary. (From Koldovsky, O., *Physiology of the Perinatal Period*, Stave, U., Ed., Plenum Publishing, New York, 1978. With permission.)

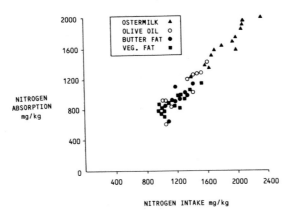

FIGURE 22.　Correlation between nitrogen intake and absorption (r = 0.94, p ≥ 0.01) in infants on four different diets.[207] (From MacLaurin, J. D., Watson, J., Stewart, M. E., Griffin, J. F., and Samuel, P. D., *Postgrad. Med. J.*, 51 (Suppl. 3), 45—51, 1975. With permission.)

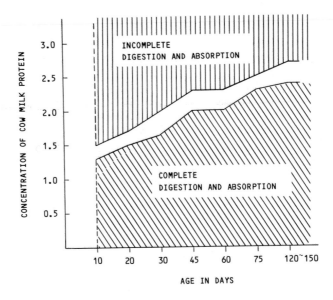

FIGURE 23.　Change of digestion and absorption of cow's milk protein in infants during four postnatal months of life.[208] Digestion and absorption was considered "complete" when analysis of ileal contents showed absence of undigested casein and both the nitrogen protein concentration and ratio nitrogen protein:total nitrogen was the same as in infants of corresponding age fed breast milk. (From Hirata, Y., Matsuo, T., and Kokubu, H., *Kobe J. Med. Sci.*, 11, 103—109, 1965. With permission.)

REFERENCES

1. Lindberg, T., *Clin. Sci.*, 30, 505—515, 1966.
2. Beneke, *Dtsch. Med. Wochenschr.*, 32, 435—436 and 448—450, 1880.
3. Zoppi, G., Andreotti, G., Pajno-Ferraro, F., Njai, D. M., and Gaburro, D., *Pediatr. Res.*, 6, 880—886, 1972.
4. Klumpp, T. G. and Neale, A. V., *Am. J. Dis. Child.*, 40, 1215—1229, 1930.
5. Gibbs, G. E., *J. Pediatr.*, 5, 941—946, 1950.
6. Delachaume-Salem, E. and Sarles, H., *Biol. Gastro-Enterol.*, 2, 135—146, 1970; *Arch. Fr. Mal. Appar. Dig.*, 59 (Suppl. 2), 10—11, 1970.
7. Hadorn, B., Zoppi, G., Shmerling, D. H., Prader, A., McIntyre, I., and Anderson, C. M., *J. Pediatr.*, 73, 39—50, 1968.
8. Auricchio, S., Della Pietra, D., and Vegnente, A., *Pediatrics*, 39, 853—862, 1967.
9. Andersen, D. H., *Am. J. Dis. Child.*, 63, 643—658, 1942.
10. Farber, S., Shwachman, H., and Maddock, C. L., *J. Clin. Invest.*, 22, 827—838, 1943.
11. Ingomar, C. J. and Terslev, E., *Arch. Dis. Child.*, 42, 289—293, 1967.
12. Vazquez, C., *Rev. Espan. Pediatr.*, 7, 75—85, 1951.
13. Véghelyi, P. V., *Pediatrics*, 3, 749—763, 1949.
14. Jirsová, V., Koldovský, O., Heringová, A., Uher, J., and Jodl, J., *Biol. Neonat.*, 13, 143—146, 1968.
15. Sheehy, T. W. and Anderson, P. R., *Am. J. Dis. Child.*, 121, 464—468, 1971.
16. Auricchio, S., Rubino, A., and Mürset, G., *Pediatrics*, 35, 944—954, 1965.
17. Dahlqvist, A. and Lindberg, T., *Clin. Sci.*, 30, 517—528, 1966.
18. Eggermont, E., *Biol. Neonat.*, 10, 266—280, 1966.
19. Fomina, L. S., *Vopr. Med. Khim.*, 6, 176—182, 1960.
20. Heilskov, N. S. C., *Acta Physiol. Scand.*, 24, 84—89, 1951.
21. Jirsová, V., Koldovský, O., Heringová, A., Uher, J., and Jodl, J., *Biol. Neonat.*, 13, 143—146, 1968.
21a. Sheehy, T. W. and Anderson, P. R., *Am. J. Dis. Child.*, 121, 464—468, 1971.
21b. Ibrahim, J., *Hoppe-Seylers Z. Physiol. Chem.*, 66, 19—36, 1910.
21c. Ibrahim, J. and Kaumheimer, L., *Hoppe-Seylers Z. Physiol. Chem.*, 66, 37—52, 1910.
22. Bolin, T. D., Davis, A. E., Seah, C. S., Chua, K. L., Yoh, V., Kho, K. M., Siak, C. L., and Jacob, E., *Gastroenterology*, 59, 76—94, 1970.
23. Cook, G. C., *Br. Med. J.*, 1, 527—530, 1967.
24. Huang, S.-S. and Bayless, T. M., *N. Engl. J. Med.*, 276, 1283—1287, 1967.
25. Jones, D. V. and Latham, M. C., *Am. J. Clin. Nutr.*, 27, 547—549, 1974.
26. Keusch, G. T., Troncale, F. J., Miller, L. H., Promadhat, V., and Anderson, P. R., *Pediatrics*, 43, 540—545, 1969.
27. Kretchmer, N., Ransome-Kuti, O., Hurwitz, R., Dungy, C., and Alakija, W., *Lancet*, 2, 392—395, 1971.
28. Olatunbosun, D. A. and Adadevoh, B. K., *Acta Paediatr. Scand.*, 61, 715—719, 1972.
29. Paige, D. M., Leonardo, E., Cordano, A., Nakashima, J., Adrianzen, B., and Graham, G. G., *Am. J. Clin. Nutr.*, 25, 297—301, 1972.
30. Reddy, V. and Pershad, J., *Am. J. Clin. Nutr.*, 25, 114—119, 1972.
31. Sahi, T., Isokoski, M., Jussila, J., and Launiala, K., *Acta Paediatr. Scand.*, 61, 11—16, 1972.
32. Woteki, C. E., Weser, E., and Young, E. A., *Am. J. Clin. Nutr.*, 29, 19—24, 1976.
32a. Shibuya, S., *J. Kurume Med. Assoc.*, 33, 1440—1446, 1970.
33. Flatz, C., Saengudom, C., and Sanguanbhokhai, T., *Nature*, 221, 758—759, 1969.
34. Boellner, S. W., Beard, A. G., and Panos, T. C., *Pediatrics*, 36, 542—550, 1965.
35. Jarrett, E. C. and Holman, G. H., *Arch. Dis. Child.*, 41, 525—527, 1966.
36. Cook, C. C., *Br. Med. J.*, 1, 527—530, 1967.
37. Anyon, C. P. and Clarkson, K. G., *N. Z. Med. J.*, 64, 694—696, 1965.
38. Jirsová, V., Koldovský, O., Heringová, A., Hôsková, J., Jirásek, J., and Uher, J., *Biol. Neonat.*, 9, 44—49, 1966.
39. Levin, R., Koldovský, O., Hôsková, J., and Jirsová, V., *Gut*, 9, 206—213, 1968.
40. Torres-Pinedo, R., Rivera, C. L., and Fernandez, S., *J. Clin. Invest.*, 45, 1916—1922, 1966.
41. James, W. P. T., *Clin. Sci.*, 39, 305—318, 1970.
42. Lugo-de-Rivera, C., Rodriguez, H., and Torres-Pinedo, R., *Am. J. Clin. Nutr.*, 25, 1248—1253, 1972.
43. Fordtran, J. S. and Ingelfinger, F. J., in *Handbook of Physiology*, Vol. 3, Washington, D.C., 1968, p. 1477.

44. Cummins, A. J., and Jussila, R., *Gastroenterology,* 29, 982—991, 1955.
45. Fordtran, J. S., Clodi, P. H., Soergel, K. H., and Ingelfinger, J., *Ann. Intern. Med.,* 57, 883—891, 1962.
46. Fordtran, J. S., Levitan, R., Bikerman, V., Barrows, B. A., and Ingelfinger, F. J., *Trans. Assoc. Am. Physicans,* 74, 195—205, 1961.
47. Gray, G. M. and Ingelfinger, F. J., *J. Clin. Invest.,* 45, 388—398, 1966.
48. Holdsworth, C. D. and Dawson, A. M., *Clin. Sci.,* 27, 371—379, 1964.
49. Schedl, H. P. and Clifton, J. A., *World Congress of Gastroenterology, 2nd, Munich,* Vol. 2, S. Karger, Basel, 1963, 728—732.
50. Talley, R. B., Schedl, H. P., and Clifton, J. A., *Gastroenterology,* 47, 382—387, 1964.
51. Vinnik, I. E., Kern, F., Jr., and Sussman, K. E., *J. Lab. Clin. Med.,* 66, 131—136, 1965.
52. Yunoszai, M. K., *J. Pediatrics,* 85, 446—448, 1974.
53. Lanzkowsky, P., Madenlioglu, M., Wilson, J. F., and Lahey, M. E., *N. Engl. J. Med.,* 268, 1441—1444, 1963.
54. Beyreiss, K., *Pädiatrie und Grenzgebiete,* 10, 151—166, 1971.
55. Meeuwisse G. W. and Dano, G., *Acta Paediatr. Scand.,* 54, 33—42, 1965.
56. Dunphy, J. V., Littman, A., Hammond, J. B., Forstner, G., Dahlquist, A., and Crane, R. K., *Gastroenterology,* 49, 12—21, 1965.
57. Townley, R. R. W., Khaw, K. T., and Shwachman, H., *Pediatrics,* 36, 911—921, 1965.
58. Kerry, K. R. and Townley, R. R. W., *Aust. Paediatr. J.,* 1, 223—235, 1965.
59. Cook, G. C., *Br. Med. J.,* 1, 527—530, 1967.
60. Keusch, G. T., Troncale, F. J., Miller, L. H., Promadhat, V., and Anderson, P. R., *Pediatrics,* 43, 540—545, 1969.
61. Antonowicz, I. and Shwachman, H., *Pediatrics,* 47, 737—743, 1971.
62. Bolin, T. D., Davis, A. E., Seah, C. S., Chua, K. L., Yoh, V., Kho, K. M., Siak, C. L., and Jacob, E., *Gastroenterology,* 59, 76—84, 1970.
63. Lebenthal, E., Tsuboi, K., and Kretchmer, N., *Gastroenterology,* 67, 1107—1113, 1974.
64. Reddy, V., and Pershad, J., *Am. J. Clin. Nutr.,* 25, 114—119, 1972.
65. Antonowicz, I., Ishida, S., Khaw, K. T., and Shwachman, H., *Pediatrics,* 45, 104—106, 1970.
66. Apollonio, T., Palumbo-Vargas, O., and Cevini, G., *Minerva Pediatr.,* 18, 2183—2185, 1966.
67. Elliot, R. B., Maxwell, G. M., and Vawser, N., *Med. J. Aust.,* 1, 46—49, 1967.
68. Cook, G. C., *Br. Med. J.,* 1, 527—530, 1967.
69. Cook, G. C., Asp, N.-G., and Dahlqvist, A., *Gastroenterology,* 64, 405—410, 1973.
70. Dunphy, J. V., Littman, A., Hammond, J. B., Forstner, G., Dahlqvist, A., and Crane, R. K., *Gastroenterology,* 49, 12—21, 1965.
71. Haemmerli, U. P., Kistler, H., Ammann, R., Marthaler, T., Semenza, G., Auricchio, S., and Prader, A., *Am. J. Med.,* 38, 7—30, 1965.
72. Kerry, K. R. and Townley, R. R. W., *Austr. Paediatr. J.,* 1, 223—235, 1965.
73. Keusch, G. T., Troncale, F. J., Miller, L. H., Promadhat, V., and Anderson, P. R., *Pediatrics,* 43, 540—545, 1969.
74. Lebenthal, E., Tsuboi, K., and Kretchmer, N., *Gastroenterology,* 67, 1107—1113, 1974.
75. Reddy, V., and Pershad, J., *Am. J. Clin. Nutr.,* 25, 114—119, 1972.
76. Townley, R. R. W., Khaw, K. T., and Shwachman, H., *Pediatrics,* 36, 911—921, 1965.
77. Welsh, J. D., Rohrer, V., Knudsen, K. B., and Paustian, F. F., *Arch. Int. Med.,* 120, 261—269, 1967.
78. Antonowicz, I., Ishida, S., Khaw, K. T., and Shwachman, H., *Pediatrics,* 45, 104—106, 1970.
79. Apollonio, T., Palumbo-Vargas, O., and Cevini, G., *Minerva Pediatr.,* 18, 2183—2185, 1966.
80. Elliot, R. B., Maxwell, G. M., and Vawser, N., *Med. J. Aust.,* 1, 46—49, 1967.
81. Andersen, D. H., *Am. J. Dis. Child.,* 63, 643—658, 1942.
82. Farber, S., Shwachman, H., and Maddock, C. L., *J. Clin. Invest.,* 22, 827—838, 1943.
83. Droese, W., *Ann. Paediatr.,* 178, 121—149 and 238—263, 1952.
84. Zoppi, G., Andreotti, G., Pajno-Ferrara, F., Njai, D. M., and Gaburro, D., *Pediatr. Res.,* 6, 880—886, 1972.
85. Hadorn, B., Zoppi, G., Shmerling, D. H., Prader, A., McIntyre, I., and Anderson, C. M., *J. Pediatr.,* 73, 39—50, 1968.
86. Delachaume-Salem, E. and Sarles, H., *Biol. Gastro-Enterol.,* 2, 135—146, 1970; *Arch. Fr. Mal. Appar. Dig.,* 59 (Suppl. 2), 10—11, 1970.
87. Klumpp, T. G. and Neale, A. V., *Am. J. Dis. Child.,* 40, 1215—1229, 1930.
88. Vazquez, C., *Rev. Espan. Pediatr.,* 7, 75—85, 1951.
89. Veghelyi, P. V., *Pediatrics,* 3, 749—763, 1949.
90. Bongiovanni, A. M., *J. Clin. Endocrinol.,* 25, 678—685, 1965.
91. Droese, W., *Annal. Paediatr.,* 178, 121—149 and 238—263, 1952.

92. Poley, J. R., Dower, J. C., Owen, C. A., and Stickler, G. B., *J. Lab. Clin. Med.*, 63, 838—846, 1964.
93. Encrantz, J.-C. and Sjövall, J., *Clin. Chim. Acta*, 4, 793—799, 1959.
94. Encrantz, J.-C. and Sjövall, J., *Acta Chem. Scand.*, 11, 1093, 1957.
95. Encrantz, J.-C. and Sjövall, J., *Clin. Chim. Acta.*, 4, 793—799, 1959.
96. Poley, J. R., Dower, J. C., Owen, C. A., and Stickler, G. B., *J. Lab. Clin. Med.*, 63, 838—846, 1964.
97. Miettinnen, T. A. and Siurala, M., *Z. Klin. Chem. Klin. Biochem.*, 9, 47—52, 1971.
98. Norman, A., Strandvik, B., and Ojamäe, O., *Acta Paediatr. Scand.*, 61, 571—576, 1972.
99. Watkins, J. B., Bliss, M., Donaldson, R. M., and Lester, R., *Pediatrics*, 53, 511—515, 1974.
100. Katz, L. and Hamilton, J. R., *J. Pediatr.*, 85, 608—614, 1974.
101. Challacombe, D. N., Edkin, S., and Brown, G. A., in *Pediatric Gastroenterolgy*, Anderson, C. M. and Burke, V., Eds., Blackwell Scientific, Oxford, 1975, 142.
102. Von Bergmann, J., Von Bergmann, K., Hadorn, B., and Paumgartner, G., *Clin. Chim. Acta*, 64, 241—246, 1975.
103. Williams, M. L., Rose, C. S., Morrow, G., Sloan, S. E., and Barness, L. A., *Am. J. Clin. Nutr.*, 23, 1322—1330, 1970.
104. Morales, S., Chung, A. W., Lewis, J. M., Messina, A., and Holt, L. E., Jr., *Pediatrics*, 6, 86—92 and 644—649, 1950.
105. Holt, L. E., Jr., *J. Pediatr.*, 46, 369—379, 1955.
106. Holt, L. E., Courtney, A. M., and Fales, H. L., *Am. J. Dis. Child.*, 17, 241—250, and 423—439, 1919.
107. Southgate, D. A. T., Widdowson, E. M., Smits, B. J., Cooke, W. T., Walker, C. H. M., and Mathers, N. P., *Lancet*, 1, 487—489, 1969.
108. Macrae, O., and Morris, N., *Arch. Dis. Child.*, 6, 75—96, 1931.
109. Lindberg, G., *Z. Kinderheil.*, 16, 90—107, 1917.
110. Holt, L. E., Courtney, A. M., and Fales, H. L., *Am. J. Dis. Child.*, 17, 241—250, 1919.
111. Malmberg, N., *Acta Paediatr. Scand.*, 2, 209—353, 1922—23.
112. Muhl, G., *Aca Paediatr. Scand.*, 2, Suppl 1, 1—41, 1924.
113. Holt, L. E., Tidwell, H. C., Kirk, C. M., Cross, D. M., and Neale, S., *J. Pediatr.*, 6, 427—480, 1935.
114. Guilbert P., Baker, D., and Barness, L. A., *J. Pediatr.*, 47, 683—689, 1955.
115. Weijers, H. A., Drion, E. F., and Van de Kamer, J. H., *Acta Paediatr.*, 49, 615—625, 1960.
116. Van de Kamer, J. H. and Weijers, H. A., 5th Intr. Congr. Nutr., *Fed. Proc. Fed. Am. Soc. Exp. Biol.*, 20 (Suppl. 7), 333—344, 1961.
117. Widdowson, E. M., *Lancet*, 2, Nov. 27, 1099—1105, 1965.
118. Southgate, D. A. T. and Barrett, I. M., *J. Nutr.*, 20, 363—372, 1966.
119. Southgate, D. A. T., Widdowson, E. M., Smits, B. J., Cooke, W. T., Walker, C. H. M., and Mathers, N. P., *Lancet*, 1, March 8, 487—489, 1969.
120. Fomon, S. J., Ziegler, E. E., Thomas, L. N., Jensen, R. L., and Filer, L. J., *Am. J. Clin. Nutr.*, 23, 1290—1313, 1970.
121. Williams, M. L., Rose, C. S., Morrow, G., Sloan, S. E., and Barness, L. A., *Am. J. Clin. Nutr.*, 23, 1322—1330, 1970.
122. Hanna, F. M., Navarrete, D. A., and Hsu, F. A., *Pediatrics*, 45, 216—224, 1970.
123. Gordon, H. H., Levine, S. Z., Wheatley, M. A., and Marples, E., *Am. J. Dis. Child.*, 54, 1030—1044, 1937.
124. Gordon, H. H. and McNamara, H., *Am. J. Dis. Child.*, 62, 328—345, 1941.
125. Droese, W., *Ann. Paediatr.*, 178, 121—149 and 238—263, 1952.
126. Joppich, G., Lohr, H., and Wolf, H., *Z. Kinderheil.*, 82, 7, 1959.
127. Droese, W. and Stolley, H., *Fette Seifen Anstrichm.*, 62, 281—285, 1960.
128. MacLaurin, J. C., Watson, J., Murphy, W., Stewart, M. E., Griffin, J. F., and Samuel, P. D., *Postgrad. Med. J.*, Suppl. 3, 51, 45—51, 1975.
129. Droese, W. and Stolley, H., *Fette Seifen Anstrichm.*, 62, 281—285, 1960.
130. Droese, W. and Stolley, H., *Dtsch. Med. Wochenschr.*, 17, 855—860, 1961.
131. Gordon, H. H., Levine, S. Z., Wheatley, M. A., and Marples, E., *Am. J. Dis. Child.*, 54, 1030—1044, 1937.
132. Gordon, H. H. and McNamara, H., *Am. J. Dis. Child.*, 62, 328—345, 1941.
133. Ocklitz, H. W. and Reinmuth, B., *Z. Kinderheil.*, 82, 321—327, 1959.
134. Signer, E., Murphy, G. M., Edkins, S., and Anderson, C. M., *Arch. Dis. Child.*, 49, 174—180, 1974.
135. Söderhjelm, L., *Acta Paediatr.*, 41, 207—221, 1952.
136. Zoula, J., Melichar, V., Novák, M., Hahn, P. and Koldovský, O., *Acta Paediatr. Scand.*, 55, 26—32, 1966.

137. Barltrop, D. and Oppe, T. E., *Arch. Dis. Child.*, 48, 496—501, 1973.
138. Davidson, M. and Bauer, C. H., *Pediatrics*, 25, 375—384, 1960.
139. Katz, L. and Hamilton, J. R., *J. Pediatr.*, 85, 608—614, 1974.
140. Milner, R. D. G., Deodhar, V., Chard, C. R., and Grout, R. M., *Arch. Dis. Child.*, 50, 654—656, 1975.
141. Morales, S., Chung, A. W., Lewis, J. M., Messina, A. and Holt, L. E., Jr., *Pediatrics*, 6, 86—92 and 644—649, 1950.
142. Senterre, J. and Lambrechts, A., *Biol. Neonat.*, 20, 107—119, 1972.
143. Snyderman, S. E., Morales, S., and Holt, L. E., Jr., *Arch. Dis. Child.*, 30, 83—84, 1955.
144. Tidwell, H. C., Holt, L. E., Jr., Farrow, H. L., and Neale, S., *J. Pediatr.*, 6, 481—489, 1935.
145. Roy, C. C., Ste.-Marie, M., Chartrand, L., Weber, A., Bard, H., and Doray, B., *J. Pediatr.*, 86, 446—450, 1975.
146. Tantibhedhyangkul, P. and Hashim, S. A., *Pediatrics*, 55, 359—370, 1975.
147. Snyderman, S. E., Morales, S., Chung, A. W., Lewis, J. M., Messina, A., and Holt, L. E. Jr., *Pediatrics*, 12, 158—163, 1953.
148. Yamashita, F., Shibuya, S., Funatsu, I., Kuno, T., and Ide, H., *Kurume Med. J.*, 16, 191—201, 1969.
149. Barnes, L. A., Morrow, G., Silverio, J., Finnegan, L. P., and Heitman, S. E., *Pediatrics*, 54, 217—221, 1974.
150. Filer, L. J., Mattson, F. H., and Fomon, S. J., *J. Nutr.*, 99, 293—298, 1969.
151. Hanna, F. M., Navarrete, D. A., and Hsu, F. A., *Pediatrics*, 45, 216—224, 1970.
152. Holt, L. E., Jr., Tidwell, H. C., Kirk, C. M., Cross, D. M., and Neale, S., *J. Pediatr.*, 6, 427—480, 1935.
153. Luther, G. and Schreier, K., *Klin. Wochenshcr.*, 41, 189—193, 1963.
154. Scheppe, K. J., Zeisel, H., Alletag, U., Habeth, E., and Kecker, H., *Med. Ernaehr.*, 6, 80—99, 1965.
155. Snyderman, S. E., Morales, S., and Holt, L. E., Jr., *Arch. Dis. Child.*, 30, 83—84, 1955.
156. Tantibhedhyangkul, P. and Hashim, S. A., *Pediatrics*, 55, 359—370, 1975.
157. Tidwell, H. C., Holt, L. E., Jr., Farrow, H. L., and Neale, S., *J. Pediatr.*, 6, 481—489, 1935.
158. Watkins, J. B., Bliss, M., Donaldson, R. M., and Lester, R., *Pediatrics*, 53, 511—515, 1974.
159. Welsch, H., Heinz, F., Lagally, G., and Stuhlfauth, K., *Klin. Wochenschr.*, 43, 902—904, 1965.
160. Williams, M. L., Rose, C. S., Morrow, G., Sloan, S. E., and Barness, L. A., *Am. J. Clin. Nutr.*, 23, 1322—1330, 1970.
161. Yamashita, F., Shibuya, S., and Funatsu, I., *Kurume Med. J.*, 16, 191—201, 1969.
162. Roy, C. C., Ste.-Marie, M., Chartrand, L., Weber, A., Bard, H., and Doray, B., *J. Pediatr.*, 86, 446—450, 1975.
163. Langworthy, C. F., *Ind. Eng. Chem.*, 15, 276—278, 1923.
164. Signer, E., Murphy, G. M., Edkins, S., and Anderson, C. M., *Arch. Dis. Child.*, 49, 174—180, 1974.
165. Lavy, U., Silverberg, M., and Davidson, M., *Pediatr. Res.*, 5, 387, 1971.
166. Lavy, U., cited in Watkins, J. B., *Pediatr. Clin. North America*, 21, 501—512, 1974.
167. Miettinen, T. A. and Siurala, M., *Z. Klin. Chem. Klin. Biochem.*, 9, 47—52, 1971.
168. Sjövall, J., *Acta Physiol. Scand.*, 46, 339—345, 1959.
169. Encrantz, J.-C. and Sjövall, J., *Clin. Chim. Acta*, 4, 793—799, 1959.
170. Norman, A., Strandvik, B., and Ojamae, O., *Acta Paediatr. Scand.*, 61, 571—576, 1972.
171. Signer, E., Murphy, G. M., Edkins, S., and Anderson, C. M., *Arch. Dis. Child.*, 49, 174—180, 1974.
172. Katz, L. and Hamilton, J. R., *J. Pediatr.*, 85, 608—614, 1974.
173. Lavy, U., Silverberg, M., and Davidson, M., *Pediatr. Res.*, 5, 387, 1971.
174. Admirand, W. H. and Small, D. M., *J. Clin. Invest.*, 47, 1043—1052, 1968.
175. Holzbach, R. T., Marsh, M., Olszewski, M., and Holan, K., *J. Clin. Invest*, 52, 1467—1479, 1973.
176. Dam, H., Kruse, I., Prange, I., Kallehauge, H. E., Fenger, H. J., and Krogh, J. M., *Z. Ernaehr.*, 10, 167—171, 1971.
177. Adler, R. D., Bennion, L. J., Duane, W. C., and Grundy, S. M., *Gastroenterology*, 68, 326—334, 1975.
178. Von Bergmann, J., Von Bergmann, K., Hadorn, B., and Paumgartner, G., *Clin. Chim. Acta*, 64, 241—246, 1975.
179. Avery, G. B., Randolph, J. G., and Weaver, T., *Pediatrics*, 37, 1005—1007, 1966.
180. Ebers, D. W., Smith, D. I., and Gibbs, G. E., *Pediatrics*, 18, 800—803, 1956.
181. Griswold, C. and Shohl, A. T., *Am. J. Dis. Child.*, 30, 541—549, 1925.
182. Harries, J. T. and Fraser, A. J., *Biol. Neonat.*, 12, 186—193, 1968.
183. Huhtikangas, H. J., *Acta Soc. Med. Fenn. Duodecim*, 24, 1—21, 1936.

184. Klumpp, T. G. and Neale, A. V., *Am. J. Dis. Child.,* 40, 1215—1229, 1930.
185. Kopel, F. B. and Barbero, G. J., *Gastroenterology,* 52, 1101, 1967.
186. Wolman, I. J., *Am. J. Med. Sci.,* 206, 770—794, 1943.
187. Ames, M. D., *Am. J. Dis. Child.,* 122—126, 1960.
188. Miller, R. A., *Arch. Dis. Child.,* 16, 22—30, 1941.
189. Vanzant, F. R., Alvarez, W. C., Berkson, J., and Eusterman, G. B., *Arch. Int. Med.,* 521, 616—631, 1933.
190. Harries, J. T. and Fraser, A. J., *Biol. Neonat.,* 12, 186—193, 1968.
191. Mason, S., *Arch. Dis. Child.,* 37, 387—391, 1962.
192. Wolman, I. J., *Am. J. Dis. Child.,* 71, 394—492, 1946.
193. Agunod, M., Yamaguchi, N., Lopez, R., Luhby, A. L., and Glass, B. G. J., *Am. J. Dig. Dis.,* 14, 400—414, 1969.
194. Ghai, O. P., Singh, M., Walia, B. N. S., and Gadekar, N. G., *Arch. Dis. Child.,* 40, 77—79, 1965.
195. Rodbro, P., Krasilnikoff, P. A., and Bitsch, V., *Scand. J. Gastroenterol.,* 2, 257—260, 1967.
196. Rodbro, P., Krasilnikoff, P. A., and Christiansen, P. M., *Scand. J. Gastroenterol.,* 2, 209—213, 1967.
197. Andersen, D. H., *Am. J. Dis. Child,* 63, 643—658, 1942.
198. Farber, S., Shwachman, H., and Maddock, C. L., *J. Clin. Invest.,* 22, 827—838, 1943.
199. Klumpp, T. G. and Neale, A. V., *Am. J. Dis. Child.,* 40, 1215—1229, 1930.
200. Veghelyi, P. V., *Pediatrics,* 3, 749—763, 1949.
201. Gibbs, G. E., *Pediatrics,* 5, 941—946, 1950.
202. Vazquez, C., *Rev. Espan. Pediatr.,* 7, 75—85, 1951.
203. Delachaume-Salem, E. and Sarles, H., *Biologie Gastro Enterol.,* 2 (Suppl. 2), 135—146, 1970.
204. Zoppi, G., Andreotti, G., Pajno-Ferrara, F., Njai, D. M., and Gaburro, D., *Pediatr. Res.,* 6, 880—886, 1972.
205. Hadorn, B., Zoppi, G., Shmerling, D. H., Prader, A., McIntyre, I., and Anderson, C. M., *J. Pediatr.,* 73, 39—50, 1968.
206. Ingomar, C. J. and Terslev, E., *Arch. Dis. Child.,* 42, 289—293, 1967.
207. MacLaurin, J. C., Watson, J., Stewart, M. E., Griffin, J. F., and Samuel, P. D., *Postgrad. Med. J.,* 51 (Suppl. 3), 45—51, 1975.
208. Hirata, Y., Matsuo, T., and Kokubu, H., *Kobe J. Med. Sci.,* 11, 103— 109, 1965.
209. Rogers, I. M., Davidson, D. C., Lawrence, J., Ardill, J., and Buchanan, K. D., *Arch. Dis. Child.,* 49, 796—801, 1974.
210. Rogers, I. M., Davidson, D. C., Lawrence, J., and Buchanan, K. D., *Arch. Dis. Child.,* 50, 120—122, 1975.
211. Hamilton, B., *Acta Paediatr.,* 2, 1—84, 1922—1923.
212. Gordon, H. H., Levine, S. Z., Wheatley, M. A., and Marples, E., *Am. J. Dis. Child.,* 54, 1030—1044, 1937.
213. Feinstein, M. S. and Smith, C. A., *Pediatrics,* 7, 19—23, 1951.
214. Zoula, J., Melichar, V., Novák, M., Hahn, P., and Koldovský, O., *Acta Paediatr. Scand.,* 55, 26—32, 1966.
215. Senterre, J. and Lambrechts, A., *Biol. Neonat.,* 20, 107—119, 1972.
216. Roy, C. C., Ste.-Marie, M., Chartrand, L., Weber, A., Bard, H., and Doray, B., *J. Pediatr.,* 86, 446—450, 1975.
217. Hamilton, B., *Acta Paediatr.,* 2, 1—84, 1922—1923.
218. Fomon, S. J., Thomas, L. N., Jensen, R. L., and May, C. D., *Pediatrics,* 22, 94—100, 1958.
219. Fomon, S. J., and May, C. D., *Pediatrics,* 22, 101—115, 1958.
220. Fomon, S. J., Thomas, L. N., and May, C. D., *Pediatrics,* 22, 935—944, 1958.
221. Fomon, S. J. and May, C. D., *Pediatrics,* 22, 1134—1147, 1958.
222. Fomon, S. J., *Pediatrics,* 26, 51—61, 1960.
223. Fomon, S. J., *Pediatrics,* 28, 347—361, 1961.
224. Widdowson, E. M., *Lancet,* 2, 1099—1105, 1965.
225. Southgate, D. A. T. and Barrett, I. M., *Br. J. Nutr.,* 20, 363—372, 1966.
226. Mac Laurin, J. C., Watson, J., Murphy, W., Stewart, M. E., Griffin, J. F., and Samuel, P. D., *Postgrad. Med. J.,* 51, 45—51, 1975.

ENDOCRINE SECRETION AND NUTRITION

James J. Jones

INTRODUCTION

Changes in endocrine secretion resulting from over- and undernutrition of energy and protein will be described. More specific hormonal effects produced by mineral and vitamin deficiencies will not be considered. In malnutrition, hormone activity is affected by changes in plasma concentration, protein binding,[1] conversion to active derivatives,[2] and target organ sensitivity.[3] Consequently, hormone determinations in plasma and urine have limited value in understanding the endocrine response to nutritional disturbances.

PROTEIN ENERGY MALNUTRITION

In young children, protein energy malnutrition (PEM) produces kwashiorkor with pitting edema, or marasmus, when the child's weight is less than 80% of expected weight for height and age.[4] Kwashiorkor usually develops rapidly often being precipitated by acute infections (particularly measles). It occurs in older children (over 12 months) who have already benefitted from a period of good nutrition (breast feeding) and developed a layer of subcutaneous fat.[5] On the other hand, marasmus shows a more gradual onset in the younger child (less than 12 months) who often has chronic diarrhea resulting from early weaning.[6]

There are four excellent reviews on the endocrine changes associated with PEM.[7-10]

Insulin

Tables 1 and 3 show that the basal (postabsorptive) plasma insulin concentration is decreased in children with either kwashiorkor or marasmus. Tables 2 and 4 show that there is a corresponding impairment of insulin secretion following stimulation tests. Since there is no consistent difference between kwashiorkor and marasmus (Tables 3 and 4), the change in insulin secretion is unlikely to be the direct result of the fall in plasma albumen or amino acid concentration.[11-13] A similar decrease in insulin secetion occurs after short periods of complete starvation in man (Tables 21 to 25) and experimental animals (Table 26).

Impaired insulin secretion has been attributed to potassium deficiency[14,15] and to a loss of "gut factors," including glucagon.[9,16,17] Insulin deficiency leads to growth failure of individual cells,[18] possibly resulting from insufficient amino acid uptake.[19] It also produces glucose intolerance[3,20] and an increase in plasma free fatty acid concentration,[21] which may lead to fatty infiltration of the liver.[22] The proportion of big insulin (proinsulin) secreted in kwashiorkor is unaltered.[23] Insulin deficiency is not the sole cause of glucose intolerance: there is also endorgan resistance to the action of insulin.[3,24]

Growth Hormone

Table 5 shows that basal (postabsorptive) plasma growth hormone concentration is raised in children with kwashiorkor, but the release of growth hormone by stimulation tests is unchanged (Table 6). The plasma half life (t½) is unaltered, showing that the increased plasma concentration is produced by a greater rate of growth hormone secretion.[42] In marasmus, basal growth hormone concentration is usually lower than in kwashiorkor (Table 7), and there is no consistent change in the rate of secretion following stimulation tests (Table 8). In adults, PEM increases plasma growth hormone concentration and the response to stimulation tests.[43,44] One to eight days of complete starvation is sufficient to raise plasma growth hormone concentration in man (Tables 30 to 32), but the effect is less constant in experimental animals. (Table 33).

In children with kwashiorkor, the activity of somatomedin is decreased by a plasma inhibitor[45,46] that prevents cell division despite the increase in growth hormone secretion.[18] Plasma somatomedin activity is also reduced by experimental PEM in rats (Table 33). The high concentration of growth hormone in PEM suggests that somatomedin controls growth hormone secretion by negative refection (feedback).[45]

In PEM, the rise in growth hormone concentration is associated with the fall in plasma amino acid concentration,[11,34] but there is no agreement as to a possible association with hypoalbuminemia.[11,12,47,48] Increased growth hormone secretion could also be caused by a loss of dopaminergic hypothalamic inhibition[49] — in kwashiorkor, urinary excretion of dopamine is depressed (Table 15).

The increased growth hormone secretion that occurs in PEM inhibits hepatic amino acid degradation,[19] produces insulin resistance,[3,24] increases plasma free fatty acids to cause fatty infiltration of the liver,[50] and decreases plasma triiodothyronine concentration (Tables 16 and 17).[51]

Cortisol

Table 9 shows that the basal (postabsorptive) plasma cortisol concentration is raised in children with kwashiorkor, although the response to stimulation tests is unchanged (Table 10). The secretion and excretion rates of cortisol and its metabolites are decreased in kwashiorkor (Table 11), showing that the increased plasma concentration is the result of a slower degradation of the hormone.[65] In severely wasted adults, the plasma half-life is similarly prolonged.[66] A rise in the plasma concentration of a hormone cannot result from a decrease in the rate of its metabolism unless the feedback control is reset. The rise in plasma cortisol represent a true change in its control, not simply defective hepatorenal inactivation.

Table 12 shows that an even greater rise in basal plasma cortisol concentration occurs in children with marasmus, although again there is no change in response to stimulation tests (Table 13). In contrast to kwashiorkor, little or no decrease in cortisol secretion and excretion rate occurs in children with marasmus (Table 14), showing that plasma cortisol is being regulated at a new and higher concentration. In PEM, plasma cortisol is increased to the greatest extent in the most severely affected children[56,57] and particularly in patients with additional hypoglycemic or septic stress.[11,68,69]

The fraction of total cortisol free and unbound to plasma protein is increased in PEM,[1,68,70,71] dexamethasone suppression is lost, and the diurnal variation becomes less evident.[65] Seven days of complete starvation is enough to increase plasma cortisol concentration although, as in kwashiorkor, both secretion and excretion rates are reduced. (Table 34). The rate of cortisol secretion and excretion are also lowered in adults with nutritional dwarfing or wasting.[64,66] Most reports indicate that starvation increases plasma corticoid concentration in experimental animals (Table 35).

In PEM, the rise in plasma cortisol concentration is an important metabolic adaptation[22,50,72] — it increases protein metabolism in muscles to provide energy and supply amino acids for hepatic protein synthesis.[19,73] The lower cortisol concentration in kwashiorkor compared with marasmus represents a less successful adaptation to PEM: it explains why plasma proteins (including lipoproteins[74]) should be lower in kwashiorkor than in marasmus, thus allowing the development of edema[75] and fatty infiltration of the liver.[50,74]

Compared with kwashiorkor, marasmus has a more gradual and earlier onset[5] that allows more opportunity for successful adaptation.[22] Kwashiorkor, on the other hand, develops more abruptly, often being precipitated by acute infections. Although the primary role of protein deficiency in the pathogenesis of kwashiorkor[8,76,77] is at present out of favor,[5,78] the relatively less severe energy deficiency in kwashiorker compared with marasmus might well explain the lower plasma cortisol concentration and consequent failure to successfully compensate for PEM.[22] Increased plasma cortisol predisposes to infection by suppressing the immune response.[71]

Catecholamine

Table 15 shows that most studies indicate that the urinary excretion of catecholamines is decreased in children with kwashiorkor, whereas three days of fasting increases catecholamine excretion in healthy people.[89] It is possible that an amino acid (tyrosine) deficiency impairs catecholamine synthesis,[90] or, alternatively, that the decrease in catecholamine formation could be a compensation for insulin deficiency.[91] The hyperglycemic effect of epinephrine is depressed in children with PEM.[92]

Thyroid Hormones

Table 16 shows that plasma thyroid hormone concentrations are decreased in children with kwashiorkor, and also, but to a lesser extent, in marasmus (Table 17). Most studies also indicate that the plasma concentration of thyroid-stimulating hormone is also lower (Tables 16 and 17), and that there is an impaired response to the hypothalamic-releasing hormone.[94,95] No consistent change in the free unbound fraction has been reported (Tables 16 and 17). The most striking finding in adults with malnutrition and edema is a fall in the plasma triiodothyronine concentration[2]; in healthy people, a short period of starvation produces a similar fall in triiodothyronine together with a rise in the proportion of the inactive "reversed" derivative (Table 36). Starvation also decreases thyroid hormone secretion in experimental animals (Table 37).

In PEM, there is a defect in iodine uptake[96] and storage;[97] thyroxine is more rapidly metabolized[98] and a greater proportion of inactive iodotyrosines is released.[99] The fall in metabolic rate that occurs in PEM[41] is the result of decreased active thyroid-hormone formation and is an important adaptation to the decreased supply of energy. In PEM, the decrease in active hormone formation may also impair the hypoglycemic release of growth hormone[8] and contribute to electrolyte disturbances[7] by depressing sodium pump activity. The rise in growth hormone concentration (Tables 5 and 7) may be responsible for the decrease in triiodothyronine formation.[51]

Sex Hormones

In kwashiorkor, plasma gonadotropin concentrations may be lowered or unaltered, and there is a poor response to the hypothalamic-releasing hormone (Table 18). Malnutrition in adult men also impairs the testicular response to endogenous gonadotropin (Table 18). No consistent change in sex-hormone secretion has been reported after starvation in man (Table 38) or in experimental animals (Table 39).

Renin and Water Balance

Table 19 shows that plasma renin activity is increased both in kwashiorkor and marasmus and that it becomes particularly high in children who later die in hospital. Although no change in juxtaglomerular granularity could be detected,[8] experimental PEM in pigs[110] and rats[111,112] confirms that plasma renin activity is often increased. Short periods (7 to 12 days) of complete starvation also increase renin activity (Table 40).

An increase in renin activity causes overhydration by producing thirst,[113] thus allowing the child to accept large volumes of overdiluted food,[78] and also by increasing renal tubular reabsorption[114] and the secretion of aldosterone[115] and antidiuretic hormone.[116]

In kwashiorkor[117,118] and experimental PEM,[119,120] the state of overhydration cannot be corrected because the kidneys are unable to excrete a water load: the balance between glomerular fileration and tubular reabsorption is lost, so that insufficient filtrate reaches the diluting segment of the nephrons (viz., the thick cortical section of the ascending limb of the loop of Henle). A loss of glomerular tubular balance (thought to be controlled by renin[121]) is considered to be the principal cause of overhydration in congestive heart failure,[122] cirrhosis,[123] and corpulmonale.[124]

A redistribution of blood flow away from outer cortical glomeruli to deeper juxtamedullary glomeruli[125] could be responsible for the change in glomerular tubular balance; it is associated with an increase of renin activity[126,127] and is induced by angiotensins.[128] Redistribution of blood flow to the deeper nephrons probably accounts for salt and water retention in cirrhotic patients with increased renin activity;[129] the same explanation may well apply to PEM.

Although overhydration with consequent electrolyte dilution is characteristic of both kwashiorkor and marasmus,[130-134] water retention in marasmus may not develop until treatment is started.[135] Clinical edema in kwashiorkor shows that subcutaneous interstitial fluid is increased; it is associated with low plasma colloid osmotic pressure,[75] heart failure,[136] increased tissue compliance (i.e., loss of elasticity),[132] and the presence of subcutaneous fat.[137] In PEM, there is a decrease in the activity of the cell membrane pump[138] leading to a movement of water from the extra- to the intracellular compartment. In the terminal stage of PEM, this redistribution becomes most pronounced[137] and produces hypovolemic circulatory failure with a decrease in plasma volume.[139,140]

Angiotensin (generated by renin) stimulates the sodium pump by providing energy from ATP.[141] This suggests that in Bartter's syndrome, renin activity is increased to compensate for inadequate sodium pump activity.[142] In the terminal stage of PEM in children[27,143] and pigs,[110] renin activity reaches its highest level, indicating that it also represents a similar attempt to compensate for sodium pump failure. Renin activity in PEM will also be stimulated by hyponatremia[144] and potassium depletion, both changes being characteristic of PEM.[134,147] Potassium deficiency per se leads to glomerular tubular imbalance with excessive proximal tubular sodium reabsorption,[148] probably mediated by changes of intrarenal renin activity.[145]

Aldosterone

Table 20 shows that plasma aldosterone concentration, secretion, and excretion are increased in PEM; a greater proportion of the hormone is free and unbound to plasma protein.[150] Aldosterone secretion is higher after 4 to 10 days complete starvation in man (Table 40) and is also increased by severe experimental PEM in pigs.[110] Aldosterone hypersecretion is probably stimulated by the renin-angiotensin system (Table 19), and it causes potassium depletion.[134]

Antidiuretic Hormone

Table 21 shows that antidiuretic activity in plasma and urine is increased in kwashiorkor. This change may result from terminal hypovolemia[139,140] with increased renin activity (Table 19). It would tend to promote overhydration and plasma hypotonicity.[134,147]

STARVATION

Insulin

Tables 22 to 26 show that almost without exception, starvation decreases the basal (postabsorptive) plasma insulin concentration and the release of insulin in response to stimulation in both man and experimental animals. This is clearly an adaptation to delay the uptake of glucose from the blood for storage and allow reserves of energy (glycogen, fat, and protein) to be mobilized. In PEM, similar changes occur (Tables 1 to 4).

Glucagon

Table 27 shows that almost without exception, starvation increases the basal (postabsorptive) plasma glucagon concentration. This is clearly an adaptation to promote the mobilization of energy reserves (glycogen, protein, and fat).[155] Starvation has no consistent effects upon the release of glucagon in response to stimulation tests: oral glucose has less effect, intravenous alanine has more, and intravenous arginine is equivocal (Table 28). Animal experiments are also inconclusive (Table 29). In PEM, there is one report of glucagon deficiency.[17]

Growth Hormone

With one possible exception, starvation invariably produces an increase in basal (postabsorptive) plasma growth hormone concentration (Tables 30 and 31). This is an adaptation that increases the mobilization of lipid from the adipose tissue and prevents the uptake of glucose from the blood into the storage tissues. A similar increase occurs in PEM (Table 5). Table 32 shows that there tends to be an increase in the growth hormone response to stimulation tests after a period of starvation. In experimental animals, most studies show an increase in growth hormone secretion after starvation (Table 33).

Somatomedin

There is a decrease in plasma somatomedin activity in both man[172] and rats (Table 33) following a short period of starvation. In PEM, the change in activity appears to be produced by a plasma inhibitor[46] that may allow growth hormone to exert its lipolytic action without stimulating cell division and without negative feedback inhibition of the hypothalamus.[45]

Cortisol

Table 34 shows that whereas the excretion of cortisol metabolites (17-hydroxycorticoids) is invariably decreased after starvation, there is often an increase in plasma concentration, indicating that the rate of degradation of cortisol is slower. A similar change occurs in experimental animals (Table 35) as also in PEM (Tables 9 to 14). A rise in plasma cortisol activity (free cortisol) represents an adaptation to starvation to allow muscle protein to be mobilized for neoglucogenesis and hepatic protein synthesis.

Thyroid

Table 36 shows that although starvation produces no consistent change in plasma thyroxine concentration, there is invariably a fall in the concentration of the active hormone, triiodothyronine, and a corresponding increase of its inactive analogue, reversed triiodothyronine. This is almost certainly the result of an adaptation of peripheral (renal) thyroxine metabolism to reduce metabolism and energy expenditure during a period of starvation. Little change occurs in plasma thyroid-stimulating hormone concentration. In experimental animals, most studies show a decrease in thyroid hormone secretion (Table 37). In PEM, thyroid activity is also reduced (Tables 16 and 17).

Sex Hormones

Tables 38 and 39 show that starvation in man and experimental animals has no clear effect on plasma sex hormone concentrations; however, urinary excretion of adrenal androgens (17 ketosteroids) is usually reduced (Table 34).

Renin and Aldosterone

Table 40 shows that starvation usually increases plasma renin activity and aldosterone secretion. Similar changes occur in experimental animals[110-112] and in PEM (Table 19). Despite the increase in renin and aldosterone, a short period of starvation typically leads to a loss of salt and water in the urine, whereas refeeding with carbohydrates causes salt and water retention. This suggests that the increase in plasma glucagon during starvation prevents the action of aldosterone[254] so that salt and water are excreted; similarly, the fall in glucagon produced by eating carbohydrates allows aldosterone to stimulate renal salt and water retention.[255]

DIET COMPOSITION

Endocrine secretion is also influenced by the relative proportions of the various foods in the diet, e.g., high carbohydrate diets lead to a greater basal and stimulated insulin secretion than low carbohydrate diets providing the same energy.[263-265] Moreover, refined carbohydrates (notably sucrose and white bread) appear to induce a greater insulin release than unrefined foods (e.g., maize meal). This may explain why hyperinsulinemic diabetes is so much more common in North America than in Africa.[266-269]

In experimental animals, low protein diets produce lower plasma insulin concentrations than diets with both a low-protein and low-carbohydrate content.[76,270] High carbohydrate diets also lower the plasma growth-hormone concentration,[210] and low carbohydrate diets augment basal and stimulated glucagon secretion.[263]

ANOREXIA NERVOSA

Many of the endocrine changes associated with anorexia nervosa appear to be simply the result of starvation itself. Table 41 shows that like starvation, anorexia increases the basal plasma growth-hormone concentration. Similarly, both starvation (Table 34) and anorexia (Table 42) increase the basal plasma cortisol concentration by decreasing the rate of cortisol degradation,[271] with little or no change in cortisol secretion or excretion rate.

Starvation (Table 36) and anorexia both lead to a lowering of plasma triiodothyronine concentration (Table 43) without change in the prohormone (thyroxine) concentration. Presumably, the decrease in triiodothyronine feedback to the pituitary accounts for the rise in plasma thyroid-stimulating hormone concentration.

Finally, anorexia like starvation is accompanied by an increase in plasma renin activity and a corresponding increase in aldosterone secretion (Table 40).[272]

Secondary amenorrhea is characteristic of anorexia nervosa, and Table 44 shows that it is probably the result of a decrease in pituitary gonadotropin secretion. A similar decrease in gonadotropins occurs after starvation (Table 38) and probably for the same reasons: either because the body weight falls below a critical value[273,274] or because an abnormal inhibitory estrin (2-hydroxy-estrone) is secreted, so that the pituitary becomes refractory to hypothalamic stimulation (Table 44).

SUMMARY OF EFFECTS OF UNDERNUTRITION

Undernutrition leads to important physiological adaptations mediated by changes in endocrine secretion:

1. Decrease of insulin secretion so as to maintain blood glucose concentration
2. Increase of glucagon concentration so as to mobilize energy reserves

3.   Decrease of somatomedin activity so that growth ceases despite increased growth hormone secretion.
4.   Decrease in cortisol inactivation so as to mobilize muscle protein as a source of energy and for hepatic protein synthesis
5.   Decreased peripheral activation of thyroxine in order to minimize basal energy requirements
6.   Water retention, possibly to compensate for a decrease in sodium pump activity (up to 45% of basal energy expenditure by the tissues is consumed by the sodium pump)
7.   Decrease in gonadotropin secretion and sexual activity

OBESITY

Insulin

Table 45 shows that the basal (postabsorptive) plasma insulin concentration and insulin secretion in response to various stimulation tests are increased by obesity. After food, insulin secretion is characteristically delayed and prolonged by obesity[186,290] and often leads to delayed (4 hr) postprandial hypoglycemia.[291] Consumption of food in excess of energy requirements, and particularly an overconsumption of refined carbohydrates,[266,267] appears to activate an intestinal "signal"[292] that stimulates beta cell hyperplasia, increases their store of insulin,[293] and causes insulin hypersecretion in obesity. The islets may also produce a "factor" responsible for end-organ (muscle, liver, and fat cell) resistance to the actions of insulin,[294-296] so that in obesity, early (2 hr) hyperglycemia tends to occur. In North America and Europe, diabetes is almost entirely a disease of the elderly and obese,[297] possibly because insulin resistance and increased metabolic clearance[183] persist in obesity, whereas insulin hypersecretion regresses with advancing age.[298] In experimental animals, obesity also produces insulin hypersecretion and resistance (Table 51).

Glucagon

Obesity has no consistent effect on glucagon secretion in man (Table 46) or experimental animals (Table 51). Glucagon resistance is produced by obesity,[307] and is accompanied by a decrease in lipolysis and ketogenesis.

Growth Hormones

Table 47 shows that basal (postabsorptive) plasma growth-hormone concentration and its release by a variety of stimulation tests are decreased by obesity. This could result from hypothalmic inhibition by hyperglycemia (i.e., insulin resistance) or increased plasma somatomedin activity.[172] The lower growth-hormone concentration would be expected to inhibit lipolysis and favor fat deposition; exactly the opposite changes occur with starvation and PEM (Tables 5 to 8 and 30 to 33). Table 51 shows that growth hormone secretion is also lower in obese experimental animals.

Cortisol

Table 48 shows that although secretion and urinary excretion rates of cortisol and its metabolites are increased by obesity, there is no change in mean plasma concentration. This indicates that obesity must increase the rate of cortisol degradation; the opposite effect occurs with starvation and PEM (Tables 9 to 14 and Table 34). The increased secretion rate could be the result of postprandial hypoglycemic hypothalamic stimulation produced by the delayed and prolonged insulin hypersecretion, or result from an increased hydration of cortisol to cortols and cortolones with a corresponding decrease in hypothalamic inhibition.[320a] Diurnal rhythmicity of cortisol secretion may also be lost.[311] Table 51 shows that corticosteroid secretion is also increased in obese mice.

Thyroid

Table 49 shows that in obesity, both the rate of secretion and inactivation of thyroid hormones are increased so that the plasma concentration remains unaltered. The rise in total metabolism that occurs as body weight becomes greater must therefore be independent of thyroid activity, body weight becoming stable when increased metabolism balances energy (food) consumption.[316]

Sex Hormone

With the possible exception of dehydroepiandrosterone, obesity has little effect on sex hormone secretion (Table 50).

Lipotropic Hormones

Pituitary liptropic hormone activity may be decreased in obesity.[322]

Animals

Effect of obesity on experimental animals is shown in Table 51.

Table 1

BASAL PLASMA-INSULIN CONCENTRATIONS (mU/*l*) IN CHILDREN WITH KWASHIORKOR (KW), AFTER RECOVERY AND IN CONTRAST GROUPS OF HEALTHY CHILDREN FROM THE SAME POPULATION

Country	Children	Number	Age (months)	Weight (% expected)	Plasma albumen (g/*l*)	Mean	SD Range	Δ[a]	Ref.
South Africa	KW	16	27±11	69±8	20±4	16	18	N[b]	25
	Recovered	16		79±11	38±6	18	14		
South Africa	KW	27	8—38		8—26	3	5	N[b]	26
	Recovered	27				4	5		
South Africa	KW	10	12—48		8—30	4	(0—8)	N[b]	23
	Recovered	10				5	(0—10)		
Rhodesia Zimbabwe	KW	22	12—30	60—81	12—36	5	(0—10)	↓[c]	27
	Recovered	22		61—95	26—39	12	(3—34)		
	Contrast	20	11—48	82—95	36—42	14	(8—22)		
Rhodesia Zimbabwe	KW died	14	22	66	20	5	2	↓[c]	28
	KW lived	12	24	69	23	7	3	↓[c]	
	Recovered	11				19	12		
	Contrast	21	18	81	40	13	5		
Uganda	KW	45	21	78		6	3	↓[c]	11
	Recovered	18				10	2		
	Contrast	140				13	14		
Uganda	KW	?[c]			<14	5	4	↓[c]	11
	Contrast	?[c]			>38	14	7	↓[c]	
Uganda	KW	5				4	(2—6)	↓[c]	29
	Recovered	5				11	(11—14)		
	Contrast	2				11	(10—11)		
Uganda	KW	24	21	72		19	(4—51)	N[b]	30
	Recovered	24				21	(5—32)		
Ethiopia	KW	21	14—45		10—25	5	(2—24)	N[b]	31
	Recovered	21				6	3		
India	KW	18	18—96	40—60	18	3	2	N[b]	32,33
	Recovered	7			35	4	3		
	Contrast	6			38	2	2		

Table 1 (continued)
BASAL PLASMA-INSULIN CONCENTRATIONS (mU/l) IN CHILDREN WITH KWASHIORKOR (KW), AFTER RECOVERY AND IN CONTRAST GROUPS OF HEALTHY CHILDREN FROM THE SAME POPULATION

Country	Children	Number	Age (months)	Weight (% expected)	Plasma albumen (g/l)	Mean	SD Range	Δ[a]	Ref.
Jamaica	KW	8	9—22	43—73		9	2	↓[c]	34
	Recovered	7				16	4		
Jamaica	KW	26	6—18	50		19	24	?↓[c]	20
	Recovered	28				19	26		
	Contrast	5				26	10		
Jamaica	KW	22	7—22	46—81		3	2	N[b]	10
	Recovered	22				3	2		
Jamaica	KW	19				7	4	↓[c]	21,35
	Recovered	19				12	6		
Mexico	KW	8	15—28	53	16—25	8	(5—10)	N[b]	36,37
	Recovered	8				5	(5—7)		
Peru	KW	3	12—30		10—36	21	(20—30)	↑[d]	38
	Recovered	4				10	(8—14)		
Peru	KW	12	16—40			8	7	?↓[c]	39
	Recovered					7	7		
	Contrast	8	13—19			11	3		

a   Δ represents the difference between the contrast group and recovered children
b   N no difference
c   ↓ decrease
d   ↑ increase
e   ? unknown

Table 2
CHANGE IN PLASMA-INSULIN CONCENTRATION (mU/l) FOLLOWING GLUCOSE, ARGININE, AND AMINO ACIDS IN CHILDREN WITH KWASHIORKOR

Test	Country	Children	Number	Age (months)	Weight (% expected)	Plasma albumen (g/l)	Change	Δ[a]	Ref.
Oral glucose (2 g/kg)	South Africa	KW	18	8—38		8—26	+11	↓[b]	17, 16
		Recovered	18				+38		
Oral glucose (2 g/kg)	South Africa	KW	4	9—34		13—24	+5	↓[b]	40
		Recovered	4				+19		
Oral glucose (2 g/kg)	South Africa	KW	5	6—27		9—24	(0.68) (Integral)	↓[b]	15
		Potassium supplement Recovered		6—27		9—24	(1.03)	↑[c]	
		Recovered	5	6—27			(9.61)		
Oral glucose (2 g/kg)	India	KW	7	18—96	40—60	18	+1	↓[b]	32, 33
		Recovered	7			35	+11		
Oral glucose (2 g/kg) and casein	Peru	KW	12	16—40			+4	↓[b]	39
		Recovered					+9		
		Contrast					+22		
I.V. glucose (0.5 g/kg)	Jamaica	KW	19	6—27			+4	↓[b]	21, 35
		Recovered					+26		
I.V. glucose (0.5 g/kg)	Jamaica	KW	26	6—18	50		+17	↓[b]	20
		Recovered	28				+53		
I.V. glucose (0.5 g/kg)	South Africa	KW	27	8—38		8—26	+15	↓[b]	17, 16
		Recovered	27				+42		
I.V. glucose (0.5 g/kg)	South Africa	KW	27	8—38		8—26	+15	↓[b]	17, 16
		Recovered	27				+42		
I.V. glucose (1 g/kg)	South Africa	KW	10	12—48		8—30	+34	↓[b]	23
		Recovered	10				+73		
I.V. glucose (1 g/kg)	South Africa	KW	18	3—27		19	+5	↓[b]	14
		Recovered	18			38	+31		

Table 2 (continued)
CHANGE IN PLASMA-INSULIN CONCENTRATION (mU/*l*) FOLLOWING GLUCOSE, ARGININE, AND AMINO ACIDS IN CHILDREN WITH KWASHIORKOR

Test	Country	Children	Number	Age (months)	Weight (% expected)	Plasma albumen (g/*l*)	Change	Δ[a]	Ref.
I.V. glucose	South Africa	KW	16	27	69	20	+70	?	25
		Recovered	16		79	38	+82		
I.V. glucose	Uganda	KW	5				+28	N[c]	29
		Recovered	5				+32		
I.V. glucose (0.5 g/kg)	Mexico	KW	8	15—28	53	<25	+7	↓[b]	36, 37
		Recovered	8				+19		
I.V. glucose (0.5 g/kg)	South Africa	KW	8	8—38		8—26	+15	↓[b]	26
		Recovered	8				+47		
I.V. glucagon (0.1 mg/kg)	Jamaica	KW	19	6—27			+11	?↓[b]	35
		Recovered					+15		
I.V. glucagon (0.1 mg/kg)	Peru	KW	3	12—30		10—36	−12	R↓[b]	38
		Recovered					+11		
I.V. arginine (0.5 g/kg)	Mexico	KW	4	15—28	53	<25	+1	↓[b]	36, 37
		Recovered	8				+7		

[a]   Δ represents the difference between recovered and contrast groups

[b]   N no difference

[c]   ↑ indicates increase

Table 3
BASAL PLASMA INSULIN CONCENTRATION (mU/l) IN CHILDREN WITH MARASMUS (MAR)

Country	Children	N	Age (months)	Weight (% expected)	Plasma albumen (g/l)	Mean	SD (Range)	Δ[a]	Δ[b] KW	Ref.
South Africa	MAR	27	8—38	<60	16—38	3	5	N[c]	N[c]	26
	Recovered	27				4	5			
Uganda	MAR	9	9±5	44		8	(4—15)	↓[d]	↓[d]	30
	Recovered	9				14	(5—24)			
India	MAR	5	18—60	30—50	32	2	3	N[c]	N[c]	32
	Recovered	6			38	2	2			
Jamaica	MAR	20	6—24	33—61		2	1	N[c]	N[c]	10
	Recovered	20				3	2			
Mexico	MAR	10	2—9	74		8	(5—10)	↓[d]	N[c]	41, 36
	Recovered	10				12	(9—14)			
Peru	MAR	3	5—16		36—40	14	(8—17)	N[c]	↓[d]	38
	Recovered	4				10	(8—14)			
Peru	MAR	9	5—11			9	5	N[c]	N[c]	39
	Recovered	8	5—11			10	10			
	Contrast	8				10	5			
Rhodesia	MAR died	4	15	53	23	6	1	↓[d]	N[c]	28
Zimbabwe	MAR lived	9	19	54	27	7	2	↓[d]	N[c]	
	Recovered	8				20	9			
	Contrast	21	18	81	40	13	5			

[a] Δ represents the difference between recovered and contrast group
[b] Δ KW represents difference from Kwashiorkor
[c] N no difference
[d] ↓ decrease

Table 4

CHANGE IN PLASMA INSULIN CONCENTRATION (mU/l) FOLLOWING GLUCOSE, ARGININE, AND GLUCAGON IN CHILDREN WITH MARASMUS (MAR)

Test	Country	Children	N	Age (months)	Weight (% expected)	Plasma albumen (g/l)	Change	Δ[a]	Δ KW[b]	Ref.
Oral glucose	South Africa	MAR	11	8—38	<60	16—38	+10	↓[c]	N[d]	17, 16
		Recovered	11				+28			
		Contrast	5				+35			
Oral glucose (2 g/kg) and casein	Peru	MAR	9	5—11			+3	↓[c]	N[d]	39
		Recovered					+7			
		Contrast					+45			
I.V. glucose (0.5 g/kg)	South Africa	MAR	9	8—38	<60	16—38	+31	N[c]	↑[e]	16, 17
		Recovered	9				+30			
		Contrast	5				+34			
I.V. glucagon	South Africa	MAR	5	8—38	<60	16—38	+12	↓[c]	N[d]	26
		Recovered	5				+29			
I.V. arginine (0.5 g/kg)	Peru	MAR	3	5—16		36—40	+4	↓[c]	↑[e]	38
		Recovered	4				+10			
I.V. arginine (0.5/kg)	Mexico	MAR	10	3—9	51		−3	↓[c]	↓[c]	41
		Recovered	10				+13			

[a] Δ represents difference in response as compared with recovery and contrast groups
[b] Δ KW represents difference from Kwashiorkor
[c] ↓ decrease
[d] N no difference
[e] ↑ increase

Table 5
BASAL PLASMA GROWTH HORMONE CONCENTRATION ($\mu g/l$) IN CHILDREN WITH KWASHIORKOR (KW)

Country	Children	N	Age (months)	Weight (% expected)	Plasma albumen (g/l)	Mean	SD (Range)	Δ[a]	Ref.
South Africa	KW	22	16—71		12—29	31	(4—65)	↑[b]	52
	Recovered	22				10	(2—35)		
	Contrast	10				7	(1—19)		
South Africa	KW	28	10—48		10—26	22	(6—46)	↑[b]	53, 54
	Recovered	16				5	(0—12)		
	Contrast	11				7	(1—21)		
South Africa	KW	17	9—36		14—20	13	8	↑[b]	47
	Recovered	17				6	6		
South Africa	KW	6	13—48			21	(13—37)	↑[b]	55
	Recovered	6				13	(8—15)		
South Africa	KW	9	9—34		13—24	20	(10—46)	? N[c]	40
	Recovered	9				16	(1—75)		
Rhodesia Zimbabwe }	KW (died)	14	12—48		20	70	10	↑[b]	56
	KW (lived)	12	12—48		23	72	6		
	Recovered	11			40	34	8		
	Contrast	21	12—24		40	29	16		
Rhodesia Zimbabwe }	KW	22	12—30	60—81	12—36	18	(8—30)	↑[b]	27
	Recovered			61—95	26—39	6	(1—9)		
Nigeria	KW	30	36			20	(7—30)	↑[b]	57
	Contrast	30	36			6	(2—12)		
Uganda	KW	9	21	>79		11	16	↑[b]	11
	KW	33	21	60—79		11	9	↑[b]	
	KW	22		<60		15	13	↑[b]	
	Recovered	5				3	2		
	Contrast	86	21			4	4		
Uganda	KW	?[d]	<48		<14	24	36	↑[b]	11
	Contrast	?[d]	<48		>30	4	6		
Uganda	KW	5	12—36		11—15	23	11	↑[b]	12
	Recovered	5			41—45	2	2		

Table 5 (continued)
BASAL PLASMA GROWTH HORMONE CONCENTRATION (μg/l) IN CHILDREN WITH KWASHIORKOR (KW)

Country	Children	N	Age (months)	Weight (% expected)	Plasma albumen (g/l)	Mean	SD (Range)	Δ[a]	Ref.
Uganda	KW	24	21	72		28		↑[b]	30
	Recovered	24				18			
India	KW	12	18—72	40—60	18	31	32	↑[b]	32, 58
	Recovered	12			29	9	10		
	Contrast	7			38	4	2		
India	KW	8	4—60	40—70		2	(0 → 12)	?N[c]	48
	Contrast	30				2	2		
Jamaica	KW	19				25	23	↑[b]	21, 35
	Recovered	19				9	5		
Jamaica	KW	10	6—19	65—81		36	16	↑[b]	10
	Recovered	10				9	5		
Jamaica	KW	8	9—22	43—73		22	15	↑[b]	34
	Recovered	8				15	6		
Mexico	KW	8	15—28	53	<25	68	(50—75)	↑[b]	36
	Recovered	8				14	(10—15)		
Chile	KW	6	8—33	61—76		26	(9—42)	↑[b]	59, 60, 61
	Recovered	5	6—15	100		4	4		
Bolivia	KW	10	5—23	<65		19	(8—38)	↑[b]	62
	Recovered	10				5	(2—7)		
	Contrast	?[d]				7	?		
Peru	KW	3	12—30		10—36	11	(8—18)	↑[b]	38
	Recovered	3				4	(0—7)		
Peru	KW	12	16—40			17	10	?N[c]	39
	Recovered					11	12		
	Contrast					21	22		
Thailand	KW	10				34	(11—80)	↑[b]	63
	Recovered	10				9	(3—17)		

[a] Δ, represents difference between recovery and contrast groups
[b] ↑, increase
[c] N, no difference
[d] ?, not known

Table 6

CHANGE IN PLASMA GROWTH HORMONE CONCENTRATION ($\mu g/l$) IN KWASHIORKOR (KW) FOLLOWING GLUCOSE, ARGININE, ETC.

Test	Country	Children	N	Age (months)	Weight (% expected)	Plasma albumen (g/l)	Change	Δ^a	Ref.
Oral glucose (2 g/kg)	South Africa	KW	4	9—36		20	−4	N[b]	47
		Recovered	4				−3		
Oral glucose (2 g/kg)	South Africa	KW	6				−10	N[b]	54
		Recovered	6				−10		
Oral glucose (2 g/kg)	South Africa	KW	4	9—34		13—24	−3	N[b]	40
		Recovered	4				−2		
Oral glucose (2 g/kg)	South Africa	KW	6				−8	N[b]	55
		Recovered	6				−9		
Oral glucose (2 g/kg)	Peru	KW	12	16—40			+5	R↓[c]	39
		Recovered					−5		
		Contrast	8				−13		
I.V. glucose (0.5 g/kg)	South Africa	KW	6	9—36		20	−5	↑[d]	47
		Recovered	6				0		
I.V. glucose (0.5 g/kg)	Jamaica	KW	19				+6	↓[c]	21, 35
		Recovered					+11		
I.V. glucose (0.5 g/kg)	Bolivia	KW	8	5—23	<65		+8	N[b]	62
		Recovered	8				+7		
I.V. glucose (0.5 g/kg)	Mexico	KW	8	15—28	53	16—25	−15	↑[d]	37
		Recovered	8				−1		
I.V. arginine (1 g/kg)	Peru	KW	3	12—30		10—36	0	↓[c]	38
		Recovered	4				+3		
I.V. arginine (0.5 g/kg)	Mexico	KW	8	15—28	53	16—25	+9	↓[c]	36, 37
		Recovered	8				+31		
I.V. arginine	Chile	KW	6	8—33	61—76		−1	↓[c]	59, 60
		Contrast	6	6—15	100		+9		61
I.V. alanine (0.2 g/kg)	South Africa	KW	5	9—34		13—24	+18	↑[d]	40
		Recovered	5				+7		

Table 6 (continued)
CHANGE IN PLASMA GROWTH HORMONE CONCENTRATION ($\mu g/l$) IN KWASHIORKOR (KW) FOLLOWING GLUCOSE, ARGININE, ETC.

Test	Country	Children	N	Age (months)	Weight (% expected)	Plasma albumen (g/l)	Change	Δ[a]	Ref.
Oral amino acids (0.5 g/kg)	Jamaica	KW	8	9—22	43—73		−10	↑[d]	34
		Recovered	7				−7		
IM Chlorpromazine (25 mg)	India	KW	6	18—72	40—60		+19	N[b]	32, 58
		Recovered	6				+18		
		Contrast	6	18—72			+16		
I.V. glucagon (0.1 mg/kg)	Jamaica	KW	19				+21	N[b]	35
		Recovered					+18		

[a] Δ represents the absolute difference in response compared with recovery and contrast groups
[b] N no difference
[c] ↓ decrease
[d] ↑ increase

Table 7

BASAL PLASMA GROWTH HORMONE CONCENTRATION ($\mu g/l$) IN CHILDREN WITH MARASMUS (MAR)

Country	Children	N	Age (months)	Weight (% expected)	Plasma albumen (g/l)	Mean	SD (Range)	Δ[a]	Δ KW[b]	Ref.
South Africa	MAR	20	10—50	37—62	10—40	26	(3—60)	↑[c]	N[d]	52, 54
	Recovered	20				7	(4—16)			
	Contrast	10				7	(1—19)			
Rhodesia	MAR died	9	12—48	<60	27	76	22	↑[c]	N[d]	56
	MAR lived	4		<60	23	63	5			
	Recovered	8	12—24		38	28	20			
	Contrast	21			40	29	16			
Uganda	MAR	3	17	<60		5	3	? N[d]	↓[e]	11
	Contrast	86		100		4	4			
Nigeria	MAR	30	23			10	(2—30)	? ↑[c]	↓[e]	57
	Contrast	30	36			6	(2—12)			
India	MAR	46	4—60	40—70		7	(0—24)	↑[c]	↑[c]	48
	Recovered	12				2	(1—5)			
	Contrast	30				2	2			
India	MAR	6	18—60	30—50	32	6	(2—10)	? N[d]	↓[e]	32, 58
	Recovered	6			36	8	(1—12)			
	Contrast	7	18—72		38	4	(1—6)			
Jamaica	MAR	25	5—24	33—61		15	10	↑[c]	N[d]	10
	Recovered	25		90		6	10			
Chile	MAR	6	6—13	41—51		4	(3—5)	↓[e]	↓[e]	59—61
	Recovered	5	6—15	100		8	(5—12)			
Mexico	MAR	10	2—9	51		7	7	↑[c]	↓[e]	36, 41
	Recovered	10				3	4			
Bolivia	MAR	13	5—23	<65		5	(2—11)	↓[e]	↓[e]	62
	Recovered	13				7	5			
Peru	MAR	4	5—16	36—40		12	(6—20)	↑[c]	N[d]	38
	Recovered	4				4	(0—7)			

Table 7 (continued)
BASAL PLASMA GROWTH HORMONE CONCENTRATION (μg/l) IN CHILDREN WITH MARASMUS (MAR)

Country	Children	N	Age (months)	Weight (% expected)	Plasma albumen (g/l)	Mean	SD (Range)	Δ[a]	Δ KW[b]	Ref.
Peru	MAR	9	5—11			21	13	? N[d]	N[d]	39
	Recovered					13	13			
	Contrast	8	5—11			32	13			
Thailand	MAR	7				66	(11—121)	↑[c]	↑[c]	63
	Recovered	7				8	(2—11)			

[a] Δ represents the difference between recovery and contrast groups
[b] Δ KW represents the difference from Kwashiorkor
[c] ↑ increase
[d] N no difference
[e] ↓ decrease

Table 8

CHANGES IN PLASMA GROWTH HORMONE CONCENTRATION ($\mu g/l$) IN CHILDREN WITH
MARASMUS (MAR) FOLLOWING ARGININE, INSULIN, AND CHLORPROMAZINE

Test	Country	Children	N	Age (months)	Weight (% expected)	Plasma albumin (g/l)	Change	Δ[a]	Δ[b] KW	Ref.
I.V. Arginine (0.5 g/kg)	Chile	MAR	6	6—13	41—51		+1	↓[c]	? N[d]	59, 60
		Contrast	5	6—15	100		+9			
I.V. Arginine	Mexico	MAR	10	2—9	51		+5	↑[e]	? N[d]	36, 41
		Recovered	10				+3			
I.V. Arginine (0.5 g/kg)	Peru	MAR	4	5—16		36—40	+6	?↑[e]	↑[e]	38
		Recovered	4				+3			
I.V. Insulin (0.1 u/kg)	USA	MAR	13	36—132	30—66		<5	↓[c]		64
		Recovered	13				+23			
IM Chlorpromazine (25 mg)	India	MAR	6	18—60	30—50	32	+7	↓[c]	↓[c]	32, 58
		Recovered	6			36	+12			
		Contrast	6			38	+16			

[a] Δ represents the absolute difference in response compared with recovery and contrast groups
[b] Δ KW represents difference from Kwashiorkor
[c] ↓ decrease
[d] N no difference
[e] ↑ increase

Table 9
BASAL PLASMA CORTISOL CONCENTRATION (μg/l) IN CHILDREN WITH KWASHIORKOR (KW)

Country	Children	N	Age (months)	Weight (% expected)	Plasma albumen (g/l)	Mean	SD (Range)	Δ[a]	Ref.
South Africa	KW	29		70	19	193	90	↑[b]	79
	Recovered	29			36	143	73		
South Africa	KW	15			20	335	154	↑[b]	71
	Contrast	10			38	102	23		
Rhodesia Zimbabwe	KW died	4	18	59	13	160		↑[b]	27
	KW lived	22	12—30	60—81	12—36	80	(50—180)	↑[b]	
	Contrast	20	12—30	82—95	36—42	10	(<10—50)		
Rhodesia Zimbabwe	KW died	14	12—48		20	163	41	↑[b]	56
	KW lived	12	12—48		23	127	45	↑[b]	
	Recovered	11			40	82	66		
	Contrast	21	12—24		40	54	24		
Uganda	KW	26	21	<60		210	75	↑[b]	11
	KW	19	21	61—70		170	65	↑[b]	
	?[d]	10	21	71—80		120	79		
	Contrast	6	21	81—90		130	37		
	Contrast	3	21	91—100		90	17		
Uganda	KW	?[d]	<48		<14	190	95	↑[b]	11
	Contrast	?[d]	<48		>30	94	105		
Nigeria	KW	30	36			220	(120—540)	↑[b]	57
	Contrast	30	36			130	(80—280)		
Egypt	KW	30	9—42	48—84		241	(60—350)	↑[b]	80
	Recovered	30				116	(80—170)		
India	KW	9	8—144	55—90	24	44	57	↓[c]	68
	Contrast					64	?[d]		
India	KW	22				249	95	↑[b]	81
	Recovered	11				170	73		
	Contrast	12				192	90		

Peru	KW	8	2—18		183	(138—232)	↑[b]	82
	Recovered	8	2—18		134	(30—244)		
	Contrast	21	2—18		120	(105—135)		
Mexico	KW	3	6—24	<60	160	(130—185)	?↑[b]	69
	KW	4	6—24	<60	320	(250—500)	↑[b]	
	stressed							
	Recovered	5	6—24		144	(104—210)		
	Contrast	24	6—24		129	22		

[a] Δ, represents the difference between recovery and contrast groups
[b] ↑, increase
[c] ↓, decrease
[d] ?, not known

Table 10

CHANGE IN PLASMA CORTISOL (C) CONCENTRATION (μg/l) OR URINE 17-HYDROXYCORTICOID (17HC) EXCRETION (mg/24 hr) FOLLOWING STIMULATION IN KWASHIORKOR (KW)

Test	Country	Children	N	Age (months)	Weight (% expected)	Plasma albumen (g/l)	Change	Δ[a]	Ref.
C after 1M Synacthen (125 μg)	India	KW	7				+327	?↑[b]	81
		Recovered	4				+244		
		Contrast	9						
C after 1M corticotropin (25 U)	Egypt	KW	15	9—42	48—84		+295	↓[c]	67
		Recovered	15				+22		
		Contrast	10				+165		
C after Piromen (0.5 μg/kg)	South Africa	KW	29	6—36	70	19	+160	N[d]	79
		Recovered	29			36	+161		
							+153		
17HC after corticotropin (20 U)	South Africa	KW	12	10—48		18	+7	N[d]	83
		Recovered	12				+9		
17HC after corticotropin (10 U)	Guatemala	KW	6	18—60			+4	N[d]	84
		Recovered	6				+2		

[a] Δ represents difference between recovery and contrast groups
[b] ↑ increase
[c] ↓ decrease
[d] N no difference

Table 11

URINE CORTICOID EXCRETION AND CORTISOL SECRETION RATE IN CHILDREN WITH KWASHIORKOR (KW)

Hormone	Country	Children	N	Age (months)	Plasma albumen (g/*l*)	Mean	SD (Range)	Δ[a]	Ref.
17 hydroxy mg/24 hr	South Africa	KW	31	10—48	18	2.0	(0.5—5.8)	?↓[b]	83
		Recovered	31			1.8	(0.3—3.6)		
		Contrast	24	2—54		2.8	(1.4—5.4)		
17 hydroxy mg/24 hr	Guatemala	KW	6	18—60		1.0	0.7	↓[b]	84
		Recovered				2.0	1.7		
17 hydroxy mg/m²/24 hr	Peru	KW	8	2—18		2.4	2.1	?↓[b]	82
		Recovered	8			2.1	2.4		
		Contrast	21	2—18		3.6	(2.6—4.6)		
17 keto µg/24 hr	India	KW	5	3—12		200	(90—780)	↓[b]	85
		Recovered	5			480	(110—160)		
		Contrast	12	3—9		410	(60—1800)		
Cortisol secretion rate µg/ 24 hr	Peru	KW	8	2—18		6.7	5.3	↓[b]	82
		Recovered	8			6.0	4.5		
		Contrast	21	2—18			(9.6—18.4)		

[a] Δ represents the difference between recovery and contrast groups

[b] ↓ decrease

Table 12

BASAL PLASMA CORTISOL CONCENTRATION ($\mu g/l$) IN CHILDREN WITH MARASMUS (MAR)

Country	Children	N	Age (months)	Weight (% expected)	Mean	SD (Range)	Δ[a]	Δ KW[b]	Ref.
Uganda	MAR	9	17	<60	230	90	↑[c]	? ↑[c]	11
	Contrast	?	<48		100	72			
Nigeria	MAR	30	23		180	(100—450)	↑[c]	↓[d]	57
	Contrast	30	36		130	(80—280)			
Rhodesia ⎱	MAR died	4	12—48		185	28	↑[c]	? N[e]	56
Zimbabwe ⎰	MAR lived	9	12—48		121	31	↑[c]	N[e]	
	Recovered	8			82	18			
	Contrast	21	12—24		54	23			
Egypt	MAR	25	8—36	30—70	224	(110—370)	↑[c]	N[e]	67
	Recovered	25			120	(90—140)			
	Contrast	20	6—36		117	(60—180)			
India	MAR	26	8—144	55—90	59	15	N[e]	↑[c]	68
	Recovered	13			123	27			
	Contrast	?			64	?			
India	MAR	8			318	150	↑[c]	↑[c]	81
	Recovered	4			148	76			
	Contrast	12			192	90			
Jamaica	MAR	28	6—24	68	282	74	↑[c]		65
	Recovered	32			115	40			
Mexico	MAR	8	6—24	<60	123	(75—180)	N[e]	N[e]	69
	MAR stressed	5	6—24		334	(235—500)	↑[c]	N[e]	
	Recovered	8			123	(100—170)			
	Contrast	24			129	22			
Peru	MAR	6	2—18		195	(155—256)	↑[c]	↑[c]	82
	Recovered	6			121	(57—174)			
	Contrast	21			120	(105—135)			
Chile	MAR	6	6—13	<50	124	75	↑[c]		86, 87
	Contrast	5	6—15	100	93	57			

[a]   Δ represents the difference between recovery and contrast groups
[b]   Δ KW represents the difference from Kwashiorkor
[d]   ↑ increase
[d]   ↓ decrease
[e]   N no difference

Table 13

CHANGE IN PLASMA CORTISOL (C) CONCENTRATION (μg/l) OR URINE 17-HYDROXYCORTICOID (17HC) EXCRETION (mg/24 hr) FOLLOWING STIMULATION IN MARASMUS (MAR)

Test	Country	Children	N	Age (months)	Weight (% expected)	Change	Δᵃ	Δ KWᵇ	Ref.
C after 1M corticotropin (25 U)	Egypt	MAR	15	8—36	30—70	+20	↓[c]	N[d]	67
		Recovered	15	6—36		+170			
		Contrast	10			+160			
C after 1M Synacthen (125 μg)	Jamaica	MAR	17	6—24	68	+304	N[d]		65, 88
		Recovered	17			+312			
C after 1M Synacthen (125 μg)	India	MAR	7			+390	↑[e]	? ↑[e]	81
		Recovered	5			+377			
		Contrast	9			+295			
C after 1M corticotropin	Chile	MAR	6	6—13	<50	+212	↓[c]		86, 87
		Contrast	5	6—15		+460			
C after I.V. insulin (0.1 U/kg)	India	MAR	5	8—144	55—90	+100	N[d]		68
		Contrast	2			+90			
17HC after corticotropin (10 U)	Guatemala	MAR	5	2—12		+0.4	↓[c]		84
		Recovered	5			+1.2			

[a] Δ represents the difference between recovery and contrast groups
[b] Δ KW represents the difference from Kwashiorkor
[c] ↓ decrease
[d] N no difference
[e] ↑ increase

Table 14

URINE CORTICOID EXCRETION AND CORTISOL SECRETION RATE IN CHILDREN WITH MARASMUS (MAR)

Hormone	Country	Children	N	Age (months)	Weight (% expected)	Mean	SD (Range)	Δ[a]	Δ KW[b]	Ref.
17 hydroxy mg/24 hr	Guatemala	MAR	5	2—12	2	3.3		↑[c]	↑[c]	84
		Recovered				1.4				
17 hydroxy mg/24 hr	South Africa	MAR	4	2—54	<67	2.0	(0.9—4.8)	?↓[d]	N[e]	83
		Contrast	24	2—54		2.8	(1.4—5.4)			
17 hydroxy mg/m²/24 hr	Peru	MAR	6	2—18		2.6	0.7	?↓[d]	N[e]	82
		Recovered	6			2.5	1.9			
		Contrast	21	2—18		3.6	(2.6—4.6)			
11 oxy μg/24 hr	Chile	MAR			<50	0		↓[d]		86
		Recovered				130				
		Contrast				120				
Cortisol secretion rate μg/24 hr	Peru	MAR	6	2—18		14.0	19.0	N[e]	↑[c]	82
		Recovered	6			10.6	6.5			
		Contrast	21	2—18		14.0	(9.6—18.4)			
Cortisol secretion rate μg/kg/24 hr	Jamaica	MAR	6	6—24	68	280	(90—460)	↓[d]		65
		Recovered	6			360	(240—520)			

[a]   Δ represents the difference between recovery and contrast groups
[b]   Δ KW represents the difference from Kwashiorkor
[c]   ↑ increase
[d]   ↓ decrease
[e]   N no difference

Table 15
URINE CATECHOLAMINES IN CHILDREN WITH KWASHIORKOR (KW) OR MARASMUS (MAR)

Hormone	Country	Children	N	Age (months)	Mean	SD (Range)	Δ[a]	Ref.
Catechol- amines μg/ m²/24 hr	Peru	KW	8	?	26	(2—95)	↑[b]	93
		Recovered			27	(11—49)		
		Contrast	21	2—18	18	(14—22)		
		Marasmus	9	?	31	(2—88)	↑[b]	
Metanephrines μg/24 hr	Mexico	KW	10	3—12	50	(30—70)	↓[c]	91
		Recovered			80	(70—120)		
		Contrast	4		110	(80—130)		
Epinephrine	Mexico	KW	8	15—28	5.3	2.5	N[d]	37, 39
		Recovered			5.3	2.5		
Epinephrine	Guatemala	KW	15		190	160	↑[b]	90
		Recovered	8		80	60		
		Contrast	12		160	110		
Norepinephine μg/24 hr	Mexico	KW	8	15—28	7.0	3.1	↓[c]	37, 49
		Recovered			20.5	21.0		
Norepinephine	Guatemala	KW	15		970	960	↓[c]	90
		Recovered	8		1130	300		
		Contrast	12		1170	1000		
Dopamine μg/ 24 hr	Mexico	KW	8	15—28	44	28	↓[c]	37, 49
		Recovered			207	30		
Dopamine μg/ hr	Guatemala	KW	15		6.5	7.7	↓[c]	90
		Recovered	8		10.3	4.6		
		Contrast	12		14.9	13.5		
3-methoxy 4- hydroxy man- delic acid mg/ 24 hr	Mexico	KW	8	15—28	1.5	1.4	N[d]	37, 49
		Recovered	8		1.5	1.4		
μg/hr	Guatemala	KW	15		43	28	↓[c]	90
		Recovered	8		60	34		
		Contrast	12		73	45		
Change in me- tanephrines after I.V. in- sulin (0.1 U/ kg) μg/mg creatinine	Mexico	KW	2	3—12	+ 1.8		↓[c]	91
		Recovered	2		+ 2.2			
		Contrast	2		+ 3.0			

[a]   Δ represents the difference between recovery and contrast groups
[b]   ↑ increase
[c]   ↓ decrease
[d]   N no difference

Table 16

PLASMA THYROID HORMONE CONCENTRATIONS IN CHILDREN WITH KWASHIORKOR (KW)

Hormone	Country	Children	N	Age (months)	Mean	SD (Range)	Δ[a]	Ref.
Thyroxine μg/ℓ	Nigeria	KW	30	36	62	(39—92)	↓[b]	57
		Recovered			117	(54—218)		
		Contrast			148	(84—275)		
Thyroxine μg/ℓ	Rhodesia Zimbabwe	KW	30	36	43	30	↓[b]	100
		Recovered	26	22	72	17		
		Contrast	11	18	76	20		
Thyroxine μg/ℓ	Peru	KW	21	23—40	46	11	↓[b]	101
		Recovered	7		75	13		
		Contrast	7	23—40	130	(99—156)		
Thyroxine μg/ℓ	Mexico	KW	27	15—28	54	11	↓[b]	37, 102
		Recovered	8		62	11		
Free thyroxine ng/ℓ	Rhodesia Zimbabwe	KW died	14	22	14	6	↓[b]	100
		KW lived	12	24	19	7	↓[b]	
		Recovered	11	18	19	3		
		Contrast	21		21	3		
Free thyroxine index	Nigeria	KW	30	36	80		↓[b]	57
		Recovered			110			
		Contrast		36	170			
Free thyroxine index	Mexico	KW	30	15—28	6.7	1.4	↑[c]	37, 102
		Recovered	8		6.1	1.7		
Free thyroxine ng/ℓ	Peru	KW	7	23—40	33	11	N[d]	101
		Recovered	7		16	21		
		Contrast	27		30	(27—37)		
Protein bound iodine μg/ℓ	India	KW	22		37	20	↓[b]	97, 103
		Recovered	18		60	21		
		Contrast	9		62	20		
Protein bound iodine μg/ℓ	Senegal	KW	39	18—30	37	14	↓[b]	104
		Recovered	29		69	15		
		Contrast			93	17		
Triiodo-thyronine ng/ℓ	Senegal	KW	43	18—30	540	(50—1880)	↓[b]	105
		Recovered	33		2330	(1130—3550)		
		Contrast			2360	(1220—3280)		

Measurement	Site	Group	n	Range	Value	(Value 2)	Δ	Ref.
Triiodo-thyronine ng/l	Rhodesia {Zimbabwe}	KW died	14	22	89	46	↓[b]	100
		KW lived	12	24	125	53	↓[b]	
		Recovered	11		1606	850		
		Contrast	21		1660	290		
Thyroid stimulating hormone mU/l	Uganda	KW	7		2.96	1.27	↓[b]	106
		Recovered		18	4.66	1.40		
Thyroid stimulating hormone mU/l	South Africa	KW	24	9—34	10.4	(3—32)	↑[c]	94, 95
		Recovered			6.0	(1—17)		
		Contrast	10	7—24	6.3	(2—10)		
Thyroid stimulating hormone mU/l	Senegal	KW	43	18—30	10.3	(2—27)	?↑[c]	105
		Recovered			8.8	(5—14)		
		Contrast	33		8.3	(3—14)		
Thyroid stimulating hormone mU/l	Mexico	KW	8	15—28	2.9	2.0	?↑[c]	37, 102
		Recovered			2.5	2.3		
Thyroid stimulating hormone U/l	Bolivia	KW			0.2	0.07	N[d]	99
		Contrast			0.19	0.05		
Thyroid stimulating hormone mU/l	Peru	KW	7			0—5.0	N[d]	101
		Recovered	27			0—3.7		
		Contrast	12			0—3.3		
Thyroid stimulating hormone mU/l	Nigeria	KW	12		5	(3—7)	↓[b]	57
		Contrast		36	12	(8—15)		
Change in thyroid stimulating hormone (mU/l) after I.V. releasing hormone (100 µg)	South Africa	KW	24	6—34	+24		↓[b]	94, 95
		Recovered			+31			
		Contrast			+35			

a   △ represents the difference between recovery and contrast groups

b   ↓ decrease

c   ↑ increase

d   N no difference

Table 17

PLASMA THYROID HORMONE CONCENTRATIONS IN CHILDREN WITH MARASMUS (MAR)

Hormone	Country	Children	N	Age (months)	Mean	SD (Range)	Δ[a]	Δ KW[b]	Ref.
Thyroxine μg/l	Nigeria	MAR	30	23	85	(42—164)	↓[c]	↑[d]	57
		Contrast	30	36	148	(85—276)			
Thyroxine μg/l	Rhodesia Zimbabwe	MAR died	4	15	54	30	↓[c]	↑[d]	100
		MAR lived	9	19	52	21			
		Recovered	8		75	28			
		Contrast	21	18	76	22			
Thyroxine μg/l	Mexico	MAR	10	2—9	103	38	↑[d]		41, 102
		Recovered			71	19			
Thyroxine μg/l	Peru	MAR	6	6—12	95	20	↓[c]	↑[d]	101, 107
		Recovered	6		90	22			
		Contrast	27		130	(99—156)			
Free thyroxine index	Nigeria	MAR	30	23	110		↓[c]	↑[d]	57
		Contrast	30	36	170				
Free thyroxine ng/l	Rhodesia Zimbabwe	MAR died	4	15	14	6	↓[c]	↑[d]	100
		MAR lived	9	19	18	24	↓[c]		
		Recovered	8		23	13			
		Contrast	21	18	21	14			
Free thyroxine index	Mexico	MAR			8.8	3.8	↑[d]		41
		Recovered			4.8	1.6			102
Free thyroxine ng/l	Peru	MAR	6	6—12	32	15	N[e]	N[e]	101, 107
		Recovered	6		21	7			
		Contrast	27		30	(27—37)			
Butanol extractable iodine μg/l	Chile	MAR	16	4—19	34	9	↓[c]		108
		Contrast	9	4—8	54	13			
Protein bound iodine μg/l	Bolivia	MAR	17	5—30	50	10	↓[c]	N[e]	99
		Contrast		1—60	70	15			
Thyroid stimulating hormone mU/l	Nigeria	MAR	11	36	7	5—11	↓[c]	↑[d]	57
		Contrast	12	36	12	8—15			

Measurement	Country	Group	n	Range	Value		p	Δ[a]	KW[b]	Ref.
Thyroid stimulating hormone mU/ℓ	Peru	MAR	6	6—12	0			N[e]	N[e]	107
		Recovered	6		0					
		Contrast	27		0	0—3.3	0.04			
Thyroid stimulating hormone U/ℓ	Bolivia	MAR	17	5—30	0.13			↓[c]	↓[c]	99
		Recovered	6		0.11					
		Contrast		1—60	0.19		0.05			
Change in butanol extractable iodine (μg/ℓ) after intramuscular thyroid stimulating hormone (1 U/kg)	Chile	MAR	16	4—19	+25			N[e]		108
		Contrast	9	4—8	+25					

[a] Δ represents the difference between recovery and contrast groups

[b] KW represents the difference from Kwashiorkor

[c] ↓ decrease

[d] ↑ increase

[e] N no difference

Table 18
PLASMA SEX HORMONES IN UNDERNOURISHED MEN AND CHILDREN, INDIAN ADULT MEN WITH EDEMA AND WASTING[109]

	PEM		Recovered		Contrast group		
	Mean	SD (Range)	Mean	SD (Range)	Mean	SD (Range)	Δ[a]
Number	28		28		16		
Age (in years)		(25—51)					
Weight (% of expected)		(65—91)					
Luteinizing hormone U/l	22.5	17.8	14.7	7.7	10.0	4.5	↑[b]
Follicle stimulating hormone U/l	17.8	14.1	14.2	9.0	13.5	6.0	↑[b]
Testosterone μg/l	3.2	1.5	5.4	1.4	5.8	1.6	↓[c]
Free testosterone ng/l	22.0	9.0	58.0	16.0			↓[c]
Estradiol ng/l	16.3	13.4	31.0	21.1			↓[c]
Free estradiol ng/l + hCG (12 kU/l)	0.30	0.27	0.34	0.25			N[d]
Δ testosterone μg/l	+4.3		+1.1				↑[b]
Δ FSH U/l	−4.3		−3.8				N[d]
Nigerian children with Kwashiorkor[57]							
Number	30				30		
Age (in months)	23				36		
Luteinizing hormone U/l	1.0	(0—9.0)			1.0	(0—8.0)	N[d]
Follicle stimulating hormone U/l	1.5	(0—5.0)			1.0	(0—12.0)	N[d]

[a]   Δ represents the difference between recovery and contrast groups
[b]   ↑ increase
[c]   ↓ decrease
[d]   N no difference

Table 19

EFFECT OF PEM ON EFFECTIVE PLASMA RENIN ACTIVITY (ANGIOTENSIN I GENERATED ng/hr/ml)

Children	Number	Age	Weight	Albumen	Mean (Median)	SD (Percentile)	Δ[a]	Ref.
KW Survived	22	12—30	60—81	12—36	(7.5)	(0.5—24.0)	↑[b]	27,149
KW Died	4	12—30	50—70	10—20	(20.0)	—	↑[b]	
KW After Recovery	22	11—48	61—95	26—39	(3.8)	(0.3—14.0)		
Contrast Group	20	12—48	82—95	36—42	(1.8)	(0.6—6.0)		27,149
KW Survived	74	12—48	62—87	16—37	(2.0)	(0.5—12.0)		
KW Died	26	12—27	49—82	14—26	(6.0)	(1.0—130.0)	↑[b]	
KW Survived	36	12—48		23	7.8	7.8	↑[b]	
KW Died	16	12—48		20	36.3	5.6	↑[b]	143
KW Recovered	18			40	2.0	5.0		
Contrast Group	21	12—24		40	4.7	5.0		
MAR Survived	24	12—48		27	10.2	6.4	↑[b]	143
MAR Died	4	12—48		23	11.8	3.0	↑[b]	
MAR Recovered	11			38	4.1	3.8		

Note: Mean (or median) is followed by SD (or 10th and 90th percentiles). Number of children (N), age (in months), weight (as percent of expected) and plasma albumin (g). All children were Africans in Rhodesia. Kwashiorkor = KW, Marasmus = MAR

[a] Δ represents the difference from recovery or contrast groups

[b] ↑ increase

Table 20
PLASMA AND URINE ALDOSTERONE AND SECRETION RATE IN PEM

Children	Country	N	Age (months)	Weight (% expected)	Plasma Albumen (g)	Mean	SD (Range)	Δ[a]	Hormone	Ref.
KW	Peru	8	23—39	70	10—24	530	(30—1440)	↑[b]	Plasma aldosterone ng L^{-1}	151, 152
KW after recovery	Peru	7			31—44	80	(10—800)			
Contrast group	Peru	8	12—19			150	70			
KW	Peru	6	23—29	70	10—21	92	(21—259)	↑?[b]	Aldosterone secretion rate μg 25 hr^{-1}	151, 152
KW after recovery	Peru	7			31—44	89	(17—216)			
Contrast group	Peru	8	12—19			75	(30—150)			
KW	South Africa	11	10—48			4.5	(0—18)	↑[b]	Urine aldosterone μg24 hr^{-1}	153
KW after recovery	South Africa	11				1.0	(0—8)			
Contrast group	South Africa	13	36—72			2.2	(0.5—5)			
KW	Jamaica	5				0.12	(0—0.4)	↓[c]	Urine aldosterone μg 24 hr^{-1}	147
KW after recovery	Jamaica	5				1.16	(0—4.3)			
KW	Uganda	6			14	78	5	↑[b]	Plasma free aldosterone % of total	150
KW after recovery	Uganda	9			20	68	9			
Contrast group	Uganda	17			32	60				
MAR	Peru	6	5—12	62	35—40	730	(570—1000)	N?[d]	Plasma aldosterone ng L^{-1}	151, 152
MAR after recovery	Peru	6	4—11			470	(330—770)			
Contrast group	Peru	8	4—11			700	300			
MAR	Peru	6	5—12	62	35—40	204	(79—452)	↑[b]	Aldosterone secretion rate μg 24 hr^{-1}	151, 152
MAR after recovery	Peru	6				91	(38—176)			
Contrast group	Peru	8	4—11			60	(20—140)			

[a] Δ represents the difference between recovery and contrast groups

[b] ↑ increase

[c] ↓ decrease

[d] N no difference

Table 21
ANTIDIURETIC HORMONE ACTIVITY IN PLASMA AND URINE IN CHILDREN WITH KWASHIORKOR (KW) AND MARASMUS (MAR)

Hormone in	Country	Children	N	Plasma (g L^{-1})	Median	Range	Δ[a]	Ref.
Plasma mU/l	India	KW	5	<20	22	17—69	↑[b]	154
		Recovered	5		<2	<2—10		
		MAR	3	>30	4	2—5	↑?[b]	
		Contrast	3		2	2—4		
Urine mU/24 hr	India	KW	5	<20	355	89—543	↑[b]	154
		Recovered	5		50	40—55		
		MAR	3	>30	38	28—68	N[c]	
		Contrast	3		50	26—52		
Urine mU/24 hr	Rhodesia Zimbabwe	KW	5	<20	73	4—151	↑[b]	28
		Contrast	5		9	3—15		

[a] Δ represents the difference between recovery and contrast groups
[b] ↑ increase
[c] N no difference

Table 22
CHANGE IN BASAL PLASMA INSULIN CONCENTRATION (mu/l) FOLLOWING A FAST IN NON-OBESE PEOPLE

Number	Duration of fast (days)	Change	Δ[a]	Ref.
6	6	−8	↓[b]	156
6	8	−6	↓[b]	157
10	3	−6	↓[b]	158
5	3	−5	↓[b]	159
8	6	−8	↓[b]	160
18	3	−10	↓[b]	161
10	4	−5	↓[b]	162
6	5	−6	↓[b]	163
9	1	−5	↓[b]	164
80	3	−8	↓[b]	165
41	3	−8	↓[b]	166
6	1	−25	↓[b]	167
12	2	−10	↓[b]	168
6	3	−3	↓[b]	169
6	3	−13	↓[b]	170
7	3	0	N[c]	171
17	3	−3	↓[b]	89

[a] Δ represents the difference from the pre-fasting concentration.
[b] ↓ decrease
[c] N no difference

Table 23
CHANGE IN BASAL PLASMA INSULIN CONCENTRATION (mu/l) FOLLOWING A FAST IN OBESE PEOPLE

N	Weight % desirable	Loss of weight (kg)	Duration of fast (days)	Change	Δ[a]	Ref.
5	128—361	8	8	−15	↓[b]	172
5	157—187	6	6	−42	↓[b]	160
9	165	40	270	−20	↓[b]	173
6	183	60	420	−9	↓[b]	174
10	93—195	30		−24	↓[b]	175
10	178		4	−9	↓[b]	162
6	171—278		14	+1	N[c]	176
16			3	−15	↓[b]	165
11		10	38	−24	↓[b]	177
15	146—218		3	−20	↓[b]	178
4	200		3	+2	N[c]	179
6	149—216		14	−27	↓[b]	180
4	150		52	−37	↓[b]	181
11	170	30	1400	−8	↓[b]	182
10	178—246		7	−10	↓[b]	183
8			21	−11	↓[b]	184
7			3	−13	↓[b]	171
9	148—244		10	−9	↓[b]	185
6	120—250		200	−10	↓[b]	186
6	115—146	5—10	90	−8	↓[b]	187

[a]   Δ represents the difference from the pre-fasting concentration.
[b]   ↓ decrease.
[c]   N no difference.

Table 24
EFFECT OF FASTING ON PLASMA INSULIN CONCENTRATION (mu/l) FOLLOWING STIMULATION TESTS IN NON-OBESE PEOPLE

Test	N	Duration of fast (days)	Change	Δ[a]	Ref.
Oral glucose 100 g at 120 min	6	3	+ 60	↑[b]	170
Oral glucose 100 g at 120 min	5	3	+ 130	↑[b]	159
I.V. glucose 0.5 g/kg	17	3	−24	↓[c]	89
I.V. glucose 0.5 g/kg	6	8	−18	↓[c]	157
I.V. glucose 0.33 g/kg	12	2	−140	↓[c]	168
I.V. arginine 0.35 g/kg	10	3	−25	↓[c]	158
I.V. arginine 10 g	18	3	−72	↓[c]	166
I.V. arginine 0.5 g/kg	7	3	−51	↓[c]	171
I.V. alanine 0.15 g/kg	10	4	−3	↓[c]	162
I.V. glucagon 30 μg/m^{-2}	6	1	−85	↓[c]	167

[a] Δ represents the difference from the pre-fasting concentration.

[b] ↑ increase.

[c] ↓ decrease.

Table 25
EFFECT OF FASTING ON PLASMA INSULIN
CONCENTRATION (mu/l) FOLLOWING
STIMULATION TESTS IN OBESE PEOPLE

Test	N	Duration of fast (days)	Change	Δ[a]	Ref.
Oral glucose					
40 g/m²	36		−70	↓[b]	188
50 g	9	55	−2800 (area)	↓[b]	189
100 g	6	270	−120	↓[b]	173
100 g	6	420	−81	↓[b]	174
100 g	10		−115	↓[b]	175
100 g	6	14	−3	N[c]	176
100 g	4	3	−3	N[c]	179
100 g	11	1400	−31	↓[b]	182
100 g	6	200	−100	↓[b]	186
100 g	6	90	−13	↓[b]	187
I.V. glucose (25 g)	9	10	+ 12	↑[d]	185
I.V. arginine	7	3	−97	↓[b]	171
I.V. alanine (4.5 g)	6	14	−6	↓[b]	180
(0.15 g/kg)	10	4	−21	↓[b]	162
I.V. tolbutamide (l g)	6	420	−60	↓[b]	174
I.V. glucagon (1 mg)	6	420	−35	↓[b]	174
(1 mg)	1	21	+ 30	↑[d]	190

[a]   Δ represents the difference from the pre-fasting response.
[b]   ↓ decrease.
[c]   N no difference.
[d]   ↑ increase.

Table 26
EFFECT OF STARVATION ON BASAL AND STIMULATED PLASMA INSULIN CONCENTRATION IN EXPERIMENTAL ANIMALS

Insulin	Species	Δ[a]	Ref.
Basal	Rat	↓[b]	191
After glucose	Rat	↓[b]	192
After tolbutamide	Rat	↓[b]	193
After aminophylline	Rat	↓[b]	192
Basal	Mouse	↓[b]	194
After tolbutamide	Mouse	↑[c]	195
Basal	Dog	↓[b]	170, 196
After glucose	Dog	↓[b]	197
After alanine	Dog	↑[c]	197
Basal	Pig	↓[b]	198
After glucose	Pig	↓[b]	198
Basal	Rabbit	↓[b]	199
After glucose	Rabbit	↓[b]	200
After glucagon	Rabbit	↓[b]	199
After glucose	Fetal rabbit	↑[c]	201
Basal	Sheep	↓[b]	202
	Sheep fetus	↓[b]	202

[a] Δ Change in basal and stimulated hormone concentration resulting from starvation.
[b]   ↓ decrease.
[c]   ↑ increase.

Table 27
CHANGE IN BASAL PLASMA GLUCAGON CONCENTRATION (ng/l) FOLLOWING A FAST

N	Weight (% desirable)	Duration of fast (days)	Change	Δ[a]	Ref.
10	100	3	+ 52	↑[b]	158
8	100	3	+ 600	↑[b]	159
18	100	3	+ 140	↑[b]	161
10	100	4	+ 58	↑[b]	162
	100	1—3	+ 40	↑[b]	203
6	100	3	+ 31	↑[b]	169
6	100	3	−190	↓[c]	170
6	165	270	− 16	↓[c]	173
8	Obese	4	+ 6	↑[b]	204
10	178	4	− 1	N[d]	162
15	146—218	3	+ 71	↑[b]	178
6	149—216	14	+ 16	↑[b]	180
4	150	3	+ 26	↑[b]	181
7	Obese	3	+ 37	↑[b]	171
8	Obese	21	− 4	↓[c]	184

[a] Δ represents the difference from the pre-fasting concentration.
[b]   ↑ increase.
[c]   ↓ decrease.
[d]   N no difference.

Table 28
EFFECT OF FASTING ON PLASMA GLUCAGON CONCENTRATION (ng/*l*) FOLLOWING STIMULATION TESTS

N	Weight (% desirable)	Duration of fast (days)	Change	Δ[a]	Test	Ref.
6	100	3	− 20	↓[b]	Oral glucose 100 g	170
8	100	3	−193	↓[b]	Oral glucose 100 g	159
5	100		+ 144	↑[c]	i.v. arginine 340 mg/kg	158
6	165	270	− 95	↓[b]	i.v. arginine 30 g	173
8	Obese	4	−550	↓[b]	i.v. arginine 250 mg/kg	204
7	Obese	3	+ 207	↑[c]	i.v. arginine	171
10	100	4	+ 270	↑[c]	i.v. alanine 150 mg/kg	162
10	178	4	+ 77	↑[c]	i.v. alanine 150 mg/kg	162
6	149—216	14	+ 18	↑[c]	i.v. alanine 4.5 g	180
6	165	270	0	N[d]	i.v. glucose 45 g	173

[a]   Δ represents the difference from the pre-fasting response.
[b]   ↓ decrease.
[c]   ↑ increase.
[d]   N no difference.

Table 29
EFFECT OF STARVATION ON BASAL AND STIMULATED PLASMA GLUCAGON CONCENTRATION IN EXPERIMENTAL ANIMALS

Glucagon	Species	Δ[a]	Ref.
Basal	Rat	N[b]	205
Basal	Rat	↑[c]	206
Basal	Rat	↓[d]	194
Basal	Dog	↓[d]	170
Basal	Dog	↑[c]	197
After glucose	Dog	↓[d]	197
Basal	Mouse	↑[c]	207

[a]   Δ difference from pre-fasting concentration.
[b]   N no difference.
[c]   ↑ increase.
[d]   ↓ decrease.

Table 30
CHANGE IN BASAL PLASMA GROWTH HORMONE CONCENTRATION (μg/*l*) FOLLOWING A FAST IN NONOBESE PEOPLE

N	Change of weight (kg)	Duration of fast (days)	Change	Δ[a]	Ref.
6	5	6	+ 8	↑[b]	156
6	5	8	+ 9	↑[b]	157
7		3	+ 5	↑[b]	208
1		2	+ 7	↑[b]	209
9		1	+ 4	↑[b]	164
15		3	+ 130%	↑[b]	210
4		2	+ 4	↑[b]	172
41		3	+ 1	↑?[b]	166
6		1	+ 8	↑[b]	167
18		3	+ 4	↑[b]	211
17	4	3	+ 3	↑[b]	89
12		years	+ 16	↑[b]	44

[a]   Δ represents the difference from the pre-fasting concentration.
[b]   ↑ increase.

Table 31
CHANGE IN BASAL PLASMA GROWTH HORMONE CONCENTRATION (μg/l) FOLLOWING A FAST IN OBESE PEOPLE

N	Change of weight (kg)	Weight (% desirable)	Duration of fast (days)	Change	Δ^a	Ref.
9	8	128—361	5	+ 2	↑[b]	172
3	>20	137—209		+ 13	↑[b]	212
6	60	183	420	+ 1	↑?[b]	174
11	13		38	−1	↓?[c]	177
13	4—10	144—295	10	+ 1	↑?[b]	213
22	>28	>160	365	+ 2	↑[b]	214
12	>35	>160	200	0	N[d]	215

[a] Δ represents the difference from the pre-fasting concentration.
[b]   ↑ increase.
[c]   ↓ decrease.
[d]   N no difference.

Table 32
EFFECT OF FASTING ON PLASMA GROWTH HORMONE (μg/l) FOLLOWING STIMULATION TESTS

N	Weight (% desirable)	Change of weight (kg)	Duration of fast (days)	Change	Δ^a	Test	Ref.
6	100	5	8	+ 1	↑[b]	i.v. glucose 0.5 g/kg	157
12	63—91		Years	+ 14	↑[b]	i.v. glucose 0.5 g/kg	44
18	100		3	−14	↓[c]	i.v. arginine 10 g	166
12	>160	>35	200	+ 10	↑[b]	i.v. arginine 30 g	215
12	63—91		Years	+ 7	↑[b]	i.v. arginine 0.5 g/kg	44
22	>160	>28	365	+ 3	↑[b]	oral glucose 100 g	214
22	>160	>28	365	+ 3	↑[b]	i.v. insulin 0.1 U/kg	214
6	183	60	420	+ 17	↑[b]	i.v. insulin 0.1 U/kg	174
13	144—295	4—10	10	−5	↓[c]	i.v. insulin 0.1 U/kg	213

[a] Δ represents the difference from the pre-fasting response.
[b]   ↑ increase.
[c]   ↓ decrease.

Table 33
EFFECT OF STARVATION ON
BASAL AND STIMULATED
PLASMA GROWTH HORMONE
CONCENTRATION IN
EXPERIMENTAL ANIMALS

Growth hormone	Species	Δ[a]	Ref.
Basal	Rat	↓[b]	216
Basal	Rat	↑[c]	217
Basal	Rabbit	↑[c]	201
After arginine	Fetal rabbit	↑[c]	201
Basal	Pig	↑[c]	218
Basal	Sheep	↑[c]	202
Basal	Mouse	↑?[c]	219
Basal	Cat	↓[b]	220
Somatomedin	Rat	↓[b]	221

[a]   Δ Difference from contrast group.
[b]   ↓ decrease.
[c]   ↑ increase.

Table 34
CHANGE IN PLASMA AND URINE CORTICOID CONCENTRATION AND EXCRETION FOLLOWING A FAST

Hormone	N	Weight (% desirable)	Change of Weight (kg)	Duration of fast (days)	Change	Δ[a]	Ref.
Plasma cortisol μg/*l*	6	100		1	0	N[b]	167
	11	Obese		14	+60	↑[c]	184
	13	130—191		7—11	+31	↑[c]	222
Plasma free cortisol μg/*l*	13	130—191		7—11	+2.7	↑[c]	222
Plasma 11 hydroxy	8	170	12	12	0	N[b]	223
Plasma 17 hydroxy μg/*l*	12	144—232	10	13	+417	?	224
Plasma dehydroepiandrosterone (μg/*l*)	8	>135	1—15	7	+330	↑[c]	225
Cortisol secretion	10	145—286	21	60	−12	↓[d]	226
rate mg/24 hr	5	138—205		7—20	−4.7	↓[d]	227
Urine free	4	140—280	4	4	+14	↑[c]	228
cortisol μg/24 hr	13	130—191		7—11	+16	↑[c]	222
Urine 11 hydroxy mg/24 hr	8	170	12	12	−55	↓[d]	223
Urine 17-hydroxycorticoids mg/24 hr	6	117		210	−16	↓[d]	229
	10	145—286	21	60	−10	↓[d]	226
	20	143	18		−4	↓[d]	230
	8	170	12	12	−3	↓[d]	223
	12	144—232	10	13	−3	↓[d]	224
	5	138—205		7—20	−5	↓[d]	227
	13	130—191		7—11	0	N[b]	222
	6	200—250	10	23	−5	↓[d]	231
Urine 17-ketosteroids	7	145—286	21	60	−6	↓[d]	226
	20	143	18		+2	?N[b]	230
	8	170	12	12	−8	↓[d]	223
	12	144—232	10	13	−6	↓[d]	224
	13	130—191		7—11	−2	?N[b]	222
	6	205—250	10	23	−5	↓[d]	231

[a] Δ represents the difference from the pre-fasting values.
[b] N no difference.
[c] ↑ increase.
[d] ↓ decrease.

Table 35
EFFECT OF STARVATION ON
PLASMA AND URINARY
CORTICOIDS IN EXPERIMENTAL
ANIMALS

Hormone	Species	Δ[a]	Ref.
Plasma Corticosterone	Rat	↑[b]	232
Plasma corticosterone	Rat	↓[c]	233
Plasma cortisol	Pig	N[d]	234
Plasma free cortisol	Pig	↑[b]	234
Plasma corticoids	Sheep	↑[b]	202
Plasma corticosterone	Rabbit	↑[b]	235
Urine 17-hydroxy	Pig	N[d]	236
Urine 17-keto	Pig	↓[c]	236
Urine 17-keto	Dog	↓[c]	196

[a] Δ Change from contrast group.
[b] ↑ increase.
[c] ↓ decrease.
[d] N no difference.

Table 36
CHANGE IN PLASMA THYROID HORMONE CONCENTRATIONS FOLLOWING
A FAST

Hormone	N	Weight (% expected)	Change of weight (kg)	Duration of fast (days)	Change	Δ[a]	Ref.
Thyroxine	10	Thin		Years	0	N[b]	2
μg/l	11	Obese	20		+2	↑[c]	237
	9	Obese		28	−5	↓[d]	238
	3	170—341		14	+8	↑[c]	239
	13	140—160	10—13	21—28	−10	↓[d]	240
	3	140	25	40	−12	↓[d]	241
	26	116—272	4—6	7	+2	↑[c]	242
	14	100		3	+6	↑[c]	243
Free thyroxine %	26	116—272	4—6	7	+0.005	↑[c]	242
Free thyroxine ng	10	Thin		Years	+16	↑[c]	2
Triiodothyronine	9	Obese		28	−790	↓[d]	238
ng/l	3	170—341		14	−800	↓[d]	239
	13	140—160	10—13	21—28	−220	↓[d]	240
	14	100		3	−640	↓[d]	243
	10	Thin		Years	−740	↓[d]	2
Reversed triiodothyronine	9	Obese		28	+180	↑[c]	244
ng/l	3	170—341		14	+200	↑[c]	239
Free triiodothyronine ng/l⁻¹	10	Thin		Years	+2.1	↑[c]	2
Thyroid stimulating	9	Obese		28	+0.4	?N[b]	238
hormone mμ/l⁻¹	13	140—160	10—13	21—28	−2.3	↓[d]	240
	9	100		1	−1.4	↓[d]	164
	10	Thin		Years	+0.5	?N[b]	2
Thyroid stimulating hormone (mU/l) after thyrotropin releasing hormone (200 μg i.v.)	9	100		1	−6.2	↓[d]	164

[a] Δ represents the difference from pre-fasting concentrations.
[b] N no difference.
[c] ↑ increase.
[d] ↓ decrease.

Table 37
EFFECT OF STARVATION ON PLASMA THYROID HORMONE CONCENTRATION IN EXPERIMENTAL ANIMALS

Hormone	Species	Δ[a]	Ref.
Thyroxine	Rat	N[b]	245
Thyroxine	Rat	↓[c]	246
Triiodothyronine	Rat	↓[c]	246
Thyroxine secretion rate	Rat	↓[c]	247

[a] Δ Change in hormone concentration after starvation.
[b] N no difference.
[c] ↓ decrease.

Table 38
CHANGES IN PLASMA SEX HORMONE CONCENTRATION DURING STARVATION

	N[a]	Weight	Δ[b] weight	Time	Change	Δ[c]	Ref.
Testosterone μg/ℓ	6	140—280	6—30	27—190	+1.3	↑?[d]	248
Luteinizing hormone U/ℓ	6	140—280	6—30	27—190	−0.7	↓?[e]	248
Follicle stimulating hormone U/ℓ	6	140—280	6—30	29—190	−1.2	↓?[e]	248
Human chorionic somatatomammotrophic hormone Δ %	3	Pregnant	3.7	3	+26	↑[d]	211
mammotrophic hormone Δ%	24	Pregnant		3	+27	↑[d]	166
Prolactin μg/ℓ	41	Pregnant		3	−2.3	↓[e]	166
Dehydroepiandrosterone μg/ℓ	8	>135	1—15	7	+330	↑[d]	225

[a] N is number, weight as % of desirable for height.
[b] Δ weight is change of weight in kg, time is duration of fast in days.
[c] Δ represents the difference from pre-fasting concentrations.
[d] ↑ increase.
[e] ↓ decrease.

Table 39
PLASMA SEX HORMONES IN ANIMALS DURING STARVATION

Hormone	Species	Δ[a]	Ref.
Follicle stimulating hormone	Rat♀	↑[b]	249
	Rat♂	↓[c]	250
	Rat♂	↓[c]	251
Luteinizing hormone	Rat♀	↑[b]	249
	Rat♂	↓[c]	250
	Rat	N[d]	251
Testosterone	Rat	↓[c]	252
Prolactin	Rat♀	↑[b]	249
	Cow	↓[c]	253

[a]   Δ change in hormone concentration following starvation difference from contrast group.
[b]   ↑ increase.
[c]   ↓ decrease.
[d]   N no difference.

Table 40

CHANGE IN PLASMA AND URINE RENIN ACTIVITY AND ALDOSTERONE
CONCENTRATION AND EXCRETION FOLLOWING A FAST

Hormone	N	Weight (% desirable)	Change of weight (kg)	Duration of fast (days)	Change	Δ^a	Ref.
Plasma renin μg/ℓ/hr	4	140—280	4	4	-1.8	↓[b]	228
activity μg/ℓ/hr	9	83—113	4—7	10—14	+2.7	↑[c]	256
U/ℓ	11	>135	8	12	+60	↑[c]	257
μg/ℓ/hr⁻¹	7	116—272	4—6	7	+73	↑[c]	258
Plasma aldesterone ng/ℓ	11	>135	8	12	+390	↑[c]	257
Aldosterone secretion rate	2	100		7	+233	↑[c]	259
μg/24 hr	9	83—113	4—7	10—14	+530	↑[c]	256
	2	150, 190	18	29, 46	-18	↓[b]	260
	1	Obese	10	21	+740	↑[c]	261
Urine aldosterone μg/24	4	140—280	4	4	+293	↑[c]	228
hr	7	Obese		4	0	N[d]	262
	6	200—250	10	23	0	N[d]	231

[a] Δ represents the difference from pre-fasting values.

[b] ↓ decrease.

[c] ↑ increase.

[d] N no difference.

Table 41

BASAL AND STIMULATED PLASMA GROWTH HORMONE AND INSULIN CONCENTRATIONS IN PATIENTS WITH ANOREXIA NERVOSA

Hormone	N	Age (years)	Mean	SD (Range)	Contrast	Δ[a]	Ref.
Growth Hormone Basal μg/ℓ	5	17—47	7	(3—13)	1—20	↑?[b]	275
	12	15—43	8	4		↑[b]	276
	5	19—43	4	(2—28)		↑?[b]	277
Growth Hormone after i.v. insulin 0.1 u/kg	5	17—47	+8	(+1—+13)	(+14—+120)	↓[c]	275
After i.v. arginine 0.5 g/kg	5	19—43	+26			N[d]	277
After oral glucose 50 g	12	15—43	+9			R	276
Insulin Basal mU/ℓ	8	17—63	26		18	?↑[b]	278
After i.v. glucose 0.33 g/kg	8	17—63	+47		+83	↓[c]	278

[a] Δ represents the difference from contrast group.
[b] ↑ increase.
[c] ↓ decrease.
[d] N no difference.

Table 42

ADRENAL CORTICOL HORMONE SECRETION IN PATIENTS WITH ANOREXIA NERVOSA

Hormone	N	Age (years)	Mean	SD (Range)	Contrast	Δ[a]	Ref.
Basal plasma cortisol μg/ℓ	15	16—28	89	(37—137)	49	↑[b]	271
Plasma cortisol after i.v. insulin 0.1 u/kg	5	17—47	+66	(0—+113)	+154	↓[c]	275
Plasma cortisol after dexamethasone 2 mg	4		−50		−110	↓[c]	279
Cortisol secretion rate, mg/24 hr	15	16—28	19	(13—32)	19	N[d]	271
Urine 17-hydroxy-corticoids mg/24 hr	16	15—43	11	6		N[d]	276
Urine 17-keto-steroids mg/24 hr	9	21—47		(3—9)	(6—18)	↓[c]	280

[a] Δ represents the difference from contrast groups.
[b] ↑ increase.
[c] ↓ decrease.
[d] N no difference.

Table 43
PLASMA THYROID HORMONES IN PATIENTS WITH ANOREXIA NERVOSA

Hormone	N	Age (in years)	Mean	SD (range)	Contrast	Δ^a	Ref.
Thyroxine μg/l	22	15—41	71	19	82	N[b]	281
Triiodothyronine ng/l	22	15—41	621	330	1152	↓[c]	281
Free thyroxine ng/l	10	16—28	19	(17—27)	16	↑?[d]	271
Thyroid stimulating hormone mU/l	10	16—28	2.1	(1—5)	1.6	↑?[d]	271
TSH after i.v. releasing hormone 500 μg	16	17—24	+10	(+4—+14)	+4	↑[d]	282
T_3 after i.v. releasing hormone 500 μg	16	17—24	+250	(+200—+600)	+280	N[b]	282

[a] Δ represents difference from contrast groups.
[b] N no difference.
[c] ↓ decrease.
[d] ↑ increase.

Table 44

PLASMA AND URINE SEX HORMONE CONCENTRATIONS IN PATIENTS WITH ANOREXIA NERVOSA

Hormone	N	Age (years)	Mean	SD (Range)	Contrast	Δ[a]	Ref.
Plasma Luteinizing Hormone uL^{-1}	15	14—26	1.9	0.5	10.3	↓[b]	283
After releasing hormone 100 μg i.v.	15	14—26	+2.1		+35.4	↓[b]	283
Follicle stimulating hormone u/ℓ	14	14—29	1.0	(0.2—2.4)	3.4	↓[b]	284
After releasing hormone 100 μg i.v.	14	14—29	+4.2		+1.8	↑[c]	284
After releasing hormone 50 μg i.v.	7	15—30	+4		+10	↓[b]	285
Plasma estradiol ng/ℓ	14	14—29	17	(12—29)	110	↓[b]	284
Plasma progesterone μg/ℓ	14	14—24	0.3	(0—0.6)	(0.2—1.3)	↓[b]	286
Plasma prolactin μg/ℓ	8	15—36	26	(11—90)	(3—16)	↑[c]	287
Urine Estradiol μg/24 hr	7	16—23	5.9	2.1	7.3	↓[b]	288
2-hydroxy estrone μg/24 hr	7	16—23	26.3	6.4	11.8	↑[c]	288
Estriol mg/24 hr	5	16—32	2.0	(0—4)	5	↓[b]	289
Dehydroepiandrosterone mg/24 hr	5	16—32	0.3	(0—0.5)	0.8	↓[b]	289

[a] Δ represents difference from contrast groups.
[b] ↓ decrease.
[c] ↑ increase.

Table 45
EFFECT OF OBESITY ON INSULIN SECRETION

Hormone	N	Age (years)	Weight (% desirable)	Mean	SD (Range)	Contrast	Δ[a]	Ref.
Basal plasma insulin mU/kg	14	15—58	126—290	41		18	↑[b]	278
Basal plasma insulin mU/kg	30	2—16	120—170	16	14	6	↑[b]	299
After oral glucose 1.75 g/kg	30	2—16	120—170	+85		+44	↑[b]	299
After i.v. glucose 8 g/kg	27	14—54	129	+36		+14	↑[b]	300
After i.v. tolbutamide 1 g	6		183	+155		+75	↑[b]	174
After i.v. glucagon 1 g	6		183	+145		+75	↑[b]	174
After i.v. arginine 30 g	9	27	166	+110		+54	↑[b]	173
After i.v. alanine 0.15 g/kg	10	24—48	178	+48		+13	↑[b]	162
After i.v. xylitol 0.38 g/kg	5	19—56	123—235	+24		+18	↑[b]	301
After oral leucine 0.2 g/kg	5		135—222	+38		+2	↑[b]	302
After oral beef 400 g	9	27	167	+28		+17	↑[b]	303
After i.v. secretin 75 u	10	15—68	120—184	+91		+53	↑[b]	304
After dexamethasone 4 mg and i.v. tolbutamide 1 g	12	14—62	138—412	+236		+116	↑[b]	305
Secretion rate mU/min	22			5.0	1.6—9.4	3.0	↑[b]	306
During glucose infusion	22			18.0	5.6	9.0	↑[b]	306

[a] Δ represents the difference from the contrast group.
[b] ↑increase.

Table 46

EFFECT OF OBESITY ON GLUCAGON SECRETION

Hormone	N	Age (in years)	Weight (% expected)	Mean	SD	Contrast	Δ[a]	Ref.
Basal plasma glucagon ng/ℓ	15		166	84	30	86	N[b]	173
After oral glucose 1.75 g/kg	13	5—15		0		+200	↓[c]	308
After i.v. glucose 45 g	15		166	−40		−20	↑[d]	173
After i.v. arginine 30 g	9	27	167	+308		+197	↑[d]	303
After i.v. alanine 0.15 g/kg	10	24—48	178	+54		+109	↓[c]	162
After oral beef 400 g	15		166	+100		+80	?↑[d]	173

[a] Δ represents the difference from contrast group.
[b] N no difference.
[c] ↓ decrease.
[d] ↑ increase.

Table 47

EFFECT OF OBESITY OR GROWTH HORMONE SECRETION

Hormone	N	Age (years)	Weight (% desirable)	Mean	SD (Range)	Contrast	Δ[a]	Ref.
Basal plasma growth hormone µg/ℓ	22	17—40	>170	0.7	0.9	3.2	↓[b]	214
	30	2—16	120—170	1.2	0.5	2.4	↓[b]	299
After i.v. insulin 0.1 u/kg	9		128—361	+8		+33	↑[b]	172
After i.v. arginine 0.5 g/kg	12	17—40	>145	+2		+15	↓[b]	215
After oral glucose 1.75 g/kg	24	5—15		+3		+25	↓[b]	309
After oral L-dopa 0.5 g	18	18—40	>140	0		+10	↓[b]	310

[a] Δ represents difference from contrast group.
[b] ↓ decrease.

Table 48
EFFECT OF OBESITY ON ADRENAL CORTEX SECRETION

Hormone	N	Age (years)	Weight (% desirable)	Mean	SD (Range)	Contrast	Δ[a]	Ref.
Basal plasma cortisol μg/ℓ	23	13—54	147—253	180	(40—260)	190	N[b]	311
After i.v. insulin 0.1 u/kg	14	8—11	139—201	+96		+148	↓[c]	312
After oral glucose 100 g	8		175	-80		-80	N[b]	313
After oral L dopa 0.5 g	18	18—40	>140	0		-43	↓[c]	310
Basal plasma free cortisol μg/ℓ	13		130—191	6.3	1.7	6.7	N[b]	222
Cortisol secretion rate mg/24 hr	32	16—67	150—279	24	(11—39)	15	↑[d]	314
Urine free cortisol μg/24 hr	13		130—191	33	11	38	N[b]	222
Urine 17 hydroxy corticoids mg/24 hr	160	3—79		4.3	(1.1—10)	2.9	↑[d]	315
Urine 11 hydroxy corticoids μg/24 hr	8		170	136	(48—295)	50—300	N[b]	223
Urine 17 ketosteroids mg/24 hr	13		130—191	5.5	2.0	10.5	↓[c]	222
Urine aldosterone μkg/24 hr	23	13—54	147—253	0.14	(0.04—0.45)	0.2	N[b]	311
Urine dehydroepiandrosterone mg/24 hr	4	19—50	>135	4.9	(0.10—9.8)	0.7	↑[d]	225
Plasma adrenocorticotropic hormone ng/ℓ	14	8—11	139—201	16.7	9.5	17.5	N[b]	312
after i.v. insulin 0.1 U/kg				+112		+211	↓[c]	312

[a]   Δ represents difference from contrast group.
[b]   N no difference.
[c]   ↓ decrease.
[d]   ↑ increase.

Table 49

EFFECT OF OBESITY ON THYROID SECRETION

Hormones in plasma	N	Weight (% desirable)	Mean	SD (Range)	Contrast	Δ^a	Ref.
Thyroxine µg/ℓ	11		81	(59—109)	(50—125)	N^b	237
Free thyroxine ng/ℓ	11		45	(20—78)	32	$?\uparrow^c$	237
Triiodothyronine ng/ℓ	23	200—300	1300	(700—1900)	(500—1600)	N^b	317
Thyroid stimulating hormone mU/ℓ	31		3.0	2.8		N^b	318
After I.V. releasing hormone 200 µg	31		+14			N^b	318
Thyronine secretion rate µg/24 hr	6		73	(63—93)	41	$\uparrow^c$	319
Thyroxine plasma half life days	10	140	4.3	(3.7—4.9)	5.5	$\downarrow^d$	241

[a] Δ represents difference from contrast group.

[b] N no difference.

[c] ↑ increase.

[d] ↓ decrease.

Table 50
EFFECT OF OBESITY ON THE SEX HORMONES ETC.

Hormone	N	Age (years)	Weight (% desirable)	Mean	SD (Range)	Contrast	Δ[a]	Ref.
Plasma								
Testosterone µg/l	6	24—70	140—270	4.0	(2.3—6)	5.3	?N[b]	248
Dehydroepiandrosterone µg	46	30	125	570	400	810	↓[c]	320
Androsterone µg	46	30	125	220	280	230	N[b]	320
Luteinizing hormone U	6	24—70	140—270	12	(5—29)	(5—30)	N[b]	248
Prolactin µg/l	9	30—45	142—215	12	5—20	3—16	?N[b]	287
Urine								
Estradiol µg/24 hr	4	14—28	>175	10.0	3.4	7.3	?↑[d]	288
Estriol µg/24 hr	4	14—28	>175	28.3	13.6	22.4	?↑[d]	288
2-hydroxyestrone µg/24 hr	4	14—28	>175	4.8	5.8	11.8	↓[c]	288
Dehydroepiandrosterone mg/24 hr	4	19—50	>135	4.9	(0.1—9.8)	0.7	↑[d]	225
Dehydroepiandrosterone production rate mg/24 hr	3			94	(49—111)	24	↑[d]	321
DHA sulfate production rate mg/24	3			17	(13—34)	18	N[b]	321
Urine noradrenaline µg/24 hr	8		175	50	14	35	?N[b]	313

[a] Δ represents difference from contrast group.

[b] N no difference.

[c] ↓ decrease.

[d] ↑ increase.

Table 51
CHANGES IN HORMONE SECRETION ASSOCIATED WITH OBESITY IN EXPERIMENTAL ANIMALS

Hormone	Species	Δ[a]	Ref.
Basal plasma insulin	Mouse	↑[b]	323
Basal plasma insulin	Rat	↑[b]	324
Basal plasma insulin	Monkey	↑[b]	325
Insulin secretion after oral glucose and arginine	Rat	↑[b]	326
Insulin secretion after intraperitoneal glucose	Mouse	↓[c]	327
Insulin receptors and insulin action	Mouse	↓[c]	328
Insulin receptors and insulin action	Rat	↓[c]	329
Glucagon secretion			
Basal plasma glucagon	Mouse	↑[b]	207
	Mouse	↓[c]	194
Basal plasma glucagon after arginine	Rat	↓[c]	326
Basal plasma growth hormone	Pig	↓[c]	330
Basal plasma growth hormone	Mouse	↓[c]	331
Basal plasma corticosteroids	Mouse	↑[b]	332
Corticosteroids after ether stress	Mouse	↑[b]	333
Basal plasma adrenocorticotropic hormone	Mouse	↓?[c]	333
Basal plasma prolactin	Mouse	↓[c]	335
Prolactin after perphenazine	Mouse	↑[b]	334
Basal plasma thyroid stimulating hormone	Rat	↑[b]	336
Basal plasma thyroxine	Rat	↓[c]	337

[a] Δ represents the difference from the contrast groups.

[b] ↑ increase.

[c] ↓ decrease.

REFERENCES

1. **Leonard, P. J. and MacWilliam, K. M.**, Cortisol binding in the serum in kwashiorkor, *J. Endocrinol.*, 29, 273—276, 1964.
2. **Chopra, I. J. and Smith, S. R.**, Circulating thyroid hormones and thyrotropin in adult patients with protein-calorie malnutrition, *J. Clin. Endocrinol. Metab.*, 40, 221—227, 1975.
3. **Bowie, M. D.**, Intravenous glucose tolerance in kwashiorkor and marasmus, *S. Afr. Med. J.*, 38, 328—329, 1964.
4. **McLaren, D. S. and Read, W. W. C.**, Classification of nutritional status in early childhood, *Lancet*, 2, 146—148, 1972.
5. **McLaren, D. S.**, The great protein fiasco, *Lancet*, 2, 93—96, 1974.
6. **Anon.**, Food fortification. Protein-calorie malnutrition, World Health Organization Technical Report Series No. 477, 1971.
7. **Gardner, L. I. and Ambacher, P.**, Eds., *Endocrine Aspects of Malnutrition*, Kroc Foundation, Santa Ynez, California, 1973.
8. **Godard, C.**, Review: the endocrine glands in infantile malnutrition, *Helv. Paediatr. Acta*, 29, 5—26, 1974.
9. **Pimstone, B.**, Endocrine function in protein-calorie malnutrition, *Clin. Endocrinol. N.Y.*, 5, 79—95, 1976.
10. **Alleyne, G. A. O., Hay, R. W., Picou, D. I., Stanfield, J. P., and Whitehead, R. G.**, *Protein-energy Malnutrition*, Arnold, London, 1976.
11. **Lunn, P. G., Whitehead, R. G., Haw, R. W., and Baker, B. A.**, Progressive change in serum cortisol, insulin and growth hormone concentrations and their relationship to the distorted amino acid pattern during development of kwashiorkor, *Br. J. Nutr.*, 29, 399—422, 1973.
12. **Kajubi, S. K. and Okel, R. M.**, Serum insulin and growth hormone after kwashiorkor, *Am. J. Clin. Nutr.*, 27, 1200—1201, 1974.
13. **Becker, D. J., Pimstone, B. L., and Hansen, J. D. L.**, The relation between insulin secretion, glucose tolerance, growth hormone, and serum proteins in protein-calorie malnutrition, *Pediatr. Res.*, 9, 35—39, 1975.
14. **Mann, M. D., Becker, D. J., Pimstone, B. L., and Hansen, J. D. L.**, Potassium supplementation, serum immunoreactive insulin concentrations and glucose tolerance in protein-energy malnutrition, *Br. J. Nutr.*, 33, 55—61, 1975.
15. **Becker, D. J., Mann, M. D., Weinkove, E., and Pimstone, B. L.**, Early insulin release and its response to potassium supplementation in protein-calorie malnutrition, *Diabetologia*, 11, 237—239, 1975.
16. **Becker, D. J., Pimstone, B. L., Hansen, J. D. L., MacHutchon, B., and Drysdale, A.**, Patterns of insulin response to glucose in protein-calorie malnutrition, *Am. J. Clin. Nutr.*, 25, 499—505, 1972.
17. **Pimstone, B. L., Becker, D. J., Weinkove, C., and Mann, M. D.**, Insulin secretion in protein-calorie malnutrition, in *Endocrine Aspects of Malnutrition*, Gardner, L. I. and Ambacher, P., Eds., Kroc Foundation, Santa Ynez, California, 1973, 289—305.
18. **Cheek, D. B. and Graystone, J. E.**, The action of insulin, growth hormone, and epinephrine on cell growth in liver, muscle, and brain of the hypophysectomized rat, *Pediatr. Res.*, 3, 77—88, 1969.
19. **Wharton, B.**, Metabolic effects of malnutrition in childhood, *J. R. Coll. Physicians London*, 7, 259—270, 1973.
20. **James, W. P. T. and Coore, H. G.**, Persistent impairment of insulin secretion and glucose tolerance after malnutrition, *Am. J. Clin. Nutr.*, 23, 386—389, 1970.
21. **Milner, R. D. G.**, Insulin secretion in human protein-calorie deficiencies, *Proc. Nutr. Soc.*, 31, 219—223, 1972.
22. **Whitehead, R. G. and Alleyne, G. A. O.**, Pathophysiological factors of importance in protein-calorie malnutrition, *Br. Med. Bull.*, 28, 72—79, 1972.
23. **Becker, D. J., Murray, P. J., Hansen, J. D. L., and Pimstone, B. L.**, Circulating "big" insulin in protein-energy malnutrition, *Br. J. Nutr.*, 30, 345—350, 1973.
24. **Alleyne, G. A. O., Trust, P. M., Flores, H. and Robinson, H.**, Glucose tolerance and insulin sensitivity in malnourished children, *Br. J. Nutr.*, 27, 585—592, 1972.
25. **Prinsloo, J. G., DeBruin, E. J. P., and Kruger, H.**, Comparison of intravenous glucose tolerance tests and serum insulin in kwashiorkor and pellagra, *Arch. Dis. Child.*, 46, 795—800, 1971.
26. **Becker, D. J., Pimstone, B. L., Hansen, J. D. L., and Hendricks, S.**, Insulin secretion in protein-calorie malnutrition. I. Quantitative abnormalities and response to treatment, *Diabetes*, 20, 542—551, 1971.
27. **Kritzinger, E. E., Kanengoni, E., and Jones, J. J.**, Effective renin activity in plasma of children with kwashiorkor, *Lancet*, 1, 412—413, 1972.
28. **Van Der Westhuysen, J. M.**, Endocrine and metabolic changes during protein-energy malnutrition, Ph.D. thesis, University of Stellenbosch, 1975.

29. **Baig, H. A. and Edozien, J. C.**, Carbohydrate metabolism in kwashiorkor, *Lancet*, 2, 662—665, 1965.

30. **Hadden, D. R.**, Glucose, free fatty acid, and insulin interrelationships in kwashiorkor and marasmus, *Lancet*, 2, 589—592, 1967.

31. **Persson, B., Habte, D., and Sterky, G.**, Plasma levels of triglycerides, FFA, D-β-hydroxybutyrate, glycerol, postheparin lipoprotein lipase (LPL), glucose and insulin, *Acta Paediatr. Scand.*, 65, 329—336, 1976.

32. **Rao, K. S. J. and Raghuramulu, N.**, Growth hormone and insulin secretion in protein-calorie malnutrition as seen in India, in *Endocrine Aspects of Malnutrition*, Gardner, L. I. and Ambacher, P., Eds., Kroc Foundation, Santa Ynez. California, 1973, 91—98.

33. **Rao, K. S. J. and Raghuramulu, N.**, Insulin secretion in kwashiorkor, *J. Clin. Endocrinol. Metab.*, 35, 63—66, 1972.

34. **Milner, R. D. G.**, Metabolic and hormonal response to oral amino acids in infantile malnutrition, *Arch. Dis. Child.*, 46, 301—305, 1971.

35. **Milner, R. D. G.**, Metabolic and hormonal responses to glucose and glucagon in patients with infantile malnutrition, *Pediatr. Res.*, 5, 33—39, 1971.

36. **Parra, A., Garza, C., Klish, W., Garcia, G., Argote, R. M., Canseco, L., Cuellar, A., and Nichols, B. L.**, Insulin-growth hormone adaptations in marasmus and kwashiorkor as seen in Mexico, in *Endocrine Aspects of Malnutrition*, Gardner, L. I. and Ambacher, P., Eds.; Kroc Foundation, Santa Ynez, Cal., 1973, 31—43.

37. **Parra, A., Klish, W., Cuellar, A., Serrano, P. A., Garcia, G., Argote, R. M., Canseco, L., and Nichols, B. L.**, Energy metabolism and hormonal profile in children with edematous protein-calorie malnutrition, *J. Pediatr.*, 87, 307—314, 1975.

38. **Graham, G. G., Cordano, A., Blizzard, R. M., and Cheek, D. G.**, Infantile malnutrition: changes in body composition during rehabilitation, *Pediatr. Res.*, 3, 579—589, 1969.

39. **Graham, G. G., Nakashima, J., Thompson, R. G., and Blizzard, R. M.**, Metabolic and hormonal responses to a protein-glucose meal in normal infants and in marasmus and marasmic kwashiorkor, *Pediatr. Res.*, 10, 832—843, 1976.

40. **Becker, D. J., Pimstone, B. L., Kronheim, S., and Weinkove, E.**, The effect of alanine infusions on growth hormone, insulin and glucose in protein-calorie malnutrition, *Metab. Clin. Exp.*, 24, 953—958, 1975.

41. **Parra, A., Garza, C., Saravia, J. L., Hazlewood, C. F., and Nichols, B. L.**, Changes in growth hormone, insulin, and thyroxine values, and in energy metabolism of marasmic infants, *J. Pediatr.*, 82, 133—142, 1973.

42. **Pimstone, B. L., Becker, D. J., and Kronheim, S.**, Disappearance of plasma growth hormone in acromegaly and protein-calorie malnutrition after somatostatin, *J. Clin. Endocrinol. Metab.*, 40, 168, 171, 1975.

43. **Alvarez, L. C., Dimas, C. O., Castro, A., Rossman, L. G., Vanderlaan, E. F., and Vanderlaan, W. P.**, Growth hormone in malnutrition, *J. Clin. Endocrinol. Metab.*, 34, 400—409, 1972.

44. **Smith, S. R., Edgar, P. J., Pozefsky, T., Chhetri, M. K., and Prout, T. E.**, Growth hormone in adults with protein-calorie malnutrition, *J. Clin. Endocrinol. Metab.*, 39, 53—62, 1974.

45. **Grant, D. B., Hambley, J., Becker, D. J. and Pimstone, B. L.**, Reduced sulphation factor in undernourished children, *Arch. Dis. Child.*, 48, 596—600, 1973.

46. **Van Den Brande, J. L., Van Buul, S., Heinrich, U., Van Roon, F., Zurcher, T., and Van Steirtegem, A. C.**, Further observations on plasma somatomedin activity in children, *Adv. Metab. Disord.*, 8, 171—181, 1975.

47. **Becker, D. J., Pimstone, B. L., Hansen, J. D. L., and Hendricks, S.**, Serum albumen and growth hormone relationships in kwashiorkor and the nephrotic syndrome, *J. Lab. Clin. Med.*, 78, 865—871, 1971.

48. **Samuel, A. M. and Deshpande, U.R.**, Growth hormone levels in protein calorie malnutrition, *J. Clin. Endocrinol. Metab.*, 35, 863—867, 1972.

49. **Parra, A., Serrano, P., Chávez, G., Garcia, G., Argote, R. M., Klish, W., Cuellar, A., and Nichols, B. L.**, Studies on daily urinary catecholamine excretion in kwashiorkor as observed in Mexico, in *Endocrine Aspects of Malnutrition*, Gardner, L. I. and Ambacher, P., Eds., Kroc Foundation, Santa Ynez, Cal., 1973, 181—190.

50. **Rao, K. S. J.**, Evolution of kwashiorkor and marasmus, *Lancet*, 1, 709—711, 1974.

51. **Lippe, B. M., Van Herle, A. J., Lafranchi, S. H., Uller, R. P., Lavin, N., and Kaplan, S. A.**, Reversible hypothyroidism in growth hormone-deficient children treated with human growth hormone, *J. Clin. Endocrinol. Metab.*, 40, 612—618, 1975.

52. **Pimstone, B. L., Barbezat, G., Hansen, J. D. L., and Murray, P.**, Studies on growth hormone secretion in protein-calorie malnutrition, *Am. J. Clin. Nutr.*, 21, 482—487, 1968.

53. **Pimstone, B. L., Wittman, W., Hansen, J. D. L., and Murray, P.**, Growth hormone and kwashiorkor. Role of protein in growth hormone homoeostasis, *Lancet*, 2, 779—780, 1966.

54. Pimstone, B. L., Becker, D. J., and Hansen, J. D. L., Human growth hormone and sulphation factor in protein-calorie malnutrition, in *Endocrine Aspects of Malnutrition,* Gardner, L. I. and Ambacher, P., Eds., Kroc Foundation, Santa Ynez, Cal., 1973, 73—90.

55. Pimstone, B. L., Barbezat, G., Hansen, J. D. L., and Murray, P., Growth hormone and protein-calorie malnutrition. Impaired supression during induced hyperglycaemia, *Lancet,* 2, 1333—1334, 1967.

56. Van Der Westhuysen, J. M., Jones, J. J., Van Niekerk, C. H., and Belonje, P. C., Cortisol and growth hormone in kwashiorkor and marasmus, *S. Afr. Med. J.,* 49, 1642—1644, 1975.

57. Olusi, S. O., Orrell, D. H., Morris, P. M., and McFarlane, H., A study of endocrine function in protein-energy malnutrition, *Clin. Chim. Acta,* 74, 261—269, 1977.

58. Raghuramalu, N., and Rao, K. S. J., Growth hormone secretion in protein-calorie malnutrition, *J. Clin. Endocrinol.,* 38, 176—180, 1974.

59. Beas, F., Contreras, I., Maccioni, A., and Arenas, S., Growth hormone in infant malnutrition: the arginine test in marasmus and kwashiorkor, *Br. J. Nutr.,* 26, 169—175, 1971.

60. Beas, F. and Muzzo, S., Growth hormone and malnutrition: the Chilean experience, in *Endocrine Aspects of Malnutrition,* Gardner, L. I. and Ambacher, P., Eds., Kroc Foundation, Santa Ynez, Cal., 1973, 1—18.

61. Beas, F., Contreras, I., Maccioni, A., and Arenas, S., Plasma growth hormone levels in severe infant malnutrition in Chile, *J. Pediatr.,* 77, 721, 1970.

62. Godard, C., Plasma growth hormone levels in severe infantile malnutrition in Bolivia, in *Endocrine Aspects of Malnutrition,* Gardner, L. I. and Ambacher, P., Eds., Kroc Foundation, Santa Ynez, Cal., 1973, 19—30.

63. Suskind, R., Amatayakul, K., Leitzmann, C., and Olson, R. E., Interrelationships between growth hormone and amino acid metabolism in protein-calorie malnutrition, in *Endocrine Aspects of Malnutrition,* Gardner, L. I. and Ambacher, P., Eds., Kroc Foundation, Santa Ynez, Cal., 1973, 99—113.

64. Powell, G. F., Brasel, J. A., Raiti, S., and Blizzard, R. M., Emotional deprivation and growth retardation simulating nypopituitrism. II. Endocrinological evaluation of the syndrome, *New Engl. J. Med.,* 276, 1279—1283, 1967.

65. Alleyne, G. A. O. and Young, V. H., Adrenocortical function in children with severe protein-calorie malnutrition, *Clin. Sci.,* 33, 189—200, 1967.

66. Cooke, J. N. C., James, V. H. T., Landon, J., and Wynn, V., Adrenocortical function in chronic malnutrition, *Br. Med. J.,* 1, 662—666, 1964.

67. Abbassy, A. S., Mikhail, M., Zeitoun, M. M., and Ragab, M., The suprarenal cortical function as measured by the plasma 17-hydroxycorticosteroid level in malnourished children, *J. Trop. Pediatr.,* 13, 87—95, 1967.

68. Samuel, A. M., Kadival, G. V., Patel, B. D., and Desai, A. G., Adrenocorticosteroids and corticosteroid binding globulins in protein-calorie malnutrition, *Am. J. Clin. Nutr.,* 29, 889—894, 1976.

69. Paisey, R. B., Angers, M., and Frenk, S., Plasma cortisol levels in malnourished children with and without superimposed acute stress, *Arch. Dis. Child.,* 48, 714—716, 1973.

70. Leonard, P. J., Cortisol binding in serum in kwashiorkor: East African studies, in *Endocrine Aspects of Malnutrition,* Gardner, L. I. and Ambacher, P., Eds., Kroc Foundation, Santa Ynez, Cal., 1973, 355—362.

71. Schonland, M. M., Shanley, B. C., Loening, W. E. K., Parent, M. A., and Coovadia, H. M., Plasma-cortisol and immunosuppression in protein-calorie malnutrition, *Lancet,* 2, 435—436, 1972.

72. Waterlow, J. C., Observations on the mechanism of adaptation to low protein intakes, *Lancet,* 2, 1091—1097, 1968.

73. Lunn, P. G., Whitehead, R. G., Baker, B. A., and Austin, S., The effect of cortisone on the course of development of experimental protein-energy malnutrition in rats, *Br. J. Nutr.,* 36, 537—550.

74. Frenk, S., Gómez, F., Ramos-Galván, F., and Cravioto, J., Fatty liver in children — kwashiorkor, *Am. J. Clin. Nutr.,* 6, 298—309, 1958.

75. Coward, W. A., Serum colloidal osmotic pressure in the development of kwashiorkor and its recovery: its relationship to albumin and globulin concentrations and oedema, *Br. J. Nutr.,* 34, 459—467, 1975.

76. Heard, C. R. C., Frangi, S. M., Wright, P. M., and McCartney. P. R., Biochemical characteristics of different forms of protein-energy malnutrition: an experimental model using young rats, *Br. J. Nutr.,* 37, 1—21, 1977.

77. Anthony, L. E. and Edozien, J. C., Experimental protein and energy deficiencies in the rat, *J. Nutr.,* 105, 631—648, 1975.

78. Naismith, D. J., Kwashiorkor in western Nigeria: a study of traditional weaning foods, with particular reference to energy and linoleic acid, *Br. J. Nutr.,* 30, 567—576, 1973.

79. **Prinsloo, J. G., Freier, E., Kruger, H., Laubscher, N. F., and Roode, H.,** Integrity of the hypothalamico-pituitary-adrenal axis in kwashiorkor as tested with Piromen, *S. Afr. Med. J.,* 48, 2303—2305, 1974.

80. **Abbassy, A. S., Mikhail, M., Zeitoun, M. M., and Ragab, M.,** The suprarenal cortical function as measured by plasma 17-hydroxycorticosteroid level in malnourished children. II. In kwashiorkor, *J. Trop. Pediatr.,* 13, 154—162, 1967.

81. **Rao, K. S. J., Srikantia, S. G., and Gopalan, C.,** Plasma cortisol levels in protein-calorie malnutrition, *Arch. Dis. Child.,* 43, 365—367, 1968.

82. **Beitins, I. A., Kowarski, A., Migeon, C. J., and Graham, G. G.,** Adrenal function in normal infants and in marasmus and kwashiorkor, *J. Pediatr.,* 86, 302—308, 1975.

83. **Lurie, A. O. and Jackson, W. P. U.,** Adrenal function in kwashiorkor and marasmus, *Clin. Sci.,* 22, 259—268, 1962.

84. **Castellanos, H. and Arroyave, G.,** Role of the adrenal cortical system in the response of children to severe protein malnutrition, *Am. J. Clin. Nutr.,* 9, 186—195, 1961.

85. **Ramachandran, M., Venkatachalam, P. S., and Gopalan, C.,** Urinary excretion of 17-ketosteroids in normal and undernourished subjects, *Indian J. Med. Res.,* 44, 227—230, 1956.

86. **Beas, F., Ferreira, E., and Rivarola, M.,** Adrenal cortical function in infants with malnutrition, as seen in Chile, in *Endocrine Aspects of Malnutrition,* Gardner, L. I. and Ambacher, P., Eds., Kroc Foundation, Santa Ynez, Cal., 1973, 343—353.

87. **Spada, E., Rivarola, M. A., and Beas, F.,** Plasma cortisol levels in infants with protein-calorie malnutrition, *J. Pediatr.,* 78, 899, 1971.

88. **Alleyne, G. A. O. and Young, V. H.,** Adrenal function in malnutrition, *Lancet,* 1, 911—912, 1966.

89. **Misbin, R. I., Edgar, P. J., and Lockwood, D. H.,** Adrenergic regulation of insulin secretion during fasting in normal subjects, *Diabetes,* 19, 688—693, 1970.

90. **Hoeldtke, R. D. and Wurtman, R. J.,** Excretion of catecholamines and catecholamine metabolites in kwashiorkor, *Am. J. Clin. Nutr.,* 26, 205—219, 1973.

91. **Bourgeois, B., Schmidt, B. J., and Bourgeois, R.,** Some aspects of catecholamines in undernutrition, in *Endocrine Aspects of Malnutrition,* Gardner, L. I. and Ambacher, P., Eds., Kroc Foundation, Santa Ynez, Cal., 1973, 163—179.

92. **Rao, K. S. J.,** Kwashiorkor and marasmus. Blood sugar levels and response to epinephrine, *Am. J. Dis. Child.,* 110, 519—522, 1965.

93. **Graham, G. G. and Placko, R. P.,** Free catecholamine excretion in the urine in normal infants and in those with marasmus or kwashiorkor, *J. Pediatr.,* 86, 965—969, 1975.

94. **Pimstone, B. L., Becker, D. J., and Hendricks, S.,** TSH response to synthetic thyrotropin-releasing hormone in human protein-calorie malnutrition, *J. Clin. Edocrinol.,* Metab., 36, 779—783, 1973.

95. **Pimstone, B. L., Becker, D. J., and Hendricks, S.,** TSH response to synthetic TRH in human protein-calorie malnutrition, in *Endocrine Aspects of Malnutrition,* Gardner, L. I. and Ambacher, P., Eds., Kroc Foundation, Santa Ynez, Cal., 1973, 243—255.

96. **El-Gholmy A., Ghaleb, H., Khalifa, A. S., Senna, A., and El-Akkad, S.,** Studies on thyroid function in malnourished infants and children in Egypt, *J. Trop. Med.,* 70, 74—80, 1967.

97. **Rao, K. S. J., Raghuramalu, N., and Srikantia, S. G.,** Thyroid function in kwashiorkor, *Indian J. Med. Res.,* 59, 1300—1304, 1971.

98. **Papazian, R. L., Iorcansky, S., and Bergada, C.,** Thyroid function in malnourished children, *J. Pediatr.,* 78, 900, 1971.

99. **Godard, C.,** Plasma thyrotropin levels in severe infantile malnutrition, in *Endocrine Aspects of Malnutrition,* Gardner, L. I. and Ambacher, P., Eds., Kroc Foundation, Santa Ynez, Cal., 1973, 221—227.

100. **Van Der Westhuysen, J. M.,** Thyroid function in protein-energy malnutrition, *Cent. Afr. J. Med.,* 22, 68—71, 1976.

101. **Graham, G. G., Baertl, J. M., Claeyssen, G., Suskind, R., Greensberg, A. H., Thompson, R. G., and Blizzard, R. M.,** Thyroid hormone studies in normal and severely malnourished infants and small children, *J. Pediatr.,* 83, 321—331, 1973.

102. **Parra, A., Klish, W., Garza, C., Argote, R. M., Garciá, G., Rodriguez, R., Cuellar, A., Canseco, L., and Nichols, B. L.,** Thyroid hormones and energy metabolism in marasmus and kwashiorkor as seen in Mexico, in *Endocrine Aspects of Malnutrition,* Gardner, L. I. and Ambacher, P., Eds., Kroc Foundation, Santa Ynez, Cal., 1973, 229—242.

103. **Rao, K. S. J. and Khan, L.,** Basal energy metabolism in malnourished children of India, in *Endocrine Aspects of Malnutrition,* Gardner, L. I. and Ambacher, P., Eds., Kroc Foundation, Santa Ynez, Cal., 1973, 307—311.

104. **Ingenbleek, Y., De Nayer, P., and De Visscher, M.,** Thyroxine binding globulin in infant protein-calorie malnutrition, *J. Clin. Endocrinol. Metab.,* 39, 178—180, 1974.

105. **Ingenbleek, Y. and Beckers, C.,** Triiodothyronine and thyroid-stimulating hormone in protein-calorie malnutrition in infants, *Lancet,* 2, 845—848, 1975.

106. Harland, P. S. E. G. and Parkin, J. M., T.S.H. levels in severe malnutrition, *Lancet,* 2, 1145, 1972.

107. Graham, G. G. and Blizzard, R. M., Thyroid hormone studies in severely malnourished Peruvian infants and small children, in *Endocrine Aspects of Malnutrition,* Gardner, L. I. and Ambacher, P., Eds., Kroc Foundation, Santa Ynez, Cal., 1973, 205—219.

108. Beas, F., Monckeberg, F., Horwitz, I., and Figuero, M., The response of the thyroid gland to thyroid-stimulating hormone (TSH) in infants with malnutrition, *Pediatrics,* 38, 1003—1008, 1966.

109. Smith, S. R., Chhetri, M. K., Johanson, A. J., Radfar, N., and Migeon, C. J., The pituitary-gonadal axis in men with protein-calorie malnutrition, *J. Clin. Endocrinol. Metab.,* 41, 60—69, 1975.

110. Van Der Westhuysen, J. M., Kanengoni, E., Mbizvo, M., and Jones, J. J., The effect of protein energy malnutrition on plasma renin and oedema in the pig, *S. Afr. Med. J.,* 51, 18—20, 1977.

111. Van Der Westhuysen, J. M., Jones, J. J., and Van Niekerk, C. H., Plasma renin activity, water excretion and the decay of injected hormones and hormonal effects in rats with protein energy malnutrition, *S. Afr. Med. J.,* 49, 1799—1803, 1975.

112. Warton, C. M. R., and Jones, J. J., Plasma renin activity in rats fed exclusively on maize (mealie) meal, *S. Afr. Med. J.,* 47, 1498—1500, 1973.

113. Fitzsimons, J. T. and Simons, B. J., The effect on drinking in the rat of intravenous infusion of angiotensin, given alone or in combination with other stimuli of thirst, *J. Physiol.,* 203, 45—57, 1969.

114. De Bono, E., Lee, G. de J., Mottram, F. R., Pickering, G. W., Brown, J. J., Keen, H., Peart, W. S., and Sanderson, P. H., The action of angiotensin in man, *Clin. Sci.,* 25, 123—257, 1963.

115. Mulrow, P. J., Ganong, W. F., Cera, G., and Kuljian, A., The nature of the aldosterone-stimulating factor in dog kidneys, *J. Clin. Invest.,* 41, 505—518, 1962.

116. Bonjour, J. P. and Malvin, R. L., Stimulation of ADH release by the renin-angiotensin system, *Am. J. Physiol.,* 218, 1555—1559, 1970.

117. Schnieden, H., Hendrickse, R. G., and Haigh, C. P., Studies in water metabolism in clinical and experimental malnutrition, *Trans. R. Soc. Trop. Med. Hyg.,* 52, 169—175, 1958.

118. Alleyne, G. A. O., The excretion of water and solute by malnourished children, *West Indian Med. J.,* 15, 150—154, 1966.

119. Srikantia, S. G. and Gopalan, C., Role of ferritin in nutritional edema, *J. Appl. Physiol.,* 14, 829—833, 1959.

120. Heller, H. and Dicker, S. E., Some renal effects of experimental dietary deficiencies, *Proc. R. Soc. Med.,* 40, 351—353, 1946.

121. Thurau, K. W. C., Dahlheim, H., Grünner, A., Mason, J., and Granger, P., Activation of renin in the single juntaglomerular apparatus by sodium chloride in the tubular fluid at the macula densa, *Cir. Res. Suppl.,* 31(2), 182—186, 1972.

122. Bell, N. H., Schedl, H. P., and Bartter, F. C., An explanation for abnormal water retention and hypoosmolality in congestive heart failure, *Am. J. Med.,* 36, 351—360, 1964.

123. Schedl, H. P. and Bartter F. C., An explanation for and experimental correction of the abnormal water diuresis in cirrhosis, *J. Clin. Invest.,* 39, 248—261, 1960.

124. Farber, M. O., Bright, T. P., Strawbridge, R. A., Robertson, G. L., and Manfredi, F., Impaired water handling in chronic obstructive lung disease, *J. Lab. Clin. Med.,* 85, 41—49, 1975.

125. Goodyer, A. V. N. and Jaeger, C. A., Renal response to nonshocking hemorrhage: role of the autonomic nervous system and of the renal circulation, *Am. J. Physiol.,* 180, 69—74, 1955.

126. Shnermann, J., Ploth, D. W., and Dahlheim, H., Interrelationship between autoregulation of glomerular filtration rate, tubulo-glomerular feedback and juxtaglomerular renin activity in normotensive and hypertensive rats, *Clin. Sci.,* 51(Suppl. 3), 105 S—107 S, 1976.

127. Abe, Y., Okahara, T., Kishimoto, T., Yamamoto, K., and Veda, J., Relationship between intrarenal distribution of blood flow and renin secretion, *Am. J. Physiol.,* 225, 319—323, 1973.

128. Itskovitz, H. D. and McGiff, J. C., Hormonal regulation of the renal circulation, *Cir. Res. Suppl.,* 34(1), 65—73, 1974.

129. Wilkinson, S. P., Smith, I. K., Clarke, M., Arroyo, V., Richardson, J., Moodie, H., and Williams, R., Intrarenal distribution of plasma flow in cirrhosis as measured by transit renography: relationship with plasma renin activity, and sodium and water excretion, *Clin. Sci.,* 52, 469—475, 1977.

130. Smith, R., Total body water in malnourished infants, *Clin. Sci.,* 19, 275—285, 1960.

131. Brinkman, G. L., Body water studies in malnutrition, *S. Afr. Med. J.,* 58, 527—573, 1964.

132. Kerpel-Fronius, F., Volume and composition of the body fluid compartments in severe infantile malnutrition, *J. Pediatr.,* 56, 826—833, 1960.

133. Alleyne, G. A. O., Studies on total body potassium in infantile malnutrition: the relation to body fluid spaces and urinary creatinine, *Clin. Sci.,* 34, 199—209, 1968.

134. Garrow, J. S., Smith, R., and Ward, E. E., *Electrolyte Metabolism in Severe Infantile Malnutrition,* Pergamon Press, London, 1968.

135. Jackman, A., in preparation, 1978.

136. **Alleyne, G. A. O.**, Cardiac function in severely malnourished Jamaican children, *Clin. Sci.*, 30, 553—562, 1966.

137. **Frenk, S., Metcoff, J., Gómez, F., Ramos-Galván, R., Cravioto, J., and Antonowicz, I.**, Intracellular composition and homeostatic mechanisms in severe chronic infantile malnutrition. II. Composition of tissues, *Pediatrics,* 20, 105—120, 1957.

138. **Patrick, J.**, Death during recovery from severe malnutrition and its possible relationship to sodium pump activity in the leucocyte, *Br. Med. J.,* 1, 1051—1054, 1977.

139. **Viart, P.**, Hemodynamic findings in severe protein-calorie malnutrition, *Am. J. Clin. Nutr.,* 30, 334—348, 1977.

140. **Viart, P.**, Blood volume changes during treatment of protein-calorie malnutrition, *Am. J. Clin. Nutr.,* 30, 349—354, 1977.

141. **Levin, K.**, The stimulating effect of angiotensin and vasopressin on adenosine triphosphatase activity in vitro, *Acta Physiol. Scand.,* 79, 37—49, 1970.

142. **Haljamäe, H., Enger, E., and Sigström, L.**, Cellular potassium transport and ATPase activity in Bartter's syndrome, *Scand. J. Clin. Lab. Invest.,* 35, 53—58, 1975.

143. **Van Der Westhuysen, J. M., Kanengoni, E., Jones, J. J., and Van Niekerk, C. H.**, Plasma renin activity in oedematous and marasmic children with protein-energy malnutrition, *S. Afr. Med. J.,* 49, 1729—1731, 1975.

144. **Holdsworth, S., McLean, A., Morris, B. J., Dax, E., and Johnston, C. I.**, Renin release from isolated rat glomeruli, *Clin. Sci.,* 51(Suppl. 3), 97 S-99 S, 1976.

145. **Brunner, H. R., Baer, L., Sealey, J. E., Ledingham, J. G. G., and Laragh, J. M.**, Influence of potassium administration and of potassium deprivation on plasma renin in normal and hypertensive subjects, *J. Clin. Invest.,* 49, 2128—2138, 1970.

146. **Himathongkam, T., Dluhy, R. G., and Williams, G. H.**, Potassium-aldosterone-renin interrelationships, *J. Clin. Endocrinol. Metab.,* 41, 153—159, 1975.

147. **Smith, R.**, Hyponatraemia in infantile malnutrition, *Lancet,* 1, 771, 1963.

148. **Lennon, E. J. and Lemann, J.**, The effect of potassium-deficient diet on the pattern of recovery from experimental metabolic acidosis, *Clin. Sci.,* 34, 365—378, 1968.

149. **Kritzinger, E. E., Kanengoni, E., and Jones, J. J.**, Plasma renin activity in children with protein-energy malnutrition (kwashiorkor), *S. Afr. Med. J.,* 48, 499—501, 1974.

150. **Leonard, P. J. and MacWilliam, K. M.**, The binding aldosterone in the serum in kwashiorkor, *Am. J. Clin. Nutr.,* 16, 360—362,1965.

151. **Beitins, I. Z., Graham G. G., Kowarski, A., and Migeon, C. J.**, Adrenal function in normal in normal infants and in marasmus and kwashiorkor: plasma aldosterone concentration and secretion rate, *J. Pediatr.,* 84, 444—451, 1974.

152. **Nigeon, C. J., Beitins, I. Z., Kowarski A., and Graham, G. G.**, Plasma aldosterone concentration and aldosterone secretion rate in Peruvian infants with marasmus and kwashiorkor, in *Endocrine Aspects of Malnutrition,* Gardner, L. I. and Ambacher, P., Eds., Kroc Foundation, Santa Ynez, Calif. , 1973, 399—424.

153. **Lurie, A. O. and Jackson, W. P. U.**, Aldosteronuria and the edema of kwashiorkor, *Am. J. Clin. Nutr.,* 11, 115—126, 1962.

154. **Srikantia, S. G. and Mohanram, M.**, Antidiuretic hormone values in plasma and urine of malnourished children, *J. Clin. Endocrinol. Metab.,* 31, 312—314, 1970.

155. **Cahill, G. F.**, Starvation in man, *N. Engl. J. Med.,* 282, 668—675, 1970.

156. **Adibi, S. A., Drash, A. L., and Livi, E. D.**, Hormone and amino acid levels in altered nutritional states, *J. Lab. Clin. Med.,* 76, 722—732, 1970.

157. **Cahill, G. F., Herrera, M. G., Morgan, A. P., Soeldner, J. S., Steinke, J., Levy, P. L., Reichard, G. A., and Kipnis, D. M.**, Hormone-fuel interrelationships during fasting, *J. Clin. Invest.,* 45, 1751—1769, 1966.

158. **Anguilar-Parada, E., Eisentraut, A. M., and Unger, R. H.**, Effects of starvation on plasma pancreatic glucagon in normal man, *Diabetes,* 18k, 717—723, 1969.

159. **Unger, R. H., Eisentraut, M., Madison, L. L., Sims, K. R., and Whissen, N.,** The effects of total starvation upon the levels of circulating glucagon and insulin in man, *J. Clin. Invest.,* 42, 1031—1039, 1963.

160. **Solomons, S. S., Ensinck, J. W., and Williams, R. H.**, Effect of starvation on plasma immunoreactive insulin and non-suppresible insulin-like activity in normal and obese humans, *Metab. Clin. Exp.,* 17, 528—534, 1968.

161. **Merimee, T. J. and Fineberg, S. E.**, Homeostasis during fasting. II. Hormone substrate difference between men and women, *J. Clin. Endocrinol. Metab.,* 37, 698—702, 1973.

162. **Wise, J. K., Hendler, R., and Felig, P.**, Evaluation of alpha-cell function by infusion of alanine in normal, diabetic, and obese subjects, *N. Engl. J. Med.,* 228, 487—490, 1973.

163. **Merimee, T. J., Felig, P., Marliss, E., Fineberg, S. E., and Cahill, G. C.**, Glucose and lipid homeostasis in the absence of human growth hormone, *J. Clin. Invest.,* 50, 574—582, 1971.

164. Vinik, A. I., Kalk, W. J., McLaren, H., Hendricks, S., and Pimstone, B. L., Fasting blunts the TSH response to synthetic thyrotropin-releasing hormone (TRH), *J. Clin. Endocrinol. Metab.*, 40, 509—511, 1975.

165. Merimee, T. J. and Tyson, J. E., Hypoglycemia in man. Pathologic and physiologic variants, *Diabetes*, 26, 161—165, 1977.

166. Tyson, T. E., Austin, K., Farinholt, J., and Fiedler, J., Endocrine-metabolic response to acute starvation in human gestation, *Am. J. Obstet. Gynecol.*, 125, 1073—1084, 1976.

167. Chaussain, J. L., Georges, P., Olive, G., and Job, J. C., Glycemic response to 24-hour fast in normal children and children with ketatic hypoglycemia. II. Hormonal and metabolic changes, *J. Pediatr.*, 85, 776—781, 1974.

168. Fink, G., Gutman, R. A., Cresto, J. C., Selawry, H., Lavine, R., and Recant, L., Glucose-induced insulin release patterns: effect of starvation, *Diabetologia*, 10, 421—425, 1974.

169. Walter, R. M., Dudl, R. J., Palmer, J. P., and Ensinck, J. W., The effect of adrenergic blockade on the glucagon responses to starvation and hypoglycemia in man, *J. Clin. Invest.*, 54, 1214—1220, 1974.

170. Vance, J. E., Buchanan, K. D., and Williams, R. H., Effect of starvation and refeeding on serum immunoreactive glucagon and insulin levels, *J. Lab. Clin. Med.*, 72, 290—297, 1968.

171. Tiengo, A., Assan, R., and Tchobroutsky, G., Metabolic and hormonal patterns after three days of total fasting in 27 obese and nonobese subjects, *Isr. J. Med. Sci.*, 8, 821—823, 1972.

172. Beck, P., Koumans, J. H. T., Winterling, C. A., Stein, M. F., Daughaday, W. H., and Kipnis, D. M., Studies of insulin and growth hormone scretion in human obesity, *J. Lab. Clin. Med.*, 64, 654—667, 1964.

173. Kalkhoff, R. K., Gossain, V. V., and Matute, M. L., Plasma glucagon in obesity. Response to arginine, glucose and protein administration, *N. Engl. J. Med.*, 289, 465—467, 1973.

174. Kalkhoff, R. K., Kim, H. J., Cerletty, J., and Ferrou, C. A., Metabolic effects of weight loss in obese subjects. Changes in plasma substrate levels, insulin, and growth hormone responses, *Diabetes*, 20, 83—91, 1971.

175. Bagdade, J. D., Porte, D., Brunzell, J. D., and Bierman, E. L., Basal and stimulated hyperinsulinism: reversible metabolic sequelae of obesity, *J. Lab. Clin. Med.*, 83, 563—569, 1974.

176. Anderson, J. W., Herman, R. H., and Newcomer, K. L., Improvement in glucose tolerance of fasting obese patients given oral potassium, *Am. J. Clin. Nutr.*, 22, 1589—1596, 1969.

177. Owen, D. E., Felig, P., Morgan, A. P., Wahren, J., and Cahill, G. F., Liver and kidney metabolism during prolonged starvation, *J. Clin. Invest.*, 48, 574—583, 1969.

178. Marliss, E. B., Aoki, T. T., Unger, R. H., Soeldner, J. S., and Cahill, G. F., Glucagon levels and metabolic effects in fasting man, *J. Clin. Invest.*, 49, 2256—2270, 1970.

179. Hoffman, R. S., Martino, J. A., Wahl, G., and Arky, R. A., Fasting and refeeding III. Antinatriuretic effect of oral and intravenous carbohydrate and its relationship to potassium excretion, *Metab. Clin. Exp.*, 20, 1065—1073, 1971.

180. Muller, W. A., Aoki, T. T., and Cahill, G. F., Effect of alanine and glycine on glucagon secretion in postabsorptive and fasting obese men, *J. Clin. Endocrinol. Metab.*, 40, 418—425, 1972.

181. Floyd, J. C., Pek, S., Fajans, S. S., Schteingart, D. E., and Conn, J. W., Effect upon plasma glucagon of severe and prolonged restriction of food intake in obese and nonobese subjects, *Diabetes*, 21(Suppl. 1), 331—332, 1972.

182. Hewing, R., Liebermeister H., Daweke, H., Gries, F. A., and Gruneklee, D., Weight regain after low calorie diet, long term pattern of blood sugar, serum lipids, ketone bodies and serum insulin levels, *Diabetologia*, 9, 197—202, 1973.

183. Genuth, S. M., Metabolic clearance of insulin in man, *Diabetes*, 21, 1003—1012, 1972.

184. Apfelbaum, M., Reinberg, A., Assan, R., and Lacatis, D., Hormonal and metabolic circadian rhythms before and during a low protein diet, *Isr. J. Med. Sci.*, 8, 867—873, 1972.

185. Bell, J. P., Donald, R. A., and Espiner, E. A., Effects of fasting on insulin secretion and glucose tolerance in obesity, *N. Z. Med. J.*, 74, 306—309, 1971.

186. El-Khodary, A. Z., Ball, M. F., Oweiss, I. M., and Canary, J. J., Insulin secretion and body composition in obesity *Metab. Clin. Exp.*, 21, 641—655, 1972.

187. Kosaka, K., Hagura, R., Odagiri, R., Saito, F., and Kuzuya, T., Effect of weight changes on serum insulin response in subjects with normal and glucose tolerance, *J. Clin. Endocrinol. Metab.*, 35, 655— 658, 1972.

188. Olefsky, J., Reaven, G. M., and Farquhar, J. W., Effect of weight reduction on obesity. Studies of lipid and carbohydrate metabolism in normal and hyperlipoproteinemic subjects, *J. Clin. Invest.*, 53, 64—76, 1974.

189. Jackson, I. M. D., McKiddie, M. T., and Buchanan, K. D., Effect of fasting on glucose and insulin metabolism of obese patients, *Lancet*, 1, 285—287, 1969.

190. Arky, R. A., Finger, M., Veverbrants, E., and Braun, A. P., Glucose and insulin response to intravenous glucagon during starvation, *Am. J. Clin. Nutr.*, 23, 691—695, 1970.

191. Millward, D. J., Nnanyelugo, D. O., James, W. P. T., and Garlick, P. J., Protein metabolism in skeletal muscle: the effect of feeding and fasting on muscle RNA, free amino acids, and plasma insulin concentrations, *Br. J. Nutr.*, 32, 127—142, 1974.

192. Weinkove, C., Weinkove, E. A., and Pimstone, B. L., Glucose tolerance and insulin release in malnourished rats, *Clin. Sci.*, 50, 153—163, 1972.

193. Bosboom, R. S., Zweens, J., and Bouman, P. R., Effects of feeding and fasting on the insulin secretory response to glucose and sulfonylureas in intact rats and isolated perfused rat pancreas, *Diabetologia*, 9, 243—250, 1973.

194. Cuendet, G. S., Loten, E. G., Cameron, D. P., Renold, A. E., and Marliss, E. B., Hormone-substrate response to total fasting in lean and obese mice, *Am. J. Physiol.*, 228, 276—283, 1975.

195. Feldman, J. M. and Lebovitz, H. E., Effect of fasting on insulin secretion and action in mice, *Endocrinology*, 86, 313—321, 1970.

196. Heard, C. R. C. and Turner, M. R., Glucose tolerance and related factor in dogs fed diets of suboptimal protein value, *Diabetes*, 16, 96—107, 1967.

197. Buckman, M. T., Conway, M. J., Seibel, J. A., and Eaton, R. P., Effect of fasting on alanine-stimulated insulin and glucagon secretion, *Metab. Clin. Exp.*, 22, 1253—1262, 1973.

198. Anderson, D. M., The effect of fasting and glucose load on insulin secretion and the Staub-Trangott phenomenon in pigs, *J. Endocrinol.*, 58, 613—125, 1973.

199. Allen, K. A., Ayres, C. E., Munday, K. A., and Turner, M. R., Effect of protein deficiency on glucagon-stimulated insulin secretion, and on glycogen storage and release in rabbits, *Proc. Nutr. Soc.*, 34, 96A—97A, 1972.

200. Turner, M. R., Allen, K. A., and Munday, K. A., Effects of age and diet on the secretion of insulin and growth hormone in rabbits, *Proc. Nutr. Soc.*, 33, 56A—57A, 1974.

201. Turner, M. R., Allen, K. A., and Munday, K. A., Insulin and growth hormone secretion in the newborn offspring of rabbits fed from mating on high-protein or low-protein diets, *Proc. Nutr. Soc.*, 33, 38A-39A, 1974.

202. Bassett, J. M. and Madill, D., The influence of maternal nutrition on plasma hormone and metabolic concentration of foetal lambs, *J. Endocrinol.*, 61, 465—477, 1974.

203. Gerich, J. E., Control of pancreatic IRG secretion in vivo — review, *Metab. Clin. Exp.*, 25, 1437—1441, 1976.

204. Gerich, J. E., Langlois, M., and Noacco, C., Glucagon secretion in obesity, *Lancet*, 1, 1323, 1973.

205. Kabardi, V. M., Eisenstein, A. B., and Strack, I., Decreased plasma insulin but normal glucagon in rats fed low protein diets, *J. Nutr.*, 106, 1247—1253, 1976.

206. Seitz, H. J., Kaiser, M., Krone, W., and Tarnowski, W., Physiologic significance of glucocorticoids and insulin in the regulation of hepatic gluconeogensis during starvation in rats, *Metab. Clin. Exp.*, 25, 1545—1555, 1976.

207. Lavine, R. L., Voyles, N., Perrino, P. V., and Recant, L., The effect of fasting on tissue cyclic cAMP and plasma glucagon in the obese hyperglycemic mouse, *Endocrinology*, 97, 615—620, 1975.

208. Merimee, T. J. and Fineberg, S. E., Growth hormone secretion in starvation: a reassessment, *J. Clin. Endocrinol. Metab.*, 39, 385—386, 1974.

209. Roth, J., Glick, S. M., Yalow, R. S., and Berson, S. A., Hypoglycemia: a potent stimulus to secretion of growth hormone, *Science*, 140, 987—988, 1963.

210. Merimee, T. J., Pulkkinen, A. J., and Burton, C. E., Diet-induced alterations of hGH secretion in man, *J. Clin. Endocrinol. Metab.*, 42, 931—937, 1976.

211. Tyson, J. E., Austin, K. L., and Farinholt, J. W., Prolonged nutritional deprivation in pregnancy: changes in human chorionic somatomammotropin and growth hormone secretion, *Am. J. Obstet. Gynecol.*, 105, 1080—1082, 1971.

212. London, J. H., Gallagher, T. F., and Bray, G. A., Effect of weight reduction, triiodothyronine, and diethylstilbestrol on growth hormone in obesity, *Metab. Clin. Exp.*, 18, 986—992, 1969.

213. Bell, J. P., Donald, R. A., and Espiner, E. A., Pituitary response to insulin-induced hypoglycemia in obese subjects before and after fasting, *J. Clin. Endocrinol. Metab.*, 31, 546—551, 1970.

214. Ball, M. F., El-Khodary, A. Z., and Canary, J. J., Growth hormone response in the thinned obese, *J. Clin. Endocrinol., Metab.*, 34, 498—511, 1972.

215. El-Khodary, A. Z., Ball, M. F., Stein, B., and Canary, J. J., Effect of weight loss on the growth hormone response to arginine infusion in obesity, *J. Clin. Endocrinol. Metab.*, 32, 42—51, 1971.

216. Trenkle, A., Effect of starvation on pituitary and plasma growth hormone in rats, *Proc. Soc. Exp. Biol. Med.*, 135, 77—80, 1970.

217. Christensson, P., Rerup, C., Seyer-Hansen, K., and Stenram, U., Elevated growth hormone in protein-deficient rats, and decreased liver RNA after hypophysectomy, *Hoppe Seyler's Z. Physiol. Chem.*, 356, 591—597, 1975.

218. Atinmo, T., Baldijao, C., Pond, W. G., and Barnes, R. H., Immunoreactive growth hormone levels in pigs fed protein or energy restricted diets during the preweaning period, *J. Nutr.*, 106, 947—951, 1976.

219. Muller, E. E., Miedico, D., Giustina, G., and Cocchi, D., Ineffectiveness of hypoglycemia, cold exposure and fasting in stimulating GH secretion in the mouse, *Endocrinology*, 88, 345—350, 1971.

220. Kokka, N., Garcia, J. F., Morgan, M., and George, R., Immunoassay of growth hormone in cats following fasting and administration of insulin, arginine, 2-deoxyglucose and hypothalamic extract, *Endocrinology*, 88, 359—366, 1971.

221. Phillips, L. S. and Young, H. S., Nutrition and somatomedin. I. Effect of fasting and refeeding on serum somatomedin activity and cartilage growth activity in rats, *Endocrinology*, 99, 303—314, 1976.

222. Galvão-Teles, A., Graves, L., Burke, C. W., Fotherby, K., and Fraser, R., Free cortisol in obesity: effect of fasting, *Acta Endocrinol. (Copenhagen)*, 81, 321—329, 1976.

223. Schachner, S. H., and Wieland, R. G., Maynard, D. E., Kruger, F. A., and Hamwi, G. J., Alterations in adrenal cortical function in fasting obese subjects, *Metab. Clin. Exp.*, 14, 1051—1058, 1965.

224. Schultz, A. L., Kerlow, A., and Ulstrom, R. A., Effect of starvation on adrenal cortical function in obese subjects, *J. Clin. Endocrinol. Metab.*, 24, 1253—1257, 1964.

225. Hendrikx, A., Heyns, W., and DeMoor, P., Influence of low-calorie diet and fasting on metabolism of dehydroepiandrosterone sulfate in adult obese subjects, *J. Clin. Endocrinol. Metab.*, 28, 1525—1533, 1968.

226. Jackson, I. M. D. and Mowat, J. I., Hypothalamic-pituitary-adrenal function in obesity and the cortisol secretion rate following prolonged starvation, *Acta Endocrinol. (Copenhagen)*, 63, 415—422, 1970.

227. Garces, L. Y., Kenny, F. M., Drash, A., and Taylor, F. H., Cortisol secretion rate during fasting of obese adolescent subjects, *J. Clin. Endocrinol. Metab.*, 28, 1843—1847, 1968.

228. Boulter, P. R., Spark, R. F., and Arky, R. A., Dissociation of the renin-aldosterone system and refractoriness to the sodium-retaining action of mineralocorticoid during starvation in man, *J. Clin. Endocrinol. Metab.*, 38, 248—254, 1974.

229. Baird, I. M., Urinary corticosteroid excretion in obese subjects, *Lancet*, 2, 10222—1026, 1963.

230. Jacobson, G., Seltzer, C. C., Bondy, P. K., and Mayer, J., Importance of body characteristics in the excretion of 17-ketosteroids and 17-ketogenic steroids in obesity, *N. Engl. J. Med.*, 271, 651—656, 1964.

231. Haag, B. L., Reidenberg, M. M., Shuman, C. R., and Channick, B. J., Aldosterone, 17-hydroxycorticosteroid, 17-ketosteroid, and fluid and electrolyte responses to starvation and selective refeeding, *Am. J. Med. Sci.*, 254, 652—658, 1967.

232. Gacs, G., The mechanism of hypoglycemia due to semistarvation in the rat, *J. Nutr.*, 106, 1557—1561, 1976.

233. Adlard, B. P. F. and Smart, J. L., Adrenocortical function in rats subjected to nutritional deprivation in early life, *J. Endocrinol.*, 54, 99—105, 1972.

234. Baldijao, C., Atinmo, T., Pond, W. G., and Barnes, R. H., Plasma adrenocorticosteroid levels in protein and energy restricted pigs, *J. Nutr.*, 106, 952—957, 1976.

235. Bouille, C. and Assenmacher, I., Effects of starvation on adrenal cortical function in the rabbit, *Endocrinology*, 87, 1390—1394, 1970.

236. Heard, C. R. C., Effects of severe protein-calorie deficiency on the endocrine control of carbohydrate metabolism, *Diabetes*, 15, 78—89, 1966.

237. Schatz, D. L., Sheppard, R. H., Palter, H. C., and Jaffri, M. H., Thyroid function studies on fasting obese subjects, *Metab. Clin. Exp.*, 6, 1075—1085, 1967.

238. Portnay, G. I., O'Brian, J. T., Bush, J., Vagenakis, A. G., Azizi, F., Arky, R. A., Ingbar, S. H., and Braverman, L. E., The effect of starvation on the concentration and binding of thyroscine and triiodothyronine in serum and the response to TRH, *J. Clin. Endocrinol. Metab.*, 39, 191—194, 1974.

239. Spaulding, S. W., Choppra, I. J., Sherwin, R. S., and Lyall, S. S., Effect of caloric restriction and diet composition on serum T_3 and reverse T_3 in man, *J. Clin. Endocrinol. Metab.*, 42, 197—200, 1976.

240. Rothenbuchner, G., Loos, U., Kiebling, W. R., Birk, J., and Pfeiffer, E. F., The influence of total starvation on the pituitary-thyroid-axis in obese individuals, *Acta Endocrinol. (Copenhagen) Suppl.*, 173, 144, 1973.

241. Benoit, F. L. and Durrance, F. Y., Radiothyroxine turnover in obesity, *Am. J. Med. Sci.*, 249, 647—653, 1965.

242. Verdy, M., Fasting in obese females. I. A study of thyroid function tests, serum proteins, and electrolytes, *Can. Med. Assoc. J.*, 98, 1031—1933, 1968.

243. Merimee, T. J. and Fineberg, E. S., Starvation-induced alterations of circulating thyroid hormone concentrations in man, *Metab. Clin. Exp.*, 25, 79—83, 1976.

244. Vagenakis, A. G., Burger, A., Portnay, G. I., Rudolph, M., O'Brian, J. T., Azizi, F., Arky, R. A., Nicod, P., Ingbar, S. H., and Braverman, L. E., Diversion of peripheral thyroxine metabolism from activating to inactivating pathways during complete fasting, *J. Clin. Endocrinol. Metab.*, 41, 191—194, 1975.

245. Strebnik, H. H., Evans, E. S., and Rosenberg, L. L., Thyroid function in female rats maintained on a protein-free diet, *Endocrinology*, 73, 267—270, 1963.

246. Shrader, R. E., Ferlatte, M. I., Hastings-Roberts, M. H., Schoenborne, B. M., Hoernicke, C. A., and Zeman, F. J., Thyroid function in prenatally protein-deprived rats, *J. Nutr.*, 107, 221—229, 1977.

247. Singh, D. V., Anderson, R. R., and Turner, C. W., Effect of decreased dietary protein on the rate of thyroid hormone secretion and food consumption in rats, *J. Endocrinol.*, 50, 445—450, 1971.

248. Suryanarayana, B. V., Kent, J. R., Meister, L., and Parlow, A. F., Pituitary-gonadal axis during prolonged total starvation in obese men, *Am. J. Clin. Nutr.*, 22, 767—770, 1969.

249. Nakanishi, Y., Mori, J., and Nagasawa, H., Recover of pituitary secretion of gonadotrophins and prolactin during re-feeding after chronic restricted feeding in female rats, *J. Endocrinol.*, 60, 329—339, 1976.

250. Howland, B. E. and Skinner, K. R., Effect of starvation on gonadotropin secretion in intact and castrated male rats, *Can. J. Physiol. Pharmacol.*, 51, 759—762, 1973.

251. Root, A. W. and Russ, R. D., Short-term effects of castration and starvation upon pituitary and serum levels of luteinizing hormone and follicle stimulating hormone in male rats, *Acta Endocrinol. (Copenhagen)*, 70, 665—675, 1972.

252. Grewal, T., Mickelsen, O., and Hafs, H. D., Androgen secretion and spermatogenesis in rats following semistarvation, *Proc. Soc. Exp. Biol. Med.*, 138, 723—727, 1971.

253. McAtee, J. W. and Trenkle, A., Effects of feeding, fasting, glucose, or arginine on plasma prolactin levels in the bovine, *Endocrinology*, 89, 730—734, 1971.

254. O'Brian, J. T., Savdek, C. D., Spark, R. F., and Arky, R. A., Glucagon induced refractoriness to exogenous mineralocorticoid, *J. Clin. Endocrinol.*, 38, 1147—1149, 1974.

255. Spark, R. F., Arky, R. A., Boulter, P. R., Saudek, C. D., and O'Brian, J. T., Renin, aldosterone and glucgon in the natriuresis of fasting, *N. Engl. J. Med.*, 292, 1335—1340, 1975.

256. Garnett, E. S., Cohen, H., Nahmias, C., and Viol, G., The roles of carbohydrate, renin, and aldosterone in sodium retention during and after total starvation, *Metab. Clin. Exp.*, 22, 867—874, 1973.

257. Chinn, R. H., Brown, J. J., Fraser, R., Heron, S. M., Lever, A. F., Murchison, L., and Roberston, J. I. S., The natriuresis of fasting: relationship to changes in plasma renin and plasma aldosterone concentrations, *Clin. Sci.*, 39, 437—455, 1970.

258. Verdy, M. and DeChamplain, J., Fasting in obese females. II. Plasma renin activity and urinary aldosterone, *Can. Med. Assoc. J.*, 98, 1034—1037, 1968.

259. Hermann, L. S., Hansen, N. C., and Gronbeck, P., Hyperaldotennism following weight reduction by complete fasting, *Ugeskr. Laeg.*, 131, 192—193, 1969.

260. Smith, R., Ross, E. J., and Marshall-Jones, P., Aldosterone and sodium excretion in obese subjects on water diet, *Metab. Clin. Exp.*, 18, 700—705, 1969.

261. Rapoport, A., From, G. L. A., and Husdan, H., Metabolic studies in prolonged fasting. I. Inorganic metabolism and kidney function, *Metab. Clin. Exp.*, 14, 31—46, 1965.

262. Katz, A. I., Hollingsworth, D. R., and Epstein, F. H., Influences of carbohydrate and protein on sodium excretion during fasting and refeeding, *J. Lab. Clin. Med.*, 72, 93—104, 1968.

263. Muller, W. A., Faloona, G. R., and Unger, R. H., The influence of antecedent diet upon glucagon and insulin secretion, *N. Engl. J. Med.*, 285, 1450—1454, 1971.

264. Hales, C. N. and Randle, P. J., Effects of low-carbohydrate diet and diabetes mellitus on plasma concentrations of glucose, nonesterified fatty acids, and insulin during oral glucose-tolerance tests, *Lancet*, 1, 780—794, 1963.

265. Grey, N. and Kipnis, D. M., Effect of diet composition on the hyperinsulinemia of obesity, *N. Engl. J. Med.*, 285, 827—831, 1971.

266. Cleave, T. L. and Campbell, G. D., Diabetes, coronary thrombosis and the saccharine disease, John Wright and Sons, Bristol, U.K., 1969, 14—65.

267. Wapnick, S., Wicks, A. C. B., Kanengoni, E., and Jones, J. J., Can diet be responsible for the initial lesion in diabetes?, *Lancet*, 2, 300—302, 1972.

268. Wicks, A. C. B. and Jones, J. J., Insulinopenic diabetes in Africa, *Br. Med. J.*, 1, 773—776, 1973.

269. Wicks, A. C. B. and Jones, J. J., Diabetes mellitus in Rhodesia: a comparative study, *Postgrad. Med. J.*, 50, 659—663, 1974.

270. Atinmo, T., Baldijao, C., Pond, W. G., and Barnes, R. H., Plasma insulin levels in weaned pigs fed protein or energy restricted diets, *J. Nutr.*, 106, 1054—1057, 1976.

271. Boyar, R. M., Hellman, L. D., Roffwarg, H., Katz, J., Zumoff, B., O'Connor, J., Bradlow, H. L., and Fukushima, D. K., Cortisol secretion and metabolism in anorexia nervosa, *N. Engl. J. Med.*, 296, 190—195, 1977.

272. Wolff, H. P., Vecsei, P., Kruck, F., Roscher, S., Brown, J. J., Dusterdieck, G. O., Lever, A. F., and Robertson, J. I. S., Psychiatric disturbance leading to potassium depletion, sodium depletion, raised plasma-renin concentration, and secondary hyperaldosteronism, *Lancet*, 1, 257—261, 1968.

273. Wilson, D. C. and Sutherland, I., The age of menarche, *Br. Med. J.,* 2, 130—132, 1949.
274. Dreizen, S., Spirakis, C. N., and Stone, R. E., A comparison of skeletal growth and maturation in under-nourished and well-nourished girls before and after menarche, *J. Pediatr.,* 70, 256—263, 1967.
275. Landon, J., Greenwood, F. C., Stamp, T. C. B., and Wynn, V., The plasma sugar, free fatty acids, cortisol, and growth hormone response to insulin, and the comparison of this procedure with other tests of pituitary and adrenal function. II. In patients with hypothalamic or pituitary dysfunction or anorexia nervosa, *J. Clinical Invest ,* 45, 437—449, 1966.
276. Kanis, J. A., Brown, P., Fitzpatrick, K., Hibbert, D. J., Horn, D. B., Nairn, I. M., Shirling, D., Strong, J. A., and Walton, H. J., Anorexia nervosa: a clinical, psychiatric, and laboratory study, *Q. J. Med.,* 43, 321—338, 1974.
277. Mecklenburg, R. S., Loriaux, D. L., Thompson, R. H., Andersen, A. E., and Lipsett, M. D., Hypothalamic dysfunction in patients with anorexia nervosa, *Medicine, (Baltimore),* 53, 147—159, 1974.
278. Stephan, F., Reville, P., Thierry, R., and Schlienger, J. L., Correlations between plasma insulin and body weight in obesity, anorexia nervosa and diabetes mellitus, *Diabetologia,* 8, 196—201, 1972.
279. Frankel, R. J. and Jenkins, J. S., Hypothalamic - pituitary function in anorexia nervosa, *Acta Endocrinol. (Copenhagen),* 78, 209—221, 1975.
280. Emanuel, R. W., Endocrine activity in anorexia nervosa, *J. Clin. Endocrinol. Metab.,* 16, 801—816, 1956.
281. Croxson, M. S. and Ibbertson, H. K., Low serum triiodothyronine (T3) and hypothyroidism in anorexia nervosa, *J. Clin. Endocrinol. Metab.,* 44, 167—174, 1977.
282. Miyai, K., Yamamoto, T., Azukizwa, M., Ishibashi, K., and Kumahara, Y., Serum thyroid hormones and thyrotropin in anorexia nervosa, *J. Clin. Endocrinol. Metab.,* 40, 334—338, 1975.
283. Beaumont, P. J. V., George, G. C. W., Pimstone, B. L., and Vinik, A. I., Body weight and the pituitary response to hypothalamic releasing hormones in patients with anorexia nervosa, *J. Clin. Endocrinol Metab.,* 43, 487—496, 1977.
284. Sherman, B. M., Halmi, K. A., and Zamudio, R., LH and FSH response to gonadotropin-releasing hormone in anorexia nervosa: effect of nutritional rehabilitation, *J. Clin. Endocrinol. Metab.,* 41, 135—142, 1975.
285. Warren, M. P., Jewelewicz, R., Dyrenfurth, I., Ans, R., Khalaf, S., and Vandenwiele, R. L., The significance of weight loss in the evaluation of pituitary response to LH-RH in women with secondary amenorrhea, *J. Clin.Endocrinol. Metab.,* 40, 601—611, 1975.
286. Palmer, R. L., Crisp, A. H., Mackinnon, P. C. B., Franklin, M., Bonnar, J., and Wheeler, M., Pituitary sensitivity to 50 mg LH/FSH-RH in subjects with anorexia nervosa in acute and recovery stages, *Br. Med. J.,* 1, 179—182, 1975.
287. Harrower, A. D. B., Yap, P. L., Nairn, I. M., Walton, H. J., Strong, J. A., and Craig, A., Growth hormone, insulin, and prolactin secretion in anorexia nervosa and obesity during bromocriptine treatment, *Br. Med. J.,* 2, 156—159, 1977.
288. Fishman, J., Boyar, R. M., and Hellman, L., Influence of body weight on estradiol metabolism in young women, *J. Clin. Endocrinol. Metab.,* 41, 989—991, 1975.
289. Bell, E. T., Harkness, R. A., Loraine, J. A., and Russell, G. F. M., Hormone assay studies in patients with anorexia nervosa, *Acta Endocrinol. (Copenhagen),* 51, 140—148, 1966.
290. Chivmello, G., Del Guercio, M. J., Carnelutti, M., and Bidone, G., Relationship between obesity, chemical diabetes and beta pancreatic function in children, *Diabetes,* 18, 238—243, 1969.
291. Nikkilä, E. A. and Taskinen, M., Ethanol-induced alterations of glucose tolerance, postglucose hypoglycemia, and insulin secretion in normal, obese and diabetic subjects, *Diabetes,* 24, 933—943, 1975.
292. Mahler, R. J., The pathogenesis of pancreatic islet hyperplasia and insulin insensitivity in obesity, *Adv. Metab. Disord.,* 7, 213—241, 1974.
293. Karam, J. H., Grodsky, G. M., Ching, K. N., Shmid, F., Burrill, K., and Forsham, P. H., "Staircase" glucose stimulation of insulin secretion in obesity; measure of beta-cell sensitivity and capacity, *Diabetes,* 23, 763—770, 1974.
294. Rabinowitz, D. and Zierler, K. L., Forearm metabolism in obesity and its response to intra-arterial insulin. Characterization of insulin resistance and evidence for adaptive hyperinsulinism, *J. Clin. Invest.,* 41, 2173—2181, 1962.
295. Harrison, L. C. and King-Roach, A. P., Insulin sensitivity of adipore tissue in vitro and the response to exogenous insulin in obese human subjects, *Metab. Clin. Exp.,* 25, 1095—1101, 1976.
296. Olefsky, J. M. The insulin receptor: its role in insulin resistance of obesity and diabetes, *Diabetes,* 25, 1154—1162, 1976.
297. Malins, J., Clinical Diabetes Mellitus and Eyre, lst ed., Spothwode, London, 1973, 23—25.
298. Johansen, K., A new principle for the comparison of insulin secretory responses, *Acta Endocrinol. (Copenhagen) ,* 74, 524—541, 1973.
299. Martin, M. M. and Martin, A. L. A., Obesity, hyperinsulinism, and diabetes mellitus in childhood, *J. Pediatr.,* 82, 192—201, 1973.

300. **Kreisberg, R. A., Boshell, B. R., Diplacido, J., and Roddam, R. F.,** Insulin secretion in obesity, *N. Engl. J. Med.,* 276, 314—319, 1967.

301. **Turner, R. C., Schneeloch, B., and Nabarro, J. D. N.,** Biphasic insulin secretory response to intravenous xylitol and glucose in normal, diabetic and obese subjects, *J. Clin. Endocrinol. Metab.,* 33, 301—307, 1971.

302. **Johnson, S., Karam, J. H., Levin, S. R., Grodsky, G. M., and Forsham, P. H.,** Hyperinsulin response to oral leucine in obesity and acromegaly, *J. Clin. Endocrinol. Metab.,* 37, 431—435, 1973.

303. **Gossain, V. V., Matute, M. L., and Kalkhoff, R. K.,** Relative influence of obesity and diabetes on plasma alpha-cell glucagon, *J. Clin. Endocrinol. Metab.,* 38, 238—243, 1973.

304. **Enk, B., Lund, B., Schmidt, A., and Deckert, T.,** Secretin induced insulin response. I. Cubital insulin concentration in normal, obese, and pancreatectomized patients, including portal insulin concentration in normals after secretin, *Acta Endocrinol. (Copenhagen),* 82, 306—311, 1976.

305. **Perley, M. and Kipnis, D. M.,** Plasma insulin response to glucose and tolbutamide of normal weight and obese diabetic and nondiabetic subjects, *Diabetes,* 15, 867—874, 1966.

306. **Nikkilä, E. A. and Taskinen, M.,** The insulin secretion rate in obesity, *Postgrad. Med. J.,* 47, (June Suppl.,) 412—417, 1971.

307. **Schade, D. S. and Eaton, R. P.** Altered tissue response to glucagon in obesity, *J. Clin. Endocrinol. Metab.,* 40, 732—735, 1975.

308. **Paulsen, E. P. and Lawrence A. M.,** Glucagon hypersecretion in obese children, *Lancet,* 2, 110, 1968.

309. **Theodoridis, C. G., Brown, G. A., Chance, G. W., and Rayner, P. H. W.,** Growth hormone response to oral glucose in children with simple obesity, *Lancet,* 1, 1068—1069, 1969.

310. **Laurian, L., Oberman, Z., Ayalon, D., Cordova, T., Herzberg, M., Horer, E., and Harell, A.,** Under-responsivenes of growth hormone secretion after L-dopa and deep sleep stimulation in obese subjects, *Isr. J. Med. Sci.,* 11, 482—487, 1975.

311. **Hankin, M. E., Theile, H. M., and Steinbeck, A. W.,** Cortisol and aldosterone excretion and plasma cortisol concentrations in normal and obese female subjects, *Clin. Sci.,* 43, 289—298, 1972.

312. **Cacciari, E., Cicognani, A., Pirazzoli, P., Tassoni, P., Zappulla, F., Salardi, S., and Bernardi, F.,** Relationships among the secretion of ACTH, GH, and cortisol during the insulin-induced hypoglycemia test in the normal and obese child, *J. Clin. Endocrinol. Metab.,* 40, 802—806, 1975.

313. **Björntorp, P., Holm, G., Jacobsson, B., Schiller-de Jounge, K., Lundberg, P., Sjöström, L., Smith, U., and Sullivan, L.,** Physical training in human hyperplastic obesity. IV. Effects on the hormonal status, *Metab. Clin. Exp.,* 26, 319—328, 1977.

314. **Schteingart, D. E., Gregerman, R. I., and Conn, J. W.,** A comparison of the characteristics of increased adrenocortical function in obesity and in Cushing's syndrome, *Metab. Clin. Exp.,* 12, 484—497, 1963.

315. **Migeon, C. J., Green, O. C., and Eckert, J. P.,** Study of adrenocortical function in obesity, *Metab. Clin. Exp.,* 12, 718—739, 1963.

316. **Payne, P. R. and Dugdale, A. E.,** Mechanisms for the control of body weight, *Lancet,* 1, 583—586, 1977.

317. **Bray, G. A., Fisher, D. A., and Chopra, I. J.,** Relation of thyroid hormones to body-weight, *Lancet,* 1, 1206—1208, 1976.

318. **Wilcox, R. G.,** Triiodothyronine, T. S. H. and prolactin in obese women, *Lancet,* 1, 1027—1029, 1977.

319. **Hung, W., Gancayco, G. P., and Heald, F. P.,** Thyroxine metabolism in obese adolescent males, *Pediatrics,* 36, 877—881, 1965.

320. **Sonka, J., Gregorova I., Tomsova, Z., Pavlova, A., Zbirkova, A., Rath, R., Urbanek, J., and Josifko, M.,** Plasma androsterone, dehydroepiandrosterone and 11-hydroxycorticoids in obesity. Effects of diet and physical activity, *Steroids Lipids Res.,* 3, 65—74, 1972.

320a. **Raith, L., Steiner, R., and Karl, H. J.,** Metabolic transformation of ^{3}H-cortisol to tetra- and hexahydrated derivatives in obesity, *Acta Endocrinol. (Copenhagen),* 66, (Suppl. 152), 97, 1971.

321. **Fehér, T. and Halmy, L.,** Dehydroepiandrosterone and dehydroepiandrosterone sulfate dynamics in obesity, *Can. J. Biochem.,* 53, 215—222, 1975.

322. **Chretien, M.,** Obesity and pituitary lipolytic hormones, *Triangle (Engl. Ed.),* 13, 63—71, 1974.

323. **Dubuc, P. U.,** The development of obesity, hyperinsulinemia, and hyperglycemia in ob/ob mice, *Metab. Clin. Exp.,* 25, 1567—1574, 1976.

324. **Zucker, L. M. and Antoniades, H. N.,** Insulin and obesity in the Zucker genetically obese rat "fatty", *Endocrinology,* 90, 1320—1330, 1972.

325. **Hamilton, C. L., Kuo, P. T., and Feng, L. Y.,** Experimental production of syndrome of obesity, hyperinsulinemia, and hyperlipidemia in monkeys, *Proc. Soc. Exp. Biol. Med.,* 140, 1005—1009, 1972.

326. **Eaton, R. P., Conway, M., and Schade, D. S.,** Endogenous glucagon regulation in genetically hyperlipemic obese rats, *Am. J. Physiol.,* 230, 1336—1341, 1976.

327. **Larkins, R. G.,** Defective insulin secretory response to glucose in the New Zealand obese mouse. Improvement with restricted diet, *Diabetes,* 22, 251—260, 1973.

328. **Soll, A. H., Kahn, C. R., Neville, D. M., and Roth, J.,** Insulin receptor deficiency in genetic and acquired obesity, *J. Clin. Invest.,* 56, 769—780, 1975.

329. **Olefsky, J., Bacon, V. C., and Baur, S.,** Insulin receptors on skeletal muscle: specific insulin binding sites and demonstration of decreased numbers of sites in obese rats, *Metab. Clin. Exp.,* 25, 179—191, 1976.

330. **Althen, T. G. and Gerrits, R. J.,** Metabolic clearance and secretion rates of porcine growth hormone in genetically lean and obese swine, *Endocrinology,* 99, 511—515, 1976.

331. **Larson, B. A., Sinha, Y. N. and Vanderlaan, W. P.,** Serum growth hormone and prolactin during and after the development of the obese-hyperglycemic syndrome in mice, *Endocrinology,* 98, 139—145, 1976.

332. **Naeser, P.,** Function of the adrenal cortex in obese-hyperglycemic mice (gene symbol ob), *Diabetologia,* 10, 449—453, 1974.

333. **Edwardson, J. A. and Hough, C. A. M.,** The pituitary-adrenal system of the genetically obese (ob/ ob) mouse, *J. Endocrinol.,* 65, 99—107, 1975.

334. **Sinha, Y. N., Salocks, C. B., and Vanderlaan, W. P.,** Control of prolactin and growth hormone secretion in mice by obesity, *Endocrinology,* 99, 881—886, 1976.

335. **Sinha, Y. N., Salocks, C. B., and Vanderlaan, W. P.,** Prolactin and growth hormone secretion in chemically induced and genetically obese mice ob/ob, *Endocrinology,* 97, 1386—1393, 1975.

336. **York, D. A., Hersham, J. M., Utiger, R. D., and Bray, G. A.,** Thyrotropin secretion in genetically obese rats, *Endocrinology,* 90, 67—72, 1972.

337. **Bray, G. A. and York, D. A.,** Thyroid function of genetically obese rats, *Endocrinology,* 88, 1095—1099, 1971.

THE EFFECTS OF NUTRITION ON ENDOCRINE FUNCTIONS

G. A. Campbell

The endocrine glands that will be considered herein are the anterior pituitary, thyroid, adrenal cortex and medulla, ovarian follicle and corpus luteum, ovarian and testicular interstitial tissue and the islets of Langerhans.

THE ANTERIOR PITUITARY GLAND

The anterior pituitary gland (AP), or adenohypophysis of higher vertebrates, is responsible for the production and release of six polypeptide hormones of major importance, namely, thyrotropin (TSH), adenocorticotropin (ACTH), follicle-stimulating hormone (FSH), luteinizing hormone (LH), prolactin (PRL), and growth hormone (GH). A variety of other synonyms have been applied to some of these hormones in an attempt to better summarize their functional role, or to define some special role for that hormone, but only the above nomenclature will be employed herein. The importance of these hormones resides in the fact that they are absolutely essential for the normal morphology and function of certain target tissues. These target tissues are themselves necessary for the fullest expression of the physiological capacities of the body. Thus, all except PRL and GH are directly and primarily responsible, in all species, for the functional integrity of target endocrine organs. PRL in most species is of primary importance for the initiation and maintenance of function of an exocrine gland, the mammary gland, and it is the supportive of at least one endocrine gland target organ, the corpus luteum, in some species. PRL is believed to be involved in a less dramatic way in the regulation of many diffuse bodily functions as well. GH is required primarily for the attainment of normal skeletal size, and as such, has its major effects during the prepubertal growth period. Like PRL, however, GH appears to be of importance for a variety of metabolic functions. The anterior lobe of the pituitary also secretes β-lipotropin (β-LPH), which has an obscure physiological role but acts as a precursor in peripheral tissues for endorphins and enkephalins.

The thyroid gland, the adrenal cortex, the follicle and corpus luteum of the ovary, and the interstitial tissue of both male and female gonads are target organ endocrines of major importance, the functions of which are regulated by AP hormone levels. Under AP control, they secrete mainly thyroxin, cortisol, estrogen, progesterone, and testosterone. The gonads and the adrenal cortex also release a number of other sex steroids and mineral and glucocorticoids, and some of these hormones are released with varying degrees of autonomy from AP control.

THE HYPOTHALAMUS

Although the AP can in certain instances exhibit a degree of its own autonomy (limited almost entirely to PRL secretion), the normal production and release of all six hormones is closely controlled by the brain, by virtue of an intimate anatomical and functional relationship with the hypothalamus. The regulatory role is accomplished by means of agents, mostly peptides, referred to as releasing factors or hypophysiotropic hormones, which are elaborated by hypothalamic neurons and which, upon being conveyed to the AP through a special hypothalamo-hypophysial portal circulation, affect the release and ultimately the production of AP hormones. The structure and primary function of three of these factors are known: TSH-releasing factor (TRH), LH- and FSH-releasing factor (GnRH), and GH-release-inhibiting factor (GIF) also known as somatostatin. There are several lines of evidence that support the idea that the biogenic amine, dopamine, may act as a PRL-release-inhibiting factor (PIF). A number of other factors are generally believed to exist, but have not as yet been isolated, i.e., PRL-releasing factor (PRF), GH-releasing factor (GRF), and ACTH-releasing factor (CRF). The hypothalamic neurons that elaborate all of these factors also can be demonstrated to have a certain degree of autonomy, but their function is doubtless highly modulated by numerous neuronal inputs from the rest of the brain and other parts of the central nervous system. In this regard, certain biogenic amines and other neurotransmitters have been implicated as regulators for changes in release of hypophysiotropic hormones. Hypothalamic function is also modulated in a feedback manner by gonadal and adrenal steroids and by the levels of hypophisiotropic hormones themselves. Some of the target hormones, especially the gonadal and adrenal steroids and thyroid hormone act directly on the AP to alter secretion as well.

THE ADRENAL MEDULLA

The adrenal medulla is composed of specialized sympathetic postganglionic neurons that do not have axonal processes, and secrete epinephrine (E) and norepinephrine (NE) directly into the blood. Two morphologically distinguishable cells are responsible for the release of these two hormones. These cells secrete E (80%) and NE (20%) when activated by preganglionic fibers reaching the medulla by way of sympathetic nerves from the sympathetic trunks. Indeed, the activity of the adrenal medulla is regulated by the sympathetic nervous system. This hormone release is not essential for continued life, but is part of the body reaction to emergencies. Both NE and E (catecholamines) have a rather short halflife in the circulation, and are then inactivated by oxidation followed by methylation and are excreted in the urine largely in this form. The nervous system is stimulated by catecholamine release as is the metabolic rate, and liver and muscle glycogenolysis and fat cell mobilization of free fatty acids are increased. The catecholamines have the potential for bringing about vasoconstriction in many regions of the body, and elevated cardiac output to elevate arterial blood pressure, but probably contribute much less than the direct activity of sympathetic nerves.

THE PANCREAS

Scattered throughout the parenchyma of the pancreas are groups of cells referred to as the islets of Langerhans. These islets are composed of three morphologically distinct cell types, α, β, and δ cells, the first two of which produce the polypeptide hormones glucagon and insulin, respectively. Glucagon release causes a rise in blood glucose by stimulating hepatic glycogenolysis. Insulin lowers blood glucose mainly by facilitating the movement of glucose into muscle and other tissues. Both hormones are regulated by blood glucose levels, such that depressed levels stimulate glucagon release and inhibit insulin release, while elevated glucose brings about the reverse effects. Both hormones are released in higher amounts in response to elevations in plasma amino acid levels. Recently the presence of at least one hypophysiotropic hormone, GIF or somatostatin, has been discovered in the pancreas. This hormone has been shown experimentally to markedly affect the release of both glucagon and insulin.

The above information has only gradually come to light as the result of innumerable investigations extending from the last half of the last century until the present. Throughout this evolution of knowledge, there has been an increasing awareness of the interrelationship between nutrition and the integrity of the endocrine system. The earlier literature has been summarized in several excellent reviews: Samuels,[244] Ershoff,[22] and Leathem.[18,20,131] The emphasis throughout all of this research has centered on the effects of various degrees of starvation, and of various specific dietary deficiencies upon the endocrine system, with very little attention diverted to the effects of overnutrition.

During the late 1960s and early 1970s, a momentous advance in the technology of measurement of circulating hormones took shape that has resulted in a revolution in endocrine research and thought: the radioimmunoassay (RIA). The RIA was developed by Berson and Yalow in the late 1950s for the detection of insulin and the techniques have since been adapted for the measurement of almost all known hormones. The acquisition of reproducible and reliable RIAs for the AP hormones has resulted in an explosive enlargement in knowledge about AP secretion and its regulation. This growth in knowledge was due to an exodus of many scientists from a world where each experiment required several tedious, expensive, often unreliable and highly variable biological assays, to one in which several findings could emerge from a single experiment based on rapid, precise, relatively cheap, and reproducible chemical assays. Although not at first in the main stream of this burgeoning information, increased knowledge about the relationships between nutrition and AP function has inevitably come to light as a result of the RIA.

Since the catalogue of information concerning nutritional influences upon the endocrine physiology, like that of other aspects of endocrinology is divisible into pre-RIA (Table 1) and post-RIA (Table 2) information, and since some pre-RIA findings have not suffered revision as a result of RIA findings, the pre-RIA documentation will be summarized, followed by a post-RIA version. Revision in thought or fact will be pointed out in the post-RIA section as needed.

Although a great many authors have contributed to many of the general findings, especially in the earlier work, only one or a few major representative references will be given in support of each item. Most of the observations documented in the following tables were made upon experimental animals, usually laboratory rodents, and are believed to apply to humans, and to mammalian species in general. Results obtained with human subjects as well will be so indicated as will those reported only in humans.

Table 1
OBSERVATIONS MADE PRIOR TO THE ADVENT OF RIA

Endocrine organ or target tissue affected	Type of dietary inadequacy	Sequelae and related findings	Ref.
Thyroid gland	Inanition	Atrophy, involution, and degeneration of the gland in lab animals and humans	1—5
		Function of gland diminished	6, 7
		Response of gland to goitrogen decreased	8, 9
		Similar findings to above with anorexia nervosa in humans	13
		Gland retains sensitivity to TSH	4
	Protein deficiency	Similar effects on the gland to those for inanition have been reported	14, 15
		Thyroid function may not be markedly decreased	16
		If protein stores are sufficiently depleted the response of the gland to goitrogens is reduced	18
		The biological value of protein (in repleting protein stores) influences the return of responsiveness to goitrogens	18
		Methionine supplement may influence return of normal function	20
		Low gland: serum I^{125} ratio	16, 17
	Iodine deficiency	Eventual hypertrophy of the gland in response to increased secretion of TSH	21
Adrenal cortex	Inanition	Hypertrophy of gland (at least relative to body weight), evidence for increased function in guinea pig	23—26
		Atrophy of gland reported (in both humans and animals)	27—29
		Decreased function of gland reported (in both humans and animals)	56
		Decreased response of gland to ACTH	56
	Protein deficiency	0% protein presents normal gland growth pattern in young rats, but not relative to body weight	32
		Diminished adrenal compensatory hypertrophy	34
		Morphology of adrenal near normal, but cortical thickness reduced	35
		Circulating 11-hydroxysteroids may be elevated due to impaired clearance	37, 38
		Dexamethasone can suppress plasma levels	38
	Vitamin C deficiency	Interfers with function of gland	36, 39
	Pantothenic acid deficiency	Causes abnormalities of the gland (as in the "exhaustion syndrome" of Selye)	40—42

Table 1 (continued)
OBSERVATIONS MADE PRIOR TO THE ADVENT OF RIA

Endocrine organ or target tissue affected	Type of dietary inadequacy	Sequelae and related findings	Ref.
	Thiamin deficiency	Leads to increased gland function above that related to anorexia	43
	Choline Deficiency	Gland response to ACTH diminished	33
	Riboflavin deficiency	Morphology of gland not altered	43
	Pyridoxine deficiency	Same as riboflavin deficiency	43
	K⁺ deficiency	May damage the adrenal cortex	44
Adrenal medulla	Protein deficiency	Adrenain excretion elevated	47
		Dopamine excretion lowered	48
		Decreased noradrenalin catabolism	48
Pancreas	Inanition	Endocrine tissues not damaged	49
Anterior pituitary	Inanition	Decreased ACTH content in pituitary gland	2
		Decreased ACTH secretion	2, 5, 31
		Diminished TSH in pituitary gland	10
		Evidence for less TSH secretion	5, 6, 9—12
		Basophiles retain active morphology	23
		Gonadotrophin content of gland normal	45, 46, 50—54
		Decreased prolactin content of gland	5
		Decreased growth hormone content	53, 54, 57
		Atrophy of gland (in both humans and animals)	30, 55, 56
		Postcastration rise in gonadotropin content of gland not blocked (in both humans and animals)	5, 55, 56, 59—61
		Damage to gland at puberty; decrease in glucose metabolism	131
		Refeeding caused decreased FSH content with return of ovarian activity	52
		AP PRL content is elevated during exposure to constant illumination, and after epinephrine administration	62
	Protein deficiency	Less ACTH release in response to cold	34
		Less ACTH release in response to partial nephrectomy or epinephrine administration	32
		Similar findings to inanition	63
		Decreased gonadotropin content of gland after 30 days in male rats	18
		Decreased gonadotropin (FSH and LH) content of gland in young male rats	64
		FSH content of gland elevated with no change in LH content	63
		Release of LH and FSH impaired	65
		Castration cells still appear after	63

Table 1 (continued)
OBSERVATIONS MADE PRIOR TO THE ADVENT OF RIA

Endocrine organ or target tissue affected	Type of dietary inadequacy	Sequelae and related findings	Ref.
		gonadectomy, normal post-castration rise in FSH and LH content occurs, plasma FSH levels were elevated sufficiently for bioassay detection	
		TSH content may or may not decrease	16, 18, 19, 66
		Decreased growth hormone secretion	16, 67, 68
Anterior pituitary	Pantothenic acid deficiency	Impaired gonadotropin release	69
	Choline deficiency	ACTH release in response to epinephrine stimulation	33
	Pyridoxine deficiency	Strongly elevated FSH content of gland, and increases LH slightly, decreases PRL content	72
	Vitamin B₁ deficiency	Increased pituitary gland TSH content	22
		Decreased gonadotropin content of gland	73
	Vitamin A deficiency	Decreased pituitary gland TSH content	22
		Increased gonadotropin content, especially in males	74
		Increased number of basophiles	75
	Vitamin E deficiency	Same effects as Vitamin A	76, 77
	Isoleucine deficiency	Decreased acidophil cell size, decreased PAS positive material in gland	70
	Fat deficiency	Increased number of acidophiles and decreased number of basophiles	71
Reproductive system (male)	Inanition	Atrophy of prostate, seminal vesicles and testis	59—60, 78—79, 80—83
		Testis — the least sensitive (in both humans and animals)	84
		Loss of Leydig Cell function first, then later spermatogenesis	59, 84, 90, 91
		Decreased seminiforous tubule size, and Leydig Cell size reported in humans after chronic underfeeding, atrophy is reversible with refeeding	56
		Prevents or delays maturition of gonadal system in young (in both humans and animals)	85—88
		More resistance in adult than young	13, 92
		Testis of rat responds to gonadotropin administration, Leydig Cells are stimulated, testis weight is restored, and spermatogenesis returns	84, 93
		Response to gonadotropins may be subnormal	84, 94—96

Table 1 (continued)
OBSERVATIONS MADE PRIOR TO THE ADVENT OF RIA

Endocrine organ or target tissue affected	Type of dietary inadequacy	Sequelae and related findings	Ref.
Reproductive system (female)	Inanition	Delays or prevents gonadal maturation, vaginal opening, and puberty	89, 97
		Ovarian atrophy, loss of regular cycles, and decreased fertility in adults (in both humans and animals)	98—101
		Amenorhea, atrophy of genitalia, and low urinary estrogens (in humans only)	56, 102, 103
		Failure of ovulation, decrease in number of large follicles, and increase in number of primary follicles	3, 104—107
		Decrease in number and morphological changes in interstitial cells	45, 108
		Corpora are present	45, 109
		Changes in reproductive system are reversed by refeeding	108, 110
		Changes in reproductive system are reversed by exposure to constant illumination	62
		Atrophic ovaries and dysfunction reversed by gonadotropin administration	60, 65, 104, 111—112
		Does not prevent the response of the vagina and uterus to estrogen, but will block the deciduoma reaction	113, 116
		Prevents growth of the mammary gland	114
		Limits the response of the mammary gland to estrogen	115
Reproductive system (Male)	Protein deficiency	Similar effects to inanition	85, 117
		Prolonged protein depletion required for a reduction in testis weight in adult male rats	85, 92, 118—120
		Testis protein decreases slower than total body protein	131
		After 1 month of protein deprivation some gonadotropins are being released from the pituitaries of adult males, in contrast to young males and females	35, 131
		Testis are needed for full repletion of protein stores	18
		Maintenance of gonads after hypophysectomy with androgen is difficult	121
		Responsiveness to PMS retained	122
		Enzyme responses after gonadotropin or androgen administration may be subnormal	92, 123
		Spermatogenesis is maintained by	85, 124

Table 1 (continued)
OBSERVATIONS MADE PRIOR TO THE ADVENT OF RIA

Endocrine organ or target tissue affected	Type of dietary inadequacy	Sequelae and related findings	Ref.
		casein even though proper growth is not	
Reproductive system (Female)		Similar effects as inanition	120—122, 125—127
		Decreases the number of ova	118, 126
		Return to normal protein intake for 3 days increases the number of vesicular follicles, and the secretion of estrogen	18
		Rate of recovery of reproductive system after stilbestrol administration depends on protein intake during, as well as after treatment	18
		Refeeding of mice after 1 month of PFD causes a rebound effect leading to an abnormally high reproductive performance	127
		Response to gonadotropins appears normal or greater than normal	128
		Response to gonadotropins may depend on degree of protein depletion	18
		Response to gonadotropins may depend on biological value of protein if receiving a small amount	121, 132
		Presence of the pituitary gland alters responsiveness	67, 117
		Minimum of 7% casein is needed for maintenance of estrus	124
		Estrogen response of uterus lessened in mice	129
		Steroid replacement (0.5 μg E + 6ng P) did not prevent the biochemical changes in the uterus during protein deprivation	131
		Minimum of 6% casein is needed for the response of the mammary gland to estrogen	115
		Less response of gonadectomized immature rat uterus to estradiol	129, 130
		Corticosterone administration does not modify the influence of diet on uterine weight of protein	131
Reproductive system (Male)	Amino acid deficiency (phenylalanine)	Causes impaired gonadal function, but the effects on gonadotropin secretion are not known	133
	(Leucine)	Similar status	134
	(Histidine)	Similar status	135
	Amino acid (tryptophan)	Similar status	136
	(Arginine)	Evidence for interference with spermatogenesis in humans and rats after 9 days, but the status of gonadotropins is not known	136, 137

Table 1 (continued)
OBSERVATIONS MADE PRIOR TO THE ADVENT OF RIA

Endocrine organ or target tissue affected	Type of dietary inadequacy	Sequelae and related findings	Ref.
	Ethionine administration	Causes severe atrophy of the seminiferous tubules and hyperplasia of the Leydig Cells	138
	Pantothenic acid deficiency	Interfers with gonadal function	163
	Biotin deficiency	Interfers with gonadal function	164
Reproductive system (Female)	Gelatin Administration	Leads to anestrum; lysine corrects this	121
	Pyridoxine deficiency	Decreased ovarian sensitivity to gonadotropins, especially FSH	168
	Nicotinic acid deficiency	Increased response of uterus and vagina to estrogen	95, 169
	Vitamin B_{12} deficiency	Decreased response of uterus and vagina to estrogen	170
	Folic acid deficiency	Decreased response of uterus and vagina to estrogen	171, 172
Reproductive system (Male)	Fat deficiency	Degeneration of seminiferous tubules and decreased spermatogenesis	139
		HCG will not reverse tubular degeneration after 29 weeks of fat deficiency compared to testosterone which will	140
Reproductive system (Female)		Can eventually lead to anestrus and sterility, leads to decreased response of uterus to stilbestrol	71, 141, 142
Reproductive system (Male)	Vitamin A deficiency	Leads to testicular degeneration	82, 143—146
		Atrophy of prostate and seminal vesicles restored by gonadotropin treatment (but all Vitamin A results are confounded by effects of anorexia)	150
		Leads to reproductive failure, but probably because of anorexia induced inanition, the effects are reversible	173, 160
		Has a specific effect on epithelium of the accessory reproductive organs	161
		Accessory organs respond normally to testosterone	165
		Gonadotropin treatment was not found to promote spermatogenesis	150
Reproductive system (Female)	Vitamin A deficiency	No changes in ovarian morphology, no changes in fecundity (so administration did not explain change in female AP)	144, 147—150
		Leads to irregular cycles	20
		Needed for normal vaginal epithelium	166
Reproductive system (Male)	Vitamin C deficiency	Causes a degeneration of the seminiferous tubules and Leydig Cells that is not due to inanition	162

Table 1 (continued)
OBSERVATIONS MADE PRIOR TO THE ADVENT OF RIA

Endocrine organ or target tissue affected	Type of dietary inadequacy	Sequelae and related findings	Ref.
Reproductive system (Female)	Vitamin C deficiency	Does not cause problems	167
Reproductive system (Male)	Vitamin E deficiency	Degeneration of seminiferous tubules, but not of interstitial tissue	82, 150—153
		(This does not apply in rabbits)	154
		(This does not apply in mice)	155
		(This does not apply in ruminants)	156
		(This does not apply in humans)	157
		Vitamin E treatment does not improve fertility	59, 82, 158, 159
		Accessory organs respond normally to testosterone	165
		Gonadotropin treatment was not found to promote spermatogenesis	150
Reproductive system (Female)		Does not result in ovarian disfunction	233
Mammary gland	Inanition	Decreased growth of mammary gland	114
		Reduced lobulo-alveolar development, which is increased after epinephrine administration or can still respond to prolactin	62
		Decreased sensitivity of gland (for growth) to estrogen	62, 173
	Protein	Needed for response of gland to estrogen	115
Pregnancy	Inanition	Decreases number and size of fetuses	121
		Estrogen and progesterone replacement restore normal pregnancy	128
	Protein deficiency	Causes effects similar to toxemia	174
		Protein free diet does not prevent implantation, but induced 86—100% embryonic loss	175
		Protein free diet during 9—10 days also brings about embryonic loss	176
		Protein free diet during last one third of pregnancy decreased maternal weight but not fetal or placental weight	176
		4 mg progesterone and 0.5 µg estrogen permit normal pregnancy in the absence of dietary protein (these are amounts of steroids needed to restore pregnancy after either hypophysectomy or ovariectomy)	128, 179
		E & P limited to days 5—9 also restores pregnancy (compared to 5—11 in hypophysectomized rats)	178
		Either estrogen alone (3 µg/day) or	128

Table 1 (continued)
OBSERVATIONS MADE PRIOR TO THE ADVENT OF RIA

Endocrine organ or target tissue affected	Type of dietary inadequacy	Sequelae and related findings	Ref.
		4—8 mg of progesterone partially maintain pregnancy	
		Reserpine which releases PRL also maintains pregnancy	177—178
		Prolactin alone will maintain pregnancy	180
		Prolactin (3—12 days) restores pregnancy by 75%	177
		Placental luteotropic or mammotropic activity is normal in the absence of dietary protein	181
		HCG given on days 3 and 12 does not restore pregnancy	177
	Fat deficiency	Produces still-birth, if deficiency is great placental injury appears	182
	Vitamin A deficiency	Can produce fetal damage and abortion	183, 184, 186 185
		Too much Vitamin A induced cleft palate	
	Vitamin E deficiency	Causes placental damage and involution of corpus luteum of pregnancy, fetal death	187
		Estrogen and progesterone or prolactin can restore function	188
	Vitamin B$_6$ deficiency	Causes fetal death with alterations resembling toxemia	189, 190
		Estrogen and progesterone can reverse these effects	191
		The pituitary hormone combination which maintains pregnancy in hypophysectomized rats cannot completely restore function, so there is some ovarian defect induced	191
	Folic acid deficiency	Required throughout pregnancy	192
		Estrogen and progesterone replacement cannot restore pregnancy	20
	Pantothenic acid deficiency	Same as folic acid	20, 193
	Choline deficiency	Induces fetal abnormalities, but hormonal aspects unknown	194
	Riboflavin deficiency	Same as choline	195
	Vitamin B$_{12}$ deficiency	Same as choline	196
Lactation	Inanition	AP hormones alone or in combination, not very effective in restoring lactational performance	197
	Protein deficiency	Adrenal corticoids alone or with GH (Prednisolone) restores lactation	198
		Evidence for low levels of PRL secretion during lactation	198
Hypothalamus	Inanition	Acute starvation decreases hypo-	53

Table 1 (continued)
OBSERVATIONS MADE PRIOR TO THE ADVENT OF RIA

Endocrine organ or target tissue affected	Type of dietary inadequacy	Sequelae and related findings	Ref.
		thalamic GH releaing activity	
		Neurohumor release in birds is blocked	22, 199
		LH releasing activity is decreased, and this content is not restored by exposure to constant illumination	18, 62
		FSH-releasing activity is decreased	19, 200
	Protein deficiency	PRL release-inhibiting activity is normal	201

Table 2
RESULTS OBTAINED SINCE THE ADVENT OF THE RIA FOR THE DETECTION OF CIRCULATING AP HORMONES

Dietary deficiency	Response	Ref.
Inanition (Males)	The synthesis of GH by AP's from starved rats were reduced in vitro, while the release increased	242
	Both synthesis and release of PRL in vitro increased	242
	12 days without food decreased serum FSH and LH, and increased AP levels of these hormones per mg AP gland	204
	Starvation 7 days after castration could not block the rise in serum LH and FSH, and AP LH levels, and the levels rose above those for well-fed animals	204
	Castration performed at the onset of starvation elicited a lessened rise in serum LH, but FSH rose as before	204
	7 days without food caused a reduction in serum LH, FSH, TSH, PRL, and GH	202
	Chronic starvation reduced LH, TSH, PRL, and GH, but permitted a return to normal % for FSH	202
	After refeeding for 7 days, GH and PRL returned to normal levels, and LH and FSH rose to levels more than twice normal, but TSH did not return to normal	202
	Fasting for 36 hr blunted the AP response to synthetic TRH administration in terms of TSH release when compared to 12 hr fasting (in humans only)	205
Inanition (Females)	Absence of feed for 1 week did not alter the rise in serum LH and FSH in rats castrated at the start of starvation, the rise in LH and FSH per mg AP gland was greater than for well-fed animals	206
	Serum levels of LH after synthetic LHRH administration were lower in patients with anorexia nervosa than that for normal individuals, and greater impairment was seen with greater weight loss	207, 208
	Serum FSH levels after weight loss were equal to or higher than that for normal patients	207, 208
	LH responses to LHRH improved with weight gain in anorexia patients, both LH responsiveness to LHRH and its return were unrelated to estrogen levels	208
	LH depressing effects of estrogen are observed with much less steroid administration	212
	The percent rise in serum LH, FSH, TSH, and PRL in response to simultaneous synthetic LHRH and TRH administration was	202

Table 2 (continued)
RESULTS OBTAINED SINCE THE ADVENT OF THE RIA FOR THE DETECTION OF CIRCULATING AP HORMONES

Dietary deficiency	Response	Ref.
	greater in rats starved for 7 days than for well-fed rats, while all except PRL behaved in this way after 2 weeks chronic inanition	
	Normal LH and FSH responses to LHRH were reported for rats under urethane anesthesia	209
	Normal LH and FSH release was observed in vitro in response to LHRH	209
Both sexes	Serum GH levels rise in response to underfeeding in humans	210
	Basal TSH levels may be normal or elevated in children and the response to TRH exaggerated and prolonged	125, 210
	Serum GH levels fall after 1 week of starvation in rats, AP levels rise for 5 days then fall	243
	T_3 administration can still lower these levels	211
	Normal TSH levels are formed in adults	213
	TBG, T_3 and T_4 levels are lower than normal in adults	213
	Short-term starvation did not decrease hypothalamic LHRH content	209
	Total starvation in obese individuals causes decreased TSH secretion and thyroid gland function, and delayed AP response to TRH	214
	Adrenal response to ACTH normal	222
	Cortisol and GH rise as serum albumin is diminished, while insulin eventually declines, in malnourished children	215, 237
	The clearance of GH is probably not impaired in children	216
	Prolonged fasting during the 1st half of human pregnancy causes a rise in serum levels of placental lactogen. This response is diminished as pregnancy progresses.	217—221
	GH levels do not change with fasting during 8—20 weeks of human gestation	217
	hPRL levels fall during 72 hr fasting at 8—20 weeks of pregnancy	217
	Alanine infusion can still elevate GH after 72 hr fasting during the first ½ of pregnancy	217
	Plasma insulin levels are lower than normal	222—228
	Plasma insulin levels respond poorly to various stimuli	228—229
	These defects may be due to diminished K^+ levels	231
	Insulin response to glucose is higher and longer than normal	232, 241
Protein deficiency	Plasma 11-hydroxycorticoids are normal	38, 240
	Results in a rise in GH in children	223, 229, 234—236
	GH will drop after oral amino acid administration	230
	GH can be further elevated by various stimuli	229
	More directly correlated with GH rise than carbohydrate deprivation	237
	Rise in GH correlated with drop in serum protein	238
	Plasma-free T_4 may be normal or elevated	239
	Adrenal response to ACTH normal	38
	Prolactin is diminished in both the pituitary and plasma of female rats after protein depletion	201, 203

REFERENCES

1. Jackson, C. M., *Am. J. Anat.*, 19, 305, 1916.
2. Morgulis, S., *Fasting and Undernutrition*, Duton, New York, 1923.
3. Mulinos, M. G. and Pomerantz, L., *J. Nutr.*, 19, 493, 1940.
4. Stephens, D. J., *Endocrinology*, 26, 485, 1940.
5. Meites, J. and Reed, J. O., *Proc. Soc. Exp. Biol. Med.*, 70, 513, 1949.
6. Meites, J. and Wolterink, L. F., *Science*, 111, 175, 1950.
7. Meites, J., *Iowa State Coll. J. Sci.*, 28, 19, 1953.
8. Gomez-Mont, F., Paschkis, K. E., and Cantarow, A., *Endocrinology*, 40, 225, 1947.
9. Meites, J. and Agrawala, I. P., *Endocrinology*, 45, 148, 1949.
10. D'Angelo, S. A., *Endocrinology*, 48, 341, 1951.
11. Meyers, A. W., *J. Med. Res.*, 36, 51, 1917.
12. Stefko, W., *Schweiz. Med. Wochenschr.*, 61, 171, 1931.
13. Perloff, W. H., Lasche, E. M., Nodine, J. H., Schneeberg, N. G., and Vieillard, C. B., *J. Am. Vet. Med. Assoc. 155, 1307, 1954.*
14. Ingle, D. J., Ward, E. O., and Kuizenga, M. H., *Am. J. Physiol.*, 149, 510, 1947.
15. Mighorst, J. C. A., *Acta Endocrinol.*, 8, 97, 1951.
16. Srebnik, H. H. and Nelson, M. M., *Endocrinology*, 70, 723, 1962.
17. Cowan, J. W. and Margossian, S., *Endocrinology*, 79, 1023, 1966.
18. Leathem, J. H., *Recent Prog. Horm. Res.*, 14, 141, 1958.
19. Warter, J., Aron, C., and Asch, L., *C. R. Soc. Biol.*, 152, 843, 1958.
20. Leathem, J. H., in *Sex and Internal Secretion*, Young, W. C., Ed., Williams & Wilkins, Baltimore, 1961, 666.
21. Griesbach, W. E., *Br. J. Exp. Pathol.*, 22, 245, 1941.
22. Ershoff, B. H., *Vitam. Horm.* N.Y., 10, 79, 1952.
23. D'Angelo, S. A., Gordon, A. S., and Charipper, H. A., *Endocrinology*, 42, 399, 1948.
24. Boutwell, R. K., Brush, M. K., and Rusch, H. P., *Am. J. Physiol.*, 154, 517, 1948.
25. Bablet, J. and Canet, J., *Ann. Inst. Pasteur*, 83, 595, 1952.
26. Platt, B. S. and Steward, R. J. C., *J. Endocrinol.*, 38, 121, 1967.
27. Quimby, F. H., *Endocrinology*, 42, 263, 1948.
28. Chatterji, A. and Sen Gupta, P. C., *Indian J. Pathol. Bacteriol.*, 27, 353, 1960.
29. Stirling, G. A., *J. Pathol. Bacteriol.*, 77, 555, 1959.
30. Mulinos, M. B. and Pomerantz, L., *J. Nutr.*, 19, 493, 1949.
31. Neilson, F. J., *Br. J. Nutr.*, 16, 387, 1962.
32. Handler, P. and Bernheim, F., *Am. J. Physiol.*, 162, 368, 1950.
33. Handler, P. and Bernheim, F., *Am. J. Physiol.*, 162, 375, 1950.
34. Moya, F., Prado, J. L., Rodriguez, R., Savard, K., and Selye, H., *Endocrinology*, 42, 223, 1948.
35. Srebnik, H. H., *Endocrinology*, 75, 716, 1964.
36. Giroud, A. and Santa, N., *C. R. Soc. Biol.*, 131, 1176, 1939.
37. Rao, K. J., Srikantia, S. G., and Gopalan, C., *Arch. Dis. Child.*, 43, 365, 1968.
38. Alleyne, G. A. O. and Young, V. H., *Clin. Sci.*, 33, 189, 1967.
39. Giroud, A., Santa, N., and Martinet, M., *C. R. Soc. Biol.*, 134, 23, 1940.
40. Morgan, A. F. and Simms, H. D., *Science*, 89, 565, 1939.
41. Deane, H. W. and McKibbin, J. M., *Endocrinology*, 38, 385, 1946.
42. Selye, H., *J. Clin. Endocrinol.*, 6, 117, 1946.
43. Deane, H. W. and Shaw, J. H., *J. Nutr.*, 34, 1, 1947.
44. Deane, H. W., Shaw, J. H., and Greep, R. O., *Endocrinology*, 43, 133, 1948.
45. Rinaldini, L. M., *J. Endocrinol.*, 6, 54, 1949.
46. Vanderlinde, R. E. and Westerfield, W. W., *Endocrinology*, 47, 265, 1950.
47. Parra, A., Serrano, P., Chavez, B., Garcia, G., Argote, R. M., Klish, W., Cuellar, A., and Nichols, B. L., in Endocrine Aspects of Malnutrition, Proc. of Symp. by Kroc. Found., Gardner, L. and Amacher, P., Eds., 181, 1973.
48. Hoeldtke, R. D. and Wurtman, R. J., *Am. J. Clin. Nutr.*, 26, 205, 1973.
49. Weinkove, C., Insulin Release and Glucose Tolerance in Malnourished Rats, Ph.D. thesis, University of Cape Town, 1974.
50. Drummond, J. C., Noble, R. L., and Wright, M. D., *J. Endocrinol.*, 1, 275, 1939.
51. Casida, L. E., in Prog. 6th Int. Cong. Nutrition, Edinburgh, 366, 1963.
52. Lamming, G. E. and Krause, J. B., in Prog. 6th Int. Cong. Nutrition, Edinburgh, 633, 1963.
53. Meites, J. and Fiel, N. J., *Endocrinology*, 77, 455, 1965.
54. Dickerman, E., Négro-Vilar, A., and Meites, J., *Endocrinology*, 84, 814, 1969.

55. Klinfelter, H. F., Jr., Albright, F., and Griswold, G. C., *J. Clin. Endocrinol.*, 3, 529, 1943.
56. Zubiran, S. and Gomez-Mont, F., *Vitamin. Horm.*, 11, 97, 1953.
57. Friedman, R. C. and Reichlin, S., *Endocrinology*, 76, 787, 1965.
58. Heard, C. R. C. and Steward, R. J. C., *Hormones*, 2, 40, 1971.
59. Mulinos, M. G. and Pomerantz, L., *Endocrinology*, 29, 267, 1941.
60. Mulinos, M. G. and Pomerantz, L., *Endocrinology*, 29, 558, 1941.
61. Gomez-Mont, F., *Protein Nutrition and Reproductive Physiology*, Rutgers University Press, New Brunswick, 1959, 58.
62. Piacsek, B. E. and Meites, J., *Endocrinology*, 81, 535, 1967.
63. Srebnik, H. H., Nelson, M. M., and Simpson, M. E., *Endocrinology*, 68, 317, 1961.
64. Leathem, J. H. and Fisher, C. J., *Anat. Rec.*, 133, 302, 1959.
65. Printz, R. H. and Greenwald, G. S., *Endocrinology*, 86, 290, 1970.
66. Srebnik, H. H., Evans, E. S., and Rosenberg, L. L., *Endocrinology*, 73, 267, 1963.
67. Srebnik, H. H., Nelson, M. M., and Simpson, M. E., *Proc. Soc. Exp. Biol. Med.*, 99, 57, 1958.
68. Srebnik, H. H., Nelson, M. M., and Simpson, M. E., *Proc. Soc. Exp. Biol. Med.*, 101, 97, 1959.
69. Granitsas, A. M. and Leathem, L. H., in *Proc. Int. Cong. Physiol.*, Brussels, 1956.
70. Scott, E. B., *Proc. Soc. Exp. Biol. Med.*, 92, 134, 1956.
71. Panos, T. C. and Finerty, J. C., *J. Nutr.*, 49, 397, 1953.
72. Wooten, E., Nelson, M. M., Simpson, M. E., and Evans, H. M., *Endocrinology*, 56, 59, 1955.
73. Evans, H. M. and Simpson, M. E., *Anat. Rec.*, 45, 216, 1930.
74. Mason, K. E. and Wolfe, J. M., *Anat. Rec.*, 45, 232, 1930.
75. Sutton, T. S. and Brief, B. J., *Endocrinology*, 25, 302, 1930.
76. Nelson, W. O., *Anat. Rec.*, 56, 241, 1933.
77. P'an, S. Y., vanDyke, H. B., Kaunitz, H., and Slanetz, C. A., *Proc. Soc. Exp. Biol. Med.*, 72, 523, 1949.
78. Jackson, C. M., *Am. J. Anat.*, 21, 321, 1917.
79. Jackson, C. M., *The Effects of Inanition and Malnutrition Upon Growth and Structure*, Balkiston, Philadelphia, 1925.
80. Steward, C. A., *J. Exp. Zool.*, 25, 301, 1918.
81. Siperstein, D. M., *Anat. Rec.*, 20, 355, 1921.
82. Mason, K. E., *Am. J. Anat.*, 52, 153, 1933.
83. Jacobs, E. C., *J. Clin. Endocrinol.*, 8, 227, 1948.
84. Moore, C. R. and Samuels, L. T., *Am. J. Physiol.*, 96, 278, 1931.
85. Horn, E. H., *Endocrinology*, 57, 399, 1955.
86. Stephens, D. J., *J. Clin. Endocrinol.*, 1, 257, 1941.
87. Davies, D. V., Mann, T., and Rowson, L. E. A., *Proc. R. Soc. London Ser. B*, 147, 322, 1957.
88. Talbert, G. B. and Hamilton, J. B., *Anat. Rec.*, 121, 763, 1955.
89. Widdowson, E. M. and Cowen, J., *Br. J. Nutr.*, 27, 85, 1972.
90. Reid, J. T., *J. Am. Vet. Med. Assoc.*, 114, 158, 1949.
91. Menze, W., *Endokrinologie*, 24, 159, 1941.
92. Leathem, J. G., Biology of the Prostate and Related Tissues, Natl. Can. Inst. Monograph 12, 201, 1963.
93. Funk, C. and Funk, I. C., *Science*, 90, 443, 1939.
94. Goldsmith, E. D., Nigrelli, R. F., and Ross, L., *Anat. Rec.*, 106, 197, 1950.
95. Kline, I. T. and Dorfman, R. I., *Endocrinology*, 48, 34, 1951.
96. Grayhack, J. T. and Scott, W. W., *Endocrinology*, 50, 406, 1952.
97. Zimmer, R., Weill, J., and Dubois, H., *N. Engl., J. Med.*, 230, 303, 1944.
98. Jackson, C. M., *Am. J. Anat.*, 18, 75, 1914.
99. Loeb, L., *J. Am. Vet. Med. Assoc.*, 77, 1646, 1941.
100. El-Sheikh, A. S., Hulet, C. V., Pope, A. L., and Casida, L. E., *J. Anim. Sci.*, 14, 919, 1955.
101. Casida, L. E., in *Reproductive Physiology and Protein Nutrition*, Leathem, J. H., Ed., Rutgers University Press, New Brunswick, New Jersey, 35, 1959.
102. Stephens, D. J., *Endocrinology*, 28, 580, 1941.
103. Rothchild, I., *Am. J. Obstet. Gynecol.*, 98, 719, 1967.
104. Marrian, G. F. and Parkes, A. S., *Proc. R. Soc. London, Ser. B*, 105, 248, 1929.
105. Stephens, D. J. and Allen, W. M., *Endocrinology*, 28, 580, 1941.
106. Guilbert, H. R., *J. Anim. Sci.*, 1, 3, 1942.
107. Bratton, R. W., *Cornell Univ. Ag. Exp. Sta. Bull.*, 924, 25, 1957.
108. Ball, Z. B., Barnes, R. H., and Visscher, M. B., *Am. J. Physiol.*, 150, 511, 1947.
109. Arvy, L., Aschkenasy, A., Aschkenasy-Lelu, P., and Gabe, M., *C. R. Soc. Biol.*, 140, 730, 1946.
110. Schultze, M. O., *J. Nutr.*, 56, 25, 1955.
111. Werner, S. C., *Proc. Soc. Exp. Biol. Med.*, 41, 101, 1939.

112. Hosoda, T., Koneo, T., Mogi, K., and Abe, T., *Proc. Soc. Exp. Biol. Med.,* 92, 360, 1956.
113. Leathem, J. H., Nocenti, M. R., and Granitsas, A., *Proc. P. Acad. Sci.,* 30, 38, 1956.
114. Reece, R. P., *Proc. Soc. Exp. Biol. Med.,* 73, 284, 1950.
115. Reece, R. P., in *Reproductive Physiology and Protein Nutrition,* Leathem, J. H., Rutgers University Press, New Brunswick, New Jersey, 1950, 23.
116. deFoe, V. J. and Rothchild, I., *Anat. Rec.,* 115, 297, 1943.
117. Leathem, J. H. and DeFoe, V. J., *Anat. Rec.,* 112, 356, 1952.
118. Aschkenasy, A., *Sang,* 25, 15, 1954.
119. Leathem, J. H., *Anat. Rec.,* 118, 323, 1954.
120. Popoff, J. S. and Okultilschew, G. Z., *Ztschr. Zuchtung B.,* 221, 1936.
121. Leathem, J. H., in *Recent Progress in the Endocrinology of Reproduction,* Lloyd, C. W., Ed., Academic Press, New York, 1959, 179.
122. Cole, H. H., Guilbert, H. R., and Goss, H., *Am. J. Physiol.,* 102, 227, 1932.
123. Leathem, J. H., in *Reproductive Physiology and Protein Nutrition,* Leathem, J. H., Ed., Rutgers University Press, New Brunswick, New Jersey, 1959, 22.
124. Guilbert, H. R. and Goss, H., *J. Nutr.,* 5, 251, 1932.
125. Ryabinina, A. Z., *Doklady Akad. Nauk. S. S. R.,* 86, 877, 1952.
126. Ishida, K., *Tohoku J. Agric. Res.,* 8, 17, 1957.
127. Courrier, R. and Raynaud, R., *C. R. Soc. Biol.,* 109, 881, 1932.
128. Nelson, M. M., in *Reproductive Physiology and Protein Nutrition,* Leathem, J. H., Ed., Rutgers University Press, New Brunswick, New Jersey, 1959, 2.
129. Lerner, L. J. and Turkheimer, A. R., *Endocrinology,* 76, 539, 1965.
130. Oslapas, R. and Leathem, J. H., *Anat. Rec.,* 151, 395, 1965.
131. Leathem, J. H., *J. Am. Sci.,* Suppl. 25, 68, 1965.
132. Yamamoto, R. S. and Chow, B. F., *Fed. Proc.,* 9, 250, 1950.
133. Maun, M. E., Cahill, W. M., and Davis, R. M., *Arch. Pathol.,* 39, 294, 1945.
134. Maun, M. E., Cahill, W. M., and Davis, R. M., *Arch. Pathol.,* 40, 173, 1945.
135. Maun, M. E., Cahill, W. M., and Davis, R. M., *Arch. Pathol.,* 41, 25, 1946.
136. Shettles, L. B., in *Proc. 3rd Ann. Cong. Bio. Sperm.,* 1942, 28.
137. Holt, L. E., Jr., Albanese, A. A., Shettles, L. B., Kajdi, C., and Wangerin, D. M., *Fed. Proc. 1,* 116, 1942.
138. Kaufman, N., Klavins, J. V., and Kinney, T. D., *Am. J. Pathol.,* 32, 105, 1956.
139. Panos, T. C. and Finerty, J. C., *J. Nutr.,* 54, 315, 1954.
140. Finerty, J. C., Klein, G. F., and Panos, T. C., *Anat. Rec.,* 127, 293, 1957.
141. Ferrando, R., Jacques, F., and Mabboux, H., *C. R. Acad. Sci.,* 241, 253, 1955.
142. Umberger, E. J. and Gass, G. H., *Endocrinology,* 63, 801, 1958.
143. Mason, K. E., *J. Exp. Zool.,* 55, 101, 1930.
144. Wolfe, J. M. and Salter, H. P., *J. Nutr.,* 4, 185, 1931.
145. Wolbach, S. B. and Howe, P. R., *Arch. Pathol.,* 5, 239, 1928.
146. Guilbert, H. R. and Hart, G. H., *J. Nutr.,* 10, 409, 1935.
147. Evans, H. M., *J. Biol. Chem.,* 77, 651, 1928.
148. Mason, K. E., *Am. J. Anat.,* 57, 303, 1935.
149. Hughes, J. S., Augel, C. E., and Lienhardt, H. F., *Kans. Agric. Exp. Stn. Bull.,* 23, 1, 1928.
150. Mason, K. E., *Sex and Internal Secretion,* Williams & Wilkins, Baltimore, 1939.
151. Mason, K. E., Vitamin E — A Symposium, *Soc. Chem. Ind., Lond.,* 1939, 31.
152. Curto, G. M., *Acta Vitaminol.,* 8, 7, 1954.
153. Mason, K. E. and Mauer, S. I., *Anat. Rec.,* 127, 329, 1947.
154. Mackenzie, C. G., *Proc. Soc. Exp. Biol. Med.,* 49, 313 1942.
155. Byran, W. L. and Mason, K. E., *Am. J. Physiol.,* 131, 263, 1941.
156. Blaxter, K. L. and Brown, F., *Nutr. Abstr. Rev.,* 21, 1, 1952.
157. Lutwak-Mann, C., *Vitamin Horm.,* 16, 35, 1958.
158. Bechmann, R., *Vitam. Horm. Fermentforsch.,* 7, 281, 1955.
159. Geller, F. C., *Arch. Gynak,* 156, 345, 1933.
160. Horn, H. W., Jr. and Maddock, C. L., *Fertil. Steril.,* 3, 245, 1952.
161. Follis, R. H., *Pathology of Nutritional Diseases,* Charles C Thomas, Springfield, Ill., 1948.
162. Mukherjee, A. K. and Banerjee, S., *Anat. Rec.,* 120, 907, 1954.
163. Barboriak, J. J., Krehl, W. A., Cowgill, G. R., and Whedon, A. D., *J. Nutr.,* 63, 591, 1957.
164. Katsh, S., Kosarick, E., and Alpern, J., *Growth,* 19, 45, 1955.
165. Mayer, J. and Truant, A. P., *Proc. Soc. Exp. Biol. Med.,* 72, 436, 1949.
166. Kahn, R. H., *Am. J. Anat.,* 95, 309, 1954.
167. Blandau, R. J., Kauntiz, H., and Slanatez, C. A., *J. Nutr.,* 38, 97, 1949.
168. Wooten, E., Nelson, M. M., Simpson, M. E., and Evans, H. M., *Endocrinology,* 63, 860, 1958.

169. Kline, I. T. and Dorfman, R. I., *Endocrinology,* 48, 345, 1951.
170. Kline, I. T., *Endocrinology,* 57, 120, 1955.
171. Hertz, R., *Endocrinology,* 37, 1, 1945.
172. Hertz, R., *Rec. Prog. Horm. Res.,* 2, 161, 1948.
173. Trentin, J. J. and Turner, C. W., *Endocrinology,* 29, 984, 1941.
174. Shipley, R. A., Chudzik, E. B., Curtiss, C., and Price, J. W., *Metabolism,* 2, 165, 1953.
175. Nelson, N. M. and Evans, H. M., *J. Nutr.* 51, 71, 1953.
176. Campbell, R. M. and Kosterlitz, H. W., *J. Endocrinol.,* 9, 45, 1953.
177. Callard, I. P. and Leathem, J. H., *Am. Zool.,* 3, 491, 1963.
178. Kinsey, W. G. and Srebnik, H. H., *Proc. Soc. Exp. Biol. Med.,* 114, 158, 1963.
179. Nelson, M. M. and Evans, H. M., *Endocrinology,* 55, 543, 1954.
180. Hays, R. L. and Kendall, K. A., *Endocrinology,* 68, 177, 1961.
181. Kinsey, W. G., *Anat. Rec.,* 148, 301, 1964.
182. Kummerow, F. A., Pay, H. P., and Hickman, H., *J. Nutr.,* 46, 489, 1952.
183. Warkany, J. and Schraffenberger, E., *Proc. Soc. Exp. Biol. Med.,* 57, 49, 1944.
184. Wilson, J. G., Roth, C. B., and Warkany, J., *Am. J. Anat.,* 92, 189, 1953.
185. Giroud, A. and Martinet, M., *C. R. Soc. Biol.,* 149, 1088, 1955.
186. Giroud, A. and Martinet, M., *C. R. Soc. Biol.,* 153, 201, 1959.
187. Cheng, D. W., Chang, L. F., and Bairson, T. A., *Anat. Rec.,* 129, 167, 1957.
188. Ershoff, B. H., *Anat. Rec.,* 87, 297, 1943.
189. Ross, M. L. and Pike, R. L., *J. Nutr.,* 60, 211, 1956.
190. Pike, R. L. and Kirksey, A., *J. Nutr.,* 68, 561, 1959.
191. Nelson, M. M., Lyons, W. R., and Evans, N. M., *Endocrinology,* 48, 726, 1951.
192. Thiersch, J. B., *Proc. Soc. Exp. Biol. Med.,* 87, 571, 1954.
193. Nelson, M. M. and Evans, H. M., *Proc. Soc. Exp. Biol. Med.,* 91, 614, 1956.
194. Dubnov, M. V., *Arch. Pathol.,* 20, 68, 1958.
195. Giroud, A., Lévy, G., LeFebvres, J., and Dupuis, R., *Vitam. Horm. Fermentforsch.,* 23, 490, 1952.
196. Nelson, M. R., Abnrich, L., and Morgan, A. F., *Proc. Soc. Exp. Biol. Med.,* 16, 394, 1957.
197. Ratner, A. and Meites, J., *Am. J. Physiol.,* 204, 268, 1963.
198. Lyons, W. R., *Endocrinology,* 78, 575, 1966.
199. Assenmacher, I., Tixier-Vidal, A., and Astier, H., *Ann. Endocrinol.,* 26, 1, 1965.
200. Négro-Vilar, A., Dickerman, E., and Meites, J., *Endocrinology,* 88, 1246, 1971.
201. Campbell, G. A., The Secretion of LtH from the Anterior Pituitary Gland in the Absence of Dietary Protein, Ph.D. thesis, University of California, Berkeley, 1973.
202. Campbell, G. A., Kurcz, M., Marshall, S., and Meites, J., *Endocrinology,* 100, 580, 1977.
203. Campbell, G. A., Grindeland, R. E., and Srebnik, H. H., *Fed. Proc.,* 29, 439, 1970.
204. Root, A. W. and Russ, R. D., *Acta Endocrinol.* 70, 665, 1972.
205. Vinik, A. I., Kalk, W. J., McLaren, H., Hendricks, S., and Pimstone, B. L., *J. Clin. Endocrinol. Metab.,* 40, 509, 1975.
206. Ibrahim, E. A. and Howland, B. E., *Can. J. Physiol. Pharmacol.,* 50, 768, 1972.
207. Sherman, B. W., Halmi, K. A., and Zamudio, R., *J. Clin. Endocrinol. Metab.,* 41, 135, 1975.
208. Warren, M. P., Jewelewicz, R., Dyrenfurth, I., Khalaj, R., and VandelWiele, R., *J. Clin. Endocrinol. Metab.,* 40, 135, 1975.
209. Root, A. W., Reiter, E. O., Duckett, G. E., and Sweetland, M. L., *Proc. Soc. Exp. Biol. Med.,* 150, 602, 1975.
210. Glick, S. M., Roth, J., Yalow, R. S., and Berson, S. A., *Rec. Prog. Horm. Res.,* 21, 241, 1965.
211. Pimstone, B., Becher, D., and Hendricks, S., *J. Clin. Endocrinol. Metab.,* 36, 779, 1973.
212. Campbell, G. A., Hodson, C., Mioduszewski, R., and Meites, J., *Endocrinol. Soc. Prog. Absts.,* 1975.
213. Rastogi, C. K., Sawhney, R. C., Panda, N. C., and Tripathy, B. B., *Horm. Metab. Res.,* 6, 528, 1974.
214. Rothenbuchner, G., Loos, U., Kressling, W. R., Birk, S., and Pfeiffer, E. F., *Acta Endocrinol. Suppl.* 173, 144, 1973.
215. Ramalingaswami, V., Lancet, *2, 733, 1969.*
216. Pimstone, B. L., Becker, D., and Kronheim, S., *J. Clin. Endocrinol. Metab.,* 40, 168, 1975.
217. Tyson, J. E., Austin, K., and Farinholt, J., *Am. J. Obstet. Gynecol.,* 125, 1073, 1976.
218. Tyson, J. E., Austin, K. E., and Farinholt, J. W., *Am. J. Obstet. Gynecol.,* 109, 1080, 1971.
219. Felig, P. and Lynch, V., *Science,* 170, 990, 1970.
220. Hare, J. W., Metzger, B. E., and Freinkel, N., *Diabetes,* 20, 338, 1971.
221. Kim, Y. J. and Felig, P., *J. Clin. Endocrinol. Metab.,* 32, 864, 1971.
222. Baig, H. A. and Edozien, J. C., *Lancet,* ii, 662, 1965.
223. Hadden, D. R., *Lancet,* ii, 589, 1967.

224. Godard, C. and Zahnd, G. R., *Helvetica Paediatr. Acta,* 26, 276, 1971.
225. Rao, K. J. and Raghuramulu, N., *J. Clin. Endocrinol. Metab.,* 35, 63, 1972.
226. James, W. P. T. and Coore, H. G., *Am. J. Clin. Nutr.,* 23, 386, 1970.
227. Milner, R. D. G., *Pediatr. Res.,* 4, 213, 1970.
228. Becker, D. J., Pimstone, B. L., Hansen, J. D. L., and Hendricks, S., *Diabetes,* 20, 542, 1971.
229. Milner, R. D. G., *Pediatr. Res.,* 5, 33, 1971.
230. Milner, R. D. G. *Arch. Dis. Child.,* 46, 301, 1971.
231. Pimstone, B., *Clin. Endocrinol.,* 5, 79, 1976.
232. Becker, D. J., Pimstone, B. L., Hansen, J. D. L., MacHutchon, B., and Drysdale, A., *Am. J. Clin. Nutr.* 25, 499, 1972.
233. Mason, K. E., *Vitam. Horm.* 2, 107, 1944.
234. Pimstone, B. L., Wittman, W., Hansen, J. D. L., and Murray, P., *Lancet,* ii, 779, 1966.
235. Pimstone, B., Barbezat, G., Hansen, J. D. L., and Murray, P., *Lancet,* ii, 1333, 1967.
236. Graham, G. G., Cordano, A., Blizzard, R. M., and Cheek, D. B., *Pediatr. Res.,* 3, 579, 1969.
237. Pimstone, B. L., Barbezat, G., Hansen, J. D. L., and Murray, P., *Am. J. Clin. Nutr.,* 21, 482, 1968.
238. Pimstone, B. L., Becker, D. J., and Hansen, J. D. L., in *Growth and Growth Hormone,* Pecile, A. and Müller, E. E., Ed., Exerpta Medica Foundation, Amsterdam, 1972.
239. Graham, G. G., Baertz, J. M., Claeyssen, G., Suskind, R., Greenberg, A. A., Thompson, R. G., and Blizzard, R. M., J. Pediatr., *83, 321, 1973.*
240. Leonard, P. J., *Lancet,* i, 845, 1965.
241. Heard, C. R. C. and Henry, P. A. J., *J. Endocrinol.,* 45, 375, 1969.
242. Akikusa, Y., *Endocrinol. Jpn.,* 18, 409, 1971.
243. Trenkel, A., *Proc. Soc. Exp. Biol. Med.,* 135, 77, 1970.
244. Samuels, L. T., in *Progress in Clinical Endocrinology,* Grune and Stratton, N. Y., 1981.

Chemical Senses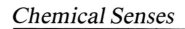

TASTE AND NUTRITION

Joseph G. Brand, Michael Naim, and Morley R. Kare

INTRODUCTION

The function of taste in nutrition is to aid in discriminating among available foods and to motivate the ingestion of those foods. The taste system of a given species may complement digestion, metabolism, and the nutrient requirements of that species. The interactions between nutrition and the chemical senses of taste and smell have received relatively little scientific attention. Progress in the field has been reported,[1,2] but in general our knowledge of this area remains incomplete. Attempts to integrate the two subjects must take into account a complex array of physiological, psychological, biochemical, and neuroendocrinological phenomena.

A framework upon which to base some initial inquiries is presented in Figure 1. The relationships outlined here are undoubtedly oversimplified and probably incomplete. The mechanisms responsible for the causitive interactions alluded to in the figure likewise, for the most part, remain obscure. Nevertheless, the figure illustrates many of the current hypotheses in this field. This review, then, will attempt to summarize the information available to date on the role of taste in nutrition. The role of olfaction in nutrition has received some previous attention (for example, see References 3 and 4).

In its present usage the word "taste" is ambiguous, and a brief look at its diverse connotations may serve to define this sense in the context of nutrition. Perhaps the most basic definition of taste concerns itself only with the reception of quality-specific, chemically evoked information via the gustatory taste bud receptors. Classically, four basic taste qualities are described: sweet, sour, salty, and bitter. Others have been argued from a psychophysical point of view (for review, see References 5 and 6), but definitive concomitant electrophysiological evidence in animals for these additional modalities is lacking. Thus the strict definition of taste is taken to denote the reception of a chemical message by oral taste bud organelles that transduce this chemical information into one of four perceptions: sweet, salty, sour, or bitter. Some of the compounds used to assess this quality perception, along with an approximate value for their detection (threshold) concentration, are presented in Table 1.

Other connotations of "taste" have arisen and are legitimate. Descriptions purporting to analyze the taste of a food, for example, generally go beyond the four primary modalities to include the realm of flavor. This definition of taste includes the perceptions derived from the overall sensory qualities that the food conveys, and it implies the use of all of our sensory capacities to describe the food.[7]

Paramount in the description of a food flavor (or a food taste, as we use the word under this definition) is its olfactory components. Some animals apparently do not use their sense of smell in diet selections (for example, see Reference 8). Others can still maintain adequate diet selection when apparently devoid of a functioning olfactory system. It is clear, however, that following bulbectomy, reinforcements necessary for learning about foods are lost.[9]

While the exact role of olfaction in food selection and food recognition is not well understood,[3] it is suggested that certain food odors in the proper context can elicit behavioral and physiological responses indicative of preparation for ingestion. A recent report has indicated that normal dometic cats form an aversion to food based on the food's odor.[10] In a well-controlled study, however, human parotid secretion flow rates were found to vary insignificantly with degree of liking and rated intensity of odorants.[11] A great deal of this behavior may be reflexive in nature or a learned re-

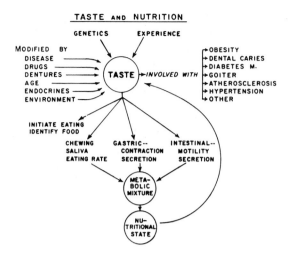

FIGURE 1.   Diagrammatic representation of some possible relationships between taste and nutrition. The figure indicates that genetic components as well as experiential factors influence taste (both sensitivity and preference) and that taste can be modified by a number of extrinsic factors as well as be involved with (but not necessarily a causative agent in) several disease states. Taste and oral stimulation have imporatnt systemic consequences which, in turn, influence the nutrition of the animal. Many of the complex interactions have been investigated or reviewed. Volumes which have information relevant to this subject are listed as References 1, 2, 7, 117, 196, and 207, as well as the volumes cited in References 3, 6, 12, 20, 26, 47, 59, 60, 72, 101, 158, 184, 186, and 188. The role played by the chemical senses (both taste and smell) in nutrition has also recently been discussed.[208] (Reprinted from Kare, M. R. and Beauchamp, G. R., in Melvin J. Swenson (ed.) *Duke's Physiology of Domestic Animals,* Ninth Edition. © 1977 by Cornell University. Used by permission of Cornell University Press.)

Table 1
SOME COMPOUNDS ELICITING A TASTE RESPONSE FROM MAN AND THEIR APPROXIMATE THRESHOLD CONCENTRATIONS[a]

Taste substance	Approximate threshold concentration *(M)*	Reference
Taste Modality: Sweet		
Sucrose	0.01	6
Glucose	0.08	6
Fructose	0.006[b] (0.013[c])	calculated from 197, 198
Saccharin (Na)	2.3×10^{-5}	6
Cyclamate (Na)	3.0×10^{-4c}	198
L-Asparty2-L-phenylalanine methyl ester	6.7×10^{-5}	calculated from 147
Beryllium Chloride	0.008	6
D-Tryptophan	2.8×10^{-4b}	calculated from 21
D-Leucine	0.002[b]	calculated from 21
D-Phenylalanine	0.001[b]	calculated from 21

Table 1 (continued)
SOME COMPOUNDS ELICITING A TASTE RESPONSE FROM MAN
AND THEIR APPROXIMATE THRESHOLD CONCENTRATIONS[a]

Taste substance	Approximate threshold concentration (M)	Reference
Taste Modality: Sweet		
Glycine	0.007[b]	calculated from 21
Thaumatin	2×10^{-7}	calculated from 22
Monellin	1×10^{-7}	calculated from 22
Taste Modality: Sour		
Hydrochloric acid	0.009	6
Nitric acid	0.011	6
Acetic acid	0.0018	6
Butyric acid	0.0020	6
Succinic acid	0.0032	6
Lactic acid	0.0016	6
Citric acid	0.0023	6
Taste Modality: Salty		
Sodium chloride	0.01	6
Lithium chloride	0.025	6
Ammonium chloride	0.004	6
Potassium chloride	0.017	6
Magnesium chloride	0.015	6
Sodium fluoride	0.005	6
Sodium iodide	0.028	6
Taste Modality: Bitter		
Quinine sulphate	4×10^{-6}	199
Quinine hydrochloride	3×10^{-6}	6
Quinidine sulphate	3×10^{-5}	199
Strychnine hydrochloride	1.6×10^{-6}	6
Nicotine	1.9×10^{-5}	6
Caffeine	7×10^{-4}	6
Phenylthiourea	2×10^{-5}	6
"tasters"		
"non-tasters"	8×10^{-3}	6
Urea	0.12	6
Brucine	7×10^{-7}	187
Theobromine	7.5×10^{-4}	187
Naringin	2.5×10^{-5}	187
L-Tryptophan	3.5×10^{-4b}	calculated from 21
L-Leucine	3.0×10^{-5b}	calculated from 21
L-Phenylalanine	1.8×10^{-4b}	calculated from 21
Magnesium sulfate	0.0046	6
Denatorium benzoate (Bitrex®)	$< 10^{-8}$	200

[a] These values are, for the most part, measures of detection threshold. For discussion of the methodologies involved in sensory testing of this type, see References 6 and 201.

[b] These values calculated from data based on equivalent intensity tests and not threshold tests, per se.

[c] Recognition threshold.

sponse.[12,13] Recent evidence indicates that the olfactory system of the human has the capacity to recognize a large number of distinct, compound odors and that this capacity to segregate a great quantity of "real odors" has heretofore been underestimated.[14] One report[4] pointed out that artificially induced hyposmia does indeed limit an individual's ability to identify food flavors, but the conclusions of this study were tempered by indicating that the olfactory system may not (by itself) be the dominant sense for flavor perception.

Additional sensory qualities of foods that are at times also considered in the purview of taste include the foods' ability to stimulate thermal and pressure receptors in the mouth. Thus some differences in the description of food "tastes" are not in fact those of taste per se but of texture. Nevertheless, even this extreme has come to be considered in the general meaning of the word "taste."[11]

The use of the taste of a food to generalize to the acceptability of that food has long been a topic of fascination. However, very little definitive research is available on this point. Distinctive food flavors are characteristic of ethnic cuisines and apparently perform functions to indicate the acceptability (safety) of the food as well as to maintain stability in cultural eating habits.[13,15] The often-avowed generalization that sweet taste denotes a potentially nutritious or utilizable substance and bitter a potentially poisonous one does not, however, stand up to critical review.

While it is true that sweetness tends to develop over time in ripening fruits, thereby apparently rendering them more attractive to foraging food seekers, it is also true that many animals that eat ripe fruits do not respond in a positive behavioral manner to the very chemicals that render the fruit sweet. Not all animals are sensitive to the same taste stimuli[16] and there is large variability among animals as to what is considered an acceptable (in human terms, sweet) taste stimulus (Reference 16 and Table 2). Clearly, other sensory cues besides taste are involved in food selection. Additionally, the fact that certain salts of lead and beryllium are perceived as sweet[6] is itself a negation of the hypothesis.

The ability of synthetic nonnutritive sweeteners to elicit a sweet perception also illustrates an overextension of this idea and, in addition, has implications for the specificity of the taste receptor system. The ready acceptance of nonnutritive sweeteners would imply that the animal can (at least initially) be confused as to the nutritive status of a food. While the concept of nonsense stimuli in receptor systems is not unique, it may be particularly disadvantageous where ingestion is concerned. The animal needs to make a rapid decision on food acceptability, and that decision is generally based on the initial chemical analyses carried out in the oral cavity. Too little nonspecificity in that analytical system could be potentially disastrous; yet too much specificity (or "fine tuning") in this receptor system may lock the animal into a narrow range of food sources, the loss of any one of which could prove nutritionally catastrophic for the species. Many animals are apparently genetically programmed to accept only specific foods and are well adapted ecologically to their surroundings, but their range is of necessity limited by the borders of their food supplies.

Sweetness alone cannot, therefore, inherently denote nutritional acceptability, but it does have an undeniably profound influence on the ontogeny of food selection. That sweet taste is apparently linked innately to ingestion is strongly suggested by studies showing that human neonates preferentially ingest sweet-tasting solutions over water controls, though they show little or no preference for or aversion to salty, sour, or bitter solutions.[17,18] As the animal matures, food taste in general can come to be associated with the acceptability or unacceptability of a particular food via a learning mechanism (for reviews, see References 13, 19, and 20).

The parallel concept that bitter taste can be equated with poisons or, at least, non-nutritious foods is equally invalid. Many compounds that have pharmacological activ-

Table 2
SPECIES VARIATION IN THE RESPONSE TO SOME CHEMICALS CONSIDERED SWEET BY MAN

Taste stimulus and response to it[a]

Animal	Saccharin	Sucrose	Lactose	Xylose	Glucose	Fructose	Ref.
Man	+	+	+	+	+	+	201
Rat	+	+	+	+ and −[b]	+	+	186
Dog[c]	+ or −[c]	+ or 0[d]			+ or 0[d]	+ or 0[d]	16
Cat	0 or −	0	0	0	0	0	16,209
Guinea pig	+				+		202,203
Pig	+[c]	+	+		+	+	16,204
Calf	0	+	0		+	+	186
Sheep	0 or −	+ or 0	0		+ or 0	0	186,205
Chicken	−	0	0	−	0		16
Porcupine	0	+		0	0	0	206

[a] Responses are indicated as follows: "+" means preference for or selection of taste substance shown in behavioral tests; "0" means indifference shown by tests; "−" means rejection shown by behavioral tests.

[b] Preference shown at concentrations below 5M; aversion shown at higher concentrations.

[c] Individual variations are pronounced with this test animal or this test solution.

[d] Test apparently not designed to segregate preference from indifference.

ity do taste bitter (e.g., many alkaloids and the goitrogenic thioureas); yet many other compounds which possess a bitter taste are important to the nutrition of the animal. For example, many amino acids and proteins have been described as bitter[21] (see Reference 22 for important exceptions). Raw and processed soy protein products can have objectionable flavors that may limit their use in bland diets.[23] While peripheral reasoning can be invoked for rationalizing the aversiveness of some of these foods (for example, raw soy contains tryptic inhibitors) much of the rationalization takes on an air of hyperbole. The parameters surrounding the ontogeny of food selection have recently been reviewed.[13,15]

Thus the concept that food palatability is a paramount determinant of consistent nutrition can be inferred, and many studies (see below) point to the validity of this concept. That taste is, at the least, an adjunct to nutrition is therefore a tenable hypothesis. That it plays a leading role in the selection and eventual efficient utilization of nutrients to insure against malnutrition is less easily argued, more difficult to conceptualize, and even harder to prove.

TASTE ANATOMY

Morphology and Distribution of Oral Taste Buds

Mammalian taste buds are multicellular, onion-shaped organelles whose apex is exposed to the environment and whose cells are generally elongated, slender-shaped structures, some of which contain villae at the apical end[24] (Figure 2). Taste bud cells are differentiated epithelial cells. They have an average life span of 8 to 13 days.[25] These slender taste bud cells are markedly different morphologically from the undifferentiated epithelial cells that surround the bud. Several types of taste bud cells have been distinguished on the basis of their morphology,[24,26] and some of these show classical synaptic relationships with innervating nerves.

Sensory neural innervation is required for morphological integrity of the taste bud (for review, see Reference 27) and presumably for the resultant biochemical function-

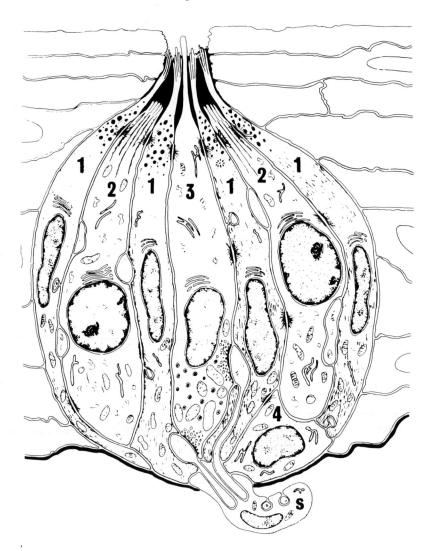

FIGURE 2.   Diagram of taste bud from the rabbit foliate region. The numbers correspond to cell types as classified by Murray.[76] Type 1 cells are the classical dark cells while type 2 cells are classical light cells. Neural elements enter from the base of the bud leaving the Schwann cell (S) and may show classical synaptic relationships with specialized type 3 cells. Basal cells (type 4) of the taste bud will eventually differentiate to a taste bud cell of slender morphology (see Reference 25). The irregularly shaped epithelial cells which surround the bud are shown in outline. (From Murray, R. G., in *The Ultrastructure of Sensory Organs*, Friedmann, I., Ed., North-Holland, Amsterdam, 1973, 43. With permission.)

ing of the bud receptor systems as well.[28-30] Taste bud integrity has been investigated prior to and following sensory nerve denervation by observing a diverse collection of histochemical reactions and correlating these with gross taste bud morphology. An elegant series of experiments[31-35] has aided our understanding of the normal histochemistry of this receptor system. Histochemical studies have demonstrated changes in phosphatase enzymes associated with the gustatory papillae following denervation.[31] For example, the concentration of adenosine triphosphatase within the bud changes in a characteristic manner following denervation.[31] Zalewski has shown that enzyme activities and normal morphology are restored following reinnervation.[33] These general observations have been confirmed by others,[36,37] and attempts have been made to implicate certain enzyme systems in quality-specific taste stimulation using the histochemical technique.[38,39] It is interesting from a mechanistic viewpoint that these studies often report changes in intracellular and not plasma membrane-associated enzyme histochemistry after incubation of the taste bud tissues with taste stimuli.

Taste buds are localized in the oral cavity and throat, usually imbedded in specialized papillae or regions of the tongue, soft palate, larynx, and pharynx. Taste buds on the tongue are located on one of three structures: the fungiform papillae clustered in the anterior two thirds of the tongue, the folliate region (grooves in the epithelium containing taste buds along the lateral posterior borders of the tongue), and circumvallate papillae located in the posterior portion of the tongue. Many animals do not have a foliate region containing taste buds, and the actual distribution of buds among the separate structures as well as the relative positions of the structures themselves varies from species to species. The interested reader is referred to a recent review on the subject.[40]

Neuroanatomy of Taste

The sense of taste is mediated by three separate sensory nerves.[30] The chorda tympani branch of the VII cranial nerve (facial) innervates taste papillae on the anterior two thirds of the tongue and has been reported to have a posterior field in the calf.[41] The glossopharyngeal nerve (the IX cranial nerve) innervates taste buds of the posterior third of the tongue, and the vagus (X cranial nerve) innervates taste buds of the epiglotis and throat. For the rat, at least, the response characteristics to gustatory stimulation (measured electrophysiologically) of the glossopharyngeal nerve are different from those of the chorda tympani. Cross-regeneration of these two nerves in the rat demonstrates that the pattern of response is characteristic of the region of the tongue being stimulated and not of the particular sensory nerve innervating that region.[42] The fact that there is vagal innervation of the taste system suggests a mechanism for taste directly influencing digestive functions of the gut (see below).

In spite of the importance of taste to the life of the well-adapted animal, the central projections of the sensory nerves innervating taste structures remain relatively unknown when compared to those of the visual and auditory systems. A recent review on this subject[43] emphasized the paucity of knowledge concerning these projections. Recent reports[44,45] indicate that the sensory nerves project via the nucleus of the solitary tract to a group of cells in the pontine tegmentum. These cells project to the thalamus and may be the link through which gustatory information projects to the limbic system.[44] Further study of the central projections of taste is obviously warranted and absolutely necessary if an understanding of the ultimate behavioral aspects of feeding and intake regulation is to be achieved.

THE ROLE OF TASTE IN FOOD SELECTION

One function of taste is to initiate the ingestion of food. This can provide a minimal cue to the animal as to the value and safety of a food and will additionally stimulate the flow of saliva. A diet is characteristic of the species. It has been suggested[46] that each animal species subsists on dietary choices dictated by the perceived relative palatability of the food. This relative palatability has species and even individual specificity and variability and, depending on the nutritional value or safety of the food, can take on both positive and negative connotations.[47] This specificity of diet selection at the species level leads to efficient use of the potential food sources in the environment.

Considerable pressure is exerted on one species when competition for available food sources arises with another species sharing the same food-producing habitat. This competition could be caused by natural calamities, such as climatic changes, or by the encrouchment by one species on another's territory. If both share the same very narrow ranges of food categories, as in the so-called specialists (see below), catastrophe for the less aggressive species is inevitable. If, on the other hand, both or one have a fairly large catalog of food sources, coexistence may be possible, at least at the gross species level.

The perceived palatability of a food source is, of course, under the purview of the animals' senses, particularly taste and smell. All individuals of the animal kingdom are programmed by genetics and/or experience to select foods which they perceive as palatable under the circumstances at the time of ingestion. It would be expected that the taste system in a particular animal species would serve to compliment the metabolic and dietary requirements of that species. This relationship, seemingly so obvious, has not received intensive investigation. There is some evidence that selection behavior based upon taste is complementary to physiologic need.[15,48,49] The best evidence is in the very specialized case of an adrenalectomized rat being able to select the sodium necessary to maintain life in a choice situation.[50,51]

An additional example illustrates the confounding influence that postingestional feedback (probably learning) has on this taste-nutrition relationship.[52] Rats deficient in vitamin B_1 are able to select the food which contains the B_1 vitamin from among several choices. The animals learn to select the proper diet by associating the sensory qualities of the B_1 diet with the beneficial effect. Only when the vitamin is added to a food source which has a distinctive taste or odor can the animal reliably select the diet containing the vitamin from among several choices. If the vitamin is removed from the now-preferred diet, the animals continue to select that diet, even though it is now deficient in vitamin B_1. Thus the animals make their initial choice based on the positive effects of the food and associate this with the overall sensory qualities of the diet, not the taste of the vitamin per se. This behavior was explored in further detail[53,54] and has recently been reviewed.[15,19]

Some animals have evolved as successful dietary specialists, forced by their genetic makeup to seek out, identify, and ingest only one or a very few types of food. All of their nutritional needs are obviously met by their food sources, and the problem of food selection can thus be solved at the receptor level. The limited food catalog of these specialists seems to be characterized by and coincident with a specialized receptor system (olfactory, gustatory, and visual) that is genetically programmed and unmodifiable, probably wired directly to the motor process of the feeding system. Species specificity in prey-attack behavior, for example, has been demonstrated for naive, newborn snakes of the genus *Thamnophis*.[55] These studies show that newborn snakes are more likely to show attack behavior to skin extracts of animals known to be preferred by the adult members of that species. That is, recognition for the attack behavior pattern is genetically programmed in the animal. These animals can, however, learn to avoid palatable prey if deletlrious postingestional consequences follow the ingestion of this prey.[56]

The generalist in food selection is able to obtain proper nutrition by feeding on a variety of substances. The most highly adaptable of these generalists is obviously the omnivore. His problems of food selection are mediated more often by availability than by specific metabolic need, and usually a trade off of one food for another can be made without obvious harm to the animal. Perhaps the extreme example of a successful generalist (omnivore) is the human, although food selection and ingestion is mediated in the human by factors other than the nutritional requirements of the body at the time of the meal. As has been recently suggested,[15] the generalist is also a specialist in at least two areas of food selections fulfilling the specific requirements for sodium and water.

Evidence for sodium "hunger" being innate is quite impressive.[57] For example, experiments have shown that given a choice, a salt (Na)-deprived animal can and will select sodium ion from a drinking tube within a matter of seconds and ingest sufficient sodium in a single feeding to compensate for prior depletion. This is undoubtedly a taste-mediated process since the preference for sodium is evident within seconds—long before postingestional consequences could have dictated the preference to the animal. Similar vitamin deficiences, for example, often take days for recovery.

Additionally, it has been shown[58] that rats made sodium deficient will preferentially ingest lithium chloride over water. Lithium chloride has a salty taste, and it is evident that the rats are fooled by the taste of the lithium and are not reinforced by the post-ingestional consequences of the lithium since these consequences are decidedly adverse. Gastrointestinal upset invariably follows LiCl ingestion. The taste of LiCl and NaCl are not exactly the same, however, since rats can discriminate Na from Li under appro-priate conditions.[51] Finally, there are taste receptors apparently uniquely adapted to mediating the quality "salty". The uniqueness of this taste is further evidenced by the (as far as we know) still unfruitful search for an acceptable salt (i.e., NaCl) substitute.

The specific aspects of water hunger are better understood both conceptually and mechanistically than are those of other hungers. These have recently been reviewed.[59] Thirst is a reaction to two sets of internal regulators: one that senses the tonicity of intracellular fluid and one that senses the volume of that fluid. Thirst initiates a search behavior which is extinguished only by successful identification and ingestion of water.

Every species studied thus far has exhibited considerable individual variability in response to taste stimuli. Calves varied from indifference to pronounced preference in their response to the common sugars.[60] In a litter of pigs, some were found to prefer markedly saccharine solutions while others rejected them.[61] In this experiment, a litter of eight pigs included six animals that showed a preference for saccharin and two that consistently rejected the sweetener. Sucrose-octaacetate at a concentration bitter to man is accepted by the fowl and by many other avian species.[8]

In humans a large number of studies have shown that there is a genetic dimorphism in the ability to taste the class of bitter compounds containing the chemical group $N-C=S$, the thioureas. The most commonly used stimulant of this class is the com-pound phenylthiourea. Individuals in a given population can be shown to be either sensitive to ("tasters") or relatively insensitive to ("non-tasters") the bitter taste of the thioureas (see Table 1). The taste sensitivity of a population to this class of com-pounds is different from that to other bitter compounds.[62] The genetic basis for this dimorphism appears to be due to an autosomal recessive inheritance. This phenome-non has been expoloited in many genetic and anthropological studies.[63-69] Many of the thioureas are goitrogenic, and a recent report[70] suggests that the ability to taste the goitrogens in food in a region of Ecuador where goiter is endemic may serve a protec-tive function by aiding the individual to avoid an overconsumption of goitrogenic com-pounds. Additional discussion of this protective function can be found in References 15 and 47.

There are substances known to modify the taste of gustatory stimuli, not by chang-ing the chemical or physical structures of the taste stimuli, but by modifying the func-tion of the taste organ itself. One of these taste modifiers is gymnemic acid (hexahy-droxy-triterpen) which appears as a glycoside with glucoronic acid. It has antisweet activity (for review, see Reference 71). That is, when the tongue is prewashed with a solution of gymnemic acid, the sweet taste normally elicited by such compounds as sucrose, glucose, or saccharin is abolished. A sugar cube literally has no taste.

Another taste modifier, miracle fruit or miraculin, is a protein which has the ability to generate a sweet-taste perception when a sour-taste stimulant is introduced into the mouth.[71,72] Miracle fruit protein is thus a true modifier in that it changes one percep-tual quality, sour, to another perceptual quality, sweet. Miracle fruit is not the only protein to have a gustatory stimulatory ability. At least two other proteins, one derived from the tropical berry *Dioscoreophyllum cumminsii* and called "monellin"[73] and the other derived from the tropical fruit *Thaumatococcus daniellii* and called "thaumatin",[74] have an intense, sweet taste themselves. That is, they are not taste modifiers but true taste stimuli. Functional and analytical comparisons have been made among these three proteins.[22]

For humans, taste sensations are generally classified by separating stimuli into categories of sweet, sour, salty, bitter, or no taste. For animals, one can only divide responses into dimensions of acceptance or selection, rejection or aversion, and indifference. Behavioral work with animals usually measures acceptance or rejection thresholds while electrophysiological recordings may be related to detection thresholds. Although some agreement has been found between behavioral and electrophysiological responses,[75] evidence to limit this observation is available. For example, the fowl indifferently consumes sucrose-octaacetate at levels evoking measurable electrophysiological responses (see discussion Reference in 8). The calf responds positively to sucrose, selecting a 1% solution in a choice situation, yet a 34% (1.0 M) solution is necessary to evoke a modest electrophysiological response.[41]

The assessment of what an animal can taste involves behavioral measures wherein the animal makes a choice based on, for example, a two-choice preference test[76] or operant conditioning techniques.[77] In the two-choice preference test, volumes of test solution and water (solvent) consumed are usually measured after their continuous availability for 24 hr. Using sugar solutions, it has generally been found that the volume of solution consumed under these general test conditions increases with increasing sugar concentration up to a maximum. Further increases in sugar concentration lead to decreased consumption and may, in some animals, actually result in the sugar solution becoming aversive, i.e., more water being consumed than sugar solution.

Brief-exposure (10-min), two-choice preference tests in rats show that sucrose is preferred over glucose.[78] Glucose, however, is the preferred sugar in long-term (24-hr), two-choice tests.[76] This difference in relative preference arises probably because the brief-exposure measure is less influenced by postingestional factors than the long-term exposure behavioral method. This would seem to indicate that the brief exposure test is a more valid measure of taste.

The definitions employed in brief-exposure and long-term preference tests are somewhat arbitrary. In some cases, even 24 hr can be shown to be a "brief" exposure time, especially if the primary determinants of selection are hypothesized to involve the total well-being (nutritional status) of the animal. Figure 3, for example, illustrates data from an experiment in which rats were permitted to make a choice between two diets differing in nutritional potential and taste. One diet contained defatted, raw soybeans as a protein source with the addition of sodium saccharin (appealing taste). The other contained defatted, heated soybeans with the addition of the aversive-tasting substance sucrose-octaacetate (2.0%). Raw soybean has a lower nutrition value than heated or cooked soy, primarily because of the lower digestibility of the raw soy protein and the presence of digestive enzyme inhibitors and other adverse physiological factors.[23,79] The data show (Figure 3) that for the first 5 to 6 days the rats preferred the diet with pleasant taste but poorer nutrition, while near days 6 and 7 they began to show a preference for the diet with "better" nutrition but poorer taste. This change in preference may be explicable by assuming that postingestional factors influenced the animals to eventually choose the diet which offered better nutrition even though it contained an aversive substance.[80]

On the other hand, it has been shown that rats, although preferring saccharin-sweetened water, tend to eat less of a saccharin-sweetened, solid diet during any given meal than a similar diet without saccharin adulteration.[81] This explanation does not, how-

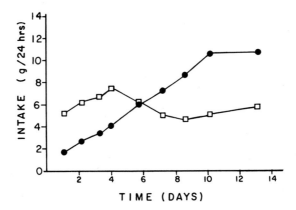

FIGURE 3.   Food intake in g/24 hr versus time in days for preference test between two diets. Diet indicated by boxes contained unground, defatted, raw soybeans plus 0.35% sodium saccharin (appealing taste), while the diet indicated by circles contained ground, defatted, heated soybean meal plus 2.0% sucrose-octaacetate (aversive taste). Both diets were continuously available over the test time period. Data points are averages from 12 rats. (Courtesy of Naim, M., Kare, M. R., and Ingle, D. E.)

ever, appear to apply to the results demonstrated by Figure 3. Here, an additional experiment with rats revealed that a diet flavored with 0.35% sodium saccharin was consistently preferred over an unflavored diet in a 2-week, 2-choice preference test. Palatability alone will not cause overeating in experimental animals, and, the theories that attempt to explain these results have been reviewed. (See, for example, References 81 to 84.)

Experiments with rats have shown that both the meal size and the intermeal intervals increase as the diet is made less palatable.[85] The total consumption by rats of a diet which contains a nonpreferred flavor is not lower than the unadulterated diet in a no-choice situation.[80] What is apparent under these conditions, then, is that the animal is literally eating to survive. The fact that his eating patterns are changing, however, indicates that he is aware of a taste problem with the food but is sufficiently motivated nutritionally that these unpalatable tastes take on secondary importance. This is not the case in all test situations, though. In some instances animals will literally starve rather than consume a diet to which they have been aversively conditioned.[86]

ASSOCIATIVE LEARNING IN TASTE AND NUTRITION

Food selection in most animals is characterized by a general neophobia, a reluctance to accept new food sources in particular. The caution displayed toward the sampling and ingestion of unique food items is in part a defensive mechanism. An animal must be certain that the food it ingests will not be poisonous. Consequently, the animal has developed rather rigid patterns of food acceptance as well as rigid standards of food quality. These deviate only as supply necessitates, and the mechanisms to carry out this deviation are for the most part inflexible.

When presented with a new food source, the animal will sample that source without ingesting a large quantity of it. Assuming the new source has a unique flavor, the animal apparently remembers that flavor when categorizing this source as novel. The ability of an animal to learn about the safety of a (new) food is well documented (for reviews, see References 15, 19, and 87; for bibliography, see Reference 88). The mechanisms involved in this learning are more obscure, although considerable progress has been made in understanding this process.[15] The learning phenomenon is generally termed "conditioned taste (or food) aversion". It is a unique form of associative learning known to occur in a wide variety of animals including man.[89,90]

The basic paradigm of food-aversion learning is quite direct. A novel taste is presented to the animal for ingestion. The novel taste might be flavored water. The animal is then exposed to an agent such as X-irradiation or the injection of a toxic drug that induces a gastrointestinal upset. The animal will subsequently avoid the novel flavor when it is next presented to him. This aversion to the flavor may last for several months, even though the pairing of the novel flavor and the sickness occurred only once. Control animals given sham irradiation or a nontoxic injection continue to ingest the flavor.

The animal has apparently associated the deleterious gastrointestinal events with the novel flavor and not with the irridiation procedure or the injection process. Similar learning has been documented to occur in humans.[90] Conditioning can be brought about with familiar foods as well as novel foods, especially if the pairing of illness with the food is made several times.[19,91]

Out of the hundreds of studies which have been performed on this learning phenomenon, several conclusions can be generated:[15]

1. Associative learning using taste as the conditioned stimulus and gastrointestinal upset as the unconditioned stimulus can occur even when the time interval between the presentation of the taste stimulus and the induction of illness is very long. This "long-delay learning" has been demonstrated for intervals of up to 12 hr,[92,93] and intervals of up to 24 hr have been reported.[94]
2. Long-delay learning involves the association of the taste or smell of the food with the gastrointestinal stimuli. No other positional or temporal factors enter into the association. This tight and unique association makes adaptive sense, since food entering via the mouth will stimulate the oral chemoreceptors and eventually produce gastrointestinal and metabolic consequences. If these consequences are deleterious, the animal needs only to associate them with the taste of the food to be able to avoid that food in the future. Association with other factors such as the food's color, position, time of day of injestion, or even temperature would only serve to unnecessarily limit the animal's choice of food sources.
3. This type of learning occurs rapidly, at times in only one trial.
4. This type of associative learning can last very long but can be eliminated (extinguished) fairly easily. For example, one can make an animal aversive to a deficient food yet can extinguish this aversion if the deficiency is corrected.

Very little experimental evidence exists indicating that humans form taste aversions as readily and via the same mechanisms as other animals. A recent paper[90] examined the frequency of food aversions in approximately 700 individuals of all ages. Food aversions were reported in 38% of all subjects. Of those reporting aversions, 87% indicated that the aversion was conditioned by a gastrointestinal upset. As in experimental animal work, visual and auditory stimuli did not serve as conditioned stimuli for this learning. In addition to showing parallels in the acquisition of this type of learning between the experimental animal literature and their survey of a human population, the authors describe additional conclusions apparently unique to the human population. Of particular interest here is their demonstration that age of the subject exerts a powerful influence on the acquisition and loss of taste aversions. Taste aversions were reported to be most common among children, and the authors delineated a critical period of ages 6 to 12 years during which aversions are acquired most readily.

Conditioned taste-aversion treatment has been attempted as a therapeutic vehicle in alcoholism and obesity. If the taste of alcohol is paired with drug-induced nausea, strong aversions have reportedly been produced.[95] As would be predicted from the experimental animal literature, pairing alcohol taste with electric shock produced no taste aversions.[90,96] Similarly, the pairing of high-caloric foods with foul odors in the treatment of obesity has reportedly produced specific aversions.[97,98] Perhaps of greater interest is the obvious parallel between the production of taste aversions in experimental animals using X-irradiation or the injection of toxic drugs and the normal course of radio- and chemotherapy in cancer treatment.[99] Is it possible that the anorexia observed so prevalently in the course of cancer[100] might at least in part be caused by disease-induced (i.e., a general visceral malaise) or therapy-induced food aversion?

THE ROLE OF TASTE IN FOOD DIGESTION

Probably because of the subjective nature of the sensory events experienced during eating, it is easy to appreciate the role that taste and smell play in food selection. Less appreciated, however, are the well-documented effects that taste and oral stimulation in general have on the systemic physiology of the organism. This interaction has received only minimal attention since the first demonstration of this phenomenon by Pavlov.[101] An outline of some of the conclusions derived from studies since then is warranted. The role of gastric and other alimentary receptors in intake regulation has recently been reviewed.[102,103]

Some of the immediate and widespread effects of oral stimulation have been documented.[104,105] These reports demonstrate that the alimentary tract, rather than being a passive canal, is actively involved in a series of anticipatory metabolic reflexes initiated by foods and fluids acting at the peripheral level. Examples of these anticipatory metabolic reflexes[104] include:

1. Changes in respiratory quotient in response to eating.
2. Hyperglycemic responses to oral stimulation with saccharin or sucrose in hungry rats (Figure 4).
3. The almost immediate (2 to 7 sec latency) increased sweating by dehydrated human subjects in a hot room when they drank fluids.
4. In rats, which were first stomach loaded with water to give a constant level of water diuresis, stimulation of the mouth with 1 to 3 ml of water, resulting in a large increase in diuresis starting within the first minute. Conversely, stimulation with 5% NaCl gave an equally immediate although much smaller inhibition of diuresis. An immediate inhibition of diuresis was also reportedly produced by eating solid foods.[106,107]

In each of the above experiments the physiological responses were extremely rapid, certainly too rapid to be due to postingestional effects. These effects were also ruled out on other grounds, such as the use of esophageal ligatures and the knowledge that the time required for metabolism of ingested glucose to carbon dioxide is on the order of hours, not minutes.[108] The metabolic changes produced by the oral stimulation were anticipatory in the sense that they preceded and were in the same direction as the changes which have been produced by the substances as a result of postabsorptive, systemic influences.

It has been recognized that oral stimulation will modify the secretory processes along the gastrointestinal tract. Pavlov and his school[101] were the first investigators to rigor-

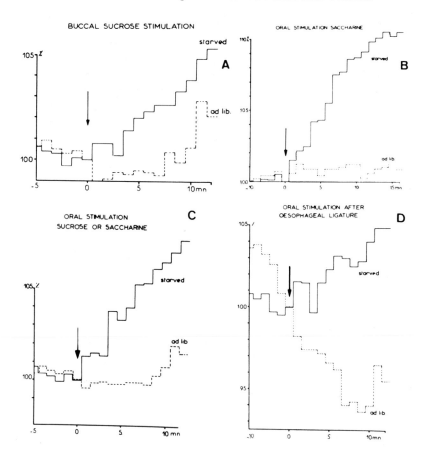

FIGURE 4.   Effect of oral stimulation by sweet-tasting substances on blood glucose
levels (as mean percent blood glucose level at zero time) in the rat. Oral stimulation
was achieved with either 30% sucrose solution (A, C, and D) or 0.01% saccharin solution (B and C) in animals fed either *ad libitum* (dashed lines) or starved for more than
5 hr (solid lines). Combined results for sucrose and saccharin are presented in graph
C. Values averaged over units of 1 min. Number of experiments: starved in A, n = 11;
in B, n = 13; in C, n = 24; in D, n = 6. *Ad lib.* in A, n = 15; in B, n = 7; in C, n = 22; in
D, n = 5. (From Nicholaidis, S., *Ann. N.Y. Acad. Sci.*, 157, 1188, 1969. With permission.)

ously study this phenomenon and demonstrated that chewing of palatable substances
by the dog initiated gastric secretion. This effect was not noted when neutral-tasting
substances were chewed. Hence it was concluded that the afferent path of the gastric
secretory reflex is similar to that for the salivary glands, namely the taste fibers.

Stimulation of gastric secretion by factors acting from the head and neck region is
termed the "cephalic phase". The stimuli for cephalic-phase release can include the
thought, expectation, sight, taste, smell, chewing, and swallowing of palatable food.
Factors evoking conditioned reflexes established by pairing of unconditioned and in-
different stimuli (light or sound) can also be effective. Interestingly, the cephalic phase
of gastric secretion is mediated entirely by the vagus. The importance of vagal nerves
was recognized by a classical demonstration in Pavlov's laboratory indicating that intact vagi were required for the cephalic-phase induction by sham feeding. Besides sham
feeding, the cephalic stimulation of gastric secretion can be elicited by insulin hypoglycemia or 2-deoxy-D-glucose glucocytopenia.[109] It was suggested that, in dogs, the
gastric response to orogastric reflexes may be excited by gustatory impulses and be
under the inhibitory control of the hypothalamic and/or tegmental areas.[110]

The stimuli-induced, neural impulses are transmitted from the cortex and subcortical area to the anterior hypothalamus, then to the medullary vagal center. These impulses then proceed via vagal nerves either directly to oxyntic glands, where they stimulate acid and pepsin secretion, or to pyloric glands where they release gastrin. The gastric secretory response to sham feeding appears after a latent period of 5 to 7 min and continues as copious acidic secretion for as long as 3 hr after the food has been eaten.[111,112] The response to sham feeding was also demonstrated in humans with an esophageal fistula and a gastric fistula, or with intubation of the esophagus by a gastrostomy tube used to drain the stomach after surgery for duodenal ulcer.[113]

It has also been shown that sham feeding of dogs and humans produces pancreatic exocrine secretions.[101,114-116] The major portion of ingested food is digested by enzymes secreted by the exocrine pancreas. These enzymes include endo- and exopeptidases, lipolytic and amylolytic enzymes, and others. Pancreatic juice is isosmotic with plasma and contains electrolytes (mainly HCO^-_3) which act in a buffering capacity against HCl from the stomach. The acidity of duodenal components is usually considered as a major controlling factor in secretin release. Secretin stimulates pancreatic flow. It is commonly assumed that oral or vagal stimulation directly results in mobilization and discharge of exocrine enzymes from the pancreas in the dog and that this response occurs 1 to 2 min after feeding and continues for approximately 30 min.[117] Pancreatic flow rate and protein output increase in dogs after sham feeding where this effect cannot be attributed to a secondary stimulation such as the passage of gastric contents into the intestine.[115]

Under normal conditions it is possible that the major effect of oral stimulation is the vagally mediated release of gastrin and acid from the stomach. For example, it has been demonstrated that gastrin can be released from the pyloric gland area by vagal activity resulting from sham feeding.[118] In addition, acidification of the antrum effectively inhibits this vagal release of gastrin.[118] The pancreatic response to vagal stimulation can also be inhibited by acidification of an innervated pouch of the pyloric gland area of the stomach in sham-fed dogs.[115]

The magnitude of a direct, neural mechanism in the pancreas remains unknown.[120] It is possible that this mechanism is relatively unimportant compared to the vagal-induced, gastric-gastrin response and other hormones that act upon the pancreas.[115,121] Perhaps both mechanisms are normally required for optimal pancreatic function.

Limited consideration has been given to the relationship between taste stimuli and gastrointestinal or pancreatic secretions. Pancreatic secretion after taste stimulation with pure compounds has recently been quantified. Various concentrations and combinations of taste stimuli have not, however, been systematically examined.

Studies of conscious dogs have indicated that both pancreatic flow and pancreatic protein output can be affected by the nature of the taste stimuli.[80,122,123] Water and a sucrose soluton mixed with a basal diet produce significantly greater stimulation of pancreatic flow and protein output than did citric acid or quinine mixed with basal diet.[122] The phenomenon of pancreatic exocrine response to appealing rather than aversive taste stimuli has been confirmed in dogs using a single taste stimulus presentation technique.[80] These results suggest that taste alone is not sufficient to affect the exocrine process. Rather, at the minimum, the swallowing process has to accompany oral stimulation in order for this mechanism to be triggered.

With respect to the regulation of the endocrine secretion of the pancreas, physiological evidence related to the disposal of ingested nutrients and direct observations obtained by means of radioimmunoassay for pancreatic hormones have revived the question of the role of the alimentary system in the regulation of pancreatic endocrine secretions. It appears that humoral and neural mechanisms involved in the control of exocrine secretion may also operate in the control of the endocrine pancreas.[124] It has been noted that glucose administered orally in man results in the development of higher blood levels of immunoreactive insulin (IRI) than those obtained when similar levels of blood glucose are produced by intravenous infusions.[125-128] In addition, the hormones important for regulating the exocrine pancreas, secretin, gastrin, and choleocystokinin were shown to cause a striking increase in insulin concentration in the pancreaticoduodenal venous plasma after their rapid, endoportal injection in anesthetized dogs.[129]

Insulin secretion during oral glucose tolerance tests in dogs occurs in several phases.[130] At least the first phase of the increase in circulating insulin (measured as IRI) at 5 to 10 min can be produced in dogs by sham feeding of glucose or tap water alone without alteration of blood glucose levels.[131] This experiment is illustrated in Figure 5. The immediate IRI increase was absent after mucosal anaesthesia of the oral cavity.[132] It was therefore assumed that at least one part of the IRI increase is initiated via receptors in the mouth.

These experiments provide dramatic evidence for the role of oral stimulation in metabolic regulation and suggest the existence of a series of "gustatory-metabolic reflexes" involved in immediate and intermediary temporal regulation of ingestion.[57,104,105] Rapid satiation of the sort provided by these reflexes is clearly functional in view of the relatively long delay before there is feedback from postabsorptive influences.

EFFECT OF CLINICAL DISEASE STATES AND AGING ON TASTE

Hypertension

A relationship between salt (primarily Na) intake and the development of or susceptibility to essential hypertension has been postulated.[133,134] This postulate has led investigators to seek a relationship between the extent of the disease and the patients' ability to taste or their disposition to select sodium chloride. An early report[135] had suggested that hypertensives consume more sodium chloride than normotensives because they cannot detect the taste of sodium chloride at levels as low as those detected by normals. This report was later confirmed and extended to include the hypothesis that genetic factors were involved in the ontogeny of essential hypertension via the development of high sodium-taste thresholds.[136] A later report on this subject[137] suggested elevated salt-recognition thresholds for hypertensives. Still other studies, however,[138-140] failed to confirm the reported differences in sodium-detection thresholds between normals and hypertensives but did show differences in salt preferences between these two groups. That is, the hypertensives as a class selected (drank) more sodium in a preference test over a 7-day period in one test and a 2-day period in another than did the normals. This preference was apparently independent of taste-detection thresholds, and limited data suggested that effective treatment for hypertension decreased the sodium preference in these patients.[140] A later study indicated that blacks as a class have higher sodium preferences than their Caucasian counterparts.[141] This finding is particularly interesting in light of the fact that blacks in the U.S. show a higher incidence of essential hypertension than do Caucasians.[142]

Cancer

Clinical evidence suggests that successful treatment of neoplastic disease is often integrally related to the diet of the patient. Agents that cause malnutrition in the cancer patient have been suggested to be general anorexia, hormonal disturbances, or other unknown mechanisms.[100] It is an accepted generalization that cancer patients who consume a nutritionally balanced diet are more likely to successfully benefit from therapy than those who remain malnourished or anorectic.[143] An alteration in taste perception

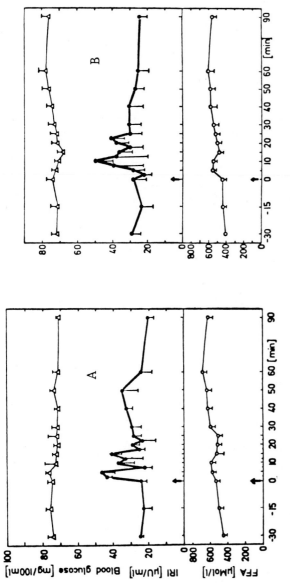

FIGURE 5.   Blood glucose levels ($\triangle$) as mg/100 ml, immunoreactive insulin ($\bullet$) as μ units/ml, and free fatty acid levels of serum ($\bigcirc$) as μ mol/l versus time before and after sham feeding of conscious dogs. Part A details the course of these three analyses with the sham feeding of 1 g of flucose per kg body weight in 50 ml of tap water (11 experiments in six animals with esophageal fistulas). Part B details the course of these three analyses with the sham feeding of 60 ml of tap water (nine experiments in five animals with esophageal fistulas). Note that sham feeding with or without taste stimuli leads to rapid, though only transitory rise in IRI and very small changes in blood glucose levels.   The arrow at zero time indicates time of stimulus delivery. (From Hommel, H., Fischer, U., Retzlaff, K., and Knöfler, H., *Diabetologia*, 8, 114, 1972. With permission.)

has been cited as a reason for the loss of interest in food often exhibited by cancer patients.[143,144]

A recent study[144,145] determined both detection and recognition thresholds for the four primary taste modalities in 50 cancer patients and 23 noncancer subjects. Decreased taste in general had been reported by 25 of the cancer patients while 16 of them reported an aversion to meat. The study found no significant differences between cancer and control patients in taste detection levels for the four primary modalities. It did report, however, that cancer patients claiming decreased taste symptom showed an elevated taste-recognition threshold for sweet, while those reporting a general meat aversion showed a lowered taste recognition threshold for bitter. A positive correlation between the extent of tumor involvement (but not tumor type) and taste abnormalities was suggested.[145] DeWys[146] has presented additional information on the involvement of taste and cancer. DeWys' results have not been confirmed.[147]

Subjective reports by cancer patients have indicated a general lessening of taste for food or at least a general reduction in the pleasurable aspects associated with food taste and eating. A model which may be applied to these patients in this instance can be suggested. A study reported that when animals are in positive energy balance, calories (i.e., metabolic properties) of ingested food take on primary importance. When an animal is in a deprived state of negative energy balance, however, the sensory properties of food (e.g., taste and smell) receive priority in regulating food intake.[82] According to this model, then, taste and other sensory properties of the food will be the primary determinants of food intake for the anorectic and cachectic cancer patient who is in negative balance. Further study on these aspects of improved nutrition for the neoplastic patient are obviously necessary.

Other Diseases

Taste problems are reportedly linked to a variety of other disease states. In many cases the single observations are unconfirmed and a significant amount of work could be carried out in the entire field of taste and clinical nutrition. Lowered thresholds have been reported in cases involving adrenal insufficiency[148,149] and cycstic fibrosis.[150] The lowered thresholds in cystic fibrosis, however, were not confirmed.[151,152] Changes in taste and smell have been reported in acute liver diseases.[153,154] Additional abnormalities in taste and smell were reported in Sjögren's syndrome (xerostomia).[155] A recent report indicates that artificially produced xerostomia in rats leads to modifications in taste preferences for salty and sour but not for sweet and bitter.[156] A congenital disorder, familia dysautonomia, has been characterized by a decrease in taste sensitivity.[157,158] General hypogusia (the lessening of the ability to taste one or more of the modalities), as well as dysgusia, is a generally reported syndrome which is apparently of multiple origin.[159] Finally, it should be noted that in general, taste thresholds in many chronic and acute debilitating diseases have been examined and found to be essentially the same as those of healthy subjects. These patients may, however, report varying changes in appetite.

Nutritional Deficiencies and Taste

The role of nutrients and their effect on taste is little understood. Since this field has recently been reviewed,[160] mention will be made here of only two deficiency states in which taste perception and food intake have been shown to be altered.

Acute vitamin A deficiency in laboratory rats leads to changes in taste preference.[161] It is suggested that this is also true for the human, but no documented evidence for this supposition has appeared. Lowered levels of zinc have also been associated with changes in and even loss of taste.[162] Hypogusia and dysgusia have reportedly been reversed in humans after therapeutic administration of zinc sulfate.[163] A recent study has shown that in a double-blind regimen, disorders of taste and smell secondary to other diseases of multiple origin did not significantly improve with zinc sulfate administration.[164] However, low systemic levels of zinc as measured in serum, urine, and saliva, were common among these patients with taste and smell abnormalities. Clearly, other mechanisms are involved in these sensory disorders,[164] and further clinical and laboratory studies should be performed to clarify these points. It is well known, for example, that zinc deficiency can produce profound changes in feeding behavior in laboratory animals, but the mechanism of this change is speculative. Systemic levels of copper have also been reportedly linked to taste changes,[160,163,165] but this is not a consistent finding.[164]

Whatever the mechanisms of these taste changes, it should be noted that both vitamin A and zinc deficiencies lead to keratinization of epithelial tissue.[166] Since taste bud cells are differentiated epithelial cells, it is likely that the overall health of these cells is likewise dependent on sufficient supplies of vitamin A and zinc. Thus taste changes associated with deficiencies of these nutrients may in fact be secondary effects of keratinization and not primary effects on the physiology of the taste mechanism. In any case, considerable study remains to be done in this area before definitive explanations of these findings are possible.

Effects of Aging on Taste

Documented evidence exists to show a dramatic decline in the number of morphologically identifiable taste buds with advancing age.[167-170] In one study, for example, the decline from middle age to old age (defined as from 74 to 85 years) was claimed to be almost 60%.[167] Evidence for a concomitant change in taste sensitivity or taste preference with advancing age is, however, contradictory. At least two studies report that while the elderly do have more complaints referrable to food and food taste than the young, these complaints could not be traced to changes in the ability of the elderly to recognize or detect the basic tastes.[171,172] Another study found changes in taste with advancing age only among a group of heavy smokers (20 cigarettes or more per day).[173] A previous study had reported no differences in taste sensitivity between smokers and nonsmokers but did report a general decline in taste sensitivity with advancing age.[174] In a recent study[175] of both detection and preference thresholds, only males in an age group of 80 to 85 showed a significant impairment relative to other groups (65 to 70 years and 40 to 45 years, male and female and 80 to 85 years, female) in the ability to detect sweet taste. No differences in preference for any of the modalities were found among the three groups. Additionally, preference ratings for sweet, sour, and bitter components of food items (commercially manufactured but varying in levels of taste-active compounds) were not significantly different among the three groups. There was, however, a slight difference in salt preference levels for the oldest male group.

Others have reported changes in taste sensitivty or preference with age. Some of these report changes in all four modalities[174,176] while others report changes in less than all four of the basic taste modalities.[141,173,178] To a large degree, much of the conflict in the literature on the subject of taste in aging can be attributed to varying testing methodologies used by the experimenters. The persistent complaints of the elderly regarding changes in food taste are well documented. Future research may attempt to relate these changes to the overall area of flavor perception, and a recent review by Schiffman addresses these problems.[179]

MECHANISMS IN TASTE RECEPTION

Knowledge of the biochemical and biophysical events that occur at the peripheral level in taste and smell is insufficient to provide complete mechanistic explanations of the phenomena. Some studies have attempted to define the biochemical and biophysical events that are linked to the transductive events of these chemoreceptive processes. One of the key ingredients necessary for the experimental verification of several contemporary theories of chemoreception[180-182] is the isolation of specific and uniquely identifiable receptor moieties. The difficulties inherent in the authentication of such receptors are appreciable.

Limited evidence to date supports the contention that a peripheral (preneural) and possibly receptor-mediated event is responsible not only for quality specificity (i.e., the ability to distinguish among sweet, sour, salty, and bitter stimuli in taste and floral, musk, sulfhydril, etc. stimuli in smell) but also quantitative intensity perceptions within a given quality, e.g., in taste, the relative sweetness of fructose versus lactose and the genetic variability in the perception of the thioureas.

One of the first experiments to deal directly with the problem of specificity was a neural cross-regeneration experiment[42] involving the two nerves that innervate the lingual taste buds: the chorda tympani which innervates the anterior portion of the tongue and the glossopharyngeal which innervates the posterior portion. The anterior portions of the (rat) tongue differ in measurable relative neural response to chemical stimuli. After cross-regeneration, electrophysiological recordings from the regenerated nerves showed that the pattern of response was characteristic of the region of the tongue being stimulated and not of the particular nerve innervating that region.

Biochemical experiments designed to measure the relative binding of ^{14}C-labeled sugars to tissue from bovine lingual papillae, one tissue type derived from taste bud material, the other from surrounding epithelium, have been reported.[183-185] The sugars bound more tightly to the materials which originated from taste papillae. In addition, the data showed that while sucrose, a highly preferred sugar behaviorally, bound tightly to taste bud tissues, lactose, a sugar to which adult cattle are less responsive,[186] bound less strongly. These studies provide direct evidence for peripheral binding specificity and suggest that the physical attachment of sweet stimuli to some peripheral entity (e.g., binding to a receptor) may be a paramount step in taste sensation. A recent report[28] has lent additional support to this hypothesis in the catfish taste system using the stimulus L—alanine.

A series of papers have reported attempts to mimic events at the receptor level by measuring various physical properties of lipid monolayers prepared from lipids extracted from bovine taste bud-containing lingual papillae. These results showed that certain physical parameters (surface tension and potentials) change as a function of either the structure of the stimulus within a quality[187,188] or as a function of the strength of a single stimulus[188,189] While some of the initial assumptions are questionable, particularly the use of bitter stimuli known to be aversive only to humans, the suggestion from this work that peripheral specificity is derived from a general rather than a specific (i.e., receptor related) property of the taste bud membrane is intriguing.

Tentative support has recently been lent to this suggestion[190] in an experiment where quinine uptake by various types of preparation of taste bud-containing and control tissue was measured. The methods used, primarily measuring quinine incorporated into a centrifuged pellet of tissue or taste bud cells, suggested a lack of binding specificity for this stimulus. This contrasts to the demonstration of binding specificity for sweet carbohydrate stimuli (see above). It is emphasized that this measure of quinine association to the tissue might be an inappropriate one, and that other, more subtle parameters such as stimulus orientation or coupled metabolic events may display peripheral specificity in bitter reception. The possibility of using fluorescent probes[191] to study the biochemical events of taste has also been suggested.[192]

Of primary interest to most studies of biochemical events of taste and smell is the question of whether there exist uniquely identifiable receptors which are responsible for initial recognition of the taste and smell stimuli. Several biochemical and electrophysiological experiments to date would suggest that these entities do exist in both taste[28,42,184,193] and smell.[194,195] A recent experiment[28] lends credence to the suggestion[29,183-185] that these receptors are contained in the plasma membrane fraction of the epithelial taste tissue. A recent volume considered some aspects of the transductive events that lead to neural discharge in taste and smell.[196]

REFERENCES

1. **Kare, M. and Maller, O., Eds.,** *The Chemical Senses and Nutrition,* Johns Hopkins Press, Baltimore, 1967.
2. **Kare, M. and Maller, O., Eds.,** *The Chemical Senses and Nutrition,* Academic Press, New York, 1977.
3. **LeMagnen, J.,** Olfaction and nutrition, in *Handbook of Sensory Physiology,* Vol. 4, Part 1, Beidler, L. M., Ed., Springer-Verlag, New York, 1971, 465—482.
4. **Mozell, M. M., Smith, B. P., Smith, P. E., Sullivan, R. L., Jr., and Swender, P.,** Nasal chemoreception in flavor identification, *Arch. Otolaryngol.,* 90, 367—373, 1969.
5. **McBurney, D. H.,** Are there primary tastes for man?, *Chem. Senses Flav.,* 1, 17—28, 1974.
6. **Pfaffmann, C., Bartoshuk, L. M., and McBurney, D. H.,** Taste psychophysics, in *Handbook of Sensory Physiology,* Vol. 4, Part 2, Beidler, L. M., Ed., Springer-Verlag, New York, 1971, 75—101.
7. **Amerine, M. A., Pangborn, R. M., and Roessler, E.,** *Principles of Sensory Evaluation of Food,* Academic Press, New York, 1965.
8. **Kare, M. R. and Rogers, J. G., Jr.,** Sense organs, in *Avian Physiology,* 3rd ed., Sturkie, P. D., Ed., Springer-Verlag, New York, 1976, 30—52.
9. **Leung, P. M. B., Larson, D. M., and Rogers, Q. R.,** Food intake and preference of olfactory bulbectomized rats fed amino acid imbalanced or deficient diets, *Physiol. Behav.,* 9, 553—557, 1972.
10. **Mugford, R.,** External influences upon the feeding of carnivores, in *The Chemical Senses and Nutrition,* Kare, M. R. and Maller, O., Eds., Academic Press, New York, 1977, 25—48.
11. **Pangborn, R. M. and Berggren, B.,** Human parotid secretion in response to pleasant and unpleasant odorants, *Psychophysiology,* 10, 231—237, 1973.
12. **Wooley, O. W., Wooley, S. C., and Williams, B. S.,** Salivation as a measure of appetite: studies of the anorectic effects of calories and amphetamine, in *Hunger: Basic Mechanisms and Clinical Implications,* Novin, D., Wyrwicka, W., and Bray, G., Eds., Raven Press, New York, 1976, 421—429.
13. **Beauchamp, G. K. and Maller, O.,** The development of flavor preferences in humans: a review, in *The Chemical Senses and Nutrition,* Kare, M. R. and Maller, O., Eds., Academic Press, New York, 1977, 291—310.
14. **Desor, J. A. and Beauchamp, G. K.,** The human capacity to transmit olfactory information, *Percept. Psychophys.,* 16, 551—556, 1974.
15. **Rozin, P.,** The selection of foods by rats, humans, and other animals, in *Advances in the Study of Behavior,* Vol. 6, Rosenblatt, J. S., Hinde, R. A., Shaw, E., and Beer, C., Eds., Academic Press, New York, 1976, 21—76.
16. **Kare, M.,** Cmparative study of taste, in *Handbook of Sensory Physiology,* Vol. 4, Part 2, Beidler, L. M., Ed., Springer-Verlag, New York, 1971, 278—292.
17. **Desor, J. A., Maller, O., and Turner, R. E.,** Taste in acceptance of sugars by human infants, *J. Comp. Physiol. Psychol.,* 84, 496—501, 1973.
18. **Desor, J. A., Maller, O., and Andrews, K.,** Ingestive responses of human newborns to salty, sour, and bitter stimuli, *J. Comp. Physiol. Psychol.,* 89, 966—970, 1975.
19. **Rozin, P. and Kalat, J.,** Specific hungers and poison avoidance as adaptive specialization of learning, *Psychol. Rev.,* 78, 459—486, 1971.
20. **Epstein, A. N.,** Oropharyngeal factors in feeding and drinking, in *Handbook of Physiology,* Vol. 1, Sect. 6, Code, C. F., Ed., American Physiological Soc., Washington, D.C., 1967, 197—218.
21. **Solms, J.,** The taste of amino acids, peptides and proteins, *J. Agric. Food Chem.,* 17, 686—688, 1969.
22. **Cagan, R. H.,** Chemostimulatory protein: a new type of taste stimulus, *Science,* 181, 32—35, 1973.
23. **Rackis, J. J., McGhee, J. E., and Hunig, D. H.,** Processing soybeans into foods: selected aspects of nutrition and flavor, *J. Am. Oil Chem. Soc.,* 52, 249A—253A, 1975.

24. **Farbman, A. I.**, Fine structure of the taste bud, *J. Ultrastruct. Res.*, 12, 328—350, 1965.
25. **Beidler, L. M. and Smallman, R. L.**, Renewal of cells within taste buds, *J. Cell Biol.*, 27, 263—272, 1965.
26. **Murray, R. G.**, The ultrastructure of taste buds, in *The Ultrastructure of Sensory Organs*, Friedmann, I., Ed., North-Holland, Amsterdam, 1973, 1—81.
27. **Guth, L.**, Degeneration and regeneration of taste buds, in *Handbook of Sensory Physiology*, Vol. 4, Part 2, Beidler, L. M., Ed., Springer-Verlag, New York, 1971, 63—74.
28. **Krueger, J. M. and Cagan, R. H.**, Biochemical studies of taste sensation. Binding of L-[^{3}H]alanine to a sedimentable fraction from catfish barbel epithelium, *J. Biol. Chem.*, 251, 88—97, 1976.
29. **Beidler, L. M.**, Taste receptor stimulation, *Prog. Biophys. Biophys. Chem.*, 12, 107—151, 1961.
30. **Oakley, B. and Benjamin, R. M.**, Neural mechanisms of taste, *Physiol. Rev.*, 46, 173—211, 1966.
31. **Zalewski, A. A.**, Changes in phosphatase enzymes following denervation of the circumvallate papilla of the rat, *Exp. Neurol.*, 22, 40—51, 1968.
32. **Zalewski, A. A.**, Role of nerve and epithelium in the regulation of alkaline phosphatase activity in gustatory papillae, *Exp. Neurol.*, 23, 18—28, 1969.
33. **Zalewski, A. A.**, Regeneration of taste buds after reinnervation by peripheral or central sensory fibers of vagal ganglia, *Exp. Neurol.*, 25, 429—437, 1969.
34. **Zalewski, A. A.**, Neurotrophic-hormonal interaction in the regulation of taste buds in the rat's vallate papilla, *J. Neurobiol.*, 1, 123—132, 1969.
35. **Zalewski, A. A.**, Regeneration of taste buds in tongue grafts after reinnervation by neurons in transplanted lumbar sensory ganglia, *Exp. Neurol.*, 40, 161—169, 1973.
36. **Kennedy, J. G.**, The effects of transsection of the glossopharyngeal nerve on the taste buds of the circumvallate papillae of the rat, *Arch. Oral Biol.*, 17, 1197—1207, 1972.
37. **Vij, S., Kanagasuntheram, R., and Krishnamurti, A.**, Enzymic changes in taste buds of monkey following transection of glossopharyngeal nerve, *J. Anat.*, 113, 425—432, 1972.
38. **Trefz, B.**, Histochemical investigation of the modal specificity of taste, *J. Dent. Res.*, 51, 1203—1211, 1972.
39. **Tsuchiya, S. and Aoki, T.**, Cholinesterase acitivities in the gustatory region of the rat tongue and their inhibition by bitter-tasting substances, *Tohoku J. Exp. Med.*, 91, 41—52, 1967.
40. **Bradley, R. M.**, Tongue topography, in *Handbook of Sensory Physiology*, Vol. 4, Part 2, Beidler, L. M., Ed., Springer-Verlag, New York, 1971, 1—30.
41. **Bernard, R.**, An electrophysiological study of taste reception in peripheral nerves of the calf, *Am. J. Physiol.*, 206, 827—835, 1964.
42. **Oakley, B.**, Altered temperature and taste responses from cross-regenerated sensory nerves in the rat's tongue, *J. Physiol.*, 188, 353—371, 1967.
43. **Burton, H. and Benjamin, R. M.**, Central projections of the gustatory system, in *Handbook of Sensory Physiology*, Vol. 4, Part 2, Beidler, L. M., Ed., Springer-Verlag, New York, 1971, 148—164.
44. **Norgren, R. and Leonard, C. M.**, Taste pathways in rat brainstem, *Science*, 173, 1136—1139, 1971.
45. **Norgren, R. and Leonard, C. M.**, Ascending central gustatory pathways, *J. Comp. Neur.*, 150, 217—237, 1973.
46. **Kare, M. R.**, Senses of animals differ from man's, *Farm Res.*, 26, 8—9, 1960.
47. **Cagan, R. H. and Kare, M. R.**, Chemical senses: influences on variability of nutritional adaptation, in *Progress in Human Nutrition, Vol. 2, The Biological and Cultural Sources of Variability in Human Nutrition*, Margen, S., and Ogan, R. A., Eds., AVI Publishing, Westport, Conn., 1978, 187—196.
48. **Maller, O.**, Specific appetite, in *The Chemical Senses and Nutrition*, Kare, M. R. and Maller, O., Eds., Johns Hopkins Press, Baltimore, 1967, 201—212.
49. **Kare, M. R. and Beauchamp, G. R.**, Taste, smell, and hearing, in *Dukes' Physiology of Domestic Animals*, 9th ed., Swanson, M., Ed., Cornell Univ. Press, Ithaca, 1977, 713—730.
50. **Richter, C. P.**, Increased salt appetitie in adrenalectomized rats, *Am. J. Physiol.*, 115, 155—161, 1936.
51. **Harriman, A. E. and Kare, M. R.**, Preference for sodium chloride over lithium chloride by adrenalectomized rats, *Am. J. Physiol.*, 207, 941—943, 1964.
52. **Harris, L. J., Clay, J., Hargreaves, F. J., and Ward, A.**, Appetite and choice of diet. The ability of the vitamin B deficient rat to discriminate between diets containing and lacking the vitamin, *Proc. R. Soc. London, Ser. B*, 113, 161—190, 1933.
53. **Rozin, P.**, Specific hunger for thiamine: recovery from deficiency and thiamine preference, *J. Comp. Physiol. Psychol.*, 59, 98—101, 1965.
54. **Rozin, P.**, Thiamine specific hunger, in *Handbook of Physiology*, Vol. 1, Sect. 6, Code, C. I. and Heidel, W., Eds., American Physiological Society, Washington, D.C., 1967, 411—431.
55. **Burghardt, G. M.**, Chemical-clue preference of inexperienced snakes: comparative aspects, *Science*, 157, 718—721, 1967.
56. **Burghardt, G. M., Wilcoxon, H. C., and Czaplicki, J. A.**, Co nditioning in garter snakes: aversion to palatable prey induced by delayed illness, *Animal Learn. Behav.*, 1, 317—320, 1973.

57. **Nachman, M. and Cole, L. P.,** Role of taste in specific hungers, in *Handbook of Sensory Physiology,* Vol. 4, Part 2, Beidler, L. M., Ed., Springer-Verlag, New York, 1971, 337—362.

58. **Nachman, M.,** Taste preferences for lithium chloride by adrenolectomized rats, *Am. J. Physiol.,* 205, 219—221, 1963.

59. **Epstein, A. N., Stellar, E., and Kissileff, H., Eds.,** *The Neurophysiology of Thirst,* Winston, Washington, D.C., 1973.

60. **Kare, M. R.,** Comparative aspects of the sense of a taste, in *Physiological Aspects of Taste,* Kare, M. R. and Halpern, B. P., Eds., Univ. Chicago Press, 1961, 6—15.

61. **Kare, M. R., Pond, W. C., and Campbell, J.,** Observations on taste reaction in pigs, *Anim. Behav.,* 13, 265—269, 1965.

62. **Fischer, R.,** Genetics and gustatory chemoreception in man and other primates, in *The Chemical Senses and Nutrition,* Kare, M. R. and Maller, O., Eds., Johns Hopkins Press, Baltimore, 1967, 61—81.

63. **Alsbirk, K. E. and Alsbirk, P. H.,** PTC taste sensitivity in Greenland Eskimos from Umanaq, *Human Hered.,* 22, 445—452, 1972.

64. **Bhalla, V.,** Variations in taste threshold for PTC in populations of Tibet and Ladakh, *Human Hered.,* 22, 453—458, 1972.

65. **Bonné, B., Ashbel, S., Berlin, G., and Sela, B.,** The habbanite isolate, *Human Hered.,* 22, 430—444, 1972.

66. **Harris, H. and Kalmus, H.,** Chemical specificity in genetical differences of taste sensitivity, *Ann. Eugen.(London),* 15, 32—45, 1949.

67. **Kalmus, H. and Smith, S. M.,** The antimode and lines of optimal separation in a genetically determined distribution with particular reference to phenylthiocarbamide sensitivity, *Ann. Hum. Gen. (London),* 29, 127—138, 1965.

68. **Kalmus, H.,** Genetics of taste, in *Handbook of Sensory Physiology,* Vol. 4, Part 2, Beidler, L. M., Ed., Springer-Verlag, New York, 1971, 165—179.

69. **Scott-Emaukpor, A. B., Uniova, J. E., and Warren, S. T.,** Genetic variation in Nigeria, *Human Hered.,* 25, 360—369, 1975.

70. **Greene, L. S.,** Physical growth and development, neurological, maturation, and behavioral functioning in two Ecuadorian Andean communities in which goiter is endemic. II. PTC taste sensitivity and neurological maturation, *Am. J. Phys. Anthropol.,* 41, 139—151, 1974.

71. **Kurihara, K.,** Taste modifiers, in *Handbook of Sensory Physiology,* Vol. 4, Part 2, Beidler, L. M., Ed., Springer-Verlag, New York, 1971, 363—378.

72. **Kurihara, K., Kurihara, Y., and Beidler, L. M.,** Isolation and mechanism of taste modifiers; taste-modifying protein and gymnemic acids, in *Olfaction and Taste, III.* Pfaffman, C., Ed., Rockefeller Univ. Press, New York, 1969, 450—469.

73. **Morris, J. A. and Cagan, R. H.,** Purification of monellin, the sweet principle of *Dioscoreophyllum cumminsii, Biochim. Biophys. Acta,* 261, 114—122, 1972.

74. **Van Der Wel, H. and Loeve, K.,** Isolation and characterization of Thaumatin I and II, the sweet-tasting proteins from *Thaumatococcus daniellii* Benth, *Eur. J. Biochem.,* 31, 221—225, 1972.

75. **Koh, S. D. and Teitelbaum, P.,** Absolute behavioral taste thresholds in the rat, *J. Comp. Physiol. Psychol.,* 54, 223—229, 1961.

76. **Richter, C. P. and Campbell, K. H.,** Taste thresholds and taste preferences of rats for five common sugars, *J. Nutr.,* 20, 31—46, 1940.

77. **Ferster, G. B. and Skinner, B. F.,** *Schedules of Reinforcement,* Appleton-Century Crofts, New York, 1957.

78. **Cagan, R. H. and Maller, O.,** Taste of sugars: brief exposure single-stimulus behavioral method, *J. Comp. Physiol. Psychol.,* 87, 47—55, 1974.

79. **Gertler, A., Birk, Y., and Bondi, A.,** A comparative study of the nutritional and physiological significance of pure soybean trypsin inhibitors and of ethanol-extracted soybean meals in chicks and rats, *J. Nutr.,* 91, 358—370, 1967.

80. **Naim, M. and Kare, M. R.,** Taste stimuli and pancreatic functions, in *The Chemical Senses and Nutrition,* Kare, M. R. and Maller, O., Eds., Academic Press, New York, 1977, 145—162.

81. **Gentile, R. L.,** Depression of intake by saccharin adulteration: the role of taste quality in the control of food intake, in *Olfaction and Taste III,* Pfaffmann, C., Ed., Rockefeller University Press, New York, 1969, 601—607.

82. **Jacobs, H. L. and Sharma, K. N.,** Taste vs. calories: sensory and metabolic signals in the control of food intake, *Ann. N.Y. Acad. Sci.,* 157, 1084—1125, 1969.

83. **Mook, D. G.,** Saccharin preference in the rat: some unplatable findings, *Psychol. Rev.,* 81, 475—490, 1974.

84. **Davis, J. D., Collins, B. J., and Levine, M. W.,** Peripheral control of meal size: interaction of gustatory stimulation and postingestional feedback, in *Hunger: Basic Mechanisms and Clinical Implications,* Novin, D., Wyrwicka, W., and Bray, G., Eds., Raven Press, New York, 1976, 395—408.

85. Gentile, R. L., The role of taste preference in the eating behavior of the albino rat, *Physiol. Behav.*, 5, 311—316, 1970.
86. Richter, C. P., Experimentally produced behavior reactions to food poisoning in wild and domesticated rats, *Ann. N.Y. Acad. Sci.*, 56, 225—239, 1953.
87. Smith, J. C., Radiation: its detection and its effects on taste preferences, in *Progress in Physiological Psychology*, Stellar, E. and Sprague, J. M., Eds., Academic Press, New York, 1971, 53—118.
88. Riley, A. L. and Baril, L. L., Conditioned taste aversions: a bibliography, *Animal Learn. Behav.*, 4, 1S—13S, 1976.
89. Seligman, M. E. P., On the generality of the laws of learning, *Psychol. Rev.*, 77, 400—418, 1970.
90. Garb, J. L. and Stunkard, A. J., Taste aversions in man, *Am. J. Psychiatry*, 131, 1204—1207, 1974.
91. Brackbill, R. and Brookshire, A., Conditioned taste aversions as a function of the number of CS—US pairs, *Psychonomic Sci. Sect. Anim. Physiol. Psychol.*, 22, 25—26, 1971.
92. Smith, J. C. and Roll, D. L., Trace conditioning with X-rays as an aversion stimulus, *Psychonomic Sci. Sect. Anim. Physiol. Psychol.*, 9, 11—12, 1967.
93. Stephens, R. M. and Etscorn, F. T., Bait-shyness in mice with a 12-hour CS-US interval, Paper presented to Kentucky Psychological Association, Barren River, Kentucky, November, 1972.
94. Etscorn, F. and Stephens, R., Establishment of conditioned taste aversions with a 24-hour CS-US interval, *Physiol. Psychol.*, 1, 251—253, 1973.
95. Lemere, F. and Voegtlin, W. L., An evaluation of the aversion treatment of alcoholism, *Q. J. Stud. Alcohol*, 11, 199—204, 1950.
96. MacCulloch, M. J., Feldman, M. P., Orford, J. F., and MacCulloch, M. L., Anticipatory avoidance learning in the treatment of alcoholism: a record of therapeutic failure, *Behav. Res. Ther.*, 4, 187—196, 1966.
97. Kennedy, W. A. and Foreyt, J. P., Control of eating behavior in an obese patient by avoidance conditioning, *Psychol. Rep.*, 22, 571—576, 1968.
98. Foreyt, J. P. and Kennedy, W. A., Treatment of overweight by aversion therapy, *Behav. Res. Ther.*, 9, 29—34, 1971.
99. Bernstein, I. L., Learned taste aversions in children receiving chemotherapy, *Science*, 200, 1302—1303, 1978.
100. Cuddy, R., *The Role of Diet in Cancer Therapy*, Report No. 17, Program Analysis and Evaluation Branch, Division of Cancer Resources and Centers, National Cancer Institute, NIH, Bethesda, MD., 1975.
101. Pavlov, I. P., *The Work of the Digestive Glands*, 2nd ed., translated by Thompson, W. H., Charles Griffin, London, 1910.
102. Sharma, K. N., Alimentary receptors and food intake regulation, in *The Chemical Senses and Nutrition*, Kare, M. R. and Maller, O., Eds., Johns Hopkins Press, Baltimore, 1967, 281—291.
103. Sharma, K. N., Jacobs, H. L., Gopal, V., and Dua-Sharma, S., Nutritional state/taste interactions in food intake: behavior and physiological evidence for gastric/taste modulation, in *The Chemical Senses and Nutrition*, Kare, M. R. and Maller, O., Eds., Academic Press, New York, 1977, 167—187.
104. Nicolaidis, S., Early systemic responses to orogastric stimulation in the regulation of food and water balance: functional and electrophysiological data, *Ann. N.Y. Acad. Sci.*, 157, 1176—1200, 1969.
105. Nicolaidis, S., Sensory-neuroendocrine reflexes and their anticipatory and optimizing role on metabolism, in *The Chemical Senses and Nutrition*, Kare, M. R. and Maller, O., Eds., Academic Press, New York, 1977, 123—140.
106. Kakolewski, J. W., Cox, V. C., and Valenstein, E. S., Short-latency antidiuresis following the initiation of food ingestion, *Science*, 162, 458—460, 1968.
107. Kakolewski, J. W. and Valenstein, E. S., Antidiuresis associated with the ingestion of food substances, in *Olfaction and Taste III*, Pfaffmann, C., Ed., Rockefeller Univ. Press, New York, 1969, 593—600.
108. Wang, C. H., Snipper, L. P., Bilen, O., and Hawthorne, B., Catabolism of glucose and gluconate in rats, *Proc. Soc. Exp. Biol. Med.*, 111, 93—97, 1962.
109. Hirschowitz, B. I. and Sachs, G., Vagal gastric secretory stimulation by 2-deoxy-D-glucose, *Am. J. Physiol.*, 209, 452—460, 1965.
110. Langlois, K. J., Lim, R. K., Rosiere, G., Stewart, D. I., and Stumpff, D. L., Unconditioned orogastric secretory reflex, *Fed. Proc.*, 11, 88—89, 1952.
111. Brooks, F. P., Central neural control of acid secretion, in *Handbook of Physiology*, Vol. 2, Sect. 6, Code, C. F., Ed., American Physiological Association, Washington, D. C., 1967, 805—826.
112. Olbe, L., Esophageal cannula dog, a simple mode of preparation for sham feeding experiments, *Gastroenterology*, 37, 460—462, 1959.
113. Knutson, U. and Olbe, L., Significance of antrum in gastric acid response to sham feeding in duodenal ulcer patients, in *Gastrointestinal Hormones and Other Subjects*, Thaysen, E. H., Ed., Munksgaard, Copenhagen, 1971, 25—28.

114. Sarles, H., Dani, R., Prezelin, G., Souville, C., and Figarella, C., Cephalic phase of pancreatic secretion in man, *Gut*, 9, 214—221, 1968.

115. Preshaw, R. M., Cooke, A. R., and Grossman, M. I., Sham feeding and pancreatic secretion in the dog, *Gastroenterology*, 50, 171—178, 1966.

116. Novis, B. H., Banks, S., and Marks, I. N., The cephalic phase of pancreatic secretion in man, *Scand. J. Gastroenterol.*, 6, 417—421, 1971.

117. Gregory, R. A., *Secretory Mechanisms of Gastrointestinal Tract*, Monogr. Physiol. Soc., No. 11, Edward Arnold, London, 1962.

118. Pe Thein, M. and Schofield, B., Release of gastrin from the pyloric antrum following vagal stimulation by sham feeding in dogs, *J. Physiol (London)*, 148, 291—305, 1959.

119. Chisholm, C. J., Young, J. D., and Lazarus, L., The gastrointestinal stimulus to insulin release, *J. Clin. Invest.*, 48, 1453—1460, 1969.

120. Crittenden, P. J. and Ivy, A. C., The nervous control of pancreatic secretion in the dogs, *Am. J. Physiol.*, 119, 724—733, 1937.

121. Brooks, F. P., The neurohumoral control of pancreatic exocrine secretion, *Am. J. Clin. Nutr.*, 26, 291—309, 1973.

122. Behrman, H. R. and Kare, M. R., Canine pancreatic secretion in response to acceptable and aversive taste stimuli, *Proc. Soc. Exp. Biol. Med.*, 129, 343—346, 1968.

123. Naim, M., Kare, M. R., and Merritt, A. M., Effects of oral stimulation on the cephalic phase of pancreatic exocrine secretion in dogs, Physiol. Behav., 20, 563—570, 1978.

124. Dupré, J., Regulation of the secretions of the pancreas, *Ann. Rev. Med.*, 21, 299—316, 1970.

125. McIntyre, N., Hodsworth, C. D., and Turner, D. S., New interpretations of oral glucose tolerance, *Lancet*, 20—21, 1964.

126. Elrick, H., Stimmler, L., Hlad, C. J., and Arai, Y., Plasma insulin response to oral and intravenous glucose administration, *J. Clin. Endocrinol.*, 24, 1076—1082, 1964.

127. Perley, M. J. and Kipnis, D. M., Plasma insulin response to oral and intravenous glucose. Studies in normal and diabetic subjects, *J. Clin. Invest.*, 46, 1954—1961, 1967.

128. Kipnis, D. M., Nutrient regulation of insulin secretion in human subjects, *Diabetes*, (Suppl.), 21, 606—616, 1972.

129. Unger, R. H., Ketterer, H., Dupré, J., and Eisentraut, A. M., The effects of secretin, pancreozymin, and gastrin on insulin and glucagon secretion in anesthetized dogs, *J. Clin. Invest.*, 46, 630—645, 1967.

130. Fischer, U., Hommel, H., Ziegler, M., and Michael, R., The mechanism of insulin secretion after oral administration. I. Multiphasic course of insulin mobilization after oral administration of glucose in conscious dogs. Differences in the behavior after intravenous administration, *Diabetologia*, 8, 104—110, 1972.

131. Hommel, H., Fischer, U., Retzlaff, L., and Knöfler, H., The mechanism of insulin secretion after oral glucose administration. II. Reflex insulin secretion in conscious dogs bearing fistulas of the digestive tract by sham-feeding of glucose or tap water, *Diabetologia*, 8, 111—116, 1972.

132. Fischer, U., Hommel, H., Ziegler, M., and Jutzi, E., The mechanism of insulin secretion after oral administration. III. Investigations on the mechanism of a reflectoric insulin mobilization after oral stimulation, *Diabetologia*, 8, 385—390, 1972.

133. Dahl, L. K. and Love, R. A., Etiological role of sodium chloride intake in essential hypertension in humans, *JAMA*, 164, 397—400, 1957.

134. Meneely, G. R. and Dahl, L. K., Electrolytes in hypertension: the effects of sodium chloride, *Med. Clin. North Am.*, 45, 271—283, 1961.

135. Fallis, N., Lasagna, L., and Tétreault, L., Gustatory thresholds in patients with hypertension, *Nature*, 196, 74—75, 1962.

136. Bisht, D. B., Krishnamurthy, M., and Rangaswamy, R., Studies on threshold of taste for salt with special reference to hypertension, *Indian Heart J.*, 23, 137—140, 1971.

137. Wotman, S., Mandel, I. D., Thompson, R. H., and Laragh, J. H., Salivary electrolytes and salt taste thresholds in hypertension, *J. Chron. Dis.*, 20, 833—840, 1967.

138. Schechter, P. J., Horwitz, D., and Henkin, R. I., Sodium chloride preference in essential hypertension, *JAMA*, 225, 1311—1315, 1973.

139. Schechter, P. J., Horwitz, D., and Henkin, R. I., Salt preference in patients with untreated and treated essential hypertension, *Am. J. Med. Sci.*, 267, 320—326, 1974.

140. Henkin, R. I., Salt taste in patients with essential hypertension and with hypertension due to primary hyperaldosteronism, *J. Chron. Dis.*, 27, 235—244, 1974.

141. Desor, J. A., Greene, L. S., and Maller, O., Preferences for sweet and salty in 9- to 15-year-old and adult humans, *Science*, 190, 686—687, 1975.

142. Stamler, J., Stamler, R., and Pullman, T., *The Epidemiology of Hypertension*, Grune and Stratton, New York, 1967.

143. Gori, G. B., The diet, nutrition, and cancer program of the NCI National Cancer Program, *Cancer Res.*, 35, 3545—3547, 1975.
144. DeWys, W. D., Abnormalities of taste as a remote effect of a neoplasm, *Ann. N.Y. Acad. Sci.*, 230, 427—434, 1974.
145. DeWys, W. D. and Walters, K., Abnormalities of taste sensation in cancer patients, *Cancer*, 136, 1888—1896, 1975.
146. DeWys, W. D., Changes in taste sensation in cancer patients: correlation with caloric intake, in *The Chemical Senses and Nutrition*, Kare, M. R. and Maller, O., Eds., Academic Press, New York, 1977, 381—389.
147. Settle, R. G., Quinn, M. R., Brand, J. G., Kare, M. R., Mullins, J. L., and Brown, R., Gustatory evaluation of cancer patients: preliminary results, in *Nutrition and Cancer*, Van Eyes, J., Seelig, M. S., and Nichols, B. L., Eds., SP Medical & Scientific Books, New York, 1979, 171—185.
148. Henkin, R. I. and Solomon, D. H., Salt-taste threshold in adrenal insufficiency in man, *J. Clin. Endocrinol. Metab.*, 22, 856—858, 1962.
149. Henkin, R. I., Abnormalities of taste and olfaction in various disease states, in *The Chemical Senses and Nutrition*, Kare, M. R. and Maller, O., Eds., Johns Hopkins Press, Baltimore, 1967, 95—113.
150. Henkin, R. I. and Powell, G. F., Increased sensitivity of taste and smell in cystic fibrosis, *Science*, 1107—1108, 1962.
151. Wotman, S., Mandel, I. D., Khotim, S., Thompson, R. H., Kutscher, A. H., Zegarelli, E. V., and Denning, C. R., Salt taste thresholds and cystic fibrosis, *Am. J. Dis. Child.*, 108, 372—374, 1964.
152. Desor, J. A. and Maller, O., Taste correlates of disease states: cystic fibrosis, *J. Pediatr.*, 87, 93—96, 1975.
153. Henkin, R. I. and Smith, F. R., Hyposmia in acute viral hepatitis, *Lancet*, 823—826, 1971.
154. Smith, F. R., Henkin, R. I., and Dell, R. B., Disordered gustatory acuity in liver disease, *Gastroenterology*, 70, 568—571, 1976.
155. Henkin, R. I., Talal, N., Larson, A. L., and Mattern, C. F. T., Abnormalities of taste and smell in Sjögren's syndrome, *Ann. Intern. Med.*, 76, 375—383, 1972.
156. Galili, D. and Maller, O., Xerostomia and taste preference, *J. Dent. Res.*, (special issue B), Abs. No. 1049, 1976.
157. Smith, A. A. and Dancis, J., Taste discrimination in familial dysautonomia, *Pediatrics*, 33, 441—443, 1964.
158. Henkin, R. I., On the mechanism of the taste defect in familial dysautonomia, in *Olfaction and Taste II*, Hayashi, T., Ed., Pergamon Press, New York, 1967, 321—335.
159. Henkin, R. I., Schechter, P. J., Hoye, R., Mattern, C. F. T., Idiopathic hypoguesia with dysgusesia, hyposmia and dysosmia: a new syndrome, *JAMA*, 217, 434—440, 1971.
160. Gershoff, S., The role of vitamins and minerals on taste and smell, in *The Chemical Senses and Nutrition*, Kare, M. R. and Maller, O., Eds., Academic Press, New York, 1977, 201—210.
161. Bernard, R. A. and Halpern, B. P., Taste changes in vitamin A deficiency, *J. Gen. Physiol.*, 52, 444—464, 1968.
162. Henkin, R. I., Patten, B. M., Re, P. K., and Bronzert, D. A., A syndrome of acute zinc loss. Cerebellar dysfunction, mental changes, anorexia, and taste and smell dysfunction, *Arch. Neurol.*, 32, 745—751, 1975.
163. Schechter, P. J., Friedewald, W. T., Bronzert, D. A., Raff, M. S., and Henkin, R. I., Idiopathic hypogeusia: a description of the syndrome and a single blind study with zinc sulfate, *Int. Rev. Neurobiol.*, Suppl. 1, Academic Press, New York, 125—140, 1972.
164. Henkin, R. I., Schecter, P. J., Friedewald, W. T., Demets, D. L., and Raff, M., A double blind study of the effects of zinc sulfate on taste and smell dysfunction, *Am. J. Med. Sci.*, 272, 285—299, 1976.
165. Henkin, R. I., Keiser, H. R., Jaffe, I. A., Sternlieb, I., and Scheinberg, I. H., Decreased taste sensitivity after D-penicillamine reversed by copper administration, *Lancet*, 2, 1268—1271, 1967.
166. Pike, R. L. and Brown, M. L., *Nutrition: An Integrated Approach*, 2nd ed., John Wiley & Sons, New York, 1975, 145—146 and 206—207.
167. Arey, L. B., Tremaine, M. J., and Monzingo, F. L., The numerical and topographical relations of taste buds to human circumvallate papillae throughout the life span, *Anat. Rec.*, 64 (Suppl. 1), 9—25, 1935.
168. Mochizuki, Y., An observation on the numerical and topographical relations of taste buds to circumvallate papillae of Japanese, *Okajimas Folia Anat. Jpn.* 15, 595—608, 1937.
169. Mochizuki, Y., Studies on the papillae foliata of Japanese. II. The number of taste buds, *Okajimas Folia Anat. Jpn.* 18, 355—369, 1939.
170. Jurisch, A., Studien über die Papillae Vallatae beim Menschen, *Z. Ges. Anat. (Abt. 1)*, 66, 1—149, 1922.
171. Cohen, T. and Gitman, L., Oral complaints and taste perception in the aged, *J. Gerontol.*, 14, 294—298, 1959.

172. Byrd, E. and Gertman, S., Taste sensitivity in aging persons, *Geriatrics,* 14, 381—384, 1959.
173. Kaplan, A. R., Glanville, E. V., and Fischer, R., Cumulative effect of age and smoking on taste sensitivity in males and females, *J. Gerontol.,* 20, 334—337, 1965.
174. Zubek, J. P., Intellectual and sensory processes in the aged, *MDSJ Med. Serv. J.* (Canada), 15, 731—733, 1959.
175. Kare, M. R., Changes in taste with age — infancy to senescence, *Food Tech.,* 29 (8), 78 (abstract), 1975.
176. Cooper, R. M., Bilash, I., and Zubek, J. P., The effect of age on taste sensitivity, *J. Gerontol.,* 14, 56—58, 1959.
177. Glanville, E. V., Kaplan, A. R., and Fischer, R., Age, sex, and taste sensitivity, *J. Gerontol.,* 19, 474—478, 1964.
178. Kalmus, H. and Trotter, W. R., Direct assessment of the effect of age on P.T.C. sensitivity, *Ann. Hum. Genet. (London),* 26, 145—149, 1962.
179. Schiffman, S., Changes in taste and smell with age: psychophysical aspects, in Sensory Systems and Communication in the Elderly, Ordy, J. M. and Brizzee, K., Eds., Raven Press, New York, 1979, 227—246.
180. Baradi, A. F. and Bourne, G. H., Localization of gustatory and olfactory enzymes in the rabbit, and the problems of taste and smell, *Nature,* 168, 977—979, 1951.
181. Beidler, L. M., A theory of taste stimulation, *J. Gen. Physiol.,* 38, 133—139, 1954.
182. Heck, G. L. and Erickson, R. P., A rate theory of gustatory stimulation, *Behav. Biol.,* 8, 687—712, 1973.
183. Cagan, R. H., Biochemical studies of taste sensation. I. Binding of ^{14}C-labeled sugars to bovine taste papillae, *Biochim. Biophys. Acta.,* 252, 199—206, 1971.
184. Cagan, R. H., Biochemistry of sweet sensation, in *Sugars in Nutrition,* Sipple, H. L. and McNutt, K. W., Eds., Academic Press, New York, 1974, 19—36.
185. Lum, C. K. L. and Henkin, R. I., Sugar binding to purified fractions from bovine taste buds and epithelial tissue, *Biochim. Biophys. Acta,* 421, 380—394, 1976.
186. Kare, M. R. and Ficken, M. S., Comparative studies on the sense of taste, in *Olfaction and Taste,* Zotterman, Y., Ed., Pergamon Press, Oxford, 1963, 285—297.
187. Koyama, N. and Kurihara, K., Mechanism of bitter taste reception: interaction of bitter compounds with monolayers of lipids from bovine circumvallate papillae, *Biochim. Biophys. Acta,* 288, 22—26, 1972.
188. Kurihara, K., Koyama, N., and Kurihara, Y., Chemical architecture and model systems of gustatory and olfactory receptor membrane, in *Olfaction and Taste IV,* Schneider, D., Ed., Wissenschafliche Verlagsgesellschaft, Stuttgart, 1972, 234—240.
189. Miyake, M., Kamo, N., Kurihara, K., and Kobatake, Y., Physico-chemical studies of taste reception. IV. Response of individual phospholipid membrane to a variety of chemical stimuli, *J. Membr. Biol.,* 22, 197—209, 1975.
190. Brand, J. G., Zeeberg, B. R., and Cagan, R. H., Biochemical studies of taste sensation. V. Binding of quinine to bovine taste papillae and taste bud cells, *Int. J. Neurosci.,* 7, 37—43, 1976.
191. Radda, G. K. and Vanderkooi, J., Can fluorescent probes tell us anything about membranes?, *Biochim. Biophys. Acta,* 265, 509—549, 1972.
192. Brand, J. G. and Cagan, R. H., Biochemical studies of taste sensation. III. Preparation of a suspension of bovine taste bud cells and their labeling with a fluorescent probe, *J. Neurobiol.,* 7, 205—220, 1976.
193. Noma, A. and Hiji, Y., Effects of chemical modifiers on taste responses in the rat chorda tympani, *Jpn. J. Physiol.,* 22, 393—401, 1972.
194. Cagan, R. H., and Zeiger, W. N., Biochemical studies of olfaction: binding specificity of radioactively labeled stimuli to an isolated olfactory preparation from rainbow trout, *Proc. Natl. Acad. Sci. U.S.A.,* 75, 4679—4683, 1978.
195. Getchell, M. L. and Gesteland, R. C., The chemistry of olfactory reception: stimulus-specific protection from sulfhydryl reagent inhibition, *Proc. Natl. Acad. Sci. U.S.A.,* 69, 1494—1498, 1972.
196. Cagan, R. H. and Kare, M. R., Eds., *The Biochemistry of Taste and Olfaction,* Academic Press, New York, 1981.
197. Morris, J. A., Sweetening agents from natural sources, *Lloydia,* 39, 25—38, 1976.
198. Stone, H. and Oliver, S. M., Measurement of the relative sweetness of selected sweetners and sweetner mixtures, *J. Food Sci.,* 34, 215—222, 1969.
199. Desor, J. A. and Brand J. G., unpublished observations, University of Pennsylvania, Philadelphia, 1973.
200. Anon., *Bitrex*^{R}, Information Sheet No. 1, Macfarlan Smith, Ltd., Edinburgh, 1967.
201. Moscowitz, H., The psychology of sweetness, in *Sugars in Nutrition,* Sipple, H. L. and McNutt, K. W., Eds., Academic Press, New York, 1974, 37—64.

202. **Jacobs, W. W. and Beauchamp, G. K.**, Glucose preferences in wild and domestic guinea pigs, *Physiol. Behav.*, 18, 491—493, 1977.
203. **Bauer, F. S.**, Glucose preference in the guinea pig, *Physiol. Behav.*, 6, 75—76, 1971.
204. **Kennedy, J. M. and Baldwin, B. A.**, Taste preferences in pigs for nutritive and non-nutritive sweet solutions, *Anim. Behav.*, 20, 706—718, 1972.
205. **Goatcher, W. D. and Church, D. C.**, Taste responses in ruminants. I. Reactions of sheep to sugars, saccharin, ethanol, and salts, *J. Anim. Sci.*, 30, 777—783, 1970.
206. **Bloom, J. C., Rogers, J. G., Jr., and Maller, O.**, Taste responses of the North American porcupine (*Erethizon dorsatum*), *Physiol. Behav.*, 11, 95—98, 1973.
207. **Denton, D. A. and Coghlan, J. P., Eds.**, *Olfaction and Taste V*, Academic Press, New York, 1975.
208. **Lepkovsky, S.**, The role of the chemical senses in nutrition, in *The Chemical Senses and Nutrition*, Kare, M. R. and Maller, O., Eds., Academic Press, New York, 1977, 413—427.
209. **Bartoshuk, L. M., Jacobs, H. L., Nichols, T. L., Hoff, L. A., and Ryckman, J. J.**, Taste rejection of non-nutritive sweetners in cats, *J. Comp. Physiol. Psychol.*, 89, 971—975, 1975.

OLFACTION AND NUTRITION

J. Le Magnen

INTRODUCTION

In the animal kingdom, nutrition, and therefore the growth and survival of animals and their species, are primarily dependent on ingestive behaviors. The ability of animals of various species to feed their young and themselves and to control in regulatory behavior the selection and consumption of an adequate amount of nutrients was and is still one of the most effective factors in selection. Such an evolutionary process led to the phylogenetic emergence in various species of sensory and central control systems of behavior finely adapted to the most efficient drive of feeding and drinking activities.

In the nutritive process, materials in the environment that are sought and eaten, and as such are defined as foods, act successively on the body at four different levels through a variety of their biochemical properties. Outside, the foodstuff acts on various sensory telereceptors, i.e., sight, nasal olfaction, through its stimulating properties with these receptors (through the receptor's sensitivity to some of the food's physical or chemical characteristics). Taken in the mouth, where it is simultaneously chewed and mixed with saliva, the food at this level is again sensorily controlled by its action on oral chemo- and mechanoreceptors. Present in the oral cavity, the food — through volatile compounds — again stimulates olfactory receptors via the retronasal or pharyngeal pathways. Reaching the gastrointestinal tract, the food, acting through a series of properties that differ from those involved in upper sensory control, begins to be digested and absorbed. Finally, as a metabolite and through its nutritive properties, the nutriment feeds the various metabolic pathways.

Three questions are raised by the interaction among these four levels:

1. What is the role of the oropharyngeal sensory receptors (particularly in this section of olfactory receptors) in a preingestive sensory analysis of the food?

2. What is the mechanism by which this sensory analysis leads to food selection and consumption adjusted to nutritional and bodily needs?

3. What is the role of postingestive events and the nutritive properties of foods in the sensory-mediated selection and consumption of foods?

OLFACTORY CHEMORECEPTION

The peripheral olfactory organs are bilaterally situated in mammals in the upper part of the nasal chamber. The sensory neuroepithelium includes the sensory cell bodies inserted between interstitial cells. From cell bodies, dendritic expansions are terminated at the surface of the neuroepithelium by ciliated vesicles. The dense layer of these olfactory cilia, bathed in aqueous mucus, is the sensory field of the chemoreception. In the brain, axons of the sensory neurons, as fibers of the olfactory nerve, reach the first synaptic relay within the olfactory bulb. Afferent and efferent fiber pathways from and to the olfactory bulbs connect the first central olfactory relay to other specific projections in the "visceral brain:" the rhinencephalon and the hypothalamus. In addition, the two olfactory bulbs are interconnected through the anterior commissure and the anterior olfactory nuclei.

A very large number of chemically defined pure molecules stimulates olfactory receptors and gives rise to an odor perception. In air-living organisms, the stimulating molecules are transported in gaseous phase up to the sensory organ either through the nasal or pharyngeal pathways.

Three functional characteristics of the olfactory chemoreception differ from, and are complementary to, the taste chemoreception:

1. The extremely low detection thresholds
2. The level of differentiation of stimuli reaching the identification of each particular odorant by its specific odor
3. The functional properties of the olfactory apparatus as telereceptor of airborne stimulants, allowing, among other consequences, some spatial localization of odor sources.

Before studying the role of these functional characteristics of odor detection and discrimination in nutrition and food selection and consumption, it is useful to review our present knowledge of the nature of odorous components of food flavors.

ODOROUS COMPOUNDS IN FOODS

Using gas-liquid chromatography associated with mass spectrography analysis, investigation into the separation and qualitative analysis of volatile fractions suspected to be the source of the specific flavor or aroma of natural foods has been carried out during the past 15 years. Such flavor analyses were conducted on fruits, vegetables, dairy and meat products, fats, and transformed foodstuffs and beverages, etc. A very important body of literature is available on this growing field of chemical investigations, and provides evidence for the following facts:

1. Most aromas of natural and processed food products are due to the combined action of a mixture of a number of volatile and more or less odorous compounds. The number of different compounds separated by the physicochemical analysis is limited with some products such as milk and some fruits; it is extremely high for others. More than 200 different peaks have been identified in the crude aroma of some fruits (strawberry, for example), and about 1000 have been identified in the aroma of coffee.
2. Most of the chemical fractions, potentially important in the global flavor, were shown to be present in the food product in very small amounts.
3. The chemical identification of these compounds pointed out their extreme variety. In addition to aldehydes, alcohols, and esters of the aromatic series, many cyclic compounds (many of them previously unknown in nature) were found.
4. These chemicals providing food flavor are not generally the nutritive components of the food products, and, from a nutritional point of view, may be considered impurities. Carbohydrates are neither volatile nor odorant. Proteins and triglycerides give rise to very odorous breakdown products. They are per se devoid of both a unique and specific odor as proteins or fats (comparable to the sweet taste of sugars) and of any individual flavor in their highly purified form.

The participation of these compounds in the flavor is dependent on both their species and the olfactory chemoreceptivity.

OLFACTORY ANALYSIS AND ODOR ASSESSMENT OF AROMAS

A distortion exists between the biochemical analysis of molecules performed by the olfactory system and a chemist's assessment of the same molecules. The odorous efficiency of a molecule is at first extrinsically dependent on its vapor pressure or relative volatility at the temperature of the source. Various odorants present in the solid or liquid food product will contribute to the active gaseous mixture in proportion to their respective volatilities. The sampling of this gaseous mixture at 37° in the head space procedure of the chromatographic technique of analysis corrects this extrinsic distortion.

As is well known, when expressed in terms of dilution in air, the odorous efficiency measured by the threshold in man is extremely variable and displays no evident correlation to physicochemical properties. Many compounds are odorless at the saturation vapor pressure; others are still active at a dilution as low as 10^{-12} to 10^{-13}. Published tables of human olfactory thresholds measured on a limited number of molecules belonging to various chemical families (200 to 300 compounds) show this wide variability of odorous efficiencies (Figure 1). Such a distribution also confirms that the olfactory threshold for many compounds is very low. Some theoretical calculation permits the inference that less than 1000 molecules of the most active compounds acting on each olfactory receptor cell are involved in stimulating the neural response at the threshold level.

Many attempts have been made to relate the odorous activity to physicochemical properties other than the uncorrelated common chemical functions. The most advanced study of this structure-activity relationship is being performed by Laffort and co-workers.[1] They have shown that it is possible to accurately predict the human olfactory threshold for more than 80 molecules by measuring four different physicochemical properties: the molecular volume, the properties of molecules as protons, donor and acceptor, and the polarizibility of an active part of the molecule. Four different chromatographic columns giving a direct and independent measure of these factors allow the computation of the olfactory threshold. The correlation between calculated and experimented thresholds reaches 0.80.

Another distortion of the olfactory system as compared to a physical count of molecules is represented by the psychophysical relation between the increasing suprathreshold concentrations of the odorous compound and the perceived intensity. This intensity does not increase in direct proportion to the number of active molecules reaching the sensory organ. A power law expresses this relation with an exponent established for about 100 molecules, varying with each of them (see Reference 2 for a compilation of data).

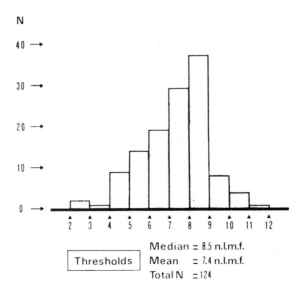

FIGURE 1. Distribution of human odor thresholds for 124 stimuli.

As a consequence of these basic physiological data, the chromatographic-spectrographic analysis of complex natural aromas has to be corrected, taking into account the relative efficiency of each compound. Another difficulty in translating the chemical analysis into terms of odor intensity is the fact that the possibility of predicting the level of perceived intensity on the basis of a quantitative assessment of the stimulus is limited to a pure compound. In a mixture, a simple additive action of the stimulating properties of each constituent is not observed. In contrast, inhibitions and synergisms, depending on associated compounds and on their relative concentration in the mixture, are empirically observed. Such effects determined in some binary mixtures[3] have not so far permitted the proposition of a generalizable law of effects. However, the model recently proposed by Berglund[4] seems to open possibilities for future solution of this practical problem of odor control.

The qualitative discrimination of odors and the assessment of their qualities in relation to food flavors raise other, more difficult questions. As mentioned above, each active molecule generates a particular and distinct odor sensation. Exceptions to this general law are identical or similar odors produced by a limited number of chemicals, often differing widely in their chemical identities. From study of the physiological mechanism involved at the receptor and central levels in odor discriminations, attempts have been made to relate molecular structures to the observed differences, similarities, or identities of odors. Despite some advances, it is currently impossible to translate the chemical identification of a molecule in terms of predicted odor quality, or the converse.

Like the intensive effects, the problem is further complicated by the combination of odors in a mixture. The basis for a prediction of the qualitative odor interaction in mixtures is lacking, and only some empirical determinations are possible.

Whatever this mechanism is, the important fact regarding food flavor distinction is the infinite possibility of sensory discriminations realized by both the complexity and variety of odorous constituents in aromas and the unlimited performance of the olfactory apparatus in discriminating pure compounds and their various mixtures. This combination explains the development in the feeding experience of specific preferences and aversions and of palatability responses to each actual food and beverage.

FOOD PALATABILITY AND ITS ROLE IN THE REGULATORY CONTROL OF FOOD INTAKE

Apart from their sensory activity, some chemicals in the environment are inactive in stimulating a feeding response. Others, named foods, are, in some conditions, accepted, taken into the mouth, chewed, and swallowed. The graded ability of foods, based on but distinct from their sensory activity, to stimulate behavioral eating responses is termed the palatability of these foods.

The sensory activity measured by, for example, the olfactory threshold is relatively constant from individual to individual and among species. In a given subject it is not dependent on the physiological state, and in particular does not vary with the nutritional status. By contrast, the palatability of food materials differs greatly among various species and within individuals of the same species. In a given subject (animals and humans), it changes over time. Typically, it is dependent on the physiological state as affected by hunger and satiety.

The palatability of foods is both sensory specific and hunger dependent. In the condition recognized as satiety associated with postingestive repletion, the food flavor is unpalatable, that is to say it has lost its efficiency to stimulate and "reward" the oral eating response. In the opposite condition, recognized as "hunger" and depending on its level, the flavor of the available food is "palatable." It stimulates the acceptance and the eating of the food. All being otherwise equal as to the level of hunger, the eating response is "sensory specific" in terms of the strength of the response and the amount eaten up to satiation, that is, it is specific of the food as a discriminable sensory cue.

In a human being, the subjective correlate of palatability and generally of the efficiency of sensory stimuli in supporting motivated and regulatory behaviors is the hedonic dimension of the sensation, its pleasantness and unpleasantness. A common characteristic of the olfactory perception is in the strength of the affective tone or hedonic value. In addition, a clear-cut division between pleasant and unpleasant odor stimuli is observed.

The origin and significance of the hedonic value of odors are obscure. Some of them are obviously unrelated to feeding. The pleasantness of floral or musky odors and the unpleasantness of putrid or fecal odors are not affected by hunger and satiety. By contrast, it is known that food-associated odors are pleasant when "palatable" in hunger and unpleasant when "unpalatable" in satiety. Using a psychophysical rating, this shift of pleasantness to unpleasantness was scored in human subjects by correlating it to the shift in palatability.[5]

Hunger dependence and sensory specificity of the palatability of foods has also been supported by the study of operant responses rewarded by food odors. Rats readily learned to press a lever delivering a puff of their food-related odor. With such food odors, the rate of the lever pressing increases in hungry rats and decreases in sated rats.[6]

Using this technique or a measure of the amount eaten in a choice between flavored vs. unflavored food, a general survey of "odor preferences" (comparable to that done on taste preferences) has not been carried out in rats or other species. In human beings, a similar investigation of odor preferences as a function of age, sex, and sociocultural background is also lacking.

A series of experiments on the animal model and in human beings confirmed the essential role of food flavors in the physiological control of feeding, and suggested its mechanism. In rats, the surgical bilateral ablation of olfactory bulbs induced a marked alteration of the normal meal pattern. Instead of discrete feeding bouts or meals separated by definite, long meal-to-meal intervals, anosmic rats exhibited a typical nibbling pattern, alternating between short episodes of feeding activity and short pauses (Figure 2).[7] It was strongly suggested that, in the absence of olfactory control of food, some essential mechanism involved in eating onset and offset was disrupted. This provided evidence for the role of olfactory projection to the lateral hypothalamic area, which appears to be critical in the control of a normal meal pattern. The brain electrolytic lesion at the level of the main olfactory-hypothalamic connection (medial forebrain bundle) was shown to reproduce the same altered meal pattern as induced by bulbectomy. The peripheral chemical lesion of the olfactory mucosa was transitorily followed by the similar abnormality.

The role of palatability of flavored food in determining meal size was demonstrated in other experiments, described next.

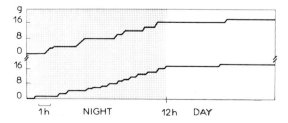

FIGURE 2. Disrupted meal pattern in olfactory bulbectomized rats. Top: meal pattern in normal rats; bottom: meal pattern in bulbectomized rats.

For 32 days, in a 2-hr morning meal daily, rats were offered a synthetic diet alternately flavored by the addition of a minute amount of an odorous compound, either A, B, C, or D. At the end of this habituation period, the amount eaten during the 2-hr meal was the same regardless of the flavored diet offered and maintained during the 2 hr. Then, every 2 days the rats were offered successively during their 2-hr morning meal the four flavored forms of the same diet, each for one-half hour. Compared to controls and to alternate days with the permanent flavor, this succession of the four different forms induced a marked increase of meal size (Figure 3).[8] However, whatever the order of presentation of flavors, the amount eaten in each successive 30-min presentation decreased, showing that cumulative postingestive satiation interacts with oral cues in determining the sensory-specific intake of food (Figure 4).[8] The simultaneous (cafeteria condition) instead of the

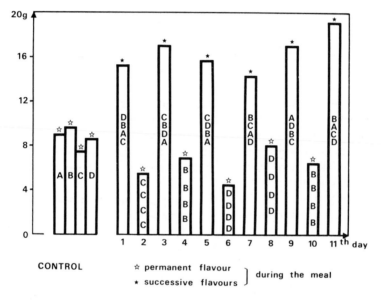

FIGURE 3.   Effect of successively presented flavored diets on meal size in rats.

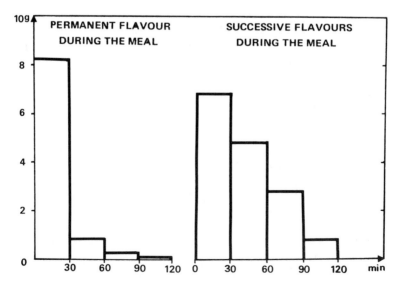

FIGURE 4.   Free consumption in four successive 30-min food presentations, with constant flavor compared to different flavors.

successive presentations of differently flavored forms of the same diet also induced an increase of the total amount eaten up to satiation (Figure 5).[9]

The recording of the speed, of eating, or intake rate, throughout the meal, taken as a measure of the strength of the feeding response provided more evidence for the role of palatability in determining meal size. Such recording in rats offered two differently flavored diets after 24 hr of food deprivation showed that the intake rate at the beginning of the meal was (1) positively correlated to the palatability of the food, and (2) increased during the first minutes of the meal. Thus, at the start of the meal, sensory properties act in a positive feedback on the feeding response. Later, the intake rate decreased until satiety with a slope again dependent on palatability. The total meal size is a result of these successive, palatability-dependent positive and negative feedbacks.

In human beings, the role of food flavors in determining the amount of food consumed is affected by trivial experiences. The cooking and sophisticated preparation of foods and the ordering of a variety of dishes within a meal (as above in the rat) commonly result in meals of excessive size in man.

Using various experimental procedures of objective measurement, the role of food palatability in human feeding behavior has been assessed in various studies. Three typical experiments are briefly described here.

Human subjects were offered a test meal composed of small pieces of bread four hours after their normal breakfast. Subjects were instructed to eat freely, one piece at a time, until satiated. In ten successive meals, the bread pieces were covered by a small layer of ten differently flavored food items (fish cream, mustard, cheese, butter, etc.). Prior to the experiment, subjects were asked to score the hierarchy of their individual preferences for the ten flavored slices. While eating, an electromyographic recording of masticatory and swallowing movements was made, documenting throughout the meal the evolution of the chewing-swallowing pattern: duration of bites, number of masticatory movements in each

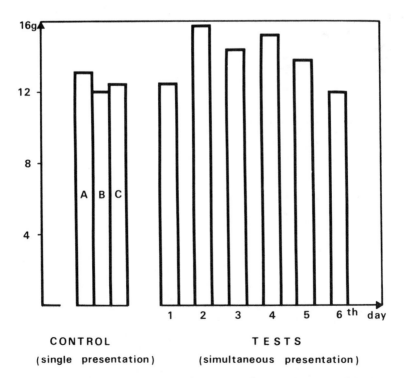

FIGURE 5.   Effect of simultaneously presented flavored diets on meal size in rats.

successive bite, etc. For each subject, it was shown that the amounts of the differently flavored items eaten were positively correlated with the level of the subject's scored preferences. Furthermore, at the beginning of the meal it was observed that some characteristics of the chewing-swallowing pattern were correlated to the palatability level of the food. For example, until each piece of bread was completely swallowed, the duration of mastication was as short and the number of masticatory movements as small as the palatability level (and therefore the amount eaten at the end of the meal) was high. Significantly, the same effect was obtained when hungry subjects (deprived of food for 6 hr), as compared to fully satiated subjects, were offered a given flavored food (Figure 6).[10]

In another experiment with human subjects, it was shown that oral cues prevail over gastrointestinal cues in determining intake (Figure 7).[11] By pressing a button, subjects took by mouth voluntarily and up to satiety, a liquid food. Simultaneously, through a tube in the stomach the pump delivered a variable proportion of the liquid food eaten by mouth. In this condition, subjects did not reduce the oral intake in proportion to the calories added in the stomach, and thus overate.

In another experiment, the prevailing importance of oral cues in determining intake was also shown.[12] Before a free meal, subjects received a drink containing either 450 or 900 cal. By addition of flavors, the two liquids, were made either highly palatable or unpalatable. The amount eaten in the subsequent meal was shown to be correlated to the respective palatabilities of the pre-feeding drinks, not to the amount of calories in the drinks. In other words, the highly palatable drink, either of high or low density, reduced the size of the subsequent meal.

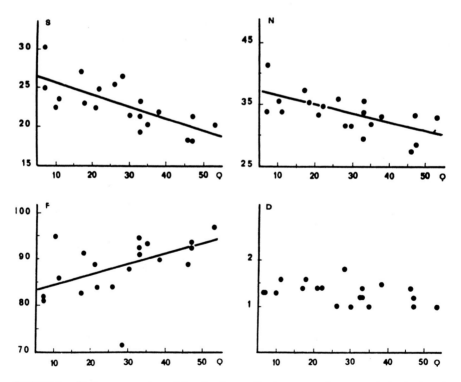

FIGURE 6.   Various parameters of the chewing-swallowing pattern in man at the beginning of the free intake of ten differently flavored diets plotted against the amount eaten of each diet at the end of the meal. S: mean duration of each bite; N: number of masticatory movements in each bite; F: frequency of mastication; D: mean number of swallowing movements in each bite.

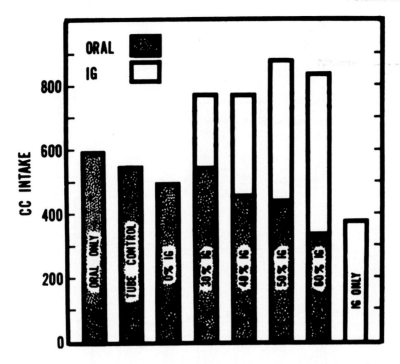

FIGURE 7.　Free oral intake of a liquid food by a human subject when various amounts of the same food are given intragastrically.

THE LEARNING OF PALATABILITY, PREFERENCES, AND AVERSIONS

The specific palatability of foods (and thus its effect on their relative acceptance and consumption) is learned. The repletive effect of various foods, related to either their respective caloric density or their specific properties as nutriments, acts as a reinforcer in a "conditioning" of palatability. Through this learning, the palatability of various foods may be roughly adjusted to their nutritive properties.

The following experiment with rats provided the first evidence that food preferences and aversions are learned and physiologically adopted.[14] Rats were presented alternately the same diet in two odorized forms. Free consumption of one of them in a short meal was supplemented by the postprandial parenteral administration of a glucose solution. A preference was so induced for the unreinforced flavored form, the other reinforced form being treated progressively by rats as if it was higher in its caloric density (Figure 8). Later, it was shown that alternate consumption of two diets differing in caloric density by addition of an inert material in one of them led to greater intake of the low caloric diet. Exhibition of the acquired and different palatability of the two diets was shown to be entirely dependent on the odor labeling of diets. After conditioning, the addition of the two flavors to a diet of an intermediary caloric density induced the same differential intake.[15] In the absence of the added odors, which had provided discriminative cues, and in anosmic rats, the "palatability learning" did not occur (Figure 9).

Despite the obvious role of education and sociocultural factors in human food habits, some data support the presumption that the same conditioning process in relation to the caloric efficiency of foods is also operative in man.[16]

In the rat model, it was shown that such learned preferences and aversions are similarly elicited by association with specific nutritive or nonnutritive effects. As early as 1933[17] and 1946,[18] it was demonstrated that the acquisition of a specific appetite for a diet containing vitamins by deficient rats was based upon the diet-associated flavor. This

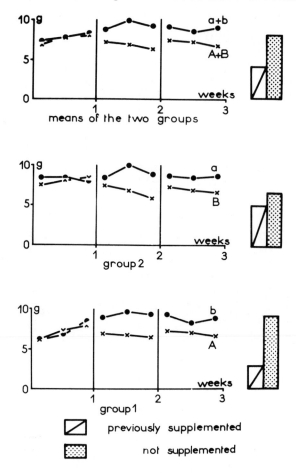

FIGURE 8.   Conditioning of the differential intake of two flavored diets by postprandial administration of a glucose solution; progressive conditioning during alternate meals finally exhibited in a choice.

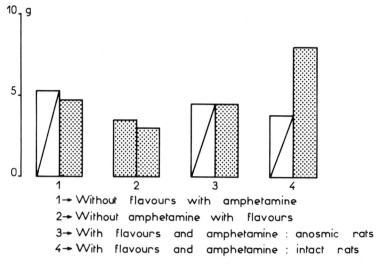

1 → Without flavours with amphetamine
2 → Without amphetamine with flavours
3 → With flavours and amphetamine : anosmic rats
4 → With flavours and amphetamine : intact rats

FIGURE 9.   Conditioning of a differential intake in rats by adding amphetamine to the diet — evidence for the role of conditioned and unconditioned stimuli.

learning process of selective appetite was extensively and elegantly studied by Rozin.[19] Recently, it was finally found that the main specific appetite represented by the selection of proteins in agreement with both the body requirement and the protein content of the food was also determined by conditioned odor preferences and aversions.[20-22] The same process is still operative in the so-called "conditioned taste aversion" due to the postingestive toxic effect of the food. Poisoning and illness acting as unconditioned stimuli induce a one-trial learning of aversion to the taste or smell of a food ingested prior to the intoxication. This process, fully described by Rzocka in 1953,[23] has again been extensively studied in recent years.

INNATE AND EXTERNAL FACTORS IN FOOD PALATABILITY

Taking these data into account, many questions remain unanswered and open to further investigations in animal species, especially in humans.

In determining the odor-mediated palatability of foods, what is the respective role of innate behavioral responses and the later ontogenic modulation by the feeding experience? In taste-mediated responses, the preference for sweet and the aversion to bitter have been shown to be genetically determined. In other areas of behavior, e.g., sexual and defensive, the responsiveness to odor attractants or repellents was also demonstrated to be inherited in various species. In some animal species, feeding responsiveness to the specific odor of the prey or host plants of the species is well documented. However, up to now, the same has not been demonstrated in man.

The role of parental education in the early development of food preferences and aversions was recently convincingly demonstrated in rats.[24-26] It is obviously of tremendous importance in human beings; in feeding as well as in other behavior, this interindividual transmission is substituted for both genetic transmission and individual learning. In this way, as is commonly recognized, sociocultural habits in man strongly influence food odor preferences and aversions and feeding habits. This important field of investigation is relatively unexplored.

Finally, in man and experimentally in animals, the "pleasure of sensations" inherited or generated by the association of stimuli with physiological reinforcements gives rise to self-rewarded and self-stimulated behavior. Such behavior develops despite possible deleterious consequences such as obesity or nutritional diseases in feeding, and the counteracting effects of these consequences through conditioning. The tasting of highly palatable foods and their refined aromas is no longer a feeding behavior. Rather, it is an aesthetic activity and the basis for a true art of food flavors.

REFERENCES

1. Laffort, P., Patte, F., and Etcheto, M., *Ann. N.Y. Acad. Sci.,* 237, 193–208, 1973.
2. Patte, F., Etcheto, M., and Laffort, P., *Chem. Senses Flavor,* 1, 283–306, 1975.
3. Koster, E. P. and MacLeod, P., in *Methods in Olfactory Research,* Moulton, D. G., Turk, A., and Johnston, J. W., Eds., Academic Press, New York, 1975, 431–444.
4. Berglund, B., Berglund, U., Lindvall, T., and Svensson, L. T., *J. Exp. Psychol.,* 100, 29–38, 1973.
5. Duclaux, R., Feisthauer, J., and Cabanac, M., *Physiol. Behav.,* 10, 1029–1034, 1973.
6. Long, C. J. and Tapp, J. T., *Psychon. Sci.,* 7, 17–18, 1967.
7. Larue, C. and Le Magnen, J., *Physiol. Behav.,* 5, 509–513, 1970.
8. Le Magnen, J., *C.R. Soc. Biol.,* 150, 32–34, 1956.
9. Le Magnen, J., *Arch. Sci. Physiol.,* 14, 411–419, 1960.
10. Pierson, A. and Le Magnen, J., *Physiol. Behav.,* 4, 61–67, 1969.
11. Jordan, H. A., *J. Comp. Physiol. Psychol.,* 68, 498–506, 1969.
12. Wooley, O. W., Wooley, S. C., and Woods, W. A., *J. Comp. Physiol. Psychol.,* 89, 619–625, 1975.
13. Le Magnen, J., *C.R. Soc. Biol.,* 153, 212–215, 1959.
14. Le Magnen, J., *Ann. N.Y. Acad. Sci.,* 157, 1126–1157, 1969.
15. Le Magnen, J., unpublished data.
16. Spiegel, T. A., *J. Comp. Physiol. Psychol.,* 84, 24–37, 1973.
17. Harris, L. J., Clay, J., Hargreaves, F. J., and Ward, A., *Proc. R. Soc. London Ser. B,* 113, 161–190, 1933.
18. Scott, E. M. and Quint, E., *J. Nutr.,* 32, 285–291, 1946.
19. Rozin, M. and Kalat, J. W., *Psychol. Rev.,* 78, 459–486, 1971.
20. Simpson, P. C. and Booth, D. A., *Q. J. Exp. Psychol.,* 25, 354–359, 1973.
21. Simpson, P. C. and Booth, D. A., *Br. J. Nutr.,* 31, 285–296, 1974.
22. Booth, D. A. and Simpson, P. C., *J. Exp. Psychol.,* 23, 135–145, 1971.
23. Rzocka, J., *Br. J. Anim. Behav.,* 1, 128–135, 1953.
24. Galef, B. G., *J. Comp. Physiol. Psychol.,* 70, 370–381, 1970.
25. Galef, B. G., Jr. and Clark, M. M., *J. Comp. Physiol. Psychol.,* 75, 341–357, 1971.
26. Galef, B. G., Jr. and Clark, M. M., *J. Comp. Physiol. Psychol.,* 78, 220–225, 1972.

Metabolism of Foreign Substances

EFFECT OF NUTRITIONAL FACTORS ON DETOXIFICATION OF ENVIRONMENTAL POLLUTANTS

W. J. Stadelman

Animals of economic importance to our food supply may become contaminated with environmental pollutants through inhalation of the air they breathe, through ingestion in feed or water, or through adsorption through the skin. The contamination is found in edible tissue of the animal as well as in milk or eggs produced. Tolerances for a number of environmental pollutants in the human food supply have been established. Without the established tolerances, the products available for human food would be greatly curtailed. Established tolerances are sufficiently below any physiological effect on test animals to give a 100-fold or greater safety factor.

Members of the animal industries have shown a keen interest in developing procedures for detoxification of contaminated animals to residue levels lower than actionable tolerances. Methods developed involve modifications in feeding and management practices to accelerate removal of the unwanted pollutant. The contaminants of greatest significance to date have been chlorinated and brominated hydrocarbons and heavy metals. All of the decontamination procedures require time to be effective.

The persistence of DDT in laying hens following a 5-day exposure to feed containing 10 to 15 ppm was reported by Stadelman[1] and by Wesley et al.[2] Significant levels of DDT or its metabolites were found in the abdominal fat 17 weeks after all detectable traces were removed from the environment of the hens. Residues detected in fatty tissue and egg yolks of hens supplied feed containing 0.1 and 0.5 ppm DDT for 30 days were reported by Liska et al.[3] The concentration in body fat was three to five times the level of DDT in the feed. With egg yolk, the level reached by hens on the 0.5 ppm feed was 1.3 ppm, just half the concentration in body fat. When the hens were subjected to a forced-molt program[2] that resulted in a cessation of egg production and a loss of body weight (fatty tissue) ranging from 10 to 20%, the depletion rate was speeded up, so that residue-free eggs were obtained 15 to 17 weeks after exposure. With continued normal feeding and management, residues were found to 19 weeks after exposure. The forced-molt program had two advantages: (a) fewer eggs to dispose of because of residues, and (b) an increased rate of lay and higher-quality eggs after the production pause.

Wesley et al.[4] attempted refinement of procedures for depletion of laying hens by using different levels of protein in the ration and an androgen injection on hens to increase lipid mobilization.[5] The hens were given the equivalent of 15 ppm DDT in the feed in the form of a capsule injected into the crop for 5 days. Residual DDT in abdominal fat declined in 16 weeks from 21.06, 18.33, and 19.22 to an average of 1.32, 1.24, and 1.43 ppm in treatments using rations containing 20% protein, 45% protein, and 75% protein respectively. The rate of depletion in the yolk samples followed a similar pattern. Residual DDT in egg yolk declined from 8.85, 8.58, and 9.18 to 0.72, 0.51, and 0.62 ppm respectively in the same treatments and in the same time period.

The relative persistence of four chlorinated hydrocarbon pesticides in laying hens was reported by Stadelman et al.[6] The pesticide, equivalent to 10 to 15 ppm in the feed, was given to the hens for 5 days by capsule in the crop. One week after exposure, residue levels were 0.7 ppm lindane, 3.6 ppm dieldrin, 0.2 ppm heptachlor, 10 ppm heptachlor epoxide, 8.8 ppm DDT, and 0.8 ppm DDE. After 10 weeks, levels were 0.1 ppm lindane, 3.9 ppm dieldrin, 0.1 ppm heptachlor, 1.0 ppm heptachlor epoxide,

1.0 ppm DDT, and 0.6 ppm DDE. After 26 weeks, there were no detectable level of lindane, heptachlor, or DDT, but there still were 1.0 ppm dieldrin, 0.3 ppm heptachlor epoxide, and 0.7 ppm DDE. Part of the reason for the wide variation in initial levels was given by Olney et al.[7] when they reported biomagnification values when pesticides were fed to broiler chicks. Values were as follows: heptachlor epoxide, 20×; dieldrin, 15×; pp′ DDT, 9×; and lindane, 3×. With the relatively short exposure of the hens,[6] the levels did not reach those of the broilers, where the pesticides were fed throughout the life of the birds.

The most effective method developed to date for reducing the level of contamination in laying hens is a forced-molt program with a high-protein (45%) ration fed for 4 to 6 weeks during the production pause. The injection of androgens was not effective. No suitable depletion procedure is available for broiler chickens or turkeys, because the times required make the possible procedures economically impractical.

Depletion procedures for other livestock have also been developed. Braund et al.[8] tried limited energy intake in combination with thryoprotein without success. Cook[9] as well as Cook and Wilson[10] reported management procedures that have been relatively successful with dairy cattle, where the residue is partially removed by maintaining the cows in heavy milk production. Slight modification of the procedure aids in residue removal from hogs, beef cattle, and sheep. The specific treatment as reported by Cook and Wilson[10] for dairy cows is as follows:

1. Check feed, water, and insecticide sprays to determine the source of contamination, then discontinue use of contaminating materials.
2. In cases of acute pesticide poisoning, cows should be drenched with 2 to 2.5 kg of activated carbon. The drench can be a slurry made of 2 to 3 parts water and 1 part activated carbon. The carbon is difficult to find. Darco S-51 activated carbon is manufactured by Atlas Chemical Company, Wilmington, Delaware.
3. If cows are in convulsions, the veterinarian may also treat them with intravenous injections of phenobarbital or some other barbiturate. When intravenous injections cease, phenobarbital should be fed at a rate of 10 mg/kg body weight/day. This amounts to about 5 g (1 tablespoon) daily. Treatment should be continued for 6 weeks or until milk tests show that the pesticides are below tolerance levels. Phenobarbital can be added to the grain ration. Milk should not be marketed until 7 days after phenobarbital feeding has stopped.
4. Activated carbon should be fed at the rate of 1 kg/head/day for 500-kg cows. The carbon can be fed successfully by mixing either with silage or grain. Some dairy cooperatives add activated carbon to the concentrate at a level of 10% and then pellet the mixture.

When both activated carbon and phenobarbital are fed, some phenobarbital may be trapped in the gut by activated carbon. It is probably best to feed the phenobarbital about 2 hr before feeding the activated carbon. The level of phenobarbital administered could undoubtedly be reduced if the drug were given by intramuscular injections. In summary, it is possible to accelerate the removal of chlorinated pesticides from livestock. At present, the combination of activated carbon and phenobarbital is the most effective treatment. The concern about pesticides in meat and milk and the development of the antidote should serve to stimulate continuing research on this problem. No doubt, more effective and less costly antidotes for pesticide poisoning in cattle can be developed.

The material discussed thus far was reviewed by Liska and Stadelman.[11] They concluded that more basic studies were needed to aid in speeding up detoxification or decontamination of food-producing animals. A number of such reports are now being published, dealing primarily with the mechanisms of metabolizing the many organic toxicants. Among these are Atallah et al.[12] on methazole, Hunt and Gilbert[13] on fertan, Quistad et al.[14] and Davison[15] on methoprene, Ruzo et al.[16] on chlorinated naphthalene, Foster and Khan[17] on atrazine, and Kacew and Singhal[18] on DDT. Hopefully, with this information now available, applications will be made to more effectively eliminate the chlorinated hydrocarbon pesticides from edible animal products.

During the last decade, additional environmental contaminants have been isolated. Most disastrous of these are the polychlorinated and polybrominated biphenyls, PCBs and PBBs. Britton and Charles[19] reported significant levels (0.13 ppm) of PCBs in tissues of broiler chickens when 0.1 ppm PCB was in the feed. With 0.5 and 1.0 ppm in the feed, tissue levels were about half the feed level, and with 5 and 10 ppm in the feed, only about 20% of these levels were found in tissues. No functional procedure for accelerated removal of PCBs have been reported thus far. Teske et al.[20] reported the half-life for residues of PCBs to be 2.93 weeks.

No really satisfactory detoxification programs have been developed. With the suggested program for laying hens or for dairy cows, they are of value to save a young flock or herd. For animals nearing the end of their productive lives, economics dictates immediate disposal.

REFERENCES

1. **Stadelman, W. J.,** Management practices for removal of residues from domestic animals, *Proc. 25th Semiannual Meeting, American Feed Manufacturers Association Nutrition Council, 1965,* pp. 35—39.
2. **Wesley, R. L., Stemp, A. R., Liska, B. J., and Stadelman, W. J.,** Depletion of DDT from commercial layers, *Poult. Sci.,* 45, 321—324, 1966.
3. **Liska, B. J., Langlois, B. E., Mostert, G. C., and Stadelman, W. J.,** Residues in eggs and tissues of chickens on rations containing low levels of DDT, *Poult. Sci.,* 43, 982—984, 1964.
4. **Wesley, R. L., Stemp, A. R., Harrington, R. B., Liska, B. J., Adams, R. L., and Stadelman, W. J.,** Further studies on depletion of DDT residues from laying hens, *Poult. Sci.,* 48, 1269—1275, 1969.
5. **Emmens, C. W. and Parkes, A. S.,** The effect of route of administration on the multiple activities of testosterone and methyl testosterone in different species, *Endocrinology,* 1, 323—331, 1939.
6. **Stadelman, W. J., Liska, B. J., Langlois, B. E., Mostert, G. C., and Stemp, A. R.,** Persistence of chlorinated hydrocarbon insecticide residues in chicken tissues and eggs, *Poult. Sci.,* 44, 435—437, 1965.
7. **Olney, J. H., Giuffrida, L., Watts, R. R., Ives, N. F., and Storherr, R. W.,** Residues in broiler chick tissues from low level feedings of seven chlorinated hydrocarbon insecticides, *J. Assoc. Off. Anal. Chem.,* 58, 785—792, 1975.
8. **Braund, D. G., Brown, L. D., Huber, J. T., Leeling, N. C., and Zabik, M. J.,** Excretion and storage of dieldrin in dairy cows fed thyroprotein and different levels of energy, *J. Dairy Sci.,* 52, 172—182, 1969.
9. **Cook, R. M.,** Pesticide removal from dairy cattle, *Ext. Bull. E-668,* Michigan State University Cooperative Extension Service, East Lansing, 1970.
10. **Cook, R. M. and Wilson, K. A.,** Removal of pesticide residues from dairy cattle, *J. Dairy Sci.,* 54, 712—718, 1971.
11. **Liska, B. J. and Stadelman, W. J.,** Accelerated removal of pesticides from domestic animals, *Residue Rev.,* 29, 51—60, 1969.
12. **Atallah, Y. H., Whitacre, D. M., and Dorough, H. W.,** Metabolism of the herbicide methazole in lactating cows and laying hens, *J. Agric. Food Chem.,* 24, 1007—1012, 1976.
13. **Hunt, L. M. and Gilbert, B. N.,** Metabolism and residues of ^{3}H- and ^{35}S-labeled ferban in sheep, *J. Agric. Food Chem.,* 24, 670—672, 1976.

14. **Quistad, G. B., Staiger, L. E., and Schooley, D. A.,** Environmental degradation of the insect growth regulator methoprene. X. Chicken metabolism, *J. Agric. Food Chem.*, 24, 644—648, 1976.
15. **Davison, K. L.,** Carbon-14 distribution and elimination in chickens given methoprene-^{14}C, *J. Agric. Food Chem.*, 24, 640—643, 1976.
16. **Ruzo, L., Jones, D., Safe, S., and Hutzinger, O.,** Metabolism of chlorinated naphthalenes, *J. Agric. Food Chem.*, 24, 581—583, 1976.
17. **Foster, T. S. and Khan, S. U.,** Metabolism of atrazine by the chicken, *J. Agric. Food Chem.*, 24, 566—570, 1976.
18. **Kacew, S. and Singhal, R. L.,** Role of cyclic adenosine $3':5'$-monophosphate in the action of 1,1,1-trichlor-2,2-bis-(*p*-chlorophenyl) ethane (DDT) on hepatic and renal metabolism, *Biochem. J.*, 142, 145—152, 1974.
19. **Britton, W. M. and Charles, O. W.,** The influence of dietary PCB on the PCB content of carcass lipid in broiler chickens, *Poult. Sci.*, 53, 1892—1893, 1974.
20. **Teske, R. H., Armbrecht, B. H., Condon, R. J., and Paulin, H. J.,** Residues of polychlorinated biphenyl in products from poultry fed Arclor 1254, *J. Agric. Food Chem.*, 22, 900—904, 1972.

NUTRITIONAL INFLUENCES ON THE TOXICITY OF PESTICIDES

Wayland J. Hayes, Jr.

FAT AND BIOENERGETICS

During the early studies of DDT, it was observed that animals that were fat or in "good condition" were somewhat less susceptible than scrawny ones to acute poisoning. This effect, observed in mammals[1] and fish,[2] is easily explained in terms of the ability of fat to store DDT so that it is not immediately available to the nervous system, the stimulation of which constitutes poisoning by this compound. Under suitable conditions, dieldrin also is less toxic in fat animals.[3] The degree of storage of chlorinated hydrocarbon insecticides in fat is not limited by their solubility,[4] but the speed with which storage occurs after a single large dose is limited by the relatively small flow of blood to fat compared to other tissues.[5] The degree of circulation to fat is proportional to its volume, however, and doubling of the amount of fat can make the difference between life and death.

At the same daily dosage, excretion of a compound does not reach maximum until its storage has reached a steady state. This undoubtedly explains the finding that dieldrin generally is excreted at a lower rate in the milk of fat cows than in that of lean ones.[6] A similar failure to reach full equilibrium probably accounts for the finding that the concentration of stored dieldrin was inversely proportional to fatness in both dogs[7] and man.[8]

Storage of chlorinated hydrocarbon insecticides rarely reaches very high levels in fat following a single dose. Following repeated, high-but-tolerated doses, storage of many of these compounds in fat reaches very high levels. For example, more DDT may be stored in the fat of a rat than would be required to kill it if the entire amount were given by mouth as a single dose. It was shown by Fitzhugh and Nelson[9] that rats may suffer tremors if they have stored high concentrations of DDT in their fat and then experience starvation so that they mobilize their fat as a source of energy. The same is true of birds under experimental conditions.[10,11]

Under natural conditions, starvation is usually partial rather than complete, and whatever food remains available is as likely to be as contaminated as the food that led to pesticide storage. With this idea in mind, Dale et al.[12] measured storage and excretion in rats before, during, and after they were put on half rations. As starvation progressed, the concentration of DDT increased not only in the decreasing volume of fat, but also in other tissues and in the blood. In response to the increased blood levels, metabolism and excretion increased even while intake of DDT was reduced to half. In most of the rats this increased excretion was sufficient to protect them from an excessive concentration of DDT, but, in a few animals, brain levels became so high that they died of DDT poisoning. When starvation was ended, both storage and excretion in the survivors eventually returned to near original levels, but before this happened both storage and excretion of metabolites decreased because the rats regained their body weight faster than they regained DDT. One or more aspects of this study have been confirmed in birds[13] or in mammals,[14-17] but not all investigators have followed the entire cycle.

It has been shown that the changes in concentration of DDT in tissue are the same whether caused by withholding food or by disease that causes partial refusal of food.[5] Whether a compound that is stored in fat will increase in concentration in all tissues when the fat is mobilized depends on several factors, notably compound, dosage, and species. Many compounds, even some that are stored in fat to a considerable degree, are metabolized rapidly enough to render their mobilization from fat so nearly matched by increased biotransformation and elimination that they never reach a toxic level. Thus it has not been possible to induce dieldrin poisoning by starving laboratory animals that have stored dieldrin.[18] In fact, after a few days of starvation, the proportion of dieldrin excreted per day is very high.[19] Dosage is crucial. Even for a compound like DDT, enough must be stored in the first place if its mobilization is to have any clinical effect.   Finally, species vary in the efficiency with which they detoxify each compound and in their bioenergetic metabolic rate; under any given set of conditions, the latter rate of small, warm-blooded animals is faster and that of large ones slower. Under these circumstances, it is not astonishing that lethal mobilization may occur in small birds.[20]

On the other hand, there is no record of a human being experiencing poisoning by a pesticide as a result of its mobilization from fat through starvation. It is unlikely that this will occur, partly because very few people store enough of any pesticide to make its rapid mobilization dangerous. Furthermore, bioenergetic metabolism is only about one fourth or one fifth as rapid in man as in the rat. A man cannot starve as fast as a rat. The slower rate of mobilizing fat in man offers a correspondingly greater opportunity for detoxication of foreign compounds released from fat.

LIPIDS: A SPECIAL FUNCTION

Because microsomal enzymes are of such great importance in the biotransformation of foreign compounds and because the importance of lipids in the function of microsomal enzymes is recognized, it might be predicted that lipids and some pesticides would interact. So far, nothing of importance outside the laboratory has been found. Diets representing the range of fats that people eat had little or no influence on the storage of a wide range of chlorinated hydrocarbon insecticides fed to rats for four generations at rates 200 times those actually found in human food.[21] On the contrary, the growth of rats receiving p,p'-DDT at the usually easily tolerated dietary level of 150 ppm was depressed if they received a diet deficient in essential fatty acids but was slightly stimulated if they received the same diet supplemented with these acids. Those with depressed growth relative to rats receiving the same deficient diet but no DDT also showed unexpected ratios of various liver lipids. All of the changes were related to the proliferation of hepatic smooth endoplasmic reticulum, and it was suggested that DDT influenced the metabolism of essential fatty acids by increasing the demand for them.[22]

VITAMIN C

Vitamin C deficiency interferes with the induction of microsmal enzymes by pesticides or other compounds. In the squirrel monkey this effect can be detected after only 2 days on a deficient diet.[23] In guinea pigs, a higher dietary level of vitamin C is required to maintain induction than to prevent scurvey.[24]

PROTEIN

The first indication that protein metabolism has a bearing on the toxicity of a pesticide was the report by Smith and Stohlman[25] to the effect that rats receiving DDT at a dietary level of 500 ppm showed greater mortality and more liver changes if their diet was deficient (8%) rather than adequate (28%) in protein. Similar results were reported for dieldrin.[26] The difference depends at least in part on microsomal enzymes. Male rats have only 24% of the normal activity of these enzymes if they receive no protein for a month, and they are incapable of generating additional enzyme activity in response to a foreign chemical.[27] McLean and McLean[28] emphasized the opposite effects of protein deficiency on the toxicity of compounds that are detoxicated and those that are toxicated by biotransformation.

Other enzymes also may be affected. For example, cholinesterase activity in serum and liver and aliesterase activity in liver were reduced in rats fed less than 15% protein. Although brain cholinesterase and aliesterase were about the same following different levels of dietary proteins, single doses of carbanolate and parathion inhibited both liver and brain cholinesterase more at the 0% casein level than at higher levels. Although not all enzymes responded differently at different protein levels, rats were more susceptible to poisoning by parathion, carbanolate, and chlordane when fed a protein-free diet.[29]

Although there is no evidence that DDT interferes with the digestion or utilization of preformed dietary protein, it has been shown[30] that DDT at a dietary level of 75 ppm interferes with the ability of calves to utilize urea as a source of nitrogen partially replacing dietary protein. Presumably, the insecticide interferes with microorganisms in the rumen, which are known to convert urea to usable protein.

A systematic study of the effect of protein on the toxicity of pesticides was the result of a concern of the World Health Organization for the health of people in underdeveloped countries where diets often are low in protein. The findings of a series of unusually careful studies are summarized briefly in Table 1 and in great detail in a book by Boyd[31] entitled *Protein Deficiency and Pesticide Toxicity*. As may be seen from the table, the degree of protein deficiency likely to exist in human food leads to no important change in the toxicity of most pesticides. In rare instances, however, extreme deficiency is associated with a tremendous increase in toxicity. The reason for the difference between compounds is unexplained except that those that produce anorexia rapidly kill animals already moribund.

For perspective, it is useful to note that, without added pesticides, weanling rats grow at about one third the normal rate if their diet contains only 8% to 9% protein but is otherwise adequate. Weanling rats fed 3.0 to 3.5% protein do not grow at all, and some die during the third month. Those fed no protein slowly lose weight and die during the second month of feeding. Excessive intake of protein has little influence on the toxicity of pesticides, and, furthermore, is unlikely to occur under practical conditions.

Presumably because both the degree of protein deficiency and the degree of exposure to pesticides are less in developing countries than those studied in the laboratory, no instance in which human poisoning by a pesticide was conditioned by protein deficiency has been reported.

The importance of the induction of microsomal enzymes in determining toxicity has already been mentioned. An illustration involves diets in which the only source of protein was either 10 or 18% glutin, an incomplete protein that reduces food intake and growth. Rats maintained on these diets were less susceptible to heptachlor than rats pair-fed diets in which the only source of protein was casein. The difference was less or even opposite, however, when the animals were permitted to eat as much of the casein diets as they wanted.[39,40] It has been suggested[5] that the lower toxicity of heptachlor in rats fed gluten depends on limited conversion to the epoxide as a result of limited activity of microsomal enzymes, whereas the even greater protection offered by a truly normal diet depends on the presence of normal fat deposits and the sequestering of both heptachlor and heptachlor epoxides in the fat.

Table 1
ESTIMATES OF THE INCREASE IN THE
ACUTE TOXICITY OF CERTAIN
PESTICIDES IN ALBINO RATS AS
RELATED TO THE CONCENTRATION OF
PROTEIN IN THEIR DIET, DURING 28
DAYS FROM WEANING UNTIL DOSING

| | Percent in diet | | | | | |
Agent	0.0	3.5	9.0	26.0	81.0	Ref.
Captan	2100.0	26.3	1.2	1.0	2.4	33
Carbaryl	8.6	6.5	1.1	1.0	1.0	34
CIPC	8.7	4.0	1.7	1.0	—	35
Diazinon	7.4	1.9	1.8	1.0	2.0	36a
DDT	4.0	2.9	1.5	1.0	3.7	37
Endosulfan	20.0	4.3	1.8	1.0	1.0	32
Lindane	12.3	1.9	1.0	1.0	1.8	36b
Monuron	11.5	3.0	1.8	1.0	—	38
Toxaphene	—	3.7	—	1.0	—	39

Modified from Boyd, E. M., Dobos, I., and Krijnen, C. J., Endosulfan toxicity and dietary protein, *Arch. Environ. Health*, 21, 18, 1970. With permission.

REFERENCES

1. **Spicer, S. S., Sweeney, T. R., Von Oettingen, W. F., Lillie, R. D., and Neal, P. A.,** Toxicological observations on goats fed large doses of DDT, *Vet. Med.,* 42, 289—293, 1947.
2. **Hoffmann, C. H. and Surber, E. W.,** Effects of feeding DDT-sprayed insects to fresh-water fish, U.S. Department of the Inter. Special Scientific Report: Fisheries, 1—9, 1949.
3. **Barnes, J. M. and Heath, D. F.,** Some toxic effects of dieldrin in rats, *Br. J. Ind. Med.,* 21, 280—282, 1964.
4. **Sedlak, V. A.,** Solubility of benzene hexachloride isomers in rat fat, *Toxicol. Appl. Pharmacol.,* 7, 79—83, 1965.
5. **Hayes, W. J., Jr.,** *Toxicology of Pesticides,* Williams and Wilkins, Baltimore, 1975.
6. **Gannon, N., Link, R. P., and Decker, G. C.,** Pesticide residue in meat and milk: storage of dieldrin in tissues and its excretion in milk of dairy cows fed dieldrin in their diets, *J. Agric. Food Chem.,* 7, 824—826, 1959.
7. **Keane, W. T. and Zavon, M. R.,** The total body burden of dieldrin, *Bull. Environ. Contam. Toxicol.,* 4, 1—16, 1969.
8. **Hunter, C. G. and Robinson, J.,** Aldrin, dieldrin, and man, *Food Cosmet. Toxicol.,* 6, 253—260, 1968.
9. **Fitzhugh, O. G. and Nelson, A. A.,** The chronic oral toxicity of DDT (2,2-bis *p*-chlorophenyl 1,1,1-trichloroethane), *J. Pharmacol. Exp. Ther.,* 89, 18—30, 1947.
10. **George, J. L. and Mitchell, R. T.,** The effects of feeding DDT-treated insects to nestling birds, *J. Econ. Entomol.,* 40(6), 782—789, 1947.
11. **Hope, C. E.,** Effect of DDT on birds and the relation of birds to the spruce budworm, 1944, Canada, Department of Lands and Forests, Division of Research Biology, Bulletin No. 2, 57—62, 1949.
12. **Dale, W. E., Gaines, T. B., and Hayes, W. J., Jr.,** Storage and excretion of DDT in starved rats, *Toxicol. Appl. Pharmacol.,* 4, 98—106, 1962.
13. **Adamczyk, E.,** Translocation of DDT in chickens under the influence of hunger, *Med. Weter.,* 27, 103—105, 1971.

14. Hukuhara, T., Distribution of DDT between the brain and fatty tissue in experimental feeding in rats and behavior of fat-stored DDT in the starvation state, *Naunyn-Schmiedebergs Arch. Pharmakol. Exp. Pathol.*, 242, 522—539, 1962.

15. Dedek, W. and Schmidt, R., Studies on the transplacental transport and metabolism of ^{3}H- and ^{14}C-labeled DDT in pregnant mice under hunger stress, *Pharmazie*, 27, 294—297, 1972.

16. Deichmann, W. B., MacDonald, W. E., Cubit, D. A., and Beasley, A. G., Effects of starvation in rats with elevated DDT and dieldrin levels, *Int. Arch. Arbeitsmed.*, 29, 233—252, 1972.

17. Shtenberg, A. E. and Diky, V. V., Changes in the metabolism of DDT deposited in the omentum of fasting albino rats, *Vopr. Pitan.*, 32, 39—43, 1973.

18. Treon, J. F. and Cleveland, F. P., Toxicity of certain chlorinated hydrocarbon insecticides for laboratory animals, with special reference to aldrin and dieldrin, *J. Agric. Food Chem.*, 3, 402—408, 1955.

19. Heath, D. F. and Vandekar, M., Toxicity and metabolism of dieldrin in rats, *Br. J. Ind. Med.*, 21, 269—279, 1964.

20. Stickel, L. F., Pesticide residues in birds and mammals, in *Environmental Pollution by Pesticides*, Edwards, C. A., Ed., Plenum Press, London, 1973, 254—312.

21. Adams, M., Coon, F. B., and Poling, C. E., Insecticides in the tissues of four generations of rats fed different dietary fats containing a mixture of chlorinated hydrocarbon insecticides, *J. Agric. Food Chem.*, 22, 69—75, 1974.

22. Tinsley, I. J. and Lowry, R. R., An interaction of DDT in the metabolism of essential fatty acids, *Lipids*, 7, 182—185, 1972.

23. Chadwick, R. W., Cranmer, M. F., and Peoples, A. J., Metabolic alterations in the squirrel monkey induced by DDT administration and ascorbic acid deficiency, *Toxicol. Appl. Pharmacol.*, 20, 308—318, 1971.

24. Wagstaff, D. J. Ascorbic acid deficiency and induction of hepatic microsomal hydroxylative enzymes by organochlorine pesticides, *Toxicol. Appl. Pharmacol.*, 19, 10—19, 1971.

25. Smith, M. I. and Stohlman, E. F., Further studies on the pharmacologic action of 2,2-bis-(p-chlorophenyl)-1,1,1-trichlorethane (DDT), *U.S. Public Health Rep.*, 60 (11), 289—301, 1945.

26. Lee, M., Harris, K., and Trowbridge, H., Effect of the level of dietary protein on the toxicity of dieldrin for the laboratory rat, *J. Nutr.*, 84, 136—144, 1964.

27. Murphy, S. D. and DuBois, K. P., The influence of various factors on the enzymatic conversion of organic thiophosphates to anticholinesterase agents, *J. Pharmacol. Exp. Ther.*, 124, 194—202, 1958.

28. McLean, A. E. M. and McLean, E. K., Diet and toxicity, *Br. Med. Bull.*, 25, 278—281, 1969.

29. Casterline, J. L., Jr. and Williams, C. H. Effect of pesticide administration upon esterase activities in serum and tissues of rats fed variable casein diets, *Toxicol. Appl. Pharmacol.*, 14, 266—275, 1969.

30. Bohman, V. R., Chi, I. A., Harris, L. E., Binns, W., and Madsen, L. L., The effect of DDT upon the digestion and utilization of certain nutrients by dairy calves, *J. Dairy Sci.*, 35(1), 6—12, 1952.

31. Boyd, E. M., *Protein Deficiency and Pesticide Toxicity*, Charles C Thomas, Springfield, Ill., 1972.

32. Boyd, E. M., Dobos, I., and Krijnen, C. J., Endosulfan toxicity and dietary protein, *Arch. Environ. Health*, 21, 15—19, 1970.

33. Krijnen, C. J. and Boyd, E. M., Susceptibility to captan pesticide of albino rats fed from weaning on diets containing various levels of protein, *Food Cosmet. Toxicol.*, 8, 35—42, 1970.

34. Boyd, E. M. and Krijnen, C. J., The influence of protein intake on the acute oral toxicity of carbaryl, *J. Clin. Pharmacol.*, 9, 292—297, 1969.

35. Boyd, E. M. and Carsky, E., The acute oral toxicity of the herbicide chlorpropham in albino rats, *Arch. Environ. Health*, 19, 621—627, 1969.

36a. Boyd, E. M., Carsky, E. and Krijnen, C. J., The effects of diets containing from 0 to 81 percent of casein on the acute oral toxicity of diazinon, *Clin. Toxicol.*, 2, 295—301, 1969.

36b. Boyd, E. M., Chen, C. P., and Krijnen, C. J., Lindane and dietary protein, *Pharmacol. Res. Commun.*, 1, 403—412, 1969.

37. Boyd, E. M. and Krijnen, C. J., Dietary protein and DDT toxicity, *Bull. Environ. Contam. Toxicol.*, 4, 256—261, 1969.

38. Boyd, E. M. and Dobos, I., Acute toxicity of monuron in albino rats fed from weaning on different diets, *J. Agric. Food Chem.*, 17, 1213—1216, 1969.

39. Boyd, E. M. and Taylor, F. I., Toxaphene toxicity in protein-deficient rats, *Toxicol. Appl. Pharmacol.*, 18, 158—167, 1971.

40. Webb, R. E. and Miranda, C. L., Effect of the quality of dietary protein on heptachlor toxicity, *Food Cosmet. Toxicol.*, 11, 63—67, 1973.

NUTRITION AND METABOLISM OF DRUGS

T. K. Basu

METABOLISM OF DRUGS

A large variety of foreign compounds are metabolized in the body in two phases of reactions:

Drug	Phase I	Oxidation	Phase II	Conjugation
	——————>	reduction	——————>	product
	Asynthetic	and/or	Synthetic	
	reaction	hydrolysis	reaction	
		product		

TYPES OF PHASE I REACTIONS CATALYZED BY DRUG-METABOLIZING ENZYMES[1]

Oxidative Reactions

Aromatic hydroxylation: aniline → *p*-aminophenol
Aliphatic hydroxylation: hexobarbital → oxohexobarbital
N-Demethylation: aminopyrine → aminoantipyrine+formaldehyde
O-Demethylation: *O*-nitroanisole → *O*-nitrophenol
S-oxide formation: chlorpromazine → chlorpromazine sulfoxide

Reductive Reactions

Nitro reduction: *p*-nitrobenzoic acid → *p*-aminobenzoic acid
Azo link reaction: 4-dimethylaminoazobenzene → aniline + *p*-dimethylaminoaniline

The enzymes involved in these reactions are localized in hepatic microsomes and require reduced nicotinamide adenine dinucleotide (NADPH), molecular oxygen and a hemoprotein, cytochrome P-450 (Figure 1).

PHASE II REACTIONS

The second phase of drug metabolism consists of synthetic reactions (or conjugation) that are concerned not only with the drugs themselves and their Phase 1 products, but also with compounds that are provided by the body and derived from materials involved in normal carbohydrate, protein, and fat metabolism. The principle conjugating agents are glycine, glutathione (cysteine), methionine, and glucuronic acid. The most common type of conjugation is the formation of an ester linkage with glucuronic acid produced from glucose:

Glucose   glucose-6-phosphate   glucose-1-phosphate   uridine-diphosphate-glucose
(UDPG)

Uridyl transferase

2 NAD ←| ←UDP-dehydrogenase

UDPGA + 2 NADH + H

(A conjugation reaction requires an 'active' intermediate compound, usually a nucleotide, and a transferring enzyme).

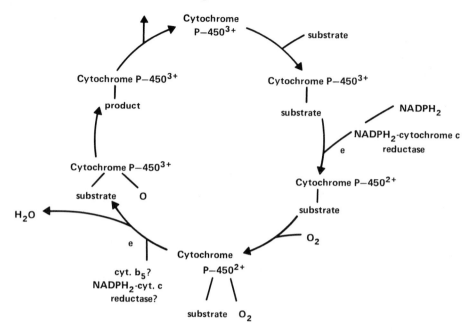

FIGURE 1.   The mechanism of hepatic microsomal hydroxylation by cytochrome P-450. (From Parke, D. V., *Enzyme Induction,* vol. 6, Plenum Press, London, 1975, 209. With permission.)

TWO-PHASE REACTIONS AND TOXICITY

An initially toxic compound may be converted to a less toxic substance, or an initially nontoxic compound may be converted into more toxic metabolites (intoxication) by Phase I reactions. The metabolite may also subsequently undergo Phase II reactions (conjugation) generally resulting in decreased toxicity. Examples of some of these processes are

Phenobarbitone (active)	Phase I → deactivation	p-hydroxy phenobarbitone (inactive)	Phase II →	p-hydroxy phenobarbitone glucuronide (inactive excretory product)
Prontosil (inactive)	Phase I → activation	sulfanilamide (active)	Phase II →	N-acetyl Sulfanilamide (inactive excretory product)

The rate at which each of the detoxicating reactions (Phase I and/or Phase II) proceeds and its relative importance may be affected by a variety of factors, including nutrition.

Table 1
EFFECT OF 72-HR STARVATION ON THE METABOLISM OF HEXOBARBITAL IN MALE RATS[2]

Animals	Hexobarbital metabolism		
	In vivo (sleeping time, min)[a]	In vitro (hexobarbital oxidase)	
		Km (mM)	Vmax
Control	14 ± 7	0.14 ± 0.03	44.6 ± 7.2
Starved	24 ± 2[b]	0.05 ± 0.01[b]	19.7 ± 2.9[b]

[a] It is the loss of righting reflex after the intraperitoneal injection of sodium hexobarbital (80 mg/kg body weight).

[b] Significantly different from control. Values represent means ± SD for at least five animals.

From Gram, T. E., Guarino, A. M., Schroeder, D. H., Davies, D. C., Reagan, R. L., and Gillette, J. R., *J. Pharmacol. Exp. Ther.*, 175, 12–21, 1970. With permission.

Table 2
EFFECT OF 72-HR STARVATION ON THE IN VITRO METABOLISM OF VARIOUS SUBSTRATES IN FEMALE AND MALE SPRAGUE-DAWLEY RATS[a,3]

Substrates	Starved male	Starved female
Aminopyrine	−51	+114
Hexobarbital	−36	+64
Pentobarbital	−47	+55
Morphine	−39	+1
Cocaine	−2	+21
Nitroanisole	+13	+90
Methylamine	+28	+43
Aniline	+64	+94
Zoxazolamine	+3	+15
Neoprontosil	−2	+102
Nitrobenzoic acid	+7	+73
Neotetrazolium	+22	+26
Dichlorophenolindophenol	0	+7

[a] The figures indicate the percentage differences from control rats.

From Kato, R., and Gillette, J. R., *J. Pharmacol. Exp. Ther.*, 150, 279–284, 1965. With permission.

Table 3
EFFECTS OF STARVATION ON THE IN VITRO METABOLISM OF DRUGS IN CASTRATED RATS[3]

		Hexobarbital		Aminopyrine		Aniline	
		Males	Females	Males	Females	Males	Females
Normal rats	Fed	3.79 ± 0.10	1.21 ± 0.17	483 ± 45	126 ± 19	437 ± 65	410 ± 55
	Starved	2.29 ± 0.23	1.67 ± 0.21	293 ± 20	377 ± 50	725 ± 73	916 ± 85
Castrated rats	Fed	1.71 ± 0.33	1.24 ± 0.11	143 ± 32	125 ± 16	443 ± 59	407 ± 60
	Starved	1.71 ± 0.18	1.67 ± 0.19	247 ± 66	370 ± 36	904 ± 94	874 ± 66

Note: Animals were starved for 72 hr. The results are expressed as the mean ± SD of the values obtained from five rats. Castration of male rats was found to impair the metabolism of hexobarbital and aminopyrine, but not aniline. However, castration of female rats did not alter the metabolism of any of these substrates.

From Kato, R. and Gillette, J. R., *J. Pharmacol. Exp. Ther.*, 150, 279—284, 1965. With permission.

Table 4
EFFECT OF 72-HR STARVATION ON THE ELECTRON TRANSPORT SYSTEM IN MALE AND FEMALE RATS[a,4]

	Starved male	Starved female
Cytochrome P-450 (nmol/mg microsomal protein)	+20	+32
NADPH-oxidase (nmol/mg microsomal protein)	-6	+20
NADPH-cytochrome c reductase (nmol/mg microsomal protein)	+4	+14
NADPH-neotetrazolium reductase (nmol/mg microsomal protein)	-12	+23

[a] The figures indicate the percentage differences from control rats.

Table 5

EFFECT OF UNDERNUTRITION DURING THE 3 WEEKS OF POSTNATAL LIFE ON THE ACTIVITY OF HEPATIC MICROSOMAL DRUG-METABOLIZING ENZYMES OF RATS[a,5]

Age (days)	Description[b]	No. of rats (no. of analyses)	Liver wt (%)	Biphenyl 4-hydroxylase (μmol/hr/g liver wt)	p-Nitrobenzoate reductase (μmol/hr/g liver wt)	4-CH$_3$ Umbelliferone glucuronyl transferase (μmol/hr/g liver wt)	Cytochrome P-450 (nmol/g liver wt)
6	UN	46 (5)	0.24 ± 0.02	1.7 ± 0.3	0.15 ± 0.02	26.0 ± 2.7	9.4 ± 0.2
	C	16 (3)	0.41 ± 0.01	1.8 ± 0.1	0.17 ± 0.03	26.0 ± 1.7	9.5 ± 0.4
12	UN	45 (10)	0.46 ± 0.04[c]	2.7 ± 0.4	0.41 ± 0.03	45.0 ± 7.6	12.6 ± 1.2
	C	9 (7)	0.81 ± 0.02	2.6 ± 0.2	0.42 ± 0.02	44.0 ± 4.4	13.0 ± 1.0
18	UN	22 (5)	0.86 ± 0.19[c]	3.6 ± 0.5	0.94 ± 0.11	57.0 ± 13.0	14.0 ± 2.7
	C	9 (5)	1.26 ± 0.15	3.5 ± 0.5	1.00 ± 0.13	69.0 ± 3.0	15.0 ± 1.3
21	UN	41 (14)	1.25 ± 0.22[c]	4.6 ± 0.4	0.70 ± 0.22	70.0 ± 7.4	21.7 ± 3.2
	C	14 (11)	2.15 ± 0.11	4.9 ± 0.3	0.90 ± 0.60	79.0 ± 7.3	23.2 ± 2.5

Note: The animals were undernourished by restricting their milk intake. This was done by establishing two groups; one group had three pups to one lactating mother, while the other had 15 pups to one lactating mother. The small groups were well nourished and served as controls for those of the larger groups which were undernourished. Litters of both groups were killed at 6, 12, 18 and 21 days after birth. It was of interest that the undernutrition during the first 3 weeks of life did not have any effect on the activity of various drug-metabolizing enzymes per gram liver weight.

[a] Each value is the mean for the number of animals shown with SD ±.

[b] C = control, UN = undernourished.

[c] Difference between UN and C, statistically significant (p <0.001).

Table 6

**EFFECT OF PHENOBARBITAL TREATMENT ON THE
PERCENTAGE INCREASE OF THE ACTIVITY OF
MICROSOMAL ENZYMES IN UNDERNOURISHED
SUCKLING RATS[5]**

	Age and description			
	12 days old		21 days old	
	Undernourished	Control	Undernourished	Control
Biphenyl 4-hydroxylase (μmol/hr/g liver wt)	185	165	93	63
p-Nitrobenzoate reductase (μmol/hr/g liver wt)	162	60	43	18
Cytochrome P-450 (nmol/g liver wt)	122	84	93	63

Note: Animals were treated with phenobarbital (10 mg/kg body weight) intra-peritoneally for 3 successive days until 24 hr before killing. The percentage induction of hepatic microsomal drug-metabolizing enzyme activities by phenobarbital treatment was higher in undernourished animals than in control animals (the increase in activity expressed as a percentage of the basal value). These findings are in agreement with other works that show younger rats being intrinsically more responsive to enzyme induction than older rats (see Tables 7 and 8).

Table 7

**EFFECT OF AGE ON THE INDUCTION OF
LIVER MICROSOMAL ENZYMES IN THE RAT[6]**

	12 days old	21 days old	52 days old
Biphenyl 4-hydroxylase	165	63	50
Biphenyl 2-hydroxylase	260	30	25
p-Nitrobenzoate reductase	60	18	8
Cytochrome P-450	84	65	30

Note: Rats were treated with phenobarbital (10 mg/kg body weight) for 3 successive days. Increase in activity is expressed as a percentage of the basal value.

Table 8
EFFECT OF AGE DIFFERENCE IN PHENOBARBITAL INDUCTION OF THE ACTIVITIES OF ELECTRON TRANSPORT SYSTEM AND DRUG OXIDATION AND REDUCTION IN RAT LIVER MICROSOMES[7]

	40 days old	100 days old	300 days old	600 days old
NADPH oxidase	181	84	46	20
NADPH-cytochrome c reductase	249	116	52	22
Cytochrome P-450	259	131	60	37
Aminopyrine *N*-demethylation	713	395	173	36
Hexobarbital hydroxylation	492	293	134	34
Aniline hydroxylation	165	94	40	31
p-Nitrobenzoate reduction	256	104	45	32

Note: The results indicate the increase by treatment with phenobarbital (60 mg/kg body wt for 3 days) expressed as a percentage of the original activity.

From Kato, R. and Takanaka, A., *J. Biochem.*, 63, 406–408, © 1968. With permission of Pergamon Press, Ltd.

Table 9
EFFECTS OF DIFFERENT CARBOHYDRATES RELATIVE TO STARCH (= 100%) ON THE ACTIVITY OF HEPATIC MICROSOMAL ENZYMES IN RATS[a,8]

Enzymes	Sucrose	Glucose	Fructose	Glucose and fructose
Biphenyl 4-hydroxylase (μmol/hr/g liver wt)	63	85	83	70
p-Nitrobenzoate reductase (μmol/hr/g liver wt)	120	170	170	130
Cytochrome P-450 (nmol/g liver wt)	75	79	90	86

Note: Animals were maintained on diets containing 60% sucrose, 60% glucose, 60% fructose, and equimolar mixture of glucose and fructose for 14 days, and the results were compared with animals fed a diet containing 60% starch.

[a] Each value is the mean of ten animals.

Table 10
EFFECTS OF CARBOHYDRATES ON THE METABOLISM OF HEXOBARBITAL IN MALE MICE[9]

	Hexobarbital metabolism	
Treatment	In vivo (sleeping time, min)[a]	In vitro (hexobarbital oxidase, nmol/mg protein/45 min)
Chow diet (control)	28.5 ± 2.5 (31)	53.4 ± 1.9 (24)
Glucose (35%)	47.2 ± 3.1[b] (32)	26.1 ± 1.9 (24)
Fructose (35%)	39.7 ± 4.8[b] (17)	40.8 ± 7.4 (10)
Sucrose (35%)	41.1 ± 3.0[b] (32)	38.7 ± 1.6[b] (24)

Note: Carbohydrates in solution were given in drinking water for 48 hr. Each value is the mean of a number of animals shown in parentheses with SE ±.

[a] It is the loss of righting reflex after the intraperitoneal injection of sodium hexobarbital (100 mg/kg body weight).
[b] Significantly different from control.

From Strother, A., Throckmorton, J. K., and Herzer, C., *J. Pharmacol. Exp. Therap.,* 179, 490–498, 1971. With permission.

Table 11
EFFECT OF DIETARY DISACCHARIDES ON THE ACTIVITY OF AROMATIC HYDROXYLASE AND THE LEVEL OF CYTOCHROME P-450[10]

Diet	Biphenyl 4-hydroxylase (μmol/hr/g liver wt)	Cytochrome P-450 (nmol/g liver wt)
Starch (control) (60%)	4.3 ± 0.2	19.8 ± 0.5
Sucrose (60%)	2.8 ± 0.1[a]	15.4 ± 0.5[a]
Lactose (60%)	6.0 ± 0.2[a]	24.2 ± 0.7[a]
Maltose (60%)	4.0 ± 0.1	19.2 ± 0.6

Note: Each value is the mean for five rats with SE ±.

[a] Statistically significant difference between animals fed starch and those fed disaccharides ($P < 0.01$).

Table 12
DIETARY PROTEIN AND METABOLISM OF DRUGS IN YOUNG AND ADULT RATS

Drugs	Ref.
Strychnine	11
Aminopyrine	11
Pentobarbital	11
Zoxazolamine	11
Ethylmorphine	12
Aniline	11, 12
Benzopyrene	13
Pyramidon	13, 14

Note: Protein deficiency was found to decrease the microsomal reaction rates *in vitro* for a variety of oxidative pathways with various substrates. The activities of microsomal enzymes, which hydroxylate benzopyrene and demethylate pyramidon, were reported to fall by over 80% in rats fed either a protein-free or a 3% casein diet for 1 week when compared with animals fed a 30% casein diet for the same period.

Table 13
DIETARY PROTEIN AND TOXICITY OF FOREIGN COMPOUNDS IN YOUNG AND ADULT RATS

Compounds	Ref.
Endosulphan	15
Diazinon	16
Dieldrin	17, 18
Endrin	19
Captan	20
Lindane	21
Dicophane	22
Carbaryl	23
Strychnine	11
Pentobarbital	11
Zoxazolamine	11
Malathion	24
Parathion	24
Phenacetin	25
Aflatoxin	26, 27

Note: The toxicity of these foreign compounds, including pesticides and drugs, was found to be increased by a protein-deficient diet in rats. The toxicities of the compounds were derived mainly from LD_{50} determinations and mortality rates. With particular reference to strychnine, pentobarbital, and zoxazolamine in rats fed a protein-deficient diet, the toxicities of these compounds were related to the rate of the metabolism of these drugs by liver microsomes in vitro.

Table 14
EFFECT OF DIETARY PROTEIN ON THE ACTIVITIES OF NADPH-LINKED ELECTRON TRANSPORT IN YOUNG AND ADULT RATS

Electron transport system	Ref.
NADPH oxidase	11
NADPH-cytochrome c reductase	11
Cytochrome P-450	11, 14
Cytochrome b_5	11

Note: The activities of the NADPH-dependent electron transport system were found to be closely related to dietary protein intake. Thus, the system involved in the metabolism of foreign compounds was found to be decreased in rats fed either a protein-deficient or a protein-free diet and increased in rats fed a high-protein diet. Marshall and McLean[14] reported that in adult rats fed a 3% casein diet and hepatic concentration of cytochrome. P-450 was reduced to one third that of the control animals. They also showed that in treatment with pheonobarbital, the cytochrome P-450 concentrations were increased in both protein-deficient and control animals, but still only one fourth of control values was observed in protein-deficient animals.

Table 15
INFLUENCE ON DIETARY PROTEIN ON THE IN VITRO METABOLISM OF HEXOBARBITAL IN IMMATURE MICE[28]

Days fed	Diet (%)	Hexobarbital metabolized (μm/hr/mg microsomal nitrogen)	Difference (%)
7	casein (27)	0.064 ± 0.008	
	casein (8)	0.087 ± 0.003[a]	+36
28	casein (27)	0.093 ± 0.003	
	casein (8)	0.067 ± 0.003[a]	−28

Note: Each value is the mean of four determinations with SD ±.

[a] Significance of difference between animals fed 27 and 8% casein diets.

From Lee, N. H. and Manthei, R. W., *Biochem. Pharmacol.*, 17, 1108–1109, © 1968. With permission of Pergamon Press, Ltd.

Table 16
EFFECT OF A PROTEIN-FREE DIET FED FOR 7 DAYS ON THE ACTIVITY OF UDP-GLUCURONYL TRANSFERASE IN MATURE AND IMMATURE RATS[28]

| | UDP-glucuronyl transferase (nmol substrate conjugated/hr/g liver) | |
	p-Nitrophenol conjugation	*o*-Aminophenol conjugation
Immature rats	+64	+71
Mature rats	+24	+56

Note: The figures indicate the percentage differences from control animals fed an 18% casein diet.

Table 17
EFFECT OF PROTEIN NUTRITION ON THE HEPATIC MICROSOMAL AROMATIC HYDROXYLASE ACTIVITY AND THE CONCENTRATION OF CYTOCHROME P-450 IN WEANLING RATS[a,30]

| | Days fed diet | | | | | |
| | 7 Days | | 14 Days | | 28 Days | |
	Group A	Group B	Group A	Group B	Group A	Group B
Biphenyl 4-hydroxylase (μmole/hr/g liver)	4.2 ± 0.1	4.7 ± 0.3	4.3 ± 0.3	7.4 ± 0.8**	3.0 ± 0.1	5.7 ± 0.5**
Cytochrome P-450 (nmol/g liver)	28.0 ± 0.6	21.0 ± 2.6*	21.0 ± 1.2	17.0 ± 0.6*	21.0 ± 1.4	17.0 ± 1.6*

Note: Male Whistar rats were weaned at 21 days. At 24 days of age, animals of similar body weight were divided into two groups: Group A, control, was fed a stock diet (Spillers) containing 21% protein ad libitum, and Group B, protein-deficient, was fed ad libitum a diet containing 7% protein made by diluting the stock diet with starch. Animals were killed after 7, 14 and 28 days. The protein-deficient diet fed for 7 days did not result in any change in the activity of biphenyl 4-hydroxylase from the control levels, but after a lag period of 14 days, the activity of the enzyme was significantly higher in the protein-deficient group. However, unlike biphenyl 4-hydroxylase, the concentration of cytochrome P-450 was reduced in the protein-deficient animals at all periods.

[a] Each value is expressed as the mean ± SD of 10 animals. Significance of difference between Groups A and B shown: *$P<0.01$; **$P<0.05$.

Table 18

EFFECT OF PROTEIN NUTRITION ON THE CONCENTRATION OF 11-HYDROXYCORTICOSTEROIDS IN THE PLASMA AND THE ACTIVITY OF BIPHENYL 4-HYDROXYLASE IN THE LIVER OF GROWING RATS[a,31]

Days fed diet	Diet	11-Hydroxycorticosteroids (mg/100 ml plasma)	Hepatic biphenyl 4-hydroxylase (μmol/mg microsomal protein/hr)
7	Control	28 ± 2	0.13 ± 0.01
	Protein deficient	28 ± 6	0.17 ± 0.01
14	Control	18 ± 2	0.14 ± 0.01
	Protein deficient	48 ± 6	0.28 ± 0.20
28	Control	17 ± 3	0.07 ± 0.01
	Protein deficient	53 ± 4	0.16 ± 0.02

Note: The concentration of 11-hydroxycorticosteroids in plasma of the protein-deficient animals did not change after 7 days on the diet, but by 14 and 28 days, the level had increased about threefold. These results were parallel to the hepatic activity of biphenyl 4-hydroxylase.

[a] Each group consisted of at least six rats. The values are means ± SE.

Table 19
LOW-PROTEIN DIET AND DECREASED TOXICITY

Compounds	Ref.
Carbon tetrachloride	13, 32
Dimethyl nitrosamine	33
Heptachlor	34
Octamethyl pyrophosphoramide	11

Note: The toxicity of a foreign compound administered to protein-deficient animals depends on whether the compound is toxic by itself or its metabolite is toxic. The best-known examples of this phenomenon are carbon tetrachloride, dimethylnitrosamine (DMN), heptachlor, and octamethyl pyrophosphoramide, the toxicity of which has been found to be decreased by a protein deficient diet. The hepatotoxicity of carbon tetrachloride has been found to be completely abolished by feeding rats a protein-free diet for 4 days and the effect is reversed by the administration of inducers of drug-metabolizing enzymes, such as DDT and phenobarbital. The hepatoxic effect of DMN has also been found to be protected in rats fed a protein-free diet for 7 days. However, unlike CCl_4, the protective effect is not reversed by treating the animals with either DDT or phenobarbital. The reason for this might be that either the rate of DMN metabolism is not affected by the inducers of microsomal enzymes or that liver damage does not depend on the rate of DMN metabolism. However, it is of interest that although protein deficiency protects liver from the toxic effect of DMN, all the survivors eventually die from malignant kidney tumors. The toxicity of heptachlor, a chlorinated hydrocarbon insecticide, has been found to be markedly reduced by low-protein diets, due to their inability to form the toxic metabolite, heptachlor epoxide. The mortality rate due to toxicity of octamethyl pyrophosphoramide has been found to be reduced in rats by feeding low-protein diets and increased by feeding high-protein diets.

Table 20
EFFECT OF DIETARY FAT CONSUMPTION ON THE HEPATIC
MICROSOMAL DRUG-METABOLIZING ENZYMES IN MALE RATS[a,35]

Enzymes	Fat-free	Corn oil (3%)	Corn oil (10%)
		Diet fed for 3 weeks	
Ethylmorphine demethylase			
Km (mmol)	0.16 ± 0.01	0.23 ± 0.01	0.23 ± 0.02
Vmax	516.9 ± 8.4	816.1 ± 14	753.7 ± 22.6
Hexobarbital oxidase			
Km (mmol)	0.18 ± 0.05	0.32 ± 0.06	0.54 ± 0.06
Vmax	369.3 ± 53.5	671.9 ± 56.0	806.0 ± 46.6
Aniline hydroxylase			
Km (mmol)	0.08 ± 0.02	0.08 ± 0.01	0.06 ± 0.01
Vmax	81.7 ± 3.8	99.3 ± 3.3	88.5 ± 1.9
Cytochrome P-450 (nmol/mg protein)	0.57 ± 0.06	0.76 ± 0.06	0.99 ± 0.10
Cytochrome b_s (nmol/mg protein)	0.42 ± 0.04	0.54 ± 0.03	0.61 ± 0.02

[a] Values represent means ± SE of at least four animals per group.

From Norred, W. P. and Wade, A. E., *Biochem. Pharmacol.,* 21, 2887–2897, © 1972. With permission of Pergamon Press, Ltd.

Table 21
EFFECT OF VARIOUS DIETARY LIPIDS ON Vmax VALUES OF THE MICROSOMAL ENZYMES OF PHENO-BARBITAL-TREATED RATS[36]

	Fat-free	Coconut Oil (3%)	Corn oil (3%)
		Diet fed for 3 weeks	
Hexobarbital oxidase (nmol/hr/mg protein)	563 ± 74	629 ± 57	857 ± 30
Aniline hydroxylase (nmol/hr/mg protein)	117 ± 13	154 ± 16	205 ± 18

Note: Values represent means ± SE of at least four animals per group. Feeding a diet containing coconut oil (largely saturated fatty acids) failed to allow increase as much as did the diet containing corn oil (largely polyunsaturated fatty acids.)

From Norred, W. P. and Wade, A. E., *Biochem. Pharmacol.,* 22, 432–436, © 1973. With permission of Pergamon Press, Ltd.

Table 22
EFFECT OF DIETARY FAT ON THE HEPATIC MICROSOMAL CONCENTRATION OF CYTOCHROME P-450 ON PHENO-BARBITAL-TREATED RATS[37]

Diet	Cytochrome P-450 (nmol/g liver)[a]
Casein (20%) (without fat)	55 ± 15 (39)
Casein (20%) + coconut oil (15%)	59 ± 15 (5)
Casein (20%) + coconut oil (10%) + linoleic acid	103 ± 8 (5)
Casein (20%) + herring oil (15%)	123 ± 19 (4)

[a] Values represent means ± SD of the number of animals shown in parentheses.

From Marshall, W. J. and McLean, A. E. M., *Biochem. J.,* 122, 569–573, 1971. With permission.

Table 23

EFFECT OF VITAMIN DEFICIENCY ON THE METABOLISM OF FOREIGN COMPOUNDS

Vitamin	Metabolism of foreign compounds			Ref.
	Reduced	Not affected	Increased	
Retinol	Aminopyrine	p-Nitrobenzoate		38
Thiamine	Hexobarbital		Heptachlor	39—41
	Zoxazolamine		Aniline	
	Aminopyrine		Ethylmorphine	
Riboflavin	Benzopyrene		Hexobarbital	
	p-Nitrobenzoate		Aniline	
	4-Dimethylamino-azobenzene		Aminopyrine	42—44
Ascorbic acid	Acetanilide			45—48
	Aniline	Meperidine		
	Zoxazolamine			49,50
	Hexobarbital			
	Pentobarbital			
	Phenacetin			
	Testosterone			
	p-Nitroanisole			
	Aminopyrine			
Tocopherol	Aminopyrine			51
	Codeine			

Table 24

EFFECT OF VITAMIN DEFICIENCY ON THE IMPAIRMENT OF HEPATIC MICROSOMAL ELECTRON TRANSPORT SYSTEM

Vitamin	Electron transport system	Ref.
Retinol	Cytochrome P-450	38
Thiamine	Cytochrome P-450	40
	Cytochrome b_5	
	NADPH-cytochrome P-450 reductase	
Riboflavin	Cytochrome c reductase	43
Ascorbic acid	Cytochrome P-450	50,52
	NADPH-cytochrome P-450 reductase	
	NADPH-cytochrome c reductase	
	Cytochrome P-450	
Tocopherol	Cytochrome P-450	53
	Cytochrome b_5	

Table 25

EFFECT OF ASCORBIC ACID ON DRUG-METABOLISM ACTIVITY IN WEANLING GUINEA PIGS[a,5,4]

Ascorbate treatment	Liver ascorbate (mg/100 g)	Cytochrome P-450[b]	P-450 reductase[c]	O-demethylase[d]	N-demethylase[e]
75 mg/day (for 8 days)	14	0.066 ± 0.006	8.9 ± 1.4	9.0 ± 0.5	15.6 ± 0.8
25 mg/day (for 8 days)	8	0.060 ± 0.004	7.5 ± 0.8	8.0 ± 0.5	15.9 ± 2.3
7 mg/day (for 8 days)	6	0.060 ± 0.004	7.0 ± 0.8	7.5 ± 0.5	14.1 ± 0.9
Ascorbate-free diet (for 8 days)	2.5	0.061 ± 0.003	5.3 ± 0.9	6.2 ± 0.6	11.8 ± 0.8
Ascorbate-free diet (for 15 days)	<1.0	0.047 ± 0.002	3.4 ± 0.4	2.6 ± 0.2	10.0 ± 0.8

a Each value is the mean of at least five animals with ± SE.
b Cytochrome P-450, μmol/100 mg of microsomal protein.
c P-450 reductase, μmol P-450 reduced/hr/100 mg microsomal protein.
d O-demethylase, μmol p-nitrophenol formed/hr/100 mg microsomal protein.
e N-demethylase, μmol formaldehyde formed/hr/100 mg microsomal protein.

From Boyd, E. M. and Boulanger, M. A., *J. Agric. Food Chem.*, 16, 834—837, 1968. With permission.

Table 26

EFFECT OF MINERAL DEFICIENCY ON THE HEPATIC MICROSOMAL DRUG-METABOLIZING ENZYMES

Mineral	Days fed mineral-deficient diets	Impaired	Not affected	Increased	Ref.
Calcium	40	Hexobarbital oxidase Aminopyrine N-demethylase p-Nitrobenzoate reductase			55
Magnesium	11–14	Aniline hydroxylase Aminopyrine N-demethylase Cytochrome P-450	p-Nitrobenzoate reductase Pentobarbital oxidase		56
Zinc	37–58	Aminopyrine N-demethylase p-Nitrobenzoate reductase Pentobarbital oxidase Cytochrome P-450	Aniline hydroxylase Zoxazolamine hydroxylase		57
Iron	—		Cytochrome P-450 Aniline hydroxylase 3,4-Benzopyrene hydroxylase p-Nitrobenzoate reductase o- and p-Aminophenol transferases	Hexobarbital oxidase Aminopyrine N-demethylase Cytochrome b_s	42

REFERENCES

1. Conney, A. H., *Pharmacol. Rev.,* 19, 317–365, 1967.
2. Gram, T. E., Guarino, A. M., Schroeder, D. H., Davies, D. C., Reagan, R. L., and Gillette, J. R., *J. Pharmacol. Exp. Ther.,* 175, 12–21, 1970.
3. Kato, R. and Gillette, J. R., *J. Pharmacol. Exp. Ther.,* 150, 279–284, 1965.
4. Kato, R., Onoda, K., and Sasajima, M., *Jpn. J. Pharmacol.,* 20, 194–209, 1970.
5. Basu, T. K., Dickerson, J. W. T., and Parke, D. V., *Biol. Neonat.,* 23, 109–115, 1973.
6. Basu, T. K., Dickerson, J. W. T., and Parke, D. V., *Biochem. J.,* 124, 19–24, 1971.
7. Kato, R. and Takanaka, A., *J. Biochem.,* 63, 406–408, 1968.
8. Basu, T. K., Dickerson, J. W. T., and Parke, D. V., *Nutr. Metab.,* 18, 302–309, 1975.
9. Strother, A., Throckmorton, J. K., and Herzer, C., *J. Pharmacol. Exp. Ther.,* 179, 490–498, 1971.
10. Basu, T. K., Ph.D. thesis, University of Surrey, England 1971.
11. Kato, R., Oshima, T., and Tomizawa, S., *Jpn. J. Pharmacol.,* 18, 356–366, 1968.
12. MgBodile, M. U. K. and Campbell, T. C., *J. Nutr.,* 102, 53–60, 1972.
13. McLean, A. E. M. and McLean, E. K., *Biochem. J.,* 100, 564–571, 1966.
14. Marshall, W. J. and McLean, A. E. M., *Biochem. Pharmacol.,* 18, 153–157, 1969.
15. Boyd, E. N. and Dubos, I., *Arch. Int. Pharmacodyn. Ther.,* 178, 153–165, 1969.
16. Boyd, E. M. and Carsky, E., *Acta Pharmacol. Toxicol.,* 27, 284–294, 1969.
17. Krishnamurthy, K., Subramanya, T. S., and Jayaraj, P., *Indian J. Exp. Biol.,* 3, 168–170, 1965.
18. Lee, M., Harris, K., and Trowbridge, H., *J. Nutr.,* 84, 136–144, 1964.
19. Boyd, E. M. and Krupa, V., *J. Agric. Food Chem.,* 18, 1104–1107, 1970.
20. Boyd, E. M. and Krijnen, C. J., *J. Clin. Pharmacol.,* 8, 225–229, 1968.
21. Boyd, E. M. and Chen, C. P., *Arch. Environ. Health,* 17, 156–160, 1968.
22. Boyd, E. M. and De Castro, E. S., *Bull. W.H.O.,* 38, 141–144, 1968.
23. Boyd, E. M. and Boulanger, M. A., *J. Agric. Food Chem.,* 16, 834–837, 1968.
24. Webb, R. E., Bloomer, C. C., and Miranda, C. L., *Bull. Environ. Contam. Toxicol.,* 9, 102–107, 1973.
25. Boyd, E. M., Boulanger, M. A., and De Castro, E. S., *Pharmacol. Res. Commun.,* 1, 15–19, 1969.
26. Madhavan, T. V. and Gopolan, C., *Arch. Pathol.,* 85, 133–137, 1968.
27. McLean, A. E. M. and McLean, E. K., *Br. Med. Bull.,* 25, 278–281, 1969.
28. Lee, N. H. and Manthei, R. W., *Biochem. Pharmacol.,* 17, 1108–1109, 1968.
29. Woodcock, B. G. and Wood, G. C., *Biochem. Pharmacol.,* 20, 2703–2713, 1971.
30. Dickerson, J. W. T., Basu, T. K., and Parke, D. V., *J. Nutr.,* 106, 258–264, 1976.
31. Basu, T. K., Dickerson, J. W. T., and Parke, D. V., *Nutr. Metab.,* 18, 49–54, 1975.
32. Campbell, R. H. and Kosterlitz, H. W., *Br. J. Exp. Pathol.,* 29, 149–159, 1948.
33. McLean, A. E. M. and Verschuuren, H. G., *Br. J. Exp. Pathol.,* 50, 22–25, 1969.
34. Weatherholtz, W. M., Campbell, T. C., and Webb, R. E., *J. Nutr.,* 98, 90–94, 1969.
35. Norred, W. P. and Wade, A. E., *Biochem. Pharmacol.,* 21, 2887–2897, 1972.
36. Norred, W. P. and Wade, A. E., *Biochem. Pharmacol.,* 22, 432–436, 1973.
37. Marshall, W. J. and McLean, A. E. M., *Biochem. J.,* 122, 569–573, 1971.
38. Becking, G. C., *Can. J. Physiol. Pharmacol.,* 51, 6–11, 1973.
39. Wade, A. E., Greene, F. E., Ciordia, R. H., Meadows, J. S., and Caster, W. O., *Biochem. Pharmacol.,* 18, 2288–2292, 1969.
40. Grosse, W. and Wade, A. E., *J. Pharmacol. Exp. Ther.,* 176, 758–765, 1971.
41. Wade, A. E., Wu, B., and Lee, J., *Biochem. Pharmacol.,* 24, 785–789, 1975.
42. Catz, C. S., Juchau, M. R., and Yaffe, S. J., *J. Pharmacol. Exp. Ther.,* 174, 197–205, 1970.
43. Shargel, L. and Mazel, P., *Biochem. Pharmacol.,* 22, 2365–2373, 1973.
44. Miller, J. A. and Miller, E. C., *Adv. Cancer Res.,* 1, 339–396, 1953.
45. Axelrod, J., Udenfriend, S., and Brodie, B. B., *J. Pharmacol. Exp. Ther.,* 111, 176–181, 1954.
46. Conney, A. H., Bray, G. A., Evans, C., and Burns, J. J., *Ann. N.Y. Acad. Sci.,* 92, 115–127, 1961.
47. Degkuritz, E. and Staudinger, H., *Hoppe-Seyler's Z. Physiol. Chem.,* 342, 63–72, 1965.
48. Kato, R., Takanaka, A., and Oshima, T., *Jpn. J. Pharmacol.,* 19, 25–33, 1969.
49. Avenia, R. W., Ph.D. thesis, Cornell University, Ithaca, N.Y., 1972.
50. Zannoni, V. G., Flynn, E. J., and Lynch, M., *Biochem. Pharmacol.,* 21, 1377–1392, 1972.
51. Carpenter, M. P., *Ann. N.Y. Acad. Sci.,* 203, 81–92, 1972.
52. Wade, A. E., Wu, B., and Smith, P. B., *J. Pharm. Sci. U.A.R.,* 61, 1205–1208, 1972.
53. Murty, H. S., Caasi, P. I., Brooks, S. K., and Nair, P. P., *J. Biol. Chem.,* 245, 5498–5504, 1970.
54. Sato, P. H. and Zannoni, V. G., *Biochem. Pharmacol.,* 23, 3121–3128, 1974.

55.   Dingell, J. V., Joiner, P. D., and Hurwitz, L., *Biochem. Pharmacol.,* 15, 971–976, 1966.
56.   Becking, G. C. and Morrison, A. B., *Biochem. Pharmacol.,* 19, 895–902, 1970.
57.   Becking, G. C. and Morrison, A. B., *Biochem. Pharmacol.,* 19, 2639–2644, 1970.

THE INFLUENCE OF DIETARY COMPOSITION ON THE METABOLISM OF NONESSENTIAL METALS

J. Quarterman

INTRODUCTION

This review describes the effects of variations in the dietary content of various nutrients or common additives, but not drugs, on the absorption, excretion, metabolism, and toxicity of a number of metals not normally considered to be essential. The composition of the diet is important because changes in it can give rise to very great differences in the fraction of the metals absorbed and in their toxic effects in experimental and practical situations.

The amount of information available differs widely from one metal to another. Those which present the greatest hazard, cadmium, lead, mercury, and strontium have been most thoroughly investigated. This review is mainly confined to the effects of diet on the metabolism of the metals, but the effects of metals on other dietary components is described when it clarifies the relationship being discussed. General features of the metabolism and toxicology of the metals are not discussed except where they are relevant to dietary effects. These topics have been reviewed elsewhere.[1,2] Some nondietary effects such as those of age and sex are mentioned where they may influence dietary interactions. It is intended that the references be comprehensive but not complete. Where a topic is very detailed, the most important or recent references are given.

MODES OF INTERACTION

Dietary components interact with metals in many ways. The metal may be bound to an indigestible material and excreted in the feces, or its absorption may be enhanced by chelation with a low molecular weight compound. There may be competition between nutritionally essential metals and toxic metals at sites of absorption or transport or in metalloenzymes. Changes in nutrient intake may regulate the content in the tissues of substances which react with the toxic metal and influence its fate and toxicity. Nutrients which modify the toxicity of a metal may do so by altering its absorption and excretion and thus the extent of its accumulation in target tissues. Alternatively, they may modify the solubility or subcellular distribution of the metal within tissues. In most cases the details of the nutrient-metal interactions described in this review are obscure. Some are unique for one metal; others, such as the dependence of retention upon dietary protein content and ascorbic acid, occur with a number of metals.

Models for some of these interactions have been suggested. In particular, a study of the electron orbital configurations of metals has given a theoretical basis for the possibility that some metals may substitute for others in biological systems and thus participate in mutually antagonistic interactions at functional sites.[3,4] While this concept has proved particularly useful in the systematic study of adverse responses arising from metal intoxication, its applicability is limited and other explanations are being sought to account for observed interactions.

ALUMINUM

The only nutrient interaction with aluminum which has received any attention is that with fluoride.[5] Aluminum salts are sometimes used to reduce the availability of dietary fluoride when this is considered to be too high.

ANTIMONY

Deprivation of water for 48 hr or intracellular dehydration, produced by giving 2% NaCl in the drinking water for 1 to 2 weeks, increased mortality in rats injected with water-soluble compounds of antimony. Raising the environmental temperature to 33.3°C for 48 hr also increased the toxicity of the antimony.[6]

ARSENIC

The toxic effects of selenium can be decreased by arsenic and those of arsenic by selenium.[7] These effects occur at low dietary levels of the elements. For example, 5 ppm sodium arsenite in the drinking water gave full protection against liver damage in rats given diets containing 15 ppm of selenium as seleniferous wheat or as sodium selenite. Several arsenic compounds are active against selenium but arsenite is the most effective.

The effect of arsenite is to inhibit the methylation of selenium and hence its expiration in a volatile form and at the same time to increase the excretion of selenium given as selenite (but not as selenate) in bile. Selenium similarly increased the biliary excretion of arsenic. In the bile these elements exist in several forms, some of which may be associated with protein, although their exact nature is not known.

BARIUM

Weanling rats absorbed about 80% of an oral tracer dose of barium but only about 7% when they were 70 days old. Barium absorption by young rats was increased by starvation for 18 hr but was not affected by the substitution of milk for a solid diet.[8] Rachitic chicks absorbed less barium than vitamin D supplemented chicks.[9]

BERYLLIUM

Vitamin D increased the deposition of oral tracer doses of beryllium in the tibia of 3- to 5-week-old chicks.[9]

CADMIUM

The metabolism and toxicology of cadmium have been reviewed and special attention given to their relationship with selenium, zinc, and copper.[4,10,11] Many features of the metabolism of cadmium and its interaction with these and other elements are related to its ability to induce the synthesis of the metal-binding protein, metallothionein.

Orally ingested cadmium was accumulated by the intestinal mucosa especially of the duodenum, which acts as a barrier to cadmium absorption.[12,13] Uptake by the mucosa was initially rapid and subsequent absorption was slow. Absorption did not require energy, was not unidirectional, and did not occur against a concentration gradient. Interaction of cadmium with other metals during absorption suggests that there is competition for binding sites.[14] However, it must be emphasized that the in vitro studies leading to most of these conclusions did not differentiate between true absorption of cadmium and adsorption onto inert structural components of the mucosa. Cadmium given parenterally was secreted into the gut contents through the gut wall and to a smaller extent in the bile; about 5% of such a dose was recovered in the feces.[15] Figures for the retention of oral doses of cadmium range from below 1 to above 10% though most are at the lower end of this range.[10] The absorption and tissue distribution of an oral dose of cadmium was similar if it was given as the chloride, sulfate, or acetate, but the fraction of the dose retained decreased as the size of the dose was increased.[16] Cadmium given to rats in the drinking water was more toxic and gave higher tissue concentrations than the same dose (5 mg Cd/kg live weight) given in the food.[17] While the fraction of cadmium retained by the body differed according to the route of administration, the rate of elimination of absorbed metal and the individual variability of retention did not depend on the route of administration.[18,19] Cadmium was accumulated by the liver and kidney whether animals were given the metal orally or parenterally.[20,21]

Pretreatment of animals with small doses of cadmium, e.g., 3 to 600 μg/kg live weight of mice, protected them against some of the effects of a later, large dose, e.g., 3 mg/kg, particularly the decreases of hematocrit and hemoglobin concentration.[10,22,23] This finding is consistent with the induction by the small dose of a cadmium-binding protein which can then bind a large cadmium dose.[10]

There is evidence that animals can adapt to continued cadmium intake. In rats and rabbits the impairment of growth and anemia due to dietary cadmium was reversed after a few weeks.[24,25]

Effect of Protein

Diets low or high in protein increase the severity of dietary cadmium poisoning.[26-28] The greater effects were due to low protein diets and included a doubling of cadmium absorption, increased tissue cadmium contents, especially of liver and kidney, and an increase in the cadmium-induced loss of body weight. There was a greater absorption of cadmium in rats even with as much as 8.5% dietary protein compared with 15.3%.

Cysteine (up to 10 mM/kg live weight) given i.p. protected rats given a subcutaneous dose of cadmium (0.02 mM/kg) against testicular damage, but produced a kidney necrosis which did not occur when cadmium was given alone.[29] Subcutaneous glutathione gave some protection against testicular damage but methionine and thiosulfate had no effect.[30] Sulfurated water also reduced cadmium toxicity.[31]

Effect of Minerals

Calcium and Vitamin D

A number of reports have now confirmed that diets containing cadmium and low in calcium can cause more severe toxic effects, including increased bone resorption, and up to twice the absorption and twice the bone, kidney, and liver contents of cadmium compared with diets containing adequate calcium.[28,32-34] When the dietary calcium of pregnant rats was reduced from 0.96 to 0.07%, the tissue cadmium contents of the dam and the young were increased and the number of dams producing litters was reduced, but the birth weight of the young was not affected.[35] The absorption of oral doses of cadmium was greater in rachitic chickens than in those given vitamin D. The vitamin treatment did not affect the uptake of parenteral cadmium by bone, so vitamin D probably affects the intestinal absorption of cadmium.[36]

Addition of cadmium to the diet reduced the absorption of calcium and the concentration of calcium bound to protein in the duodenal mucosa.[37] Earlier reports found that the hydroxylation of vitamin D by kidney mitochondria was inhibited by cadmium and the reduced absorption of calcium in cadmium poisoning could follow from this.[38] A later report, however, showed that the hydroxylation of vitamin D in vivo is not impaired by cadmium poisoning. In this case the mitochondria may be protected by the prior formation of metallothionein. If the cadmium-binding protein metallothionein is added to kidney mitochondria in vitro, the hydroxylation of vitamin D is no longer inhibited by cadmium.[39] The possible involvement of the kidney and endocrine organs in this interaction has been discussed.[40,41]

Iron

Anemia is a frequent consequence of cadmium ingestion in man and animals, and its severity can be reduced by parenteral or oral doses of iron.[10,42] Cadmium reduced the intestinal absorption of iron but not its subsequent utilization.[43-48] A more detailed examination in mice has shown that low levels of cadmium inhibited iron uptake by the intestinal mucosa but higher levels inhibited both uptake and transfer.[49] Cadmium had a similar effect on cobalt absorption. When iron absorption was enhanced by a low-iron diet, cadmium absorption was increased, apparently by the enhanced activity of a mucosal uptake step common to both metals. In conditions of low-iron absorption, cadmium absorption was concentration dependent.

Selenium

It was first observed in 1960 that small amounts of selenite protect male gonads against necrosis produced by cadmium.[50] Since then all the other toxic effects of cadmium have been shown to be prevented by selenite or selenomethionine. The topic is under investigation by many groups and has been frequently reviewed.[4,10,11,51] Most of these investigations have involved parenteral injections of large doses of one or both elements into rats and have shown a complex effect of selenium on cadmium metabolism. In one experiment, for example, labeled cadmium (1.1 mg/kg live weight) was given to rats subcutaneously with or without labeled selenite (0.8 mg/kg) also given subcutaneously. In the rats given selenite, while toxic effects were reduced, cadmium concentration in blood and testes increased, but that in liver and kidneys decreased. The soluble fraction of these tissues contained most of the cadmium. Selenium diverted this soluble cadmium from low molecular weight proteins to larger ones. The authors conclude that selenite has modified the properties of an existing protein or proteins such that they now find cadmium in a less toxic form than before the administration of selenite. When cadmium is given by mouth the toxic symptoms are different from when it is given by injection, but there is evidence that some interaction occurs. Thus while cadmium decreases weight gain and increases mortality on a selenium-free diet, it has no effect with a diet containing a toxic level (40 ppm) of selenium.[52]

The converse situation, that is the possible effect of cadmium on selenium, has been investigated.[53] Injected cadmium, unlike mercury, did not potentiate dimethylselenide toxicity.[51] When rats were depleted of selenium and vitamin E, the resulting liver necrosis was made worse by silver but not by cadmium.[54] The appearance of white muscle disease in lambs was not affected by the addition of 1 ppm cadmium to the diet.[55]

Zinc

Zinc and cadmium occur together in nature and interact with each other in many ways at the biochemical and the nutritional level. Relatively large doses of zinc, given orally or parenterally, will protect against the toxic manifestations of cadmium except where these involve cadmium-induced disturbances of copper metabolism.[4,10,56] Cadmium can produce symptoms of zinc deficiency which can be corrected by zinc administration.[57] Intraperitoneal doses of zinc cause a redistribution of tissue cadmium by a mechanism as yet unknown.[58]

High levels of dietary cadmium (350 ppm) given to calves reduced the absorption and tissue content of oral ^{65}Zn and increased the total fecal excretion of the labeled zinc.[59] Later work with rats with smaller levels of cadmium showed that cadmium decreased the uptake of zinc by the mucosa of the gut with a range of dietary zinc levels but that zinc transport from the lumen to the carcass was not affected by cadmium in zinc-deficient rats and hamsters and was decreased in zinc-supplemented animals.[60,61]

Both zinc and cadmium stimulate the synthesis of metallothionein, a low molecular weight, metal-binding protein, and many of their interrelationships may be explained by their effects on the concentration of this protein and their binding to it.[10,62]

Copper

Cadmium is known to decrease tissue copper content and to reduce the passage of copper across the placenta without being transported in any significant quantity itself.[5,56,57] For example, when the dietary cadmium of pregnant ewes was increased from 0.7 to 3.5 ppm, the liver copper content of the ewes was unchanged but that of the lambs was reduced from 100 to 22 ppm.[63]

There is very little information about the effects of dietary copper on cadmium metabolism. One report shows that i.p. copper increased the concentration of cadmium in the liver, decreased it in kidney, and had no effect on blood cadmium.[58]

Copper is bound strongly by metallothionein and exchanges with zinc and cadmium bound to that protein, but it is not clear how these properties relate to the effects observed in vivo.[4,62]

Other Metals

Mercury, given i.p., alters the concentration of cadmium differently in tissues.[58] Lead and arsenic exacerbate the teratogenic effect of cadmium.[64,64a] Manganese reduced the anemia produced by cadmium.[22]

EFFECT OF VITAMINS

The anemia and other toxic effects of cadmium were reduced as dietary *pyridoxine* was increased from 0 to 44 ppm. The authors believe that pyridoxine modifies the metabolism of cadmium rather than that it counters the changes in iron metabolism produced by cadmium.[25] The anemia produced by cadmium was also prevented by prior administration of *thiamine*.

Ascorbic acid synthesis is decreased by cadmium poisoning.[65,66] The anemia and decreased tissue ascorbate concentrations produced by cadmium were reversed by ascorbate administration, but the histological damage to the liver and failure of ascorbate and xylulose synthesis were not altered.[67] The improvement of the anemia in quail given 75 ppm cadmium following doses of ascorbate may have been due to the increased absorption of iron from the intestinal tract.[68] In chicks given 50 or 100 ppm cadmium in the food, hematocrit was not affected and the decreased body weight and tibia weight were not improved by 1% dietary ascorbate.[69]

CESIUM

As in the case with many other metals the absorption of cesium decreased markedly after weaning.[70,71] The retention of cesium however was less in weanling than in suckling or adult mice.[72] Retention was also increased if suckling was prolonged.[73]

Diets high in fat, carbohydrate, or protein, or a restricted supply of food, increased the absorption and retention of cesium but the effects on tissue concentrations varied from tissue to tissue.[74]

Increases of dietary potassium decreased cesium absorption.[70,71,73] Dietary supplements of rubidium had a lesser effect than potassium. Beet pulp (20%), fluoride (70 ppm), ferriferrocyanide (1%), and vitamin D decreased cesium retention.[76,77] Lactose increased it and vitamin A was without effect.[73,77]

LEAD

The influence of the diet on the absorption and metabolism of lead has been investigated more thoroughly than that of any other nonessential element.

When data from different experiments are compared, account must be taken of a number of nonnutritional factors which can have a major influence on lead metabolism and which may affect conclusions drawn from dietary studies. For example, suckling rats had a very high absorption of several elements including lead, and young, weaned rats retained more of oral and intraperitoneal doses of ^{203}Pb than did older rats.[78-82] The fraction of lead absorbed from the food decreased with age, and at maturity there were important species differences in the fractional absorption and retention of dietary lead. Man retained about 10% of orally ingested lead, the sheep, rabbit, and rat about 1%.[83-85] In rats and sheep the retention of lead differed between the sexes, and sex differences also existed in the sensitivity to lead. Pregnant sheep were more sensitive to lead than nonpregnant ewes.[86-88] In a study of agricultural workers, males had higher blood lead levels than females.[89] Administration of methandrostenolone to rats and of ACTH or 6 α-methylprednisolone to human subjects reduced the retention of lead.[90,91]

The amount of lead in the diet had no effect on the fraction of ingested lead which was retained over a wide range of dietary lead in rats and sheep.[82,84,92] The fraction of intraperitoneal doses of ^{203}Pb ranging from 1 to 5000 μg/kg body weight retained by rats was also found to be constant.[93,94] This behavior of lead is in marked contrast to that of other metallic elements. The fraction of lead retained depends also on the form in which it is presented. Thus metallic lead is poorly absorbed (14% of the retention of lead given as acetate) while lead administered as carbonate is well absorbed (164% of lead as acetate).[82] Lead given to rats in the divalent or hexavalent form is found in tissues as the divalent ion.[95] There is evidence of considerable individual variability in the absorption of an oral dose of lead.[96]

The metabolism of lead is affected by the extent and duration of prior exposure to it. Thus in rats, sheep, and cattle given lead continuously in the food or water the concentration of lead in blood and other tissues is at a maximum at 6 to 8 months from the start of lead ingestion.[87,95-97] In sheep, tissue lead concentrations rise steeply when lead is first given and are then nearly constant until they begin to decrease after about 8 months exposure.[87,96] A single dose of 10 mg lead/kg body weight given intraperitoneally to rats 2 days before an intraperitoneal dose of 50 mg/kg produced no significant changes in lead metabolism, growth, or hematology.[98] A similar intraperitoneal injection of lead to mice reduced the toxicity of an injection of 200 mg lead/kg 4 days later but did not protect them against the toxic effects of a diet containing 4% PbCO$_3$. The decrease of hematocrit and ALAD* activity which followed ingestion of this diet was increased by prior lead injection.[99] The absorption and excretion of ^{203}Pb were not affected by the inclusion of 20 ppm lead in the food for the previous 3 months. The only effect of prior feeding of lead was to increase the total activity/g in the liver.[100]

There is some evidence that lead could be an essential nutrient.[101]

Dietary Effects

Level of Total Food and Water Intake**

When the total intake of a nutritionally complete diet for rats was restricted so that

---

*   ∂-aminolaevulinate dehydrase.

** More recent experiments by the author have modified the above ideas about the effects of protein and fat on lead retention. When a reduction in dietary protein is not accompanied by reductions in food intake or growth rate of rats, then lead retention decreased as dietary protein decreased.[101a]

The described effects of dietary fat content on lead retention have been demonstrated in experiments lasting 2 to 4 days. Over 3 to 5 weeks, no effect of fat on lead retention was observed.

the rats continued to grow but more slowly than a control group given the same diet to appetite, the retention of dietary lead was increased by over 100%.[92] In fasting humans, the absorption of lead was as high as 50% while in nonfasting subjects it was 6 to 14%.[102] Such observations illustrate the importance of allowing for possible effects arising from changes in food intake when the influence of changes in dietary composition under lead retention is being investigated.

When mice were deprived of water to the extent that they lost 12% of their body weight, they died more rapidly after a dose of lead. They were also more susceptible to lead toxicity at 96° or 60° than at 72°F, and at 95° lead excretion in urine and feces was lower than at 72°.[103]

Effect of Protein and Amino Acid Content of the Diet

Tissue lead concentrations were increased and the toxic effects of dietary lead worse when dietary protein was less than about 10%.[104-108] With low-protein diets, kidney lead concentration was increased less than that of other tissues.[106,107] When the dietary protein was increased to 40% or over, lead retention was also increased in the whole body, kidneys, and femur, but not in blood and liver.[106,109] In some of these experiments the food intake was controlled.[106] The results of the others may have been influenced by a possible reduction of food intake by the experimental rats.

Supplementation of the diet with amino acids can produce changes in lead metabolism. The addition of 0.5% or less methionine to a diet reduced the lead content of tissues.[100,105,107,110-112] In some cases these effects occurred in the presence of supplementary cystine.[100,107,110] Reduction of tissue lead uptake also occurred in response to intraperitoneal or oral doses of methionine.[100]

Cystine supplements increased total carcass and kidney lead concentrations without increasing those of blood or liver.[30,31] The absorption of lead has been shown to be influenced by dietary supplements of several other amino acids and in this respect resembles calcium.[100,113] The effect of particular amino acids in the retention of the two metals is not always in the same direction; for example, methionine decreased lead but increased calcium retention. It must be noted however that experiments with calcium tested only the absorption by the gut, whereas in the lead experiments tissue lead concentrations were affected even when methionine was given intraperitoneally.

Thus the effect on the retention and tissue distribution of lead of changes in dietary protein content may be a result of a complex of effects due to food restriction and changes in the supply of amino acids which in turn differ in their individual effects.

Effect of Lipid Content of the Diet

Very large increases in lead uptake, up to ten times, have been found when the dietary fat was increased from 5 or 10% or more.[109,114] Reducing the dietary fat to very low levels did not alter lead uptake from that observed at 5 to 10%.[109] Rats given lead and 40% dietary fat died in a few days with degeneration and fatty infiltration of the liver. With 5% fat, they lived longer and had no liver damage.[115]

This effect of fat may be particularly important for suckling and other animals or humans who are receiving most of their food in the form of milk, since rats which were given dried or liquid milk absorbed 30 to 50 times more lead than those given commercial rat food.[116] The milk diet was low in iron (see below) but the most significant difference from the commercial diet was the fat content (25% $\sim$ 4%). Lactose had only a small effect on lead absorption (see below).[100] The effects of milk on lead metabolism have been reviewed.[117]

Bile probably plays an important role in the mechanism by which fat increases lead absorption. When bile was present in the gut, the absorption of lead was much greater than when the bile duct was cannulated and bile flow diverted.[118] In these experiments the increased absorption due to bile was much smaller than that produced by changes of dietary fat but the rats were starved before the experiment. When bile salts (0.5%), lecithin (0.5%), or choline (1%) were added to a semipurified diet containing either 5% or 20% fat, [203]Pb absorption was increased.[100] Bile and bile salts affect calcium absorption in a similar way to that of lead. Lecithin may have an important role since phospholipids are a major component of bile, are involved in fat absorption, and the compound of lead with lecithin is fat soluble.[100,119-120] Further involvement of lead with phospholipids has been suggested in erythrocyte and bacterial membrane lipids.[121,122]

Effect of Carbohydrates

An alginate preparation, high in guluronic acid, given to human subjects with an oral dose of [203]Pb, had no effect on the absorption of the isotope.[123] The same alginate was given to rats for 3 or 4 days before an oral dose of [203]Pb. When the rats were receiving a commercial diet, the addition of 10% alginate increased the absorption of lead. When the alginate was added to a diet containing mainly cellulose, sucrose, and dried milk, lead absorption was decreased.[124] The addition of alginate to a whole milk diet for rats also decreased lead absorption.[125]

Pectin, unlike the high guluronic acid-alginate discussed above, reduced lead absorption and its toxic effects in rats and humans offered either crude or semipurified diets. In rats, 0.2 to 0.5 g apple pectin/kg body weight reduced the toxic effects of lead and 5% in the diet decreased the retention and urinary excretion of lead.[126,127] In humans and rats, diets high in vegetables or cabbage pectin reduced the severity of clinical lead toxicity.[128]

Dietary fructose modified the effect of lead on tissue-free amino acid patterns, alkaline phosphatase activity, and histochemical changes induced by lead; and 10% lactose in a semipurified diet increased retention by about 50%.[100,129]

Effect of Major Minerals: Calcium, Phosphate, and Vitamin D

The best-documented dietary influence on lead metabolism is that of calcium. Early work, much of it on human patients, established the main features of the changes in blood lead concentration and lead excretion to high or low dietary calcium, intravenous calcium gluconate, and parathyroid hormone (which increased lead excretion). Though some of the results were conflicting, calcium treatment was not always distinguished from other treatments, and dietary calcium and phosphate levels were not always controlled independently.[130-134]

When the dietary calcium of rats was reduced to levels below requirement, lead retention was greatly increased, sometimes by a factor of ten.[85,109,135-138] In sheep, pigs, and horses, low dietary calcium increased the lead content of tissues or the severity of lead poisoning.[96,139,140] Early observations that calcium supplements given to human subjects orally or by intravenous infusion increased the rate of accretion of lead have not been repeated.[131]

Low dietary phosphate content influenced lead retention and tissue lead levels in the same way as did low dietary calcium; its effect was independent of dietary calcium and additive with it.[85,138]

When the dietary content of calcium or phosphate was increased above the requirement, the retention of lead by rats was decreased.[100,141,142] Increasing the dietary phosphorus content of a lamb's diet from 0.3 to 1.3% reduced the lead content of bone but not that of liver and kidney.[143] Vitamin D supplementation increased lead absorption in rats.[142]

Low dietary contents of calcium and phosphate and supplements of vitamin D all increase the concentration of calcium binding protein (CaBP) in the intestinal mucosa.[144] The way in which these nutrients affect the absorption of lead is compatible with the idea that lead can be transported by CaBP. The idea is further supported by the observation that lead absorption in rats and the stimulating effect of vitamin D were greatly reduced by prior treatment with cycloheximide, a drug which inhibits protein synthesis.[85]

The release and excretion of lead which has already been incorporated into the tissues are also affected by these dietary components. A low dietary Ca/P ratio or vitamin D supplementation reduced blood lead concentration and lead release from bone.[145] Low dietary calcium almost completely prevented lead loss from rats; low dietary phosphate had a lesser effect.[85] In human subjects, calcium supplementation of the diet or intravenous administration of calcium has been reported to increase lead excretion.[131,146] In rats, there are conflicting reports about the effect of high dietary calcium on lead release.[141,145]

The absorption of calcium and lead is influenced by dietary calcium, phosphate, and vitamin D in similar ways but the movement of the two elements is not always similar. Thus an increased rate of calcification is not necessarily accompanied by increased lead deposition.[147] The loss of lead from bones in a period of severe resorption during weaning depended on the composition of the diet and not on the degree of resorption.[138] When the diet was low in calcium, the increase in the lead content of the liver in rats and sheep was large relative to the increase in lead content of other tissues, while there was no change in calcium content.[85,96]

The concentration of lead in the fetus of the rat was modified by the calcium and phosphate content of the diet to the same extent as other soft tissues of the pregnant rat were affected.[138]

A further important effect of low calcium diets in rats and monkeys is that the animals developed a pica and that they chose diets or water containing lead in preference to lead-free food or water.[148,149] These effects occurred in monkeys with diets containing 84% of the recommended dietary calcium content and were not prevented in rats by intraperitoneal administration of lead.

Magnesium

Omission of a magnesium supplement from a semipurified diet caused a small increase in the absorption of an oral dose of ^{203}Pb during 48 hr.[109]

Sulfur Compounds

A variety of sulfur compounds has been used to mitigate the toxic effects of lead. Many have been administered by injection but oral doses of hydrogen sulfide-water, and calciulate, a mineral containing calcium and sulfur, promoted lead excretion or reduced toxic effects of lead.[150,151] Sodium sulfate given to rats in the food did not reduce lead retention, but lead sulfide was retained less well than lead acetate.[109,112] The effects of dietary sulfur-amino acids have been mentioned above.

Sheep given a diet low in sulfur (about 0.1%) containing 200 or 400 ppm lead lost appetite and weight and some died within a few weeks. These symptoms were prevented or reduced by the addition to the diet of 0.15 or 0.3% sulfur as sodium sulfate.[87,152] This supplement also reduced histological signs of damage in the liver and kidney. The anemia and osteoporosis which occurred in males, but not in castrates, as a result of lead poisoning were prevented. Blood lead concentrations were reduced by the sulfate supplement initially but after about 3 months were fairly constant and not influenced by dietary treatment.

In the ruminant, dietary sulfate is converted into a variety of sulfur compounds in the rumen. Sulfide and methionine may reduce the availability or retention of lead. The small amount of evidence so far available suggests that cystine may increase lead retention but reduce its toxicity.

Trace Elements

Iron, selenium, zinc, copper, cobalt, and fluoride have been reported to influence lead metabolism.

Iron

In lead-poisoned rabbits, intramuscular administration of iron saccharate reduced tissue lead contents and some of the toxic effects of the lead.[153] Rats given lead in the drinking water and made iron-deficient by consuming a diet containing 5 ppm iron for 10 weeks had greater tissue lead contents, greater urinary lead concentrations, and more severe signs of toxicity than rats given lead and adequate iron.[154] The intestinal transport of ^{210}Pb was increased when rats became iron deficient.[155] In contrast to these results with rabbits and rats, iron supplementation over a 6-month period of urban children with serum iron less than 80 μg/100 ml caused a small increase in blood lead concentrations.[156]

Lead is known to be bound to ferritin in several tissues, and it had been suggested that lead bound to ferritin in the gut mucosa is not absorbed and that variations in the concentration of ferritin may influence lead absorption.[155,157] In a typical 3-week experiment with rats the amount of lead absorbed can be increased by 1000 μg by iron deficiency. The gut tissue, however, contains only about 20 μg lead and whether or not this is absorbable is not significant.[100] Lead is also bound to transferrin and this protein may have a role in the transport of lead.[158]

Iron-deficient rats exposed to lead ate less and grew less well than iron-repleted rats, but the reduction of food intake did not account for all the increased lead absorption resulting from iron deficiency.[100]

Selenium

In an experiment in which rats were given 0 or 200 ppm lead in the food, urine ALA and tissue lead concentrations tended to be lower and blood ALAD higher when the diet contained 0.05 or 0.5 ppm selenium than when it contained 0.015 or 1.0 ppm selenium.[159] This observation confirmed observations by other workers who found that more severe toxic effects of lead were produced in the presence of diets deficient in vitamin E (see below).[160] The addition of 1 ppm selenium to a quail diet of unstated selenium content had no effect on lead metabolism except to increase kidney lead content.[161]

Zinc

When dietary zinc in rats was increased from 8 to 50 and 200 ppm the retention, tissue concentrations, and toxic effects of lead decreased by up to half.[162] Other workers have used much higher levels of both metals. Young horses were given diets with or without 800 ppm lead and 5400 ppm zinc.[163] The addition of zinc greatly mitigated the symptoms of lead poisoning but increased the lead content of liver and kidney. Brain and muscle lead contents were not affected by zinc. In pigs given diets with or without 1000 ppm lead and 4000 ppm zinc, addition of zinc to a diet containing lead decreased growth, food intake, serum calcium bone density, and ash content, and increased kidney, liver, and bone lead contents. Blood lead was not affected.[164]

It is not clear how far these differing effects of dietary zinc on lead metabolism are related to the different levels of zinc used or to different species. Most of the lead in liver and kidney is bound to a high molecular weight protein and very little with proteins of similar weight to metallothioneins whose concentration could be affected by zinc.[165]

Copper and Cobalt

Oral doses of copper (0.3 mg $CuCl_2$/kg body weight per day) and cobalt (0.8 mg $CoCl_2$/kg body weight per day) prevented weight loss, deaths, and changes in buccal mucosa produced in rats by oral doses of lead acetate (10 mg/kg body weight per day).[166] Cobalt decreased urinary excretion of lead and increased liver lead concentration but prevented a decrease in hematocrit and hemoglobin concentration. Copper had opposite effects on these three parameters.

When rats were given a diet with 5000 ppm lead, ceruloplasmin but not hemoglobin concentration or hematocrit was reduced if the diet had 2.5 ppm copper. If the copper content was as low as 0.5 ppm, hemoglobin concentration and hematocrit were also reduced by the lead supplement. Blood lead concentrations were lower with 2.5 ppm than with 0.5 ppm copper.[167]

Fluoride

The addition of 300 ppm fluoride to a diet containing 200 ppm lead increased mortality and lead concentrations in blood and femur but not in kidney.[168] Hematological parameters were not affected by the addition of fluoride and the authors conclude that the increased toxicity was not related to the increased lead retention.

Vitamins

B Vitamins

Nicotinic acid, given orally or intravenously, reduced the toxic effects of lead, in particular the increased porphyrin concentrations in blood and urine, the inhibition of pyridine coenzyme synthesis, disturbed gastrointestinal movements, and increased tissue adrenaline concentrations.[169-171] These ameliorating effects of nicotinic acid have been observed in humans, rabbits, and dogs but not in rats.[172,173] Nicotinic acid synthesis by rabbits following a dose of tryptophan was reduced by lead poisoning. The production of xanthurenic acid and other metabolites of tryptophan was also reduced and it was concluded that there was no evidence for the inhibition by lead of reactions involving pyridoxine.[172]

Other workers found that heme synthesis in lead-poisoned rats was improved by injections of nicotinic acid or vitamin C, but not by a tenfold increase of dietary nicotinic acid.[174]

Intramuscular injections of pyridoxine and vitamin B_{12} reduced disturbances of porphyrin metabolism produced by lead, but there were contradictory reports of the effects of AMP and inosine on rabbits.[175-178]

Vitamin C

Large oral doses of vitamin C decreased the severity of lead poisoning. Five mg of the vitamin per day improved the weight of guinea pigs but increased liver (but not kidney) lead concentrations; 0.5 mg/day had little effect.[179] In rabbits, urinary excretion of ALA and bone lead contents were decreased by vitamin C, and in sheep stiffness and poor growth due to lead poisoning were improved by 200 or 800 mg vitamin C per day.[111,180,181]

Vitamin E

Vitamin E deficiency in rats exacerbated the decreased hematocrit, increased reticulocyte count and splenic enlargement due to lead poisoning. The resistance to mechanical trauma of red blood cells from vitamin E deficient, lead-poisoned rats was reduced and the authors believe that vitamin E deficiency potentiates the anemia of lead poisoning by rendering the erythrocyte more susceptible to splenic sequestration.[182,183]

Other Nutritional Factors
Alcohol

When lead-poisoned rats were given ethyl alcohol in the drinking water, they lost weight, had an increased kidney weight, and increased lead concentrations in kidneys and bones. Blood lead, hemoglobin, and hematocrit were not affected.[184] The depression of blood ALAD was less when both lead and alcohol were given to human subjects than with either alone. It is believed that these agents have opposite effects on the concentration of reduced glutathione in the erythrocyte and this in turn affects the activity of ALAD.[185]

Acidosis and Alkalosis

Early reports that infusion of ammonium chloride or sodium bicarbonate increased lead excretion have not been followed up.[131]

Citric Acid

Although citrate increased the gastrointestinal absorption of lead most reports claim that large doses of citrate decrease lead retention.[117,186,187] Negative reports of the effect of citrate on retention may be because its stimulating effects on absorption and excretion are balanced or because it is rapidly metabolized.

Chelating Agents

Chelating agents can influence both the absorption and excretion of lead and their effect is influenced by age.[94,187] Some of them, particularly EDTA and penicillamine, are used in the treatment of lead poisoning because they cause a rapid excretion of the metal. This property is probably a reflection of their ability to chelate lead. Similar processes may account for the modifying effects of cystine, citrate, or alginate upon lead toxicity.

LITHIUM

Lithium salts are used in the treatment of various psychiatric disorders, but there was considerable individual variability in the degree to which an oral dose of lithium (given as carbonate) was retained.[188] One report states that lithium as carbonate, citrate, or acetate was equally well absorbed and that normal and achlorhydric patients absorbed lithium equally well; but another report finds that lithium as chloride, given orally, was less well absorbed than oral lithium as carbonate.[189,190] Lithium given after a meal was completely absorbed and produced no side effects but given on an empty stomach there was diarrhea and incomplete absorption.[191]

The growth retardation and polyuria produced in rats by lithium salts were reduced by oral doses of potassium chloride and, to a lesser extent, by sodium chloride, although these supplements did not alter serum lithium concentration.[192] Potassium deficiency altered the distribution of lithium within the tissues.[193] Renal lithium excretion was decreased by doses of ammonium chloride or potassium chloride, by a low-sodium chloride diet, sodium bicarbonate, or by osmotic diuresis produced by urea.[194]

The effects of iodine deficiency on the thyroid in rats and humans were exacerbated by lithium.[195,196] Choline stimulated the transport of lithium in cattle tissues.[197]

MERCURY

The toxicity and metabolism of mercury depend greatly on its chemical form: metallic, inorganic salt, or alkyl or aryl compound. The metabolism of these various forms of mercury has been reviewed, but the literature contains much less evidence of dietary effects than is the case with lead or cadmium.[4,198] This may be partly because most experiments have involved parenteral administration of mercury compounds and partly because the gastrointestinal absorption of organic mercury compounds is very efficient, usually well over 50%.[199,200] Inorganic mercury compounds are less well absorbed than are alkyl or aryl compounds. Interconversion of the forms of mercury may occur in the body; for example, there is evidence that mercuric salts may be methylated in the gut and that metallic mercury is oxidized to mercuric form by erythrocytes.[201-203] There is an enterohepatic circulation of mercury, and the subsequent absorption of mercury secreted by bile varied with the form in which the mercury was originally administered.[204,205] The mercury in bile secreted after oral administration of inorganic mercury was less well absorbed than the inorganic mercury, but that derived from methyl mercury and present in bile as a mercury-cysteine complex was very well absorbed.[206,207] Attempts have been made to decrease the toxicity of mercury by reducing the reabsorption of the metal secreted into the gut. For example, the toxicity was decreased and the fecal excretion of a parenteral dose of methyl mercury in mice was increased by feeding 3.3% of hair powder which had been reduced by thioglycollate.[208]

The percentage retention by chickens of oral or intramuscular doses of mercuric chloride or phenylmercuric acetate was independent of the size of the dose between 2 and 75 mg/kg.[209] Protection against a normally lethal dose of mercury was conferred by a prior smaller dose.[210] This may be an example of the same adaptive process which makes chronic administration of mercury less severe than acute treatment.

Susceptibility to mercury poisoning was also influenced by ambient temperature, genetic constitution, and hormone treatment.[211-214]

Effects of Organic Nutrients

Oral doses of glutamic acid protected against mercury poisoning.[215]

There is a complex relationship between mercury and vitamin C.[216] Oral mercuric chloride (8 mg/kg body weight) decreased the concentration of ascorbic acid in brain, adrenals, and spleen of guinea pigs given a maintenance dose of the vitamin. Vitamin C (5 mg/kg per day or 1% in the drinking water) did not affect the decrease of growth and weight of liver and kidney due to mercury. It increased the deposition of mercury in liver and kidney but prevented mercury-induced adrenal hypertrophy.

Folic acid had no effect on acute toxic effects of mercury in rats.[217]

Ethanol given to rats by mouth increased the rate of exhalation of metallic mercury given intravenously and reduced the mercury content of the whole body, lungs, heart, and brain but increased that of gut and liver. Ethanol dosing inhibited the rate of oxidation of metallic mercury to mercuric ion by erythrocytes.[203]

Effects of Minor Elements
Selenium

The protective effect of small amounts of selenium against the toxicity of a number of metals, including mercury, has received a great deal of interest and been the subject of several reviews.[4,218,219] Most of the work has been done with parenteral injections of one or both elements, but recently the basic findings have been confirmed in dietary experiments. On the basis of earlier work which had shown that selenium compounds were highly effective against the toxicity of cadmium and that parenteral mercuric salts could protect against selenium, it was predicted and was subsequently shown that when selenite or selenomethionine was injected with or after mercury, the toxic effects of the mercury were absent or greatly decreased. Concentrations of mercury were decreased in liver and kidney but increased in blood and testes. Selenite also reduced the transfer of mercury to fetal and suckling rats. The mechanism of these interactions is not understood but it seems likely that a metal-binding protein is involved such as has been found in the antagonisms among copper, zinc, cadmium, and selenium.

If selenite is administered before the mercury compound a more severe toxic effect is obtained than by either substance alone, and these toxic effects are more severe in males than in females. It is believed that selenite is converted by the body into the more toxic dimethylselenide and that once this has been formed its toxicity is increased and its respiratory excretion inhibited by mercury.

Selenium, 0.5 or 5 ppm in the food of rats, reduced the toxicity of methyl mercury or mercuric chloride given in the food or the water.[220-222] Dietary mercury (500 ppm) also prevented the growth failure due to 40 ppm dietary selenium in chicks, but 0.5 ppm dietary mercury given to ewes eating a selenium-deficient diet (<0.04 ppm selenium) did not influence the severity of the selenium deficiency syndrome, white muscle disease, in their lambs.[223,224]

An association between selenium and mercury in nontoxic states is suggested by correlations between the concentrations of these two elements in samples of tuna fish and of human tissues.[225,226]

Prior doses of cadmium and cobalt protect against mercury poisoning.[30] The uptake of mercury by rat intestine in vitro is increased by zinc, copper, and manganese, but the absorption by intact rats is not affected by iron deficiency.[204,227]

RUBIDIUM

Rubidium can replace potassium in the diets of rats or chicks for about 2 weeks before toxic effects begin to appear. Thus the growth retardation produced by diets deficient in potassium was reversed by the addition of 0.1 or 0.2% rubidium, but if rubidium was added to a diet adequate in potassium, growth was decreased and the animals became hyperirritable and spastic.[228,229]

Oral administration or addition to the diet of vitamin E or selenium (to rats previously given a vitamin E deficient diet) stimulated the uptake of rubidium-86 by liver slices that had previously been depleted of their potassium by cooling. This stimulation was not found in kidneys, hemidiaphragms, or erythrocytes. It was suggested that vitamin E and selenium may affect transcellular cation gradients and hence rubidium uptake by stabilizing membrane structures.[230]

SILVER

Silver, given in the drinking water at concentrations of 130 to 1000 ppm, is a strong liver poison, but its hepatic necrogenic effects in rats and chicks given a diet containing lard could be reversed by increased dietary vitamin E, selenium, and cyanocobalamin but not methionine.[231] When chicks were given a fat-free, casein-gelatin diet and 1500 ppm silver pectoral exudates were produced. This effect was not prevented by vitamin E or selenium but only by vitamin E together with methionine.

Conversely, the growth of chicks which was reduced by the addition of 5 ppm selenium to the diet was increased by the addition of 40 ppm silver.[232] Silver is believed to reduce selenium toxicity both by interfering with selenium absorption and by causing the accumulation of a nontoxic selenium compound in the tissues.

Silver is also a strong antagonist of copper. Dietary silver (900 ppm) produced cardiac enlargement, decreased aortic elastin and decreased concentrations of copper in blood, liver, spleen, and brain in chicks. All of these effects were reversed by the addition of 50 ppm copper to the diet.[233]

STRONTIUM

The influence of diet on strontium metabolism has received a great deal of attention because of the importance of strontium-90 in radioactive fallout, and is the subject of a number of articles in a book on strontium metabolism.[234]

Stable strontium at dietary levels comparable with those of calcium produces toxic effects, including bone deformities and uncoordination.[235]

Absorption of strontium by rats is very high up to weaning (over 80%) and then decreases to adult values (about 8%) at 90 days of age.[236] Most strontium is absorbed from the ileum in the first 2 hr after ingestion and about twice as much is absorbed from a liquid diet as from a solid diet.[237] Bile salts and sodium lauryl sulfate, which increase the lipid solubility of strontium, increase its absorption from ligated ileal loops in vivo in the chick.[238]

The retention of a single parenteral dose of strontium was decreased from about 80% to about 10% in rats that had previously been given a diet containing 6% strontium lactate for 6 days.[239]

In many respects the metabolism of strontium is similar to that of calcium. Nutrients which modify the metabolism of calcium have similar effects on strontium, but the organism also discriminates against strontium in favor of calcium in processes in which both metals take part. Some nutrients can modify the extent of this discrimination.

Effects of Protein, Fats, and Carbohydrates

About 45% more strontium was absorbed by rats given a diet with 20% casein than by those given a diet with casein replaced by zein. The absorption and deposition in bone of tracer doses of calcium and strontium were influenced to a similar extent by dietary protein but the increase of ^{89}Sr in serum was about five times as great as that of ^{45}Ca. The addition of 10% cellulose decreased strontium absorption, but 8% corn oil had no effect. Males absorbed less strontium than females.[240] In one report, increased dietary fat and the addition of soya decreased strontium absorption but in another, fat had no effect.[241,242]

Alginates, added at about 5 to 10% of the diet, have been used to reduce the absorption of a number of toxic metals including strontium.[243-245] Alginates with a high guluronic acid content inhibit strontium uptake much more strongly than calcium uptake.[246] In some physical forms alginates may have no effect on strontium absorption.[247]

The blood level of ^{85}Sr after an oral dose of the isotope was not influenced by the addition of lactose or lysine to the diet.[234,242,248]

Effects of Calcium, Phosphate, and Vitamin D

Increased dietary contents of calcium or phosphate or both decreased the absorption of strontium.[234,249,250] Phosphates are believed to reduce strontium retention both by reducing transport from the gut and by increasing excretion through the kidney.[251] Parenteral polyphosphates were effective only in large doses.[252]

The discrimination of the gut against strontium in favor of calcium decreases with age in human infants.[253] Dietary phosphate given to lactating rats decreased the amount of strontium transferred to the young in milk.[254] The fraction of the strontium in the body of pregnant rats which was transferred to the young increased with each successive pregnancy.[255]

Chronic administration of strontium can cause a syndrome very like rickets that is brought about by reduction of intestinal calcium absorption and by inhibition of bone calcification.[256-258] A major factor in the production of "strontium rickets" is inhibition by strontium of vitamin D hydroxylation.[259] The condition was improved by 1,25-dihydroxycholecalciferol (DHCC) but not by vitamin D. The substance in *Solanum malacoxylon* which mimics the action of DHCC also prevents the rachitic effects of strontium poisoning.[260] Strontium may also affect calcium metabolism by stimulating the secretion of calcitonin.[261,262]

Effect of Magnesium

Dietary supplements of magnesium salts increased the discrimination of the gut against strontium absorption in favor of calcium.[263] The retention of strontium in the body was reduced by the administration of magnesium perfused into the gut or given in the diet, in the drinking water, or parenterally.[241,264,265] Dietary magnesium also decreased the transfer of strontium to the young of pregnant rats.[266]

Effects of Other Minerals

When the drinking water of rats contained 100 ppm fluoride, strontium retention in the skeleton was increased by about 30%; 1 ppm fluoride had no effect.[267] In contrast to this observation, water containing 3 ppm fluoride decreased the uptake of ^{90}Sr by rats.[268] In areas of the USSR where the water contained between 0.8 and 4.0 ppm fluoride the accumulation of strontium in the skeleton of humans was less and the discrimination against strontium in favor of calcium was greater than in areas where the water contained 0.6 ppm fluoride or less.[234]

Lead (20 to 200 ppm) decreased the transport of ^{85}Sr by everted duodenal sacs.[269]

A mixture of barium sulfate and sodium sulfate has been used to reduce strontium uptake.[270,271] So also has aluminum phosphate gel and ammonium chloride.[272,273]

Effects of Vitamins

Oral doses of vitamin A decreased the absorption of strontium by rats and increased the discrimination in favor of calcium.[274,275] Large doses of vitamins A, D, B_6, or pantothenic acid all promoted loss of strontium from bone.[276]

The inhibition of vitamin B_{12} absorption by chelators could be counteracted by oral dosing with a number of metal salts, including strontium.[277]

THALLIUM

Dietary supplements of potassium given to rats, dogs, and sheep increased the urinary, but not the fecal, excretion of thallium. The excreted thallium was mobilized from the tissues, and the supplements afforded slight protection against the mortality due to thallium dosing.[278] The transport of thallium across the placenta of the rat is small and potassium deficiency of the dam had no effect on the toxicity of maternal thallium to the fetus.[279]

THORIUM

A complex of thorium with EDTA was absorbed and deposited in bone up to fifty times more efficiently than the oxide, chloride, or nitrate. The absorption of all compounds was increased about three times if rats were starved for 12 hr before the thorium was given.[280] Dietary tetracycline reduces thorium and plutonium deposition in bone by about 40%.[281]

TIN

There is some evidence that tin is an essential nutrient, in that the growth of rats that were given a highly purified diet increased by about 50% when the diet was supplemented with 100 ppm tin.[282]

The decreases in hemoglobin and serum iron induced by 150 ppm tin were prevented by increasing the dietary copper from 6 to 50 ppm and were less marked when the iron content was increased from 35 to 250 ppm. The growth depression due to tin could not be completely prevented by copper or iron.[283]

TITANIUM

Reduction of dietary sodium chloride or calcium carbonate progressively increased the tissue content and altered the distribution among the tissues of titanium and vanadium in the rat.[284]

ADDENDUM OF MORE RECENT OBSERVATIONS ON NUTRIENT-METAL INTERACTIONS

The metabolism of some metals, especially those considered to be important environmental pollutants, has continued to be the subject of intensive study and some general reviews have appeared.[285-288]

ALUMINUM

The value of aluminum salts in reducing fluoride toxicity has been shown in several species with varying degrees of success.[289,290] A new observation which may have important applications is that aluminum reduced the absorption and retention of iron.[291] Aluminum has also been shown to increase phosphate balance, possibly alter plasma parathyroid hormone levels,[292] and to reverse the inhibition by lead of δ-aminolevuilinic acid dehydratase.[293]

ANTIMONY

Cysteine alleviated antimony toxicity, but, unlike penicillamine, decreased its anti-schistosomal activity.[294]

ARSENIC

The inhibition by arsenic of succinic acid dehydrogenase in various tissues was influenced by the diet.[295]

CADMIUM

Recent reviews have included discussions of interactions of cadmium with nutrients and adventitious dietary contaminants.[285,296-299]

The fraction of ingested cadmium retained by rats decreased with increasing age, and the distribution among the tissues changed.[300,301] Chronic underfeeding did not affect cadmium toxicity.[302] Pretreatment of rats with small doses of cadmium or zinc protected them against subsequent larger doses of cadmium,[303] although this protective effect was limited in capacity.[304] This pretreatment with cadmium altered the intracellular distribution of the metal in the liver and decreased the biliary excretion of copper, mercury, zinc, silver, and lead, but not of arsenic, manganese, or methylmercury.[305] Milk increased cadmium absorption,[300,306] and the increased toxic effects due to a reduction of dietary protein from 17.9 to 8.8 g/100 g could be reversed almost completely by the addition of 0.5 g methionine/100 g diet.[306]

Calcium and Vitamin D

The means by which low dietary calcium decreases the absorption and toxic effects of orally ingested cadmium continue to be investigated,[297,308-310] though there are some conditions in which this effect was not observed.[311,312] In this and the reverse effect, the reduction of calcium absorption by dietary cadmium,[311,313,314] there is evidence that the two metals compete for binding sites on mucosal calcium-binding protein.

There is further evidence that cadmium inhibited the 1-hydroxylation of 25-hydroxycholecalciferol in the kidney,[315] but that 1,25-dihydroxycholecalciferol did not influence cadmium retention.[316]

Trace Elements

In iron-deficient rats there was increased absorption of cadmium and deposition of cadmium in the duodenal mucosa.[317,318] Iron supplementation reduced tissue cadmium levels and symptoms of toxicity.[318-320]

Selenium-deficient rats have been found to be more sensitive to inhaled cadmium,[321] and a number of hepatic and pancreatic changes induced by cadmium can be prevented by dietary selenium or zinc,[322,323] though selenium did not affect the induction by cadmium of metallothionein in the liver and kidney.[324]

Cadmium increased the uptake of copper by the rat mucosa but decreased its absorption.[325] Conversely, copper, zinc, and manganese given to quail decreased the absorption of cadmium but not its uptake by the duodenal mucosa.[326] The relation of copper and zinc to cadmium toxicity has been discussed.[327]

LEAD

The absorption and retention of orally ingested lead has now been shown to decrease for up to 9 months after weaning.[328] A considerable fraction of maternal lead can appear in the suckling litter, and there is evidence for the active secretion of lead from blood into milk.[329-331] Work with everted gut sacs has shown that absorption of lead is a passive process related to water flow and occurs at a similar rate in all parts of the gut,[332-334] but work with *in situ* preparations found that the absorption from the jejunum was greater than that from duodenum or colon.[335]

Lead ingestion has now been associated with a reduced water intake and urine production,[336,337] urinary kallikrein excretion,[338] and increased renal insufficiency.[339] Metabolic acidosis decreased and alkalosis increased urinary lead excretion.[340]

Protein

Diets low in protein increased some signs of lead toxicity and blood lead concentrations but not the concentration of lead in other tissues.[341] It is possible, however, that low protein diets as such may have no effect or even decrease lead retention, the increased lead toxicity observed with these diets being due to the associated reduction in growth.[342]

Lipid

The addition of 5 g of lecithin or mixed bile salts to 1 kg semipurified diet doubled the absorption of lead, while exteriorization of the bile duct almost completely prevented any lead absorption, suggesting that agents which simulate bile or stimulate bile flow are essential for lead absorption.[343] Lead in the form of a purified phospholipid complex was absorbed no better than the acetate.[344]

Calcium and Vitamin D

Vitamin D stimulated the absorption of lead from the small intestine, but only in the distal parts,[345] in contrast to the effect of the vitamin on calcium absorption which occurs principally in the duodenum. One report claims that the dietary calcium level affects the excretion of lead rather than its absorption,[346] while another finds the concentration of calcium in the gut, not that in the blood, is the determining factor influencing lead retention.[347] Excess dietary calcium reduced the deposition of lead in the body, but also tended to reduce the release of lead already incorporated in the tissues.[348]

Calcitonin decreased blood lead concentrations and the uptake of lead by bone,[349,350] whereas parathyroid hormone reduced the retention of dietary lead by some process which did not involve its absorption by the gut.[351]

In human infants aged 14 to 746 days lead retention was over 30% and was related directly to lead intake and inversely to dietary calcium content.[352] In a large survey of lead-burdened children, blood lead was inversely related to blood calcium and calcium intake and directly to serum 25-hydroxycholecalciferol, suggesting that lead toxicity is related to a relative vitamin D deficiency.[353] A source of bone meal, used as a dietary calcium supplement, has been reported to produce severe lead poisoning.[354]

Autistic and atypical children who often exhibit pica had blood lead levels higher than normal.[355] Lead pica was induced in rats by calcium deficiency and to a smaller extent by dietary deficiencies of zinc and magnesium.[356]

Magnesium

Dietary supplements of magnesium decreased the severity of the symptoms of lead poisoning, mobilized lead from bone, and increased urinary lead excretion, although the lead content of some soft tissues was increased.[357]

Iron

Several reports have shown that iron deficiency increases and iron excess decreases the retention of lead.[320,358-361] This seems to be due to changes in absorption by the gut in which competitive binding by a high-molecular-weight protein plays a part. In some conditions this interaction was not observed.[362] In weanling rats, lead has been shown to increase iron absorption.[363] In humans, the relation of serum iron to blood lead depended on the sex of the subjects.[364]

Selenium

If selenium is given along with subcutaneously administered lead naphthenate, the toxic effects of the lead are mitigated but tissue contents of both elements are greater than when either is given alone.[365]

Zinc

The inhibition by lead of δ-aminolevuilinic acid dehydratase has been shown to be reversed by zinc in vitro and in vivo in several species.[366-369] At low concentrations cadmium has a similar effect to zinc, but inhibits the enzyme at higher concentrations.[370] Zinc supplements given to pregnant lead-poisoned rats increased the weight of the pups and decreased their lead content.[371]

Copper
The reports on the interactions among copper, iron, and lead are conflicting.[372-374] The effects may be important and deserve further study.

Ascorbic Acid
Ascorbic acid alone[375] or in combination with zinc,[376] iron,[377] or EDTA[378] is effective in promoting excretion of lead or reducing the severity of its toxicity. Lead in turn affected tissue ascorbic acid concentrations and some enzymes involved in ascorbic acid metabolism.[375]

Vitamin E and Selenium
Vitamin E deficiency and lead toxicity both decrease the deformability and hence increase the fragility of erythrocytes.[379,380] Exhaled ethane, an indicator of tissue lipid peroxidation, was increased by lead poisoning, and increased further when the diets were also deficient in vitamin E and selenium.[381]

Other Dietary Constituents
The absorption of lead from semipurified diets is greater than from commercial diets,[382] and the inclusion of tannic acid in rat diets decreased the toxicity of lead acetate.[383]

LITHIUM

Lithium is believed to decrease the ability of the body to conserve sodium.[384] Its toxicity was increased by a low intake of sodium[385] but decreased by reduced food intake,[386] by a supplement of potassium,[387] or by supplements of trace minerals, chelators, and vitamins.[388]

MERCURY

Mercury was found to be absorbed from all parts of the gut including the stomach.[389] Fish[390] and vegetables[391] reduced the availability of mercury compared with other foods. Chronic salt loading[392] or other means of promoting high urine flow[393] prevented the acute renal failure of mercury poisoning.

Ascorbic acid increased the intestinal absorption of mercury[394,395] and had no effect in reducing the toxicity of the metal.[396] Mercury reduced tissue concentrations and synthesis of the vitamin and inhibited l-glucuronolactone oxidase activity.[396]

Selenium decreased the toxicity of mercury in eggs.[397,398] In rats, selenium reduced the toxicity of the metal but increased tissue mercury concentration and reduced mercury excretion, perhaps by facilitating metallothionein synthesis.[399,400] Pretreatment with cadmium and zinc produced similar effects to selenium dosing, again probably due to induction of metallothionein synthesis.[401,402]

RUBIDIUM

Ascorbic acid ameliorated the toxic effects of rubidium on the liver and kidney, but did not improve the anemia or poor growth.[403] The rubidium and cesium uptake of cattle depended on the type of pasture and the season of the year.[404]

SILVER AND TELLURIUM

α-Tocopherol, but not selenium, prevented lesions of silver poisoning,[405] but both nutrients reduced tellurium toxicity.[406]

STRONTIUM

The importance of vitamin D and its metabolites in strontium absorption and the antagonistic effect of calcium have been emphasized.[407-409] The inhibition of calcium absorption by strontium was reversed by vitamin D.[407] Strontium absorption was decreased in diabetes[410] and by dietary alginate.[411]

TIN

Tin absorption is believed to occur passively from all parts of the gut, and is decreased by the presence of organic acids such as ascorbic and citric,[412] although a variety of other food components had no effect on retention.[413] Tin inhibited the secretion of gastric acid[414,415] and caused an accumulation of calcium in the kidneys with a decreased concentration of urine calcium.[416-418] The kidney calcification was prevented by simultaneous administration of lead[416] or citrate.[419] Tin also inhibited the stimulation of calcium absorption by vitamin D.[419]

TITANIUM

Tissue retention of titanium was increased in rats when the diets were deficient in protein, fat, or carbohydrates.[420]

REFERENCES

1. **Browning, E.,** *Toxicology of Industrial Metals,* 2nd ed., Butterworths, London, 1969.
2. **Monier-Williams, G. W.,** *Trace Elements in Food,* Chapman and Hall, London, 1949.
3. **Hill, C. H. and Matrone, G.,** Chemical parameters in the study of in vivo and in vitro interactions of transition elements, *Fed. Proc. Fed. Am. Soc. Exp. Biol.,* 29, 1474—81, 1970.
4. **Bremner, I.,** Heavy metal toxicities, *Q. Rev. Biophys.,* 7, 75—125, 1974.
5. **Underwood, E. J.,** *Trace Elements in Human and Animal Nutrition,* 3rd ed., Academic Press, London, 1971.
6. **Baetjer, A. M.,** Effects of dehydration and environmental temperature on antimony toxicity, *Arch. Environ. Health,* 19, 784—792, 1969.
7. **Levander, O. A.,** Factors that modify the toxicity of selenium, in *Newer Trace Elements in Nutrition,* Mertz, W. and Cornatzer, W. E., Eds., Marcel Dekker, New York, 1971, 57—83.
8. **Taylor, D. M., Bligh, P. H., and Duggan, M. H.,** The absorption of calcium, strontium, barium and radium from the gastrointestinal tract of the rat, *Biochem. J.,* 83, 25—29, 1962.
9. **Worker, N. A. and Migicovsky, B. B.,** Effect of vitamin D on the utilization of beryllium, magnesium, calcium, strontium and barium in the chick, *J. Nutr.,* 74, 490—494, 1961.
10. **Friberg, L., Piscator, M., Nordberg, G. F., and Kjellstrom, T.,** *Cadmium in the Environment,* Chemical Rubber Co., Cleveland, Ohio, 1974.
11. **Parízek, J., Ošťádalová, I., Kaloušková, J., Babický, A., and Beneš, J.,** The detoxifying effects of selenium. Interrelations between compounds of selenium and certain metals, in *Newer Trace Elements in Nutrition,* Mertz, W. and Cornatzer, W. E., Eds., Marcel Dekker, New York, 1971, 85—124.
12. **Jacobs, R. M., Fox, M. R. S., Fry, B. E., and Harland, B. F.,** The effect of a two-day exposure to dietary cadmium on the concentration of elements in duodenal tissue of Japanese quail, Hoekstra, W. G., Suttie, J. W., Ganther, H. E., and Mertz, W., Eds., in *Trace Element Metabolism in Animals-2,* University Park Press, Baltimore, 1974, 684—686.
13. **Sahagian, B. M., Harding-Barlow, I., and Perry, H. M.,** Uptake of zinc, manganese, cadmium and mercury by intact strips of rat intestine, *J. Nutr.,* 90, 259—267, 1966.
14. **Sahagian, B. M., Harding-Barlow, I., and Perry, H. M.,** Transmural movements of zinc, manganese, cadmium and mercury by rat small intestine, *J. Nutr.,* 93, 291—300, 1967.
15. **Cikrt, M. and Tichy, M.,** Excretion of cadmium through bile and intestinal wall in rats, *Br. J. Ind. Med.,* 31, 134—139, 1974.

16. Moore, W., Stara, J. F., and Crocker, W. C., Gastrointestinal absorption of different compounds of ¹¹⁵Cadmium and the effect of different concentrations in the rat, *Environ. Res.,* 6, 159—164, 1973.

17. Pribblie H.-J. and Wesweig, P. H., Effects of aqueous and dietary cadmium on rat growth and tissue uptake, *Bull. Environ. Contam. Toxicol.,* 9, 271—275, 1973.

18. Moore, W., Stara, J. F., Crocker, W. C., Malanchuk, M., and Iltes, R., Comparison of ¹¹⁵Cadmium retention in rats following different routes of administration, *Environ. Res.,* 6, 473—478, 1973.

19. Ithakissios, D. S., Kessler, W. V., Arvesen, J. N., and Baen, G. S., Variability of cadmium-109 uptake in rats as affected by route of administration and manner of expressing results, *Bull. Environ. Contam. Toxicol.,* 12, 281—288, 1974.

20. Gunn, S. A., Gould, T. C., and Anderson, W. A. D., Selectivity of organ response to cadmium injury and various protective measures, *J. Pathol. Bacteriol.,* 96, 89—96, 1968.

21. Shaikh, Z. A. and Lucis, O. J., Biological differences in cadmium and zinc turnover, *Arch. Environ. Health,* 24, 410—418, 1972.

22. Abe, T., Itokawa, Y., and Inoue, K., Experimental cadmium poisoning. I. Effect of preadministration of heavy metals and vitamins on acute cadmium poisoning in mice, *Jpn. J. Hyg.,* 26, 498—504, 1972.

23. Yoshikawa, H., Preventive effects of pretreatment with small doses of metals upon acute metal toxicity. IV. Cadmium, *Med. Biol.,* 79, 211—214, 1969.

24. Stowe, H. D., Wilson, M., and Goyer, R. A., Clinical and morphologic effects of oral cadmium toxicity in rabbits, *Arch. Pathol.,* 94, 389—405, 1972.

25. Stowe, H. D., Goyer, R. A., Medley, P., and Cates, M., Influence of pyridoxine on cadmium toxicity in rats, *Arch. Environ. Health,* 28, 209—216, 1974.

26. Sujuki, S., Taguchi, T., and Yokohashi, G., Dietary factors influencing the retention rate of orally administered ¹¹⁵CdCl₂ in mice with special reference to calcium and protein concentrations in the diet, *Ind. Health,* 7, 155—159, 1969.

27. Abe, T., Seisuke, T., and Itokawa, Y., Experimental cadmium poisoning. II. Effect of protein and calcium deficiency in chronic cadmium rat poisoning, *Jpn. J. Hyg.,* 27, 308—315, 1972.

28. Sakamoto, N., Experimental studies of cadmium absorption, effects of protein and calcium deficiencies, *Jpn. J. Hyg.,* 30, 78, 1975.

29. Kennedy, A., The effect of l-cysteine on the toxicity of cadmium, *Br. J. Exp. Pathol.,* 49, 360—364, 1968.

30. Gunn, S. A., Gould, T. C., and Anderson, W. A. D., Protective effect of thiol compounds against cadmium-induced vascular damage to testes, *Proc. Soc. Exp. Biol. Med.,* 122, 1036—1039, 1966.

31. Geraci, V., Action of sulphurated water on experimental heavy metal poisoning, *Gazz. Int. Med. Chir.,* 69, 2324—2326, 1964.

32. Larsson, S.-E. and Piscator, M., Effect of cadmium on skeletal tissue in normal and calcium-deficient rats, *Isr. J. Med. Sci.,* 7, 495—498, 1971.

33. Kobayashi, J., Nakahara, H., and Hasegawa, Y., Accumulation of cadmium in organs of mice fed on cadmium polluted rice, *Jpn. J. Hyg.,* 26, 401—409, 1971.

34. Piscator, M. and Larsson, S.-E., Retention and toxicity of cadmium in calcium deficient rats, *Proc. 17th Int. Cong. Occup. Health,* 1974 (see ref. 10).

35. Pond, W. G. and Walker, E. F., Effect of dietary calcium and cadmium level of pregnant rats on reproduction and on dam and progeny tissue mineral concentrations, *Proc. Soc. Exp. Biol. Med.,* 148, 665—668, 1975.

36. Worker, N. A. and Migicovsky, B. B., Effect of vitamin D on the utilisation of zinc, cadmium and mercury in the chick, *J. Nutr.,* 75, 222—224, 1961.

37. Sugawara, N., Sugawara, C., and Niyake, K., Effect of cadmium on calcium absorption of rat duodenum, *Jpn. J. Hyg.,* 30, 79, 1975.

38. Feldman, S. L. and Cousins, R. J., Influence of cadmium on the metabolism of 25-hydroxy cholecalciferol in chicks, *Nutr. Rep. Int.,* 8, 251—260, 1973.

39. Suda, T., Horiuchi, N., Ogata, E., Ezawa, I., Otaki, N., and Kimura, M., Prevention by metallothionein of cadmium-induced inhibition of vitamin D activation reaction in kidney, *FEBS Lett.,* 42, 23—26, 1974.

40. Washko, P. W. and Cousins, R. J., Effect of low dietary calcium on chronic cadmium toxicity in rats, *Nutr. Rep. Int.,* 11, 113—127, 1975.

41. Piscator, M. and Larsson, S.-E., Effects of long-term cadmium exposure in calcium-deficient rats, in *Trace Element Metabolism in Animals-2,* Hoekstra, W. E., Suttie, J. W., Ganther, H. E., and Mertz, W., Eds., University Park Press, Baltimore, 1972, 687—689.

42. Pond, W. G., Walker, E. F., and Kirtland, D., Cadmium-induced anemia in growing pigs: protective effect of oral or parenteral iron, *J. Anim. Sci.,* 36, 1122—1124, 1973.

43. **Berlin, M. and Friberg, L.,** Bone marrow activity and erythrocyte destruction in chronic cadmium poisoning , *Arch. Environ. Health,* 1, 478—480, 1960.
44. **Doyle, J. J. and Pfander, W. H.,** Interactions of cadmium with copper, iron, zinc and manganese in ovine tissues, *J. Nutr.,* 105, 599—606, 1975.
45. **Bunn, C. R. and Matrone, G.,** In vitro interactions of cadmium, copper, zinc and iron in the mouse and rat, *J. Nutr.,* 90, 395—399, 1966.
46. **Banis, R. J., Pond, W. G., Walker, E. F., and O'Connor, J. R.,** Dietary cadmium, iron and zinc interactions in the growing rat, *Proc. Soc. Exp. Biol. Med.,* 130, 802—806, 1969.
47. **Freeland, J. H. and Cousins, R. J.,** Effect of dietary cadmium on anaemia, iron absorption and cadmium-binding protein in the chick, *Nutr. Rep. Int.,* 8, 337—347, 1973.
48. **Weber, C. W. and Reid, B. L.,** Effect of toxic levels of cadmium and its interrelationship to iron, zinc and ascorbic acid in growing chicks, in *Trace Element Metabolism in Animals-2,* Hoekstra, W. G., Suttie, J. W., Ganther, H. E., and Mertz, W., Eds., University Park Press, Baltimore, 1974, 694—695.
49. **Hamilton, D. L. and Walberg, L. S.,** Relationship between cadmium and iron absorption, *Am. J. Physiol.,* 227, 1033—1037, 1974.
50. **Kar, A. B., Das, R. P., and Mukerji, F. N. I.,** Prevention of cadmium-induced changes in the gonads of rats by zinc and selenium — a study in antagonism between metals in the biological system, *Proc. Nat. Inst. Sci. India,* 26B (suppl. 40), 1960.
51. **Parízek, J., Kalousková, J., Babický, A., Beneš, J., and Pavlík, L.,** Interaction of selenium with mercury, cadmium, and other toxic metals, in *Trace Element Metabolism in Animals-2,* Hoekstra, W. G., Suttie, J. W., Ganther, H. E., and Mertz, W., Eds., University Park Press, Baltimore, 1974, 119—131.
52. **Chen, R. W., Whanger, P. D., and Weswig, P. H.,** Selenium-induced redistribution of cadmium binding to tissue-proteins: a possible mechanism of protection against cadmium toxicity, *Bioinorg. Chem.,* 4, 125—133, 1975.
53. **Hill, C. H.,** Reversal of selenium toxicity in chicks by mercury, copper and cadmium, *J. Nutr.,* 104, 593—598, 1974.
54. **Ganther, H. E., Wagner, P. A., Sunder, M. L., and Hoekstra, W. G.,** Protective effects of selenium against heavy metal toxicities, *Trace Subs. Environ. Health,* 6, 247—258, 1972.
55. **Whanger, P. D., Weswig, J. A., and Oldfield, J. E.,** Effects of cadmium, mercury, tellurium, arsenic, silver, and cobalt on white muscle disease, *Nutr. Rep. Int.,* 14, 63—72, 1976.
56. **Petering, H. G.,** The effect of cadmium and lead on copper and zinc metabolism, in *Trace Element Metabolism in Animals-2,* University Park Press, Baltimore, 1974, 311—325.
57. **Mills, C. F.,** Trace element interactions: effects of dietary composition on the development of imbalance and toxicity, in *Trace Element Metabolism in Animals-2,* Hoekstra, W. G., Suttie, J. W., Ganther, H. E., and Mertz, W., University Park Press, Baltimore, 1974, 79—90.
58. **Shank, K. E. and Vetter, R. J.,** Effects of copper, mercury and zinc on the uptake and distribution of cadmium-115 in the albino rat, *Environ. Lett.,* 6, 13—18, 1974.
59. **Roberts, K. R., Miller, W. J., Stoke, P. E., Gentry, R. P., and Neathery, M. W.,** High dietary cadmium on zinc absorption and metabolism in calves fed for comparable nitrogen balances, *Proc. Soc. Exp. Biol. Med.,* 144, 906—908, 1973.
60. **Evans, G. W., Grase, C. I., and Hahn, C.,** The effect of copper and cadmium on ^{65}Zn absorption in zinc-deficient and zinc-supplemented rats, *Bioinorg. Chem.* 3, 115—120, 1974.
61. **Miller, D. W., Vetter, R. J., Hullinger, R. L., and Shaw, S. L.,** Uptake and distribution of cadmium-115 in calcium-deficient and zinc-deficient golden hamsters, *Bull. Environ. Contam. Toxicol.,* 13, 40—43, 1975.
62. **Webb, M. and Verschoyle, R. D.,** An investigation of the role of metallothioneins in protection against the acute toxicity of the cadmium ion, *Biochem. Pharmacol.,* 25, 673—679, 1976.
63. **Mills, C. F. and Dalgarno, A. C.,** The influence of dietary cadmium concentration on liver copper in ewes and their lambs, *Proc. Nutr. Soc.,* 31, 73—74A, 1972.
64. **Ferm, V. H.,** Synteratogenic effect of lead and cadmium, *Experientia,* 25, 58, 1969.
64a. **Holmberg, R. E. and Ferm, V. H.,** Interrelation of selenium, cadmium, and arsenic in mammalian teratogenesis, *Arch. Environ. Health,* 18, 873—877, 1969.
65. **Chatterjee, G. C., Banerjee, S. K. and Pal, D. R.,** Cadmium administration and l-ascorbic acid metabolism in the rat: effect of l-ascorbic acid supplementation, *Int. J. Vitam. Nutr. Res.,* 43, 370—377, 1973.
66. **Patnaik, B. K.** Effect of cadmium chloride on the ascorbic acid concentration in the testes of rat, *Ind. J. Exp. Biol.,* 9, 500—501, 1971.
67. **Chatterjee, G. C., Banerjee, S. K., and Pal, D. R.,** Cadmium administration and l-ascorbic acid metabolism in rats, *Int. J. Vitam. Nutr. Res.,* 43, 370—377, 1973.
68. **Fox, M. R. S., Fry, B. E., Harland, B. F., Schertal, M. E., and Weeks, C. E.,** Effect of ascorbic acid on cadmium toxicity in the young *coturmix, J. Nutr.,* 101, 1295—1299, 1971.

69. **Weber, C. W. and Reid, B. L.**, Effect of toxic levels of cadmium and its interrelationship to iron, zinc, and ascorbic acid in growing chicks, in *Trace Element Metabolism in Animals-2,* Hoekstra, W. G., Suttie, J. W., Ganther, H. E., and Mertz, W., Eds., University Park Press, Baltimore, 1974, 694—695.

70. **Lengermann, F. W.**, Retention of radiocesium by rats before and after weaning, *J. Nutr.,* 99, 419—424, 1969.

71. **Mahlum, D. D. and Sikov, M. R.**, Comparative metabolism of ^{137}Cs by adult, suckling and prenatal rats, *Comp. Biochem. Physiol.,* 30, 169—175, 1969.

72. **Matsusaka, N. and Inaba, J.**, Whole-body retention of caesium-137 in suckling and weaning mice, *Nature (London),* 214, 303—304, 1967.

73. **Inaba, J., Matsusaka, N., and Ichikawa, R.**, Effect of potassium, lactose and thyroxine administration on radiocesium retention in young rats, *J. Radiat. Res.,* 10, 94—100, 1969.

74. **Snipes, M. B. and Reidesel, M. L.**, Studies of diet as a factor in ^{137}Cs metabolism in rats, *J. Nutr.,* 97, 212—218, 1969.

75. **Johnson, J. E., Garner, D., and Ward, G. M.**, Influence of dietary potassium, rubidium and sodium on the retention of radiocesium in rats, *Proc. Soc. Exp. Biol. Med.,* 127, 857—860, 1968.

76. **Wolsieffer, J. R. and Stookey, G. R.**, Effect of dietary factors on Cs-137 retention in rats, *J. Dent. Res.,* 52, 844—847, 1973.

77. **Szot, Z., Geisler, J., Zylicj, E., and Klocjewick, M.**, Retention in rats following injections of vitamin D or vitamin D, *Acta Physiol. Pol.,* 24, 577—586, 1973.

78. **Forbes, G. B. and Reino, J. C.**, Effect of age on gastrointestinal absorption (Fe, Sr, Pb) in the rat, *J. Nutr.,* 102, 647—652, 1972.

79. **Kostial, K., Šimonovic, I., and Pišonić, C.**, Reduction of lead absorption from the intestine in new-born rats, *Environ. Res.,* 4, 360—363, 1971.

80. **Kostial, K., Kello, D., and Harrison, G. H.**, Comparative metabolism of lead and calcium in young and adult rats, *Int. Arch. Arbeitsmed.,* 31, 159—161, 1973.

81. **Momčilović, B. and Kostial, K.**, Kinetics of lead retention and distribution in suckling and adult rats, *Environ. Res.,* 8, 214—220, 1974.

82. **Barltrop, D. and Meek, F.**, Absorption of different lead compounds, *Postgrad. Med. J.,* 51, 805—809, 1975.

83. **Kehoe, R. A.**, The metabolism of lead in man in health and disease. I. The normal metabolism of lead, *J. R. Inst. Public Health,* 24, 81—97, 1961.

84. **Blaxter, K. L.**, Lead as a nutritional hazard to farm livestock. II. The absorption and excretion of lead by sheep and rabbits, *J. Comp. Pathol. Ther.,* 60, 140—159, 1950.

85. **Quarterman, J. and Morrison, J. N.**, The effects of calcium and phosphorus on the retention and excretion of lead in rats, *Br. J. Nutr.,* 34, 351—362, 1975.

86. **Kostial, K., Maljković, T., and Jugo, S.**, Lead acetate toxicity in rats in relation to age and sex, *Arch. Toxicol.,* 31, 265—269, 1974.

87. **Quarterman, J., Morrison, J. N., Humphries, W. R., and Mills, C. F.**, The effect of dietary sulphur and castration on lead poisoning in lambs, *J. Comp. Pathol. Ther.,* 87, 405—416, 1977.

88. **Allcroft, R. and Blaxter, K. L.**, Lead as a nutritional hazard to farm livestock. V. The toxicity of lead to cattle and sheep and an evaluation of the lead hazard under farm conditions, *J. Comp. Pathol. Ther.,* 60, 209—218, 1950.

89. **Hutchinson, T. C., Guba, M., and Cunningham, L.**, Lead, calcium, zinc, copper and nickel distributions in vegetables and soils of an intensively cultivated area and levels of copper, lead and zinc in the growers, *Trace Subs. Environ. Health,* 8, 81—93, 1974.

90. **Ghelberg, N. W. and Nagy, S.**, Protective effect of methandrostenolone on lead retention in experimental intoxication, *Rev. Roum. Med. Interne,* 8, 557—562, 1971.

91. **Essing, H.-G., Szadkowski, D., Schaller, K.-H., and Laake, R.-W.**, Blood levels and renal efflux of some inorganic substances relevant to occupational medicine with respect to glucocorticoid-active drugs, *Arzneim.- Forsch.,* 25, 231—235, 1971.

92. **Quarterman, J., Morrison, J. N., and Humphries, W. R.**, The effects of dietary lead content and food restriction on lead retention in rats, *Environ. Res.,* 12, 180—187, 1976.

93. **Kostial, K. and Momcilović, B.**, Transport of ^{203}Pb and ^{47}Ca from mother to offspring, *Arch. Environ. Health,* 29, 28—30, 1974.

94. **Jugo, S., Maljkovic, T., and Kostial, K.**, The effect of chelating agents on lead excretion in rats in relation to age, *Environ. Res.,* 10, 271—279, 1975.

95. **Moore, M. R., Meridith, P. A., Goldberg, A., Carr, K., Toner, P., and Lawrie, T. D. V.**, Cardiac effects of lead in drinking water of rats, *Clin. Sci. Mol. Med.,* 49, 337—341, 1975.

96. **Quarterman, J., Morrison, J. N., and Humphries, W. R.**, The effect of dietary calcium and phosphate on lead poisoning in lambs, *J. Comp. Pathol. Ther.,* 87, 417—429, 1977.

97. Kelliher, D. J., Hilliard, E. P., Poole, D. B. R., and Collins, J. D., Chronic lead intoxication in cattle: preliminary observations on its effects on the erythrocyte and on porphyrin metabolism, *Irish J. Agric. Res.,* 12, 61—69, 1973.

98. Sanai, G. H., Hasegawa, T., and Yoshikawa, H., Pretreatment of rats with lead in experimental acute lead poisoning, *J. Occup. Med.,* 14, 301—305, 1972.

99. Garber, B. and Wei, E., Adaptation to the toxic effects of lead, *Amer. Ind. Hyg. Assoc. J.,* 33, 756—760, 1972.

100. Quarterman, J., Morrison, J. N., and Humphries, W. R., unpublished observations.

101. Schwarz, K., New essential trace elements (Sn, V, F, Si): progress report and outlook, in *Trace Element Metabolism in Animals-2,* Hoekstra, W. G., Suttie, J. W., Ganther, H. E., and Mertz, W., Eds., University Park Press, Baltimore, 1974, 355—380.

101a. Quarterman, J., Morrison, E., Morrison, J. N., and Humphries, W. R., Dietary protein and lead retention, *Environ. Res.,* 17, 68—77, 1978.

102. Robinowitz, M., Wetherill, G. W., and Kopple, J. D., Human uptake of dietary and atmospheric lead: stable isotope and balance study, *Proc. 2nd Ann. NSF-RANN Trace Contam. Conf.,* 1973, 308—315.

103. Baetjer, A. M., Jourdar, S. N. D., and McQuary, W. A., Effect of environmental temperature and humidity on lead poisoning in animals, *Arch. Environ. Health,* 1, 463—477, 1960.

104. Baernstein, H. D., Grand, J. A., and Neal, P. A., The effect of protein intake on lead poisoning, *J. Biol. Chem.,* 140, viii, 1941.

105. Gontzea, I., Sutzesco, P., Dumitracke, S., and Bistriceanu, E., Recherches sur le rôle de l'apport protéique sur les moyens de défense de l'organisme envers quelques toxiques chimiques, *Arch. Mal. Prof. Med. Trav. Secur. Soc.,* 31, 471—480, 1970.

106. Gontzea, I., Sutzesco, P., Coccora, D., and Lungu, D., Importance of dietary proteins on the resistance of the organism to lead poisoning, *Arch. Sci. Physiol.,* 17, 211—218, 1964.

107. Milev, N., Sattler, E.-L., and Menden, E., Aufnahme und Einlagerung von Blei im Körper unter veschiedenen Ernährungsbedingungen, *Med. Ernähr.,* 11, 29—32, 1970.

108. Der, R., Fahim, Z., Hilderbrand, D., and Fahim, M., Combined effect of lead and low protein diet on growth, sexual development and metabolism in female rats, *Res. Commun. Chem. Pathol. Pharmacol.,* 9, 723—738, 1974.

109. Barltrop, D. and Khoo, H. E., The influence of nutritional factors on lead absorption, *Postgrad. Med. J.,* 51, 795—800, 1975.

110. Baernstein, H. D. and Grand, J. A., The relation of protein intake to lead poisoning in rats, *J. Pharmacol. Exp. Therap.,* 74, 18—24, 1942.

111. Yun, H. C., Influence of ascorbic acid and methionine on the ALAD activity in lead poisoning, *Yakhok Hoe Chi,* 19, 21—29, 1975; *Chem. Abstr.,* 84, 13115, 1976.

112. Quarterman, J., Humphries, W. R., and Morrison, J. N., The influence of sulphur compounds on the availability of lead to rats, *Proc. Nutr. Soc.,* 35, 34—35A, 1976.

113. Wasserman, R. H., Comar, C. L., and Nold, M. M., The influence of amino acids and other compounds on the gastrointestinal absorption of ^{45}Ca and ^{89}Sr in the rat, *J. Nutr.,* 59, 371—383, 1956.

114. Weyrauch, F. and Necke, A. Zur Feige der Milch-Schleimsuppen — und Fettprophylaxe bei der Bleivergiftung, *Z. Hyg. Infektionskr.,* 14, 629—634, 1933.

115. Chiochi, H. and Cardeza, A. F., Hepatic lesions produced by lead in rats fed a high fat diet, *Arch. Path.,* 48, 395—404, 1949.

116. Kello, D. and Kostial, K., The effect of milk diet on lead metabolism in rats, *Environ. Res.,* 6, 355—360, 1973.

117. Stephens, R. and Waldron, H. A., The influence of milk and related dietary constituents on lead metabolism, *J. Nutr.,* 59, 371—383, 1956.

118. Cikrt, M. and Tichy, M., Role of bile in intestinal absorption of ^{203}Pb in rats, *Experientia,* 31, 1320—1321, 1975.

119. Wasserman, R. H. and Taylor, A. N., Some aspects of the intestinal absorption of calcium with special reference in vitamin D, in *Mineral Metabolism,* Comar, C. L. and Bronner, F., Eds., Academic Press, New York, 1969, 379—386.

120. O'Doherty, P. J. A., Kakis, G., and Kuksis, A., Role of luminal lecithin in intestinal fat absorption, *Lipids,* 8, 249—255, 1973.

121. Westerman, M. P. and Jensen, W. N., $^{32}PO_4$ incorporation into phosphatidic acid of lead-poisoned and normal red cells, *Fed. Proc. Fed. Am. Soc. Exp. Biol.,* 149, 325—329, 1975.

122. Tornabene, T. G. and Peterson, S. L., Interaction of lead and bacterial lipids, *Appl. Microbiol.,* 29, 680—684, 1975.

123. Harrison, G. E., Carr, T. E. F., Sutton, A., Humphreys, E. R., and Rundo, J., Effect of alginate on the absorption of lead in man, *Nature (London),* 224, 1115—1116, 1969.

124. **Carr, T. E. F., Nolan, J., and Durakovic, A.**, Effect of alginate on the absorption and excretion of [203]Pb in rats fed milk and normal diets, *Nature (London)*, 224, 1115, 1969.
125. **Kostial, K., Šimonović, I., and Pišonic, M.**, Reduction of lead absorption from the intestine in newborn rats, *Environ. Res.*, 4, 360—363, 1971.
126. **Chaika, S. A.**, Protective effect of pectins in the poisoning of animals with lead aerosols, Gigiena Truda i Prof. Zabol., 10, 47—49, 1966; *Chem. Abstr.*, 65, 1286a, and 4518, 1966.
127. **Murer, H. K. and Crandell, L. A.**, Effect of pectin on the retention of dietary lead (radium D), *J. Nutr.*, 23, 249—258, 1942.
128. **Livshits, O. D.**, Effect of local pectin-containing foods on the removal of lead from an organism, *Tr. Permsk, Gos. Med. Inst.*, 99, 92—94, 1970; *Chem. Abstr.*, 78, 80461, 80462, 1973; see also *Chem. Abstr.*, 71, 59126, 99967, 1969.
129. **Pletscher, A., Richterlich, R., Thoelen, H., Ludin, H., and Staub, H.**, Uber das Verhalten von Aminosauren und Fermenten bei Schwermetall-Vergiftung. II. Mitteilung und die virkung von Calcium und Läwulose bei der experimentellen Bleivergiftung, *Helv. Physiol. Pharmacol. Acta*, 10, 328—338, 1952.
130. **Hunter, D. and Aub, J. C.**, Lead studies. XV. The effect of parathyroid hormone on the excretion of lead and of calcium in patients suffering from lead poisoning, *Q. J. Med.*, 20, 123—140, 1927.
131. **Aub, J. C.**, The biochemical behaviour of lead in the body, *JAMA*, 104, 87—90, 1935.
132. **Schmitt, F. and Basse, W.**, Beeinflussung des Bleispiegels im Blut und der Bleiausscheidung in Urin durch verschiedene Kelkpräparate und seine Beziehung zum Phosphatstoffwechsel, *Arch. Exp. Pathol. Pharmakol.*, 184, 541—546, 1936.
133. **Tompsett, S. L. and Chalmers, J. N. M.**, Studies in lead mobilization, *Br. J. Exp. Pathol.*, 20, 408—416, 1939.
134. **Lederer, L. G. and Bing, F. C.**, Effect of calcium and phosphorus on retention of lead, *JAMA*, 114, 2457—2461, 1940.
135. **Shields, J. B. and Mitchell, H. H.**, The effect of calcium and phosphorus on the metabolism of lead, *J. Nutr.*, 21, 541—552, 1941.
136. **Six, K. M. and Goyer, R. A.**, Experimental enhancement of lead toxicity by low dietary calcium, *J. Lab. Clin. Med.*, 76, 933—942, 1970.
137. **Mahaffey, K. R., Goyer, R. A., and Haseman, J. K.**, Dose-response to dietary calcium, *J. Lab. Clin. Med.*, 82, 92—100, 1973.
138. **Quarterman, J., Morrison, J. N., and Carey, L. F.**, The influence of calcium and phosphate on lead metabolism, *Trace Subs. Environ. Health*, 7, 347—352, 1974.
139. **Hsu, F. S., Krook, L., Pond, W. G., and Duncan, J. R.**, Interactions of dietary calcium with toxic levels of lead and zinc in pigs, *J. Nutr.*, 105, 112—118, 1975.
140. **Willoughby, R. A., Thirapatsakun, T., and McSherry, B. J.**, Influence of rations low in calcium and phosphate on blood and tissue lead concentrations in the horse, *Am. J. Vet. Res.*, 23,
141. **Quarterman, J., Morrison, J. N., and Humphries, W. R.**, The influence of high dietary intakes of calcium on lead retention and release in rats, *Proc. Nutr. Soc.*, 34, 89A—90A, 1975.
142. **Fleischman, A. I., Yacowitz, H., Hayton, T., and Bierenbaum, M. L.**, Effect of calcium and vitamin D upon the fecal excretion of some metals in the mature male rats fed a high fat, cholesterol diet, *J. Nutr.*, 95, 19—22, 1968.
143. **Morrison, J. N., Quarterman, J., and Humphries, W. R.**, Lead metabolism in lambs and the effect of phosphate supplements, *Proc. Nutr. Soc.*, 33, 88A, 1974.
144. **Wasserman, R. H. and Corradino, R. A.**, Vitamin D, calcium and protein synthesis, *Vitam. Horm.*, 31, 50—61, 1973.
145. **Sobel, A. E. and Burger, M.**, Calcification. XIII. The influence of calcium, phosphorus and vitamin D on the removal of lead from blood and bone, *J. Biol. Chem.*, 212, 105—110, 1955.
146. **Litzner, S., Weyrauch, F., and Barih, E.**, Untersuchungen uber Bleiausscheicheng durch bestimmte Kostformen und Arzneimittel beim Menschen, *Arch. Gewerbepathol. Gewerbehyg.*, 2, 330—335, 1931.
147. **Sobel, A. E., Yuska, H., Peters, D. D., and Kramer, B.**, The biochemical behavior of lead. I. The influence of calcium, phosphorus and vitamin D on lead in blood and bone, *J. Biol. Chem.*, 132, 239—265, 1940.
148. **Snowdon, C. T. and Sanderson, B. A.**, Lead pica produced in rats, *Science*, 183, 92—94, 1974.
149. **Jacobson, J. L. and Snowdon, C. T.**, Increased lead ingestion in calcium-deficient monkeys, *Nature (London)*, 262, 51—52, 1976.
150. **Uzbekov, G. A.**, Hydrogen sulphide as an antidote against heavy metal poisoning and the mechanism of its prophylactic action, *Chem. Abstr.*, 60, 8543d, 1964.
151. **Banciu, T., Georgesen, L., Sirbu, Z., Constantinescu, C., and Banciu, M.**, Hepatoprotective effect of a sulphur-calcium hydromineral agent (calciulata) in liver lesions due to lead poisoning, *Minerva Med.*, 61, 966—969, 1970.

152. Morrison, J. N., Quarterman, J., Humphries, W. R., and Mills, C. F., The influence of dietary sulphate on the toxicity of lead to sheep, *Proc. Nutr. Soc.*, 34, 77—78A, 1975.
153. Pecora, L., Vecchione, C., and Fati, S., Rapporti tra ferro e piombo ell' intossicazione saturina, *Folia Med. (Naples)*, 43, 776—784, 1960.
154. Six, K. M. and Goyer, R. A., The influence of iron deficiency on tissue content and toxicity of ingested lead in the rat, *J. Lab. Clin. Med.*, 79, 128—136, 1972.
155. Kochen, J. and Greener, Y., Interaction of ferritin with lead and cadmium, *Pediatr. Res.*, 9, 323; (abstr.) 399, 1975.
156. Angle, C. R., Stelmak, K. L., and McIntire, M. S., Lead and iron deficiency, *Trace Subs. Environ. Health*, 9, 377—385, 1975.
157. Rüssel, H. A., Über die Bindung von Blei an Eisenhydroxidhältige Stoffe in Leber, Niere und und Milz vergifteter Rinder, *Bull. Environ. Contam. Toxicol.*, 5, 115—124, 1970.
158. Kochen, J. and Greener, Y., Lead binding by transferrin, *Pediatr. Res.*, 9, 323, (abstr.) 400, 1975.
159. Cerclewski, F. L. and Forbes, R. M., Influence of dietary selenium on lead toxicity in the rat, *J. Nutr.*, 106, 783—788, 1976.
160. Levander, D. A., Morris, V. C., Higgs, D. J., and Ferretti, R. J., Contrasting effects of vitamin E and selenium in poisoned rats, *Proc. 10th Int. Cong. Nutr.*, 134; (abstr.) 1517, 1975.
161. Stone, C. L. and Soares, J. H., The effect of dietary selenium level on lead toxicity in the Japanese quail, *Poult. Sci.*, 55, 341—349, 1976.
162. Cerklewski, F. L. and Forbes, R. M., Influence of dietary zinc on lead toxicity in the rat, *J. Nutr.*, 106, 689—696, 1976.
163. Willoughby, R. A., MacDonald, E., McSherry, B. J., and Brown, G., Lead and zinc poisoning and the interaction between lead and zinc poisoning in the foal, *Can. J. Comp. Med.*, 36, 348—359, 1972.
164. Hsu, F. S., Krook, L., Pond, W. G., and Duncan, J. R., Interactions of dietary calcium with toxic levels of lead and zinc in pigs, *J. Nutr.*, 105, 112—118, 1975.
165. Bolanowska, W. and Sapota, A., Binding of lead by liver and kidney proteins and subcellular fractions, *Bromatol. Chem. Toksykol.*, 8, 91—98, 1975.
166. Chaika, P. A., Effect of cobalt and copper salts during the toxic action of lead on animals, *Vopr. Pitan.*, 27, 29—33, 1968.
167. Klauder, D. S., Murthy, L., and Petering, H. G., Effect of dietary intake of lead acetate on copper metabolism in male rats, *Trace Subs. Environ. Health*, 6, 131—136, 1972.
168. Mahaffey, K. R. and Stone, C. L., Effect of high fluorine intake on tissue lead concentrations, *Fed. Proc. Fed. Am. Soc. Exp. Biol.*, 35, 256, (Abstr. 283), 1976.
169. Silvestroni, A. and Balletta, A., Nicotinic acid in the erythrocytic biosynthesis of the nicotinic nucleotide during experimental lead poisoning, *Folia Med.* 47, 1121—1129, 1964.
170. Pecora, L., Silvestroni, A., and Brancaccis, A., Relations between the porphyrin metabolism and the nicotinic acid metabolism in saturine poisoning, *Panminerva Med.*, 8, 284—288, 1966.
171. Mambeeva, A. A., *Disturbance of the Gastrointestinal Tract during Lead Poisoning*, Kazakhstan, Alma-Ata, 1975.
172. Tenconi, L. T. and Acocella, G., Chemotherapy of lead poisoning. I. Effects of lead poisoning on the metabolism of tryptophan to nicotinic acid in the rat, *Acta Vitaminol.*, 20, 189—194, 1966.
173. Acocella, G., Chemotherapy of lead poisoning. II. Effects of nicotinic acid on coproporphyrinuria in lead poisoned rats, *Acta Vitaminol.*, 20, 195—202, 1966.
174. Kao, R. L. and Forbes, R. M., Lead and vitamin effects on synthesis, *Arch. Environ. Res.*, 27, 31—35, 1973.
175. Pokotilenko, G. M., Vitamin B_6 therapy in experimental lead poisoning with lead and with benzene, *Farmakol. Toksikol.*, 27, 88—89, 1964.
176. Evalshko, Yu. P., Influence of complexion treatment and of vitamin B_{12} on the porphyrin turnover during chronic lead poisoning, *Chem. Abstr.*, 65, 1285h, 1966.
177. Pecora, L., Mole, R., Balletta, A., Daniele, E., and Pesaresi, C., Action of adenosine 5-monophosphate and inosine on porphyrin metabolism in experimental saturnism, *Folia Med.*, 46, 349—360, 1963.
178. Gajdos, A., Gajdos-Torok, M., Danchev, D., and Benord, H., Effect of adenosine 5-monophosphatic acid on the anemia and the factors that control it in the rabbit poisoned with lead, *Nouv. Rev. Fr. Hematol.*, 4, 385—394, 1964.
179. Gontea, I., Sutescu, P., Stanciu, V., and Lungu, D., Vitamin C in lead poisoning in the guinea pig, *Iguiena*, 13, 501—509, 1964.
180. Clegg, F. G. and Rylands, J. M., Osteoporosis and hydronephrosis of young lambs following the ingestion of lead, *J. Comp. Pathol.*, 76, 15—22, 1966.
181. Granata, A. and Quattrocchi, A., Chronic occupational saturnism. The peripheral hemolytic changes induced by ascorbic acid and their importance in the evaluation of the severity of the condition, *Med. Lavoro*, 56, 50—57, 1965.

182. Levander, O. A., Morris, V. C., Higgs, D. J., and Ferritti, R. J., Lead poisoning in vitamin E-deficient rats, *J. Nutr.*, 105, 1481—1485, 1975.

183. Levander, D. A., Factors that influence the deformability of red blood cells from vitamin E-deficient lead-poisoned rats, *Fed. Proc. Fed. Am. Soc. Exp. Biol.*, 35, 741, (Abstr.) 2953, 1976.

184. Mahaffey, K. R. and Goyer, R. A., Influence of ethanol ingestion on lead toxicity in rats fed isocaloric diets, *Arch. Environ. Health*, 28, 217—222, 1974.

185. Moore, M. R., Lead, ethanol and δ-aminolaevulinate dehydratase, *Biochem. J.*, 129, 43-44P, 1972.

186. Garber, B. T. and Weig, E., Influence of dietary factors on the gastrointestinal absorption of lead, *Toxicol. Appl. Pharmacol.*, 27, 685—691, 1974.

187. Jugo, S., Maljkovic, T., and Kostial, K., Influence of chelating agents on the gastrointestinal absorption of lead, *Toxicol. Appl. Pharmacol.*, 34, 259—263, 1975.

188. Sherry, M., Lithium retention and response, *Lancet*, 1, 1267—1268, 1969.

189. Schou, M., Amidsen, A., and Thornsen, K., Clinical and experimental observations concerning the absorption and elimination of lithium and on lithium poisoning, *Acta Psychiatr. Scand. Suppl.*, 203, 153—155, 1968.

190. Morrison, J. M., Pritchard, H. D., Braude, M. C., and D'Aguanno, W., Plasma and brain lithium levels after lithium carbonate and lithium chloride administration by different routes in rats, *Proc. Soc. Exp. Biol. Med.*, 137, 889—892, 1971.

191. Jeppsson, J. and Sjögren, J., The influence of food on side effects and absorption of lithium, *Acta Psychiatr. Scand.*, 51, 285—288, 1975.

192. Olsen, O. V., Jensen, J., and Thornsen, K., Effect of potassium on lithium-induced growth retardation and polyuria in rats, *Acta Pharmacol. Toxicol.*, 36, 161—171, 1975.

193. Lode, H., Senft, G., and Losert, W., Influence of potassium deficiency on the distribution of lithium between the intra- and extra-cellular spaces, *Naunym-Schmiederbergs Arch. Pharmakol. Exp. Pathol.*, 258, 418—429, 1967.

194. Thomsen, K. and Schon, M., Renal lithium excretion in man, *Am. J. Physiol.*, 215, 823—827, 1968.

195. Cooper, T. B., Wagner, B. M., and Kline, N. S., Mode of action of lithium on iodine metabolism, *Biol. Psychiatry*, 2, 273—278, 1970.

196. Jensen, S. E., Amidsen, A., and Olsen, T., Iodine metabolism in lithium therapy, *Ugeskr. Laeg.*, 130, 1518—1520, 1968.

197. Corper, W. R., Stoddard, D. D., and Martin, D. F., Choline activation of lithium transport, *Experientia*, 29, 1249—1250, 1973.

198. Aaronson, R. M. and Spiro, H. M., Mercury and the gut, *Am. J. Dig. Dis.*, 18, 583—594, 1973.

199. Taguchi, Y., Microdetermination of total mercury and the dynamic aspects of the methylmercury compounds in animal organisms. II. Behavior of low concentration methylmercury compounds in vivo, *Nippon Eiseigaku Zasshi*, 25, 156—164, 1968.

200. Ellis, R. W. and Fang, S. C., Elimination, tissue accumulation and cellular incorporation of mercury in rats receiving an oral dose of ^{203}Hg-labelled phenylmercuric acetate and mercuric acetate, *Toxicol. Appl. Pharmacol.*, 11, 101—113, 1967.

201. Abdulla, M., Arnesjö, R., and Ihse, I., Methylation of inorganic mercury in experimental jejunal blind loops, *Scand. J. Gastroenterol.*, 8, 565—567, 1973.

202. Rowland, I. R., Davies, M. J., and Grasso, P., The methylation of mercury by the gastrointestinal contents of the rat, *Biochem. Soc. Trans.*, 3, 502—504, 1975.

203. Magas, L., Clarkson, T. W., and Greenwood, M. R., Depression of pulmonary retention of mercury vapour by ethanol: identification of site of action, *Toxicol. Appl. Pharmacol.*, 26, 180—183, 1973.

204. Sahagian, B. M., Harding-Barlow, I., and Perry, H. M., Uptakes of zinc, manganese, cadmium and mercury by intact strips of rat intestine, *J. Nutr.*, 90, 259—267, 1966.

205. Cikrt, M., Enterohepatic circulation of copper-64, manganese-54 and mercury-203 in rats, *Arch. Toxicol.*, 31, 51—59, 1973.

206. Norseth, T., Biliary excretion and intestinal reabsorption of mercury in the rat after injection of methylmercuric chloride, *Acta Pharmacol. Toxicol.*, 33, 280—288, 1973.

207. Norseth, T. and Clarkson, T. W., Biotransformation of methylmercury salts in the rat by specific determination of inorganic mercury, *Biochem. Pharmacol.*, 19, 2775—2783, 1970.

208. Takahashi, H. and Hirayama, K., Accelerated elimination of methylmercury from animals, *Nature (London)*, 232, 201—202, 1971.

209. Miller, V. L., Larkin, D. V., Bearse, G. E., and Hamilton, C. M., The effects of dosage and administration of two mercurials on mercury retention in two strains of chickens, *Poult. Sci.*, 46, 142—145, 1967.

210. Yoshikawa, H., Preventive effect of pretreatment with low dose of metals in acute toxicity of metals in mice, *Ind. Health*, 8, 184—191, 1970.

211. Trakhtenberg, I. M., Savitskii, I. V., and Shterengarts, R. Ya., Effect of low mercury concentrations on the organism (problem of combined action of toxic and thermal factors), *Chem. Abstr.*, 64, 20505h, 1966.

212. Miller, V. L., Bearse, G. E., and Csonka, E., Mercury retention in several strains and strain crosses of chickens, *Poult. Sci.*, 49, 110—114, 1970.

213. Jelinek, J., Mikulaskova, J., and Pelc, B., The action of some steroid compounds on $HgCl_2$ nephrosis in mouse and rat kidney, *Acta Biol. Med. Ger.*, 13, 204—208, 1964.

214. Klinkmann, H. and Hübel, A., Testosteron-Behandlung bei schwerer extravenoser Sublimat-Intoxication, *Muench. Med. Wochenschr.*, 106, 1466—1468, 1964.

215. Souvard, S., Stanescu, C., Nitelea, I., Nestorescu, B., and Vrejoitt, G., The protective action of glutamic acid in experimental mercury poisoning, *Arch. Environ. Health*, 16, 626—632, 1968.

216. Blackstone, S., Hurley, R. J., and Hughes, R. E., Some interrelationships between vitamin C and mercury in the guinea pig, *Food Cosmet. Toxicol.*, 12, 511—516, 1974.

217. Taraba, I. and Bull, G. M., Failure of folic acid to influence mortality of rats with acute tubular necrosis caused by mercury, *Postgrad. Med. J.*, 44, 116—117, 1968.

218. Parizek, J., Ostádalová, I., Kalonsková, J., Babický, A., and Beneš, J., The detoxifying effects of selenium. Interrelations between compounds of selenium and certain metals, in *Newer Trace Elements in Nutrition*, Mertz, W. and Cornatzer, W. E., Eds., Marcel Decker, New York, 1971, 85—122.

219. Parizek, J., Kalouskavá, J., Babický, A., Beneš, J., and Pavlík, L., Interaction of selenium with mercury, cadmium and other toxic metals, in *Trace Element Metabolism in Animals-2*, Hoekstra, W. G., Suttie, J. W., Ganther, H. E., and Mertz, W., Eds., University Park Press, Baltimore, 1974, 119—131.

220. Potter, S. and Matrone, G., Effect of selenite on the toxicity of dietary methylmercury and mercuric chloride in the rat, *J. Nutr.*, 104, 638—647, 1974.

221. Ganther, H. E., Wagner, P. A., Sunde, M. L., and Hoekstra, W. G., Protective effects of selenium against heavy metal toxicities, *Trace Subs. Environ. Health*, 6, 247—252, 1972.

222. El-Begearmi, H. M., Gondie, C., Ganther, H. E., and Sunde, M. L., Attempts to quantitate the protective effect of selenium against mercury toxicity using Japanese quail, *Fed. Proc. Fed. Am. Soc. Exp. Biol.*, 32, (Abstr.) 3756, 1973.

223. Hill, C. H., Reversal of selenium toxicity in chicks by mercury, copper and cadmium, *J. Nutr.*, 104, 593—598, 1974.

224. Ganther, H. E., Goudie, C., Sunde, M. L., Kopecky, M. J., Wagner, P., Oh, S.-H., and Hoekstra, W. G., Selenium: relation to decreased toxicity of methylmercury added to diets containing tuna, *Science*, 175, 422—424, 1972.

225. Kosta, L., Bryne, A. R., and Zelenko, V., Correlation of selenium and mercury in man, *Nature (London)*, 254, 238—239, 1975.

226. Gabbiani, G., Baic, D., and Deziel, C., Studies on tolerance and ionic antagonism for cadmium or mercury, *Can. J. Physiol. Pharmacol.*, 45, 443—450, 1967.

227. Pollack, S., George, J. N., Reba, R. C., Kaufman, R. M., and Crosby, W. H., The absorption of non-ferrous metals in iron deficiency, *J. Clin. Invest.*, 44, 1470—1473, 1965.

228. Glendening, B. L., Shrenk, W. G., and Parrish, D. B., Effects of rubidium in purified diets fed to rats, *J. Nutr.*, 60, 563—579, 1956.

229. Sasser, L. P., Keinholz, E. W., and Ward, G. M., Interaction of rubidium and potassium in chick diets, *Poult. Sci.*, 49, 114—118, 1969.

230. Levander, D. A. and Morris, V. C., Effects of vitamin E and selenium on rubidium-68 uptake by rat liver slices, *J. Nutr.*, 101, 1013—1022, 1971.

231. Bunyan, J., Diplock, A. T., Gawthorne, M. A., and Green, J., Vitamin E and stress. VIII. Nutritional effects with dietary stress with silver in vitamin E-deficient chicks and rats, *Br. J. Nutr.*, 22, 165—182, 1968.

232. Jensen, L. S., Modification of a selenium toxicity in chicks by dietary silver and copper, *J. Nutr.*, 105, 769—775, 1975.

233. Peterson, R. P. and Jensen, L. S., Interrelationship of dietary silver with copper in the chick, *Poult. Sci.*, 54, 771—775, 1975.

234. Leinham, J. M. A., Loutit, J. F., and Martin, J. H., Eds., *Strontium Metabolism*, Academic Press, London, 1967.

235. Bartley, J. C. and Reber, E. F., Toxic effects of stable strontium in young pigs, *J. Nutr.*, 75, 21—28, 1961.

236. Forbes, G. B. and Reina, J. C., Effect of age on gastrointestinal absorption (Fe, Sr, Pb) in the rat, *J. Nutr.*, 102, 647—652, 1972.

237. Marcus, C. S. and Lengemann, F. W., Absorption of ^{45}Ca and ^{85}Sr from solid and liquid food at various levels of the alimentary tract of the rat, *J. Nutr.*, 77, 155—160, 1962.

238. **Webling, D. D. and Holdsworth, E. D.**, Bile and the absorption of strontium and iron, *Biochem. J.*, 100, 661—663, 1966.
239. **Teru, T. M., Gusmano, E. A., and Cohn, S. H.**, Decrement in radiostrontium retention following stable strontium prefeeding in the growing rat, *J. Nutr.*, 87, 399—406, 1965.
240. **Hartsook, E. W., Cowan, R. L., Chanoller, P. T., and Whelan, J. B.**, Effect of dietary protein source and corn oil and cellulose level on strontium-calcium discrimination in growing rats, *J. Nutr.*, 97, 95—103, 1969.
241. **Dubrovina, Z. V., Malkin, P. M., and Andreeva, L. P.**, Effects of calcium, magnesium, phosphate and fat on assimilation of strontium, *Radiobiology*, 5, 183—189, 1965.
242. **Waibel, P. E. and Mraz, F. R.**, Calcium, strontium and phosphate in the chick as influenced by nutritional and endocrine variations, *J. Nutr.*, 84, 58—64, 1964.
243. **Skoryna, S. C., Tanaka, Y., Moore, W., and Stara, J. F.**, Prevention of of gastrointestinal absorption of excessive trace element intake, *Trace Subs. Environ. Health*, 6, 3—11, 1973.
244. **Gibbons, R. A., Sansom, B. F., and Sellwood, R.**, The passage of calcium and strontium across the gut of the anaesthetized goat, *J. Physiol. (London)*, 222, 397—406, 1972.
245. **Sutton, A.**, Reduction of strontium absorption in man by the addition of alginate to the diet, *Nature (London)*, 216, 1005—1006, 1967.
246. **Patrick, G.**, Inhibition of strontium and calcium uptake by rat duodenal slices: comparison of polyuronides and related substances, *Nature (London)*, 216, 815—816, 1967.
247. **Milin, L. and Anderson, J. J. B.**, Whole body retention of strontium-89 in swine given sodium alginate or barium and sodium sulphates, *J. Nutr.*, 97, 181—184, 1969.
248. **Fournier, P.**, Effect of lactose on strontium absorption, *Isr. J. Med. Sci.*, 7, 389—391, 1971.
249. **Palmer, R. F. and Thomson, R. C.**, Strontium-calcium interrelationships in the growing rat, *Am. J. Physiol.*, 207, 561—566, 1964.
250. **Morrison, G. E., Howells, G. R., Pollard, J., Kostial, K., and Manitašenić, R.**, Effect of dietary phosphorus supplementation on the uptake of radioactive strontium in rats, *Br. J. Nutr.*, 21, 561—569, 1966.
251. **Gruden, N., Rabadjija, L., and Kostial, K.**, Effect of phosphates on strontium and cadmium metabolism in control, parathyroidectomised and parathormone-treated rats, *Arh. Hig. Rada. Toksikol.*, 19, 25—32, 1968.
252. **Bates, T. H. and Smith, H.**, Influence of polyphosphates on retention of radioactive strontium in rat and mouse, *Nature (London)*, 212, 925—926, 1966.
253. **Anon.**, Calcium, phosphate and strontium metabolism in infants, *Nutr. Rev.*, 27, 254—256, 1969.
254. **Kostial, K., Šimonović, I., and Pišonić, M.**, Effect of calcium and phosphates on gastrointestinal absorption of strontium and calcium in newborn rats, *Nature (London)*, 215, 1181—1182, 1967.
255. **Buldakov, L. A. and Erokhin, R. A.**, Metabolism of ^{90}Sr in rats fed high calcium diets, *Fed. Proc. Fed. Am. Soc. Exp. Biol.*, 25, T99—102, 1966.
256. **Schmidt, B. and Lang, K.**, Effect of lipid soluble vitamins on the metabolism of ^{90}Sr and calcium in growing rats. I. The influence of vitamin D, *Klin. Wochenschr.*, 42, 942—948, 1964.
257. **Corradino, R. A. and Wassermann, R. H.**, Strontium inhibition of vitamin D_3-induced calcium binding protein and calcium absorption in the chick, *Proc. Soc. Exp. Biol. Med.*, 133, 960—963, 1970.
258. **Stoney, E.**, Calcium and strontium changes in bone associated with continuous administration of stable strontium to rats, *Arch. Biochem. Biophys.*, 124, 575—581, 1968.
259. **Omdahl, J. L. and De Luca, H. F.**, Strontium induced rickets: metabolic basis, *Science*, 174, 949—951, 1971.
260. **Wasserman, R. H.**, Calcium absorption and calcium binding protein synthesis: Solanum Malacoxylon reverses strontium inhibition, *Science*, 143, 1092—1094, 1974.
261. **Pento, J. T.**, Relative influence of calcium, strontium and magnesium on calcitonin secretion in the pig, *Endocrinology*, 94, 1176—1180, 1974.
262. **Bates, R. F.**, Stimulation of calcitonin secretion by strontium, *J. Physiol.*, 238, 76P, 1964.
263. **Ebel, J. G. and Comar, C. L.**, Effect of dietary magnesium on strontium-calcium discrimination and incorporation into bone of rats, *J. Nutr.*, 96, 403—408, 1968.
264. **Mraz, F. R.**, Intestinal absorption of ^{45}Ca and ^{89}Sr as affected by calcium, strontium and magnesium, *Poult. Sci.*, 52, 1288—1289, 1973.
265. **Clark, I.**, Effects of magnesium on strontium absorption, *Proc. Soc. Exp. Biol. Med.*, 116, 984—987, 1964.
266. **Annenkov, B. N.**, Influence of calcium, magnesium and strontium on the transfer of ^{90}Sr from female rat to descendants, *Radiobiologia*, 6, 455—458, 1966.
267. **Lengemann, F. W. and Comar, C. L.**, Fluoridated water and the skeletal uptake of ^{85}Sr and ^{45}Ca by young rats, *J. Nutr.*, 79, 195—199, 1963.
268. **Knizhnikov, N. A., Grozovskaya, V. P., Vlasov, P. A., Belousova, D. and Sedov, V. V.**, Role of calcium and fluoride in food and water on the protection of rats from the effects of Sr-90, *Gig. Sanit.*, 33, 38—44, 1968.

269. Gruden, N., Stantic, M., and Buben, M., Influence of lead on calcium and strontium transfer through duodenal wall in rats, *Environ. Res.*, 8, 203—206, 1974.

270. Milin, L. and Anderson, J. J. B., Whole-body retention of strontium-85 in swine given sodium alginate or barium and sodium sulphates, *J. Nutr.*, 97, 181—184, 1969.

271. Kostial, K., Maljoković, T., Kadić, M., Manitašević, R., and Morrison, G. E., Reduction of the absorption and retention of strontium in rats, *Nature (London)*, 215, 182, 1967.

272. Carr, T. E. F. and Nolan, J., Inhibition of the absorption of dietary radiostrontium by aluminium phosphate gel and sodium alginate in the rat, *Nature (London)*, 219, 500—501, 1968.

273. Spencer, H., Samachson, J., Hardy, E. P., and Rivera, J., Effect of intravenous calcium and of orally-administered ammonium chloride on strontium-90 excretion in man, *Radiat. Res.*, 25, 695—705, 1965.

274. Schmidt, B. and Lang, K., Effect of lipid soluble vitamins on the metabolism of ^{29}Sr and calcium in growing rats. II. Effects of vitamin A, *Klin. Wochenschr.*, 43, 375—382, 1965.

275. Spreng, P., Effect of parathyroid hormone and vitamin A on the retention of radiostrontium in the rat, *Nature (London)*, 214, 513—514, 1967.

276. Cordelli, F., Corvaglia, E., Bracci, R., and Benedetti, P. A., Effects of high dosages of vitamins A, D, B$_6$ and pantochemic acid on the metabolism of ^{85}Sr in young rats, *Riv. Clin. Pediatr.*, 77, 271—278, 1966.

277. Okuda, K. and Sasayama, K., Effects of EDTA and metal ions in intestinal absorption of vitamin B$_{12}$ in man and rats, *Proc. Soc. Exp. Biol. Med.*, 120, 17—20, 1965.

278. Gehring, P. J. and Hammond, P. B., The inter-relationship between thallium and potassium in animals, *J. Pharmacol. Exp. Therap.*, 155, 187—201, 1967.

279. Gibson, J. E. and Becker, B. A. Placental transfer, embryotoxicity and teratogenicity of thallium in normal and potassium-deficient rats, *Toxic. Appl. Pharm.*, 15, 120—132, 1970.

280. Pavlovskoya, N. A., Provotorov, A. V., and Makeeva, L. G., Thorium resorption from the gastrointestinal tract by the blood and its accumulation in organs and tissues of rats, *Gig. Sanit.*, 36, 47—51, 1971.

281. Taylor, D. M., Chipperfield, A. R., and James, A. C., Effects of tetracycline on deposition of plutonium and related elements in rat bone, *Health Phys.*, 21, 197—204, 1971.

282. Schwarz, K., Milne, D. B., and Vinyard, E., Growth effects of tin compounds in rats maintained in a trace element-controlled environment, *Biochem. Biophys. Res. Commun.*, 40, 22—29, 1970.

283. De Groot, A. P., Subacute toxicity of inorganic tin as influenced by dietary levels of iron and copper, *Food Cosmet. Toxicol.*, 11, 955—962, 1973.

284. Krutikova, N. A., Effect of sodium chloride and calcium carbonate limitation on titanium and vanadium content of rat organs, *Vopr. Pit.*, 32 (5), 59—61, 1973.

285. Nordberg, G. F., Ed.,*Effects and Dose-Response Relationships of Toxic Metals*, Elsevier, Amsterdam, 1976.

286. Brown, S. S., Ed.,*Clinical Chemistry and Chemical Toxicology of Metals*, Elsevier/North-Holland, Amsterdam, 1977.

287. Levander, O. A., Nutritional factors in relation to heavy metal toxicants, *Fed. Proc. Fed. Am. Soc. Exp. Biol.*, 36 (5), 1683—1687, 1977.

288. Webb, M., Ed., Chemicals in food and environment, *Br. Med. Bull.*, 31, 181—260, 1975.

289. Said, A. N., Slagsvold, P., Bergh, H., and Laksesvela, B., High fluorine water to Wether sheep maintained in pens. Aluminium chloride as a possible alleviator of fluorosis, *Nord. Vet. Med.*, 29, 172—180, 1977.

290. Cakir, A., Sullivan, T. W., and Mather, F. B., Alleviation of fluoride toxicity in starting turkeys and chicks with aluminium, *Poult. Sci.*, 57, 498—505, 1978.

291. Rastogi, S. P., Padilla, F., and Boyd, C. M., Effect of aluminium hydroxide on iron absorption, *J. Arkansas Med. Soc.*, 73 (3), 133—134, 1976.

292. Cam, J. M., Luck, V. A., Eastwood, J. B., and de Wardener, H. E., The effect of aluminium hydroxide orally on calcium phosphorus and aluminium metabolism in normal subjects, *Clin. Sci. Mol. Med.*, 51, 407, 1976.

293. Meredith, P. A., Moore, M. R., and Goldberg, A., Effects of aluminium, lead and zinc on δ-aminoleucilinic acid dehydratase, *Enzyme*, 22 (1), 22—27, 1977.

294. Samira, S. and Khayyal, M. T., Effect of cysteine on the hepatic toxicity and antischistosomal activity of antimonyl potassium tartrate, *Bull. W.H.O.*, 53, 379—384, 1976.

295. Tsutsumi, S., Usui, Y., and Matsumoto, Y., Arsenic metabolism. 8. Influence of different diets on the inhibition of succinic acid dehydrogenase activity in rats, *Nippon Yakurigaku Zasshi*, 70 (4), 515—522, 1974.

296. Neathery, M. W. and Miller, W. J., Metabolism and toxicity of cadmium, mercury and lead in animals: a review, *J. Dairy Sci.*, 58, 1767—1781, 1975.

297. **Bremner, I.**, The toxicity of cadmium, zinc and molybdenum and their effects on copper metabolism, *Proc. Nutr. Soc.*, 38, 235—242, 1979.

298. **Webb, M.**, Cadmium, *Br. Med. Bull.*, 31, 246—250, 1975.

299. **Bremner, I.**, Cadmium toxicity, *Wld. Rev. Nutr. Diet.*, 32, 165—197, 1978.

300. **Kello, D. and Kostial, K.**, Influence of age and milk diet on cadmium absorption from the gut, *Toxicol. Appl. Pharmacol.*, 40, 277—282, 1977.

301. **Kello, D. and Kostial, K.**, Influence of age on whole body retention and distribution of ^{115}m Cd in the rat, *Environ. Res.*, 14, 92—98, 1977.

302. **Cousins, R. J., Squibb, K. S., Feldman, S. L., de Bari, A., and Silbon, B. L.**, Biomedical responses of rats to chronic exposure to dietary cadmium in ad libitum and equalized regimes, *J. Toxicol. Environ. Health*, 2, 929—943, 1977.

303. **Leber, A. P. and Miya, T. S.**, A mechanism for cadmium and zinc-induced tolerance to cadmium toxicity: involvement of metallothionein, *Toxicol. Appl. Pharmacol.*, 37, 403—414, 1976.

304. **Irons, R. D. and Smith, J. C.**, Prevention by copper of cadmium sequestration by metallothionein in liver, *Chem. Biol. Interact.*, 15, 289—294, 1976.

305. **Klaasen, C. D.**, Effect of metallothionein on hepatic disposition of metals, *Am. J. Physiol.*, 234, E47—53, 1978.

306. **Engström, B. and Nordberg, G.**, Effects of milk diet on gastrointestinal absorption of cadmium in adult mice, *Toxicology*, 9, 195—203, 1978.

307. **Gontzea, I. and Popescu, F.**, The effect of body protein on resistance to cadmium, *Br. J. Ind. Med.*, 35, 154—160, 1979.

308. **Washko, P. W. and Cousins, R. J.**, Role of dietary calcium and calcium binding protein in cadmium toxicity in rats, *J. Nutr.*, 107, 920—928, 1977.

309. **Hamilton, D. L. and Smith, M. W.**, Inhibition of intestinal calcium uptake by cadmium and the effect of a low calcium diet on cadmium retention, *Environ. Res.*, 15, 175—184, 1978.

310. **Washko, P. W. and Cousins, R. J.**, Metabolism of ^{109}Cd in rats fed normal and low-calcium diets, *J. Toxicol. Environ. Health*, 1, 1055—1066, 1976.

311. **Hamilton, D. L. and Smith, M. W.**, Cadmium inhibits absorption by rat intestine, *J. Physiol.*, 265, 54—55P, 1977.

312. **Yuhas, E. M., Miya, T. S., and Schnell, R. C.**, Influence of cadmium on calcium absorption from the rat intestine, *Toxicol. Appl. Pharmacol.*, 43, 23—31, 1978.

313. **Ando, M., Sayato, Y., Tonomura, M., and Osawa, T.**, Studies on excretion and uptake of calcium by rats after continuous oral administration of cadmium, *Toxicol. Appl. Pharmacol.*, 39, 321—327, 1977.

314. **Ando, M., Sayato, Y., and Osawa, T.**, Studies on the disposition of calcium in bones of rats after continuous oral administration of cadmium, *Toxicol. Appl. Pharmacol.*, 46, 625—632, 1978.

315. **Lorentzon, R. and Larsson, S. E.**, Vitamin D metabolism in adult rats at low and normal calcium intake and the effect of cadmium exposure, *Clin. Sci. Mol. Med.*, 53, 439—446, 1977.

316. **Loretnzon, R. and Larsson, S.-E.**, Intestinal absorption and tissue retention of cadmium and calcium in normal rats and rats given an active metabolite of vitamin D (1,25-dihydroxycholecalciferol), *Clin. Sci. Mol. Med.*, 55, 195—198, 1978.

317. **Valberg, L. S., Sorbie, J., and Hamilton, D. L.**, Gastrointestinal metabolism of cadmium in experimental iron deficiency, *Am. J. Physiol.*, 231, 462—467, 1976.

318. **Flanagan, P. R., McLellan, J. S., Haist, J., Cherian, G., Chamberlain, M. J., and Valberg, L. S.**, Increased dietary cadmium absorption in mice and human subjects with iron deficiency, *Gastroenterology*, 74, 841—846, 1978.

319. **Suzuki, T. and Yoshida, A.**, Long-term effectiveness of dietary iron and ascorbic acid in the prevention and cure of cadmium toxicity in rats, *Am. J. Clin. Nutr.*, 31, 1491—1498, 1978.

320. **Ragan, H. A.**, Effects of iron deficiency on the absorption and distribution of lead and cadmium in rats, *J. Lab. Clin. Med.*, 90, 700—706, 1977.

321. **Reddy, K. A., Omaye, S. T., Hasegawa, G. K., and Cross, C. E.**, Enhanced lung toxicity of intratracheally instilled cadmium chloride in selenium-deficient rats, *Toxicol. Appl. Pharmacol.*, 43, 249—257, 1978.

322. **Merali, Z. and Singhal, R. L.**, Protective effect of selenium on certain hepatotoxic and pancreotoxic manifestations of sub-acute cadmium administration, *J. Pharmacol. Exp. Ther.*, 195, 58—66, 1975.

323. **Merali, Z. and Singhal, R. N.**, Prevention by zinc of cadmium-induced alterations in pancreatic and hepatic functions, *Br. J. Pharmacol.*, 57, 573—579, 1976.

324. **Pitrowski, J. K., Bern, E. M., and Werner, A.**, Cadmium and mercury binding to metallothionein as influenced by selenium, *Biochem. Pharmacol.*, 26, 2191—2192, 1977.

325. **Davies, N. T. and Campbell, J. K.**, The effect of cadmium on intestinal copper absorption and binding in the rat, *Life Sci.*, 20, 955—960, 1977.

326. Jacobs, R. M., Jones, A. O. L., Fox, M. R. S., and Fry, B. E., Retention of dietary cadmium and the amelioratve effect of zinc, copper and manganese in Japanese quail, *J. Nutr.,* 108, 22—32, 1978.

327. Bremner, I. and Campbell, J. K. Effect of copper and zinc status on susceptibility to cadmium intoxication, *Environ. Health Perspect.,* 25, 125—128, 1978.

328. Quarterman, J. and Morrison, E., The effect of age on the absorption and excretion of lead, *Environ. Res.,* 17, 78—83, 1978.

329. Mocilovic, B., The effect of maternal dose on lead retention in suckling rats, *Arch. Environ. Health,* 33, 115—117, 1978.

330. Mocilovic, B., Lead metabolism in lactation, *Experientia,* 35, 517, 1979.

331. Lorenzo, A. V., Gewirtz, M., Morher, C., and Davidowski, L. I., The equilibration of lead between blood and milk of lactating rabbits, *Life Sci.,* 21, 1679—1684, 1977.

332. Gruden, N. and Stantic, M., Transfer of lead through the rats intestinal wall, *Sci. Total Environ.,* 3, 288—292, 1975.

333. Coleman, I. P. L., Hilburn, M. E., and Blair, J. A., The intestinal absorption of lead, *Biochem. Soc. Trans.,* 6, 915—917, 1978.

334. Blair, J. A., Coleman, I. P. L., and Hilburn, M. E., The transport of the lead cation across the intestinal membrane, *J. Physiol.,* 286, 343—350, 1979.

335. Gerher, G. B. and Deroo, J., Absorption of radioactive lead (^{210}Pb) by different parts of the intestine in young and adult rats, *Environ. Physiol. Biochem.,* 5, 314—318, 1975.

336. Quarterman, J. , Morrison, J. N., and Morrison, E., Changes in water intake, urine production and salt metabolism in lead-poisoned sheep, *Proc. Nutr. Soc.,* 36, 102A, 1977.

337. Johnson, D. R. and Kleinmann, L. I., Effects of lead exposure on renal function in young rats, *Toxicol. Appl. Pharmacol.,* 48, 361—367, 1979.

338. Boseals, P., Salimei, E., Adams, A., and Porcelli, G., Effects of environmental lead levels on the urinary kallikrein excretion of exposed workers, *Life Sci.,* 20, 1715—1722, 1977.

339. Campbell, B. C., Beattie, A. D., Moore, M. R., Goldberg, A., and Reid, A. C., Renal insufficiency associated with excessive lead exposure, *Br. Med. J.,* 482—485, 1977.

340. Victery, W., Vander, A. J., and Mouw, D. R., Effect of acid-bace status on renal excretion and accumulation of lead, *Fed. Proc. Fed. Am. Soc. Exp. Biol.,* 37, (Abstr.) 3727, 1978.

341. Mylroie, A. A., Moore, L., and Erogbogbo, V., Influence of dietary factors on blood and tissue lead concentrations and lead toxicity, *Toxicol. Appl. Pharmacol.,* 41, 361—367, 1977.

342. Quarterman, J., Morrison, E., Morrison, J. N., and Humphries, W. R., Dietary protein and lead retention, *Environ. Res.,* 17, 68—77, 1978.

343. Quarterman, J., Morrison, J. N., and Humphries, W. R., The role of phospholipids and bile in lead absorption, *Proc. Nutr. Soc.,* 36, 103A, 1977.

344. Ku, Y., Alvary, G. H., and Mahaffey, K. R., Comparative effects of feeding lead acetate and phospholipid-bound lead on blood and tissue lead concentrations in young and adult rats, *Bull. Environ. Contam. Toxicol.,* 20, 561—567, 1978.

345. Smith, C. M., DeLuca, H. F., Tanoka, Y., and Mahaffey, K. R., Stimulation of lead absorption by vitamin D administration, *J. Nutr.,* 108 843—847, 1978.

346. Barton, J. C., Conrad, M. E., Harrison, L., and Nuby, S., Effects of calcium on the absorption and retention of lead, *J. Lab. Clin. Med.,* 91, 366—376, 1978.

347. Meredith, P. A., Moore, M. R., and Goldberg, A., The effect of calcium on lead absorption in rats, *Biochem. J.,* 166, 531—537, 1977.

348. Quarterman, J., Morrison, J. N., and Humphries, W. R., The influence of high dietary calcium and phosphate on lead uptake and release, *Environ. Res.,* 17, 60—67, 1978.

349. Norimatsu, H. and Talinage, R. V., Influence of calcitonin on the initial uptake of lead and mercury by bone, *Proc. Soc. Exp. Biol. Med.,* 161, 94—98, 1979.

350. Rosen, J. F., Actions of calcitonin and parathyroid hormone in lead-intoxicated rats, *Clin. Res.,* 4, 755, 1972.

351. Mouw, D. R., Wagner, J. G., Kalitis, K., Vander, A. J., and Major, G. H., The effect of parathyroid hormone on the renal accumulation of lead, *Environ. Res.,* 15, 20—27, 1978.

352. Ziegler, E. E., Edwards, B. B., Jensen, R. L., Mahaffey, K. R., and Fomon, S. J., Absorption and retention of lead by infants, *Pediatr. Res.,* 12, 29—34, 1978.

353. Sorrell, M., Rosen, J. F., and Roginsky, M., Interactions of lead, calcium, vitamin D and nutrition in lead-burdened children, *Arch. Environ. Health,* 32, 160—164, 1977.

354. Crosby, W. H. Lead contaminated health food. Association with lead poisoning and leukemia, *JAMA,* 237, 2627—2629, 1977.

355. Cohen, D. J., Johnson, W. T., and Caparulo, B. K., Pica and elevated blood lead level in autistic and atypical children, *Am. J. Dis. Child.,* 130, 47—48, 1976.

356. Snowdon, C. T., A nutritional basis for lead pica, *Physiol. Behav.,* 18, 885—893, 1977.

357. Singh, N. P., Thind, I. S., Vitale, L. F., and Pawlow, M., Intake of magnesium and toxicity of lead: an experimental model, *Arch. Environ. Health,* 34, 168—173, 1979.

358. **Conrad, M. E. and Barton, J. C.,** Factors affecting the absorption and excretion of lead in the rat, *Gastroenterology,* 74, 731—740, 1978.

359. **Hamilton, D. L.,** Interrelationships of lead and iron retention in iron-deficient mice, *Toxicol. Appl. Pharmacol.,* 46, 651—661, 1978.

360. **Barton, J. C., Conrad, M. E., Nuby, S., and Harrison, L.,** Effects of iron on the absorption and retention of lead, *J. Lab. Clin. Med.,* 92, 536—547, 1978.

361. **Angle, C. R., McIntire, M. S., and Brivik, G.,** Effect of anaemia on blood and tissue lead in rats, *J. Toxicol. Environ. Health,* 3, 557—563, 1977.

362. **Robertson, I. K. and Wormwood, M.,** Lead and iron absorption from rat small intestine: the effect of iron deficiency, *Br. J. Nutr.,* 40, 253—260, 1978.

363. **Dobbins, A., Johnson, D. R., and Nathan, P.,** Effect of exposure to lead on maturation of intestinal iron absorption of rats, *J. Toxicol. Environ. Health,* 4, 541—550, 1978.

364. **Wisbowo, A. A. E., Castilho, P., Del. Herber, R. F. M., and Ziehuis, R. L.,** Blood lead and serum iron levels in non-occupationally exposed males and females, *Int. Arch. Occup. Environ. Health,* 39, 113—120, 1977.

365. **Rastogi, S. C., Clausen, J., and Srivastava, K. C.,** Selenium and lead: mutual detoxifying effects, *Toxicology,* 6, 377—388, 1976.

366. **Borden, E. A., Contrell, A. C., and Kilroe-Smith, T. A.,** The in vitro effect of zinc on the inhibition of human δ-aminoleucolinic acid dehydratase by lead, *Br. J. Ind. Med.,* 33, 85—87, 1976.

367. **Contrell, A. C., Kilroe-Smith, T. A., Simoes, M. M., and Border, E. A.,** The effect of zinc and pH on the behavior of δ-aminoleucilinic acid dehydratase activity in baboons exposed to lead, *Br. J. Ind. Med.,* 34, 110—113, 1977.

368. **Haeger-Aronsen, B., Schutz, A., and Abdulla, M.,** Antagonistic effect in vivo of zinc on inhibition of δ-aminoleucilinic acid dehydratase by lead, *Arch. Environ. Health,* 31, 215—220, 1976.

369. **Thomasino, J. A., Zuroweste, E., Brooks, S. M., Petering, H. G., Lerner, S. I., and Finelli, V. N.,** Lead, zinc and erythrocyte δ-aminoleucilinic acid dehydratase relationships in lead toxicity, *Arch. Environ. Health,* 32, 244—247, 1977.

370. **Davis, J. R. and Auram, M. J.,** A comparison of the stimulatory effects of cadmium and zinc on normal and lead-inhibited human erythrocyte δ-aminoleucilinic acid dehydratase activity in vitro, *Toxicol. Appl. Pharmacol.,* 44, 181—190, 1978.

371. **Cerklowski, F. L.,** Influence of dietary zinc on lead toxicity during gestation and lactation in the female rat, *J. Nutr.,* 109, 1703—1709, 1979.

372. **Klauder, D. S. and Petering, H. G.,** Protective value of dietary copper and iron against some toxic effects of lead in rats, *Environ. Health Perspect.,* 12, 77—80, 1975.

373. **Klauder, D. S. and Petering, H. G.,** Anaemia of lead intoxication: a role for copper, *J. Nutr.,* 107, 1779—1785, 1977.

374. **Cerklewski, F. L. and Forbes, R. M.,** Influence of dietary copper on lead toxicity in the young male rat, *J. Nutr.,* 107, 143—146, 1977.

375. **Pal, D. R., Chatterjee, J., and Chatterjee, G. C.,** Influence of lead administration on l-ascorbic acid metabolism in rats: effect of l-ascorbic acid supplementation, *Int. J. Vit. Nutr. Res.,* 45, 429—437, 1975.

376. **Papaionnou, R., Sohler, A., and Pfeiffer, C. C.,** Reduction of blood lead levels in battery workers by zinc and vitamin C, *J. Orthomolec. Phych.,* 7, 1—13, 1978.

377. **Suzuki, T. and Yoshida, A.,** Effect of dietary supplementation of iron and ascorbic acid on lead toxicity in rats, *J. Nutr.,* 109, 928—938, 1979.

378. **Goyer, R. A. and Cherian, M. G.,** Ascorbic acid and EDTA treatment of lead toxicity in rats, *Life Sci.,* 24, 433—438, 1979.

379. **Anon.,** Interactions of lead poisoning and vitamin E deficiency, *Nutr. Rev.,* 36, 156—158, 1978.

380. **Levander, O. A., Morris, V. C., and Ferretti, R. J.,** Comparative effects of selenium and vitamin E in lead-poisoned rats, *J. Nutr.,* 107, 378—382, 1977.

381. **Sifri, M. and Hoekstra, W. G.,** Effect of lead on lipid peroxidation in rats deficient or adequate in selenium and vitamin E, *Fed. Proc. Fed. Am. Soc. Exp. Biol.,* 37, 757, 1978.

382. **Mylroie, A. A., Moore, L., Olyai, B., and Anderson, M.,** Increased susceptibility to lead toxicity in rats fed semipurified diets, *Environ. Res.,* 15, 57—64, 1978.

383. **Peaslee, M. H. and Einhellig, F. A.,** Protective effect of tannic acid in mice receiving dietary lead, *Experientia,* 33, 1206, 1977.

384. **Jensen, J. and Olesen, O. V.,** Lithium induced loss of body sodium and the development of severe intoxication in rats, *Acta Pharmacol. Toxicol.,* 35(4), 337—346, 1974.

385. **Dolman, D. and Edmonds, C. J.,** Lithium transport by colon of normal and sodium-depleted rats, *J. Physiol.,* 259, 759—770, 1976.

386. **Smith, D. F.,** The role of sodium in the effect of food intake on renal lithium clearance in rats, *Toxicol. Appl. Pharamcol.,* 33, 276—280, 1975.

387. Olesen, O. V. and Thomsen, K., A preventive effect of potassium against fatal lithium intoxication in rats, *Neuropsychobiology,* 2, (2—3), 112—117, 1976.
388. Isaacs, J. P., Ballich, N. L., and Lamb, J. C., Non-toxic therapy of endogenous manic depression, *Trace Subs. Environ. Res.,* 9, 349—354, 1975.
389. Sasser, L. B., Jarboe, G. E., Walter, B. K., and Kelman, B. J., Absorption of mercury from ligated segments of the rat gastrointestinal tract, *Proc. Soc. Exp. Biol. Med.,* 157, 57—60, 1978.
390. Chang, C. W. J., Nakanuera, R. M., and Brooks, C. C., Effect of varied dietary levels and forms of mercury on swine, *J. Anim. Sci.,* 45, 279—285, 1977.
391. Koscheev, A. K. and Lioshits, O. D., The effect of vegetables on the glycogen forming and decontaminating function of the liver in chronic mercury poisoning, *Vopr. Pit.,* (6), 69—72, 1976.
392. Lamerie, N., Ringoir, S., and Leusen, I., Effect of variation in dietary NaCl on total and fractional renal blood flow in the normal and mercury-intoxicated rat, *Cir. Res.,* 39, 506—511, 1976.
393. Thiel, G., Protection of rat kidneys against HgCl$_2$-induced acute renal failure by induction of high urine flow without renin suppression, *Kidney Int.,* 10, S191—200, 1976.
394. Murray, D. R. and Hughes, R. E., The influence of dietary ascorbic acid on the concentration of mercury in guinea pig tissues, *Proc. Nutr. Soc.,* 35, 118A—119A, 1976.
395. Blackstone, S., Hurley, R. J., and Hughes, R. E., Some inter-relationships between vitamin C and mercury in the guinea pig, *Food Cosmet. Toxicol.,* 12, 511—516, 1974.
396. Chatterjee, G. C. and Pal, D. R., Metabolism of l-ascorbic acid in rats under in vivo administration of mercury: effect of l-ascorbic acid supplementation, *Int. J. Vit. Nutr. Res.,* 45, 284—292, 1975.
397. Yuhara, S., Sastrohadinoto, S., and Haeruman, H., Effect of selenium and mercury on survival of chick embryos, *Poultry Sci.,* 55, 1423—1428, 1976.
398. Yuhara, S., Sastrohadinoto, S., and Budiarso, I. T., Effect of selenium and mercury on gross morphology and histopathology of chick embryos, *Poultry Sci.,* 55, 2424—2433, 1976.
399. Bark, R. F., Jordan, H. E., and Kiker, K. W., Some effects of selenium status on inorganic mercury metabolism in the rat, *Toxicol. Appl. Pharmacol.,* 40, 71—82, 1977.
400. Piotrowski, J. K., Bern, E. M., and Werner, A., Cadmium and mercury binding to metallothionein as influenced by selenium, *Biochem. Pharmacol.,* 26, 2191—2192, 1977.
401. Webb, M. and Magos, L., Cadmium thionein and the protection by cadmium against the neprhotoxicity of mercury, *Chem. -Biol. Interact.,* 14, 357—369, 1976.
402. Yamane, Y., Fukino, H., and Inagawa, M., Suppressive effect of zinc on the toxicity of mercury, *Chem. Pharmacol. Bull.,* 25, 1509—1518, 1977.
403. Chatterjee, G. C., Chatterjee, S., Chatterjee, K., Sahn, A., Bhattacharyga, A., Chakraborty, D., and Das, P. K., Studies on the protective effect of ascorbic acid in rubidium toxicity, *Toxicol. Appl. Pharmacol.,* 51, 47—58, 1979.
404. Heine, K., Wiechen, A., and Finger, H., Caesium and rubidium metabolism in cows, *Naturwissenschaften,* 64 (10), 531—532, 1977.
405. Van Vleet, J. F., Induction of lesions of selenium-vitamin E deficiency in pigs fed silver, *Am. J. Vet. Res.,* 37, 1415—1420, 1976.
406. Van Vleet, J. F., Protection by various nutritional supplements against lesions of selenium-vitamin E deficiency induced in ducklings fed tellurium or silver, *Am. J. Vet. Res.,* 38, 1393—1398, 1977.
407. Rousselet, F., El Solh, N., Maurat, J. P., Gruson, M., and Girard, M. L., Calcium metabolism and strontium:strontium vitamin D interaction, *C. R. Seances Soc. Biol. Paris,* 169, 322—329, 1975.
408. Escanero, J., Carre, M., and Miravet, L., Effect of various vitamin D$_3$ metabolites and calcium on intestinal strontium absorption, *C.R. Seances Soc. Biol. Paris,* 170, 47—53, 1976.
409. Spencer, H., Kramer, L., and Hardy, E. P., Effect of phosphate or ^{90}Sr balance in man, *Health Phys.,* 33(5), 417—423, 1977.
410. Miler, D. L. and Schedl, H. P., Effects of experimental diabetes on intestinal strontium absorption in rats, *Proc. Soc. Exp. Biol. Med.,* 152, 589—592, 1976.
411. Van Barnveld, A. A., Van Puymbroeck, S., and Vanderborght, O., The action of sodium alginate in food on a ^{85}Sr body burden in mice, *Health Phys.,* 33, 533—537, 1977.
412. Kojima, S., Saito, K., and Kiyozumi, M., Studies on poisonous metals. IV. Absorption of stannic chloride from rat alimentary tract and effect of various food components on its absorption, *Yakugaku Zasshi,* 98 (4), 495—502, 1978.
413. Fritsch, P., de Saint Blanquat, G., and Derache, R., Effect of various dietary components on absorption and tissue distribution of orally administered inorganic tin in rats, *Food Cosmet. Toxicol.,* 15, 147—149, 1977.
414. Yamaguchi, M., Endo, T., and Yamamoto, T., Action of tin on the secretory effect of agents which stimulate gastric acid secretion in rats, *Toxicol. Appl. Pharm.,* 43, 417—423, 1978.
415. Yamaguchi, M. and Yamamoto, T., Decrease of gastric secretion in rats orally administered stannous chloride, *Nippon Eiseigaky Zasshi,* 31 (3), 453—456, 1976.

416. **Yamaguchi, M., Sato, H., and Yamamoto, T.**, Effect of lead on development of calcium metabolic disturbances in rats treated with stannous chloride, *Nippon Eiseigaku Zasshi,* 30 (6), 615—618, 1976.
417. **Yamamoto, T., Yamaguchi, M., and Sato, H.**, Accumulation of calcium in kidney and decrease of calcium in serum of rats treated with tin chloride, *J. Toxicol. Environ. Health,* 1 (5), 749—756, 1976.
418. **Webb, M., Ed.**, Decrease of calcium concentration in urine of rats treated with stannous chloride, *Chem. Pharm. Bull.,* 24 (12), 3199—3201, 1976.
419. **Webb, M., Ed.**, Effects of vitamin D_3 on serum calcium concentration in rats treated with stannous chloride, *Nippon Eiseigaku Zasshi,* 30 (5), 536—542, 1975.
420. **Krutikova, N. A. and Popov, V. V.**, Distribution of Titanium in the body during qualitatively and quantitatively incomplete nutrition, *Vopr. Pit.,* 4, 83—85, 1978.

THE EFFECT OF DIETARY FACTORS ON TOXICITY AND DISPOSITION OF DRUGS AND OTHER XENOBIOTICS*

Eino Hietanen, M.D.

INTRODUCTION

Drugs, certain endogenous substances (hormones, bile acids, and bilirubin), and environmental compounds are metabolized by the enzyme system leading to the inactivation or activation of the original compound, changing its water solubility and influencing its excretion. The term nutrition includes major nutrients, i.e., proteins, carbohydrates, and fats, as well as noncaloric nutrients, i.e., vitamins, minerals, and trace elements. However, the human diet contains many other compounds used either as intentional food additives or substances entering the diet nonintentionally and called contaminants. In this presentation the word "nutrition" with be dealt with broadly and will include food additives and contaminants.

Numerous factors are known to influence drug metabolism both in man and animals, including age, sex, pregnancy, species and strain variation, diseases, environmental pollutants, and other drugs in the diet.[1-11] The diet may change the rate of elimination of drugs and result in altered therapeutic response in an individual. Moreover, it may change the metabolic pattern of foreign, nontherapeutic compounds in the body. In extreme cases dietary factors may modify the metabolism of potentially harmful (e.g., carcinogenic) compounds to a more carcinogenic form. This will be mediated through the changes in the activity of the drug-metabolizing enzyme system on the one hand and, on the other, food may introduce harmful compounds to the body. Nutrition may influence or contribute to 40 to 60% of all human cancers; however, human cancer may in 80 to 90% of all cases have its origin in environmental factors.[12-15] In this article the influence of diet (including both nutrients and contaminants) on the disposition and metabolism of xenobiotics and the tissue responses to these metabolites will be discussed.

BIOTRANSFORMATION OF XENOBIOTICS

Reaction Types

The biological effects of drugs and other xenobiotics are regulated by their metabolic rates in the liver and extrahepatic tissues. The activities of drug-metabolizing enzymes are also regulated by nutrients and other dietary components.[16] But dietary constituents may themselves be metabolized through these enzymes to biologically more active forms or to inactive, easily excretable, derivatives. The metabolic pathway can be divided into first and second phase reactions (Figure 1).[17-22] The first-phase reactions are composed of two enzyme systems. The mixed function oxidase or monooxygenase system catalyzes numerous oxidative reactions and produces unstable epoxides from aromatic and olefinic compounds ready to react with tissue macromolecules.[18,19,21,23] These intermediates will be further metabolized by epoxide hydrases catalyzing the enzymatic conversion of epoxides to biologically less active hydroxylated products.[24]

The products of the first-phase reactions and compounds, containing in their native structure carboxyl and amino groups, are substrates for the second-phase reactions.

* The original research by the author cited in this review has been supported by grants from NIH (ROI ES 01684) and from the J. Vainio and Y. Jahnsson Foundations.

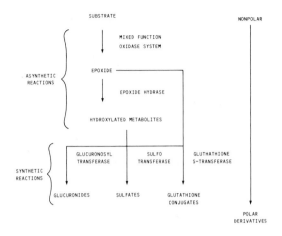

FIGURE 1.   The principal pathways in the biotransformation reactions. The substrate can be a drug, an environmental xenobiotic, or an endogenous compound. The right-hand arrow illustrates the increase in the polarity (water solubility) in the metabolic processes.

These reactions include enzymes catalyzing the conjugation of the substrate with glucuronic acid, sulfate, or glutathione (Figure 1).[17,25,26] The conjugated metabolites are usually very polar and easily excreted either to the urine or bile, depending on their molecular structure and weight.[17,22,27] Even the polar metabolites are not always excreted from the body but may be split in to unconjugated biologically active metabolites and reenter the circulation.[28-31]

Tissue Distribution

The enzymes of the drug-metabolizing system are located in various subcellular compartments. The mixed function oxidase system is isolated as microsomes in the endoplasmic reticulum after ultracentrifuge separation although low activity may also be found in other subcellular compartments.[32-35] The epoxide hydrase is also a microsomal enzyme complex.[36] The UDPglucuronosyltransferase enzyme catalyzing the conjugation of endogenous and exogenous compounds with glucuronic acid is located deep in the endoplasmic reticulum.[32,35] The sulfotransferase and glutathione transferases are in the cytoplasm, and glycine conjugation takes place in mitochondria.[25,30,37] For a detailed description of the drug-metabolizing enzyme system recent reviews are recommended.[19,21,23,38-40]

Reactive Intermediates

For a better understanding of how nutrition may interact with the toxicity of drugs and other xenobiotics it is necessary to have a view of the mechanisms by which these toxic metabolites are formed. It is known that the metabolites may yield toxic reactions from allergy to cancer. Mycotoxins and cycasin are known to cause liver cancer; nitrate, nitrite, and nitrosamides, gastric cancer; and nitrosamine liver and colon cancers, at least.[15,41-47]

The formation of reactive intermediates from some compounds either present in the diet as contaminants or upon whose metabolism dietary factors will have an influence is shown in Figure 2.[48-53] A typical example of a compound which is not in itself carcinogenic but which yields carcinogenic metabolites in the body is 2-acetylaminofluorene, a colon carcinogen. The compound is first metabolized by microsomal mixed

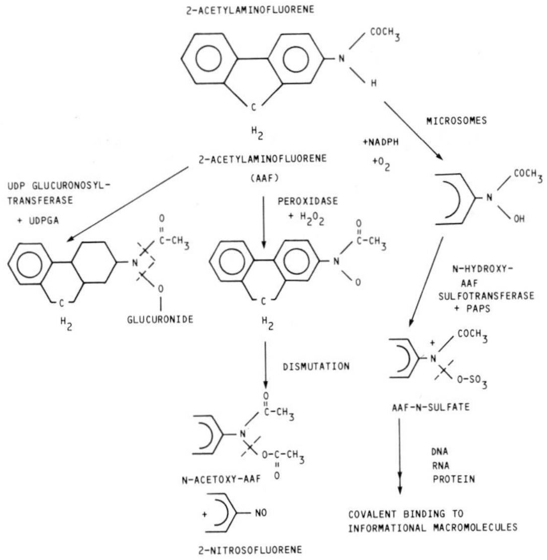

FIGURE 2A.   The metabolism of 2-acetylaminofluorene by the drug-metabolizing enzymes and the production of toxic, covalently binding sulfate-metabolite. UDPGA = uridine diphosphoglucuronic acid; NADPH = nicotine adenine dinucleotide; PAPS = 3′-phosphoadenosine-5′-phosphosulfate.

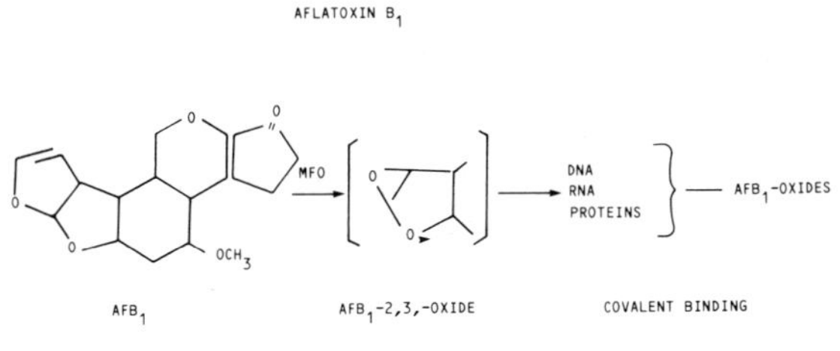

FIGURE 2B.   The metabolism of aflatoxin B₁ (AFB₁) by mixed function oxidase (MFO) enzymes and the production of the reactive intermediate, aflatoxin B₁ oxide.

function oxidase system to *N*-hydroxy-acetylaminofluorene. This intermediate is sulfated in the cytosolic compartment. Exceptionally the conjugated form, sulfate, will be bound covalently to informational macromolecules leading to the carcinogenic transformation.[53] As an example of compounds where epoxides are toxic intermediates, the metabolism of aflatoxin is shown in Figure 2B. Aflatoxin is first metabolized to the epoxide by a mixed function oxidase system. These epoxides are very labile and will be further metabolized by epoxide hydrases followed by the conjugation reactions with glucuronic acid, glutathione, or sulfate.

Of great interest and biological significance is the proportion of epoxides not conjugated but combining with tissue nucleophilic adducts resulting in carcinogenic transformation in the cell.[16] Later in this chapter further examples of the formation of toxic metabolites are given. In this context one should notice also the production of active metabolites from therapeutic drugs and industrial chemicals, which metabolites may cause drug-induced tissue damage and toxic reactions.[54-57] The hepatic as well as extrahepatic drug metabolism can be altered, e.g., due to the nutritional deficiency or due to the excess of some nutrients, as is shown later.[58] The changes are not in harmony in all drug-metabolizing enzymes but they may even be in the opposite directions as a result of the same nutritional change. Thus, the consequences may also change accordingly, emphasizing the importance of knowing nutritional effects on the drug metabolism, step by step.

THE EFFECT OF DIETARY FACTORS ON DRUG-METABOLIZING ENZYME ACTIVITIES

The activities of hepatic microsomal drug-metabolizing enzymes are influenced by the nutritional status, and extensive metabolism of drugs and other xenobiotics may modify nutritional demands.[59] In addition to the hepatic drug metabolism the extra-hepatic drug metabolism may in some cases be of high significance and this activity may be even more dependent on dietary modifications than hepatic drug metabolism.[3,21,60] Many aspects of nutritional influences on drug metabolism have been acknowledged, but much needs to be done — in particular the evaluation of the nutritional significance in drug metabolism needs to be established clinically.

Starvation

The response of drug metabolism to starvation is markedly dependent on the substrate, sex, and species (Table 1). In male rats starvation decreases the hexobarbitone metabolism but increases aniline metabolism.[61] Reidenberg found in man that fasting had only slight effects on half-lives of drugs and obesity does not markedly change them.[64] Electron microscopic studies have shown that in starved animals there were changes in the structure of the hepatic endoplasmic reticulum as the amount of ergastoplasm was reduced.[65] This might be due to compositional changes as during fasting relative proportions of oleic and linoleic acids decrease and arachidonic acid and total phospholipids increase in the subcellular fractions of the liver.[65] The influence of starvation on drug metabolism seems to be dependent on the sex of the animal.[62,63] Hydroxylation of barbiturates decreases during starvation in male rats while in female rats it increases.[63] In male rats the hydroxylation of hexobarbitone and pentobarbitone is threefold as compared to female animals when fed *ad libitum*. After a 72-hr starvation period, a 50% increase is present in the hepatic activity of female rats while a 50% decrease is found in male rats.[5,63] In later studies Kato has established that the differences in the hepatic response to starvation are due to the dependence of the hydroxylation of these barbiturates on androgenic hormones.[5] Low barbiturate metabolism was found in castrated rats, where starvation had no influence on enzyme activities, while the administration of methyltestosterone again caused the sex differences in response to starvation.[5] Refeeding of starved female rats decreased the aminopyrine, hexobarbitone, and aniline metabolism, to the control level.[5] The activity of UDP glucose dehydrogenase activity is decreased in the livers of starved animals while β-glucuronidase activity is enhanced in the livers of fasted rats.[5] The response of conjugation reactions to starvation is highly dependent on the substrate (Table 1). Most of the glucuronidation reactions decrease during starvation.[66,67]

The effect of starvation on the activities of the drug-metabolizing enzymes is substrate specific and shows interspecies variation. Moreover, there is a significant sex dependence even in the way that the response to starvation may be quite opposite depending on the sex and species.

Lipids

Lipids form an integral part in the composition and structure of subcellular mem-

Table 1
DRUG METABOLISM DURING STARVATION[1,61-63]

Nonsynthetic reactions						Synthetic Reactions	
Decreased		No changes		Increased			
Substrate	Species	Substrate	Species	Substrate	Species	Substrate	Change
Hexobarbitone	Mouse, rat	p-Nitroanisole	Rat	Aniline	Rat	p-Nitrophenol	Decrease
Pentobarbitone	Mouse, rat	Zoxazolamine	Rat	Neoprontosil	Rat, female		
Chlorpromazine	Mouse, rat	Aminopyrine	Rat	p-Nitrobenzoic acid	Rat, female		
Acetanilide	Mouse, rat	Cytochrome P-450	Rat	p-Dimethylaminoazobenzene	Rat	Testosterone	Decrease
Aminopyrine	Mouse, rat	NADPH cyt, c Reductase	Rat	Aminopyrine	Rat, female	Chloramphenicol	Decrease
p-Nitrobenzoic acid	Mouse, rat			Aniline	Rat, female		
3,4-Benzpyrene	Rat			Hexobarbitone	Rat, female	Bilirubin	Increase
Ethylmorphine	Mouse			Ethylmorphine	Mouse		
				p-Nitroanisole	Rat		

branes.[32-34,68-71] When many drug-metabolizing enzymes are located in this membrane matrix one might well expect that changes in the membrane structure will also influence enzyme activities. Joly et al.[69] studied the effect of dietary fat on hepatic drug-metabolizing enzyme activities combined with ethanol administration. They fed rats either 35% or 2% fat diets (on caloric basis). The high-fat diet with ethanol increased the cytochrome P-450 and microsomal phospholipid contents per gram of liver while with a low-fat diet the increase in the cytochrome P-450 content was less and no difference was found in the microsomal phospholipid content.[69] Ethanol increased the cytochrome P-450 content in the high-fat group from 0.95 to 1.70 nmol/mg protein while the increase in the low-fat group was only from 0.80 to 1.05. The high-fat diet contained a corn oil-olive oil mixture while the low-fat diet contained 2% fat as linoleate.[69] McLean and co-workers have widely studied the effects of various dietary fats on the hepatic cytochrome P-450 contents.[72-74] They found that a fat-free diet depressed hepatic phenobarbitone-induced cytochrome P-450 concentration to 36% from the value found in rats fed stock pellets. A preparation of 10% corn oil, herring oil, and coconut oil, supplement by 5% linoleic acid, enhanced the concentration twofold from the fat-free level but not to the level found in rats fed stock pellets.[73] It is thus possible that the induction is lower in rats fed a fat-free diet than in controls, but this study does not justify conclusions on the basal activity levels since the rats had phenobarbitone in their drinking water.

The activities of the mixed-function oxidase enzymes decrease during fat deficiency when rats are fed a fat-free diet.[75] The composition of dietary fats, fatty acids, and cholesterol all influence the drug-metabolizing enzyme activities.[76-93] The amounts of each lipid component are also of high importance in the regulation of biotransformation rates both in the liver and gastrointestinal tract,[78,80] even in the way that intestinal response to dietary lipids is higher than hepatic response.[79,82] The enzyme induction is enhanced by polyunsaturated fatty acids,[73,93,94] giving a reason to expect that the unsaturated fatty acids modify the membrane components.[79] The dietary phosphatidylcholine regulates the substrate binding to cytochrome P-450, which might partially explain the interaction of dietary lipids and drug metabolism.[89,90]

A fat-free diet decreases the hepatic cytochrome P-450 content to some extent when compared to rats fed stock pellets, but the addition of herring oil in the fat-free diet did not enhance the cytochrome P-450 content.[7] However, after phenobarbitone induction the cytochrome P-450 content was much lower in the livers of rats fed a fat-free diet than in those supplemented by the herring oil. The addition of linoleic acid (50 g/kg) to the fat-free diet caused a full induction by phenobarbitone. This might prove the essential role of linoleic acid in the regulation of the drug-metabolizing enzyme activities.

Feeding a high-fat diet (butter fat and cholesterol) to rats induces fatty liver, increases liver enzymes in serum, and causes degenerative cardiomyopathy and bradycardia.[95] The toxicity of adrianomycin is also increased due to the lowered excretion possibly because of the decreased metabolic rate.[95] When rats were fed a 10% saturated-fat diet from the last week of pregnancy up to 3 to 4 months of age a reduction of the cytochrome P-450 concentration and the benzpyrene hydroxylase activity was found while no change was present in aniline hydroxylase activity.[76] Crude rapeseed and sunflower seed oils enhanced aniline hydroxylation while there was no change in the cytochrome P-450 concentration.[76] Moreover, microsomal compositional changes of lipids followed the dietary changes.[76] In young mice, the feeding of rapeseed oil decreased hexobarbital metabolism by 44%, while no difference was found in adults.[88] On a caloric basis, a 30% rapeseed-oil diet for 3 days prolonged the hexobarbital sleeping time in young males compared to mice having a comparable amount of peanut oil in their diet.[88] This difference might be due to the large proportion of erucic acid in the rapeseed oil.

Lambert and Wills studied the effect of various lipid diets on the metabolism of benzo(a)pyrene in the rat liver.[86,87] They found no difference between a fat-free and a 10% lard diet while a 10% corn-oil diet increased the hydroxylation of benzo(a)pyrene about 35%. On the other hand, herring oil did not enhance the metabolism. A 5% lard diet, supplemented with 5% methyl linoleate, enhanced the metabolism of benzo(a)pyrene, suggesting the essential role of linoleate in the diet in enhancing the oxidative metabolism of xenobiotics.

Dietary lipids may change the membrane-bound drug-metabolizing enzyme activities by changing the membrane fluidity,[71,96,97] and the effect of exposure of active sites of enzymes to substrates. This might also have an influence on the substrate affinity.

Lipids seem to be of high significance in the regulation of the drug-metabolizing enzyme activities both in the liver and extrahepatic organs. As lipids are integral, structural, and compositional parts of the subcellular membranes, dietary lipids also influence the membrane-bound enzyme activities. Nutritional lipids change the membrane fluidity and thus regulate the substrate penetration. Various lipids seem to have different effects on the drug metabolism. A fat-free diet quite uniformly depresses monooxygenase activities and apparently increases UDPglucuronosyltransferase activity. Also, saturated fats seem to depress hydroxylation reactions while essential fatty acids and cholesterol are necessary to maintain the monooxygenase activity. The induction of drug-metabolizing enzymes is dependent on the lipoidal microenvironment of the enzymes and thus on the dietary lipids.

Proteins

In man, quite a few studies have been completed on the effect of various protein diets on drug metabolism.[98-102] Malnutrition changes the half-lives of many drugs and steroid hormones.[100] Alvares, Conney, and co-workers found that a change of regular home diet in man to a high-protein — low-carbohydrate diet decreased the half-life of antipyrine 41% and that of theophylline 36% in 2 weeks while a further change to a low-protein — high-carbohydrate diet for 2 weeks increased the half-lives 63% and 46%, respectively. (Table 2).[98,99] Thus, the half-lives of drugs metabolized both through cytochrome P-450 as antipyrine and through cytochrome P-448 as theophylline were changed in man by dietary manipulation.[98]

A low-protein diet produces morphological and compositional changes in the rat liver. The microsomal protein content decreases, liver DNA content per gram of wet weight is lowered, while cell volume increases, and the total hepatic lipid content increases in rats fed a low-protein diet.[103] Table 3 summarizes the influence of the low-protein diet on the drug metabolism. Feeding the protein-deficient diet from weanlings onward decreases total cytochrome P-450 content, its specific concentration and the specific activities of mixed-function oxidase enzymes, and increases the UDPglucuronosyltransferase activity, these effects being mediated possibly through glucocorticoids.[60]

Variation in the dietary protein content also influences enzyme induction.[106] An 8% protein diet for 3 weeks decreased in postsuckling rats the N-demethylation rate of aminopyrine, the azo-reduction of neoprontosil, sulfokinase activity, and increased the glucuronidation of p-nitrophenol.[105] No changes were found in the hydroxylation of hexobarbitone.[105] Also, the cytochrome P-450 content in the liver was decreased but no difference was found in the NADPH cytochrome c reductase activity. Hexobarbitone sleeping time was nearly threefold in protein-deficient rats.[11,106] Refeeding returned the enzyme activities to normal but not the body weights.[106]

Table 2
EFFECT ON NUTRITIONAL VARIATION ON
DRUG ELIMINATION IN MAN[98,99]

Dietary				
Protein (%)	Fat (%)	Carbohydrates (%)	Antipyrine	Theophylline
44	21	35	1.48	1.44
10	20	70	0.91	0.99
15	35	50	1	1

Note: Dietary protein, fat, and carbohydrate contents are shown. Voluntary test persons were on each diet for 2 weeks. The data show the elimination rates as compared to control diet shown by 1.

Table 3
THE EFFECT OF LOW-PROTEIN DIET ON
HEPATIC BIOTRANSFORMATION
REACTIONS[5,16,60,72,73,103-111]

Nonsynthetic reactions

	Species	Change
Aminopyrine demethylation	Rat	↓
Aniline hydroxylase	Rat	↓
Biphenyl 4-hydroxylase	Rat	↓
Cytochrome P-450	Rat	↓
Ethylmorphine demethylase	Rat	↓
N-Methylaniline demethylation	Rat	↓
NADPH cytochrome c reductase	Rat	↓
p-Nitrobenzoate reductase	Rat	↑
Hexobarbitone hydroxylase	Rat	⇌

Synthetic reactions

Substrate	Species	Conjugation	Change
4-Methylumbelliferone	Rat	Glucuronidation	↑
p-Nitrophenol	Rat	Glucuronidation	↑
o-Aminophenol	Rat	Glucuronidation	↑
Bilirubin	Rat	Glucuronidation	⇌
Chloramphenicol	Guinea pig	Glucuronidation	↑
Chloramphenicol	Man	Glucuronidation	↓
p-Nitrophenol	Rat	Sulfatation	⇌

Dickerson and Walker studied the induction of drug-metabolizing enzymes in malnutrition during development.[2] They and others found that the induction by phenobarbitone, for example, was greater in the liver of malnourished than in well-nourished animals.[1,112] It seems that immature rats are more susceptible to xenobiotics than adults. During the development of the central nevous system the changes in the cellular metabolism caused by malnutrition may not be reversible.[113-115]

Marshall and McLean fed rats a 3% casein diet for 15 days and found a decrease in the hepatic cytochrome P-450 concentration, while the phenobarbitone administration induced cytochrome P-450 but not to the control level.[72,116] It seemed that the low-protein diet increased the toxicity of those compounds not needing metabolic activation while the toxicity of those needing to be activated metabolically was lower.[72,117]

A 7-day feeding of protein-free diet caused a 70% increase of the p-nitrophenol and o-aminophenol conjugation in the livers of immature rats.[111] Also, some of the first-phase reactions were induced by a low-protein diet. Feeding a 7% casein diet for 14 to 28 days caused an increase in the biphenyl 4-hydroxylase and p-nitrobenzoate reductase activities as well as in the conjugation of 4-methylumbelliferone.[104] The biochemical basis for the behavior of drug-metabolizing enzymes in protein deficiency is not yet clear. It might be due to the conformational changes or to the increase in corticosteroid excretion. The enzymatic adaptation to a low-protein diet may take place as soon as in 4 days.[7] Marshall and McLean found that the inducing response to phenobarbitone was severely reduced in rats given a low-protein diet.[116] There are also tissue-specific responses to dietary protein. The lungs seem to be quite sensitive to dietary protein variation but no such alteration can be seen in the renal enzyme activities.[118]

Campbell compared the effects of a 5% and a 20% protein diet on the hepatic drug-metabolizing enzyme activities by feeding the rats 2 weeks of these diets.[16] The binding of aflatoxin B_1 to DNA was depressed by 70%. The cytochrome P-450 concentration was only 30% in the 5% group of that found in the 20% group as was also the NADPH cytochrome P-450 reductase activity.[16,103] The ethylmorphine N-demethylase and aniline hydroxylase activities were also markedly decreased by a 5% protein diet. The activity after phenobarbitone induction was also decreased although the induction was as many-fold in the low-protein group as in the 20% protein group.

Sachan fed rats for 1 month with either a low (3.5%), normal, (26%), or high (42%), protein diet and also induced hepatic drug-metabolizing enzyme activities by administering phenobarbitone 10 mg/kg intraperitoneally three times.[108] A low-protein diet decreased the biphenyl-4-hydroxylase activity as did also a high-protein diet, while both diets enhanced p-nitrobenzoate reductase activity and had no effects on the cytochrome P-450 concentration and conjugation of 4-methylumbelliferone.[108] The low-protein diet abolished the sex difference of cytochrome P-450 and biphenyl-4-hydroxylase. Wood and Woodcock found that a protein-free diet enhanced the UDPglucuronosyltransferase activity in the liver when either p-nitrophenol or o-aminophenol were used as aglycones. No increase in sulfotransferase was found and the activities of oxidative reactions were decreased.[110]

Carbohydrates

The variation of dietary carbohydrates may also interact with biotransformation reactions. Table 4 shows those substrates whose metabolism was decreased in rat or mouse by feeding a high-carbohydrate diet. Nash and Bender studied the effect of dietary sucrose on the metabolism of pentobarbitone.[120] Basu and co-workers studied the effect of dietary substitution of starch by sucrose, glucose, fructose, or equimolar mixture of glucose and fructose on drug metabolism.[119] They found the lowest biphenyl-4-hydroxylase activity in the livers of rats fed either by sucrose or by a mixture of glucose and fructose, while starch and glucose and fructose had higher activities. Respective changes were found in the cytochrome P-450 concentration and after the induction by phenobarbitone. Feeding a 60% sucrose diet to weanling rats reduced the specific and total activities of biphenyl hydroxylase when compared to the respective starch diet.[2,119] However, in adult rats a 70% sucrose diet decreased the sleeping time by pentobarbitone.

Table 4
THE DECREASE OF DRUG METABOLISM
BY A HIGH CARBOHYDRATE
DIET[2,7,119,120]

Carbohydrate	Species	Substrate
Sucrose	Mouse	Phenobarbitone
	Rat	Biphenyl
		Pentobarbitone
		Aniline
		p-Dimethylaminoazobenzene
		p-Nitrobenzoic acid
		Neoprontosil
		Cytochrome P-450
		NADPH cytochrome
		Carisoprodol
Glucose	Mouse	Hexobarbitone
	Rat	Dimethylnitrosamine
		Biphenyl
		Cytochrome P-450

Vitamins

Vitamins may serve as cofactors in the drug-metabolizing enzyme systems and the justification to expect that they may also regulate the metabolic rate of drugs (Tables 5 and 6). Vitamin C regulates the integrity of mixed-function oxidase enzymes.

Severe vitamin C deficiency decreases the cytochrome P-450 concentration and causes a typical binding spectrum of Type II substrates.[134] In guinea pigs the ascorbic acid deficiency was produced by feeding ascorbic acid-poor diet for 10 days, whereafter the ascorbic acid levels were only 10% of those in control animals.[124] The hepatic cytochrome P-450 concentration was 30% lower than in control animals; in the pulmonary cytochrome P-450 concentration, a respective decrease was present. Also, the ethoxycoumarine *O*-deethylase activity was decreased (about 50%) but the benzpyrene hydroxylase and epoxide hydrase activities were unchanged.[124] The enzyme induction by phenobarbitone behaved comparably, i.e., the activity of enzymes decreased by the ascorbic acid deficiency was lower after the enzyme induction than in controls, and the activity of those enzymes not responsive to the ascorbic acid deficiency also had equal activity to the livers of control guinea pigs after the phenobarbitone induction. Ascorbic acid supplementation in guinea pigs slightly decreased the glucuronidation of *o*-aminophenol while no effect was found on hydroxylative reactions and increase in the glutathione conjugation.[132]

However, *p*-nitroanisole and aminopyrine metabolism were enhanced by ascorbic acid supplementation (Table 6). Induction of drug-metabolizing enzymes increased excretion of ascorbic acid in rats to the urine, and in man and guinea pigs the excretion of glucaric acid.[129,139] Ascorbic acid-deficient guinea pigs are more responsive to zoxazolamine than normal guinea pigs (Table 6).[129] Inducers of the drug-metabolizing enzymes stimulate the synthesis of L-ascorbic acid in the rat and elevate the urinary excretion of D-glucaric acid in man and guinea pigs, stimulating the enzymes of the glucuronic acid pathway.[139]

Vitamin A deficiency in the rat decreases the hepatic cytochrome P-450 contents and drug-metabolizing enzyme activities (Table 6).[128] Retinoid deficiency also decreases the cytochrome P-450 content, ethylmorphine hydroxylation, and aniline hydroxylation.[60,128] Vitamin A and its synthetic analogs, retinoids, are potent agents for the control of cell differentiation in epithelial tissues.[140-143] They may interact with the

Table 5
DRUG METABOLISM DURING VITAMIN OR MINERAL DEFICIENCIES[1,5,121-135]

	Cytochrome P-450	Aminopyrine metabolism	NADPH cytochrome c reductase	Pentobarbitone/ hexobarbitone metabolism	Pentobarbitone sleeping time	Aniline metabolism	p-Nitrobenzoic acid metabolism	Codeine metabolism	Conjugation bilirubin	Ethoxycoumarin O-deethylation	Benzo(a)pyrene hydroxylation	Epoxidation
Vitamin Deficiencies												
E	0.57—0.94	0.53										
K	0.95	0.95—1.12	0.95—1.14			0.58—0.62		0.59				
Ascorbic acid (guinea pig)	0.69	1.16			1.58	0.91—1.02	0.91—0.95		1.29—1.30	0.50	1.0	1.0
Mineral Deficiencies												
Iron	1.04	1.53—1.55	1.30	1.19—1.21	1.37	1.69—1.79						
Mg	0.74		0.68			0.54						

Note: Control values are denoted by 1.

Table 6
THE EFFECT OF DIETARY VITAMINS ON HEPATIC DRUG METABOLISM AND DRUG-METABOLIZING ENZYME COMPONENTS[1,5,124-138]

Vitamin	Metabolic rate		
	Decreased	Unchanged	Increased
Vitamin A			
Deficiency	Aminopyrine	NADPH Cytochrome c	
	Aniline	Reductase	
	Cytochrome P-450		
Vitamin C (Guinea pig)			
Excess			*p*-Nitroanisole
			Aminopyrine
Deficiency	Acetanilide		
	Aniline		
	Antipyrine		
	Hexobarbitone		
	Zoxazolamine		
	Coumarin		
	Cytochrome P-450		
Vitamin E			
Deficiency	Aminopyrine		
	Codeine		
	Aniline		
Thiamin			
Excess	Zoxazolamine	Hexobarbitone	
	Heptachlor		
	Aniline		
	Cytochrome P-450		
	NADPH Cytochrome c reductase		
Deficiency		Hexobarbitone	Aniline
			Heptachlor
Riboflavin			
Deficiency	Benzpyrene	Aminopyrine	Aniline
	Ethylmorphine	Hexobarbitone	
	NADPH Cytochrome c reductase	Cytochrome P-450	
	Glucuronidation		

Note: Experiments have been conducted with mice if not stated otherwise.

initiation or progression phase of the development of the cancer. In the trachea and bronchi potentially premalignant lesions have been found in the absence of retinoids.[140,142,143] Similar effects of retinoid deficiency have been found in the stomach, intestine, testis, uterus, kidney, bladder, and skin.[144]

In prostate cultures the hyperplastic and anaplastic lesions induced by chemical carcinogens can be reversed by the addition of retinoids.[145,146] It is evident that retinoid deficiency enhances susceptibility to chemical carcinogenesis in the respiratory system,[147] bladder,[148] and colon.[149] A relationship has been found between the low dietary intake of vitamin A and high incidence of lung cancer.[150] In retinoid deficiency a fourfold binding of benzo(*a*)pyrene metabolites takes place to the tracheal epithelial DNA, as compared to controls.[151]

The specific activities of drug-oxidation enzymes are depressed in microsomes from livers of rats and rabbits fed vitamin E-deficient diet (Table 5 and 6).[127] Treatment of rats with α-tocopherol normalized the activities. Specific activities of the drug-metabolizing enzymes were decreased by castration in vitamin E-deficient rats, while in the vitamin E-supplemented rats, no decrease was present, indicating the interaction of vitamins and hormones in the regulation of drug metabolism.[127] This was further confirmed when in vitamin E-deficient rats the effect of castration could be reversed with α-tocopherol and testosterone. A decrease in the hepatic cytochrome P-450 level and the drug-metabolizing enzyme activities has been found in vitamin E-deficient rats,[126] while α-tocopherol administration increases the activities of the drug-metabolizing enzymes.[124-126,130] Apparently this increase is due to the increased synthesis of cytochrome P-450, which is inhibited by actinomycin D.[126,152] This is also to judge that α-tocopherol deficiency decreases heme synthesis and by this mechanism decreases enzyme activities.

Vitamin K deficiency increases pentobarbitone-induced sleeping time, while no significant decrease in in vitro enzyme activities was found (Table 5).

Riboflavin deficiency decreases the cytochrome c reductase activity, and azoreductase and benzpyrene hydroxylase activities, and has no effect on the cytochrome P-450 concentration (Table 5).[131] Excessive amounts of thiamin in the diet may decrease the metabolism of numerous compounds while deficiency increases the metabolism of aniline and heptachlor (Table 6).

Minerals

In addition to the function of minerals, as cofactors, they participate in other ways in the regulation of drug-metabolizing enzyme activities. Feeding the calcium-free diet to rats decreases the activities of drug-metabolizing enzymes.[1,153] Feeding a calcium-free diet for 40 days decreases the hepatic drug-metabolizing enzyme activities in the weanling rats and increases the sleeping time of hexobarbitone.[1] Diets deficient in zinc or magnesium cause a decrease in hepatic cytochrome P-450 concentration and in the activities of the mixed function oxidase enzyme system (Table 5).[122,123,154]

Iron deficiency stimulates hepatic metabolism of Type I (aminopyrine) and Type II (aniline) substances (Table 5); however, in the intestinal mucosa, iron deficiency depresses cytochrome P-450 levels.[155,156] Magnesium deficiency in rats decreases hepatic drug metabolism (Table 5).[121] Nickel, cobalt, and iron impair cellular heme-dependent metabolism both by inhibiting heme biosynthesis and by inducing heme degradation.[157] These metals depress cellular respiration and reduce indirectly the biotransformation activity. They perturb cellular glutathione content and may alter the activity of glutathione-dependent enzymes. Levander found that the toxicity of lead was increased in rats by feeding a diet low in calcium or iron.[158] Copper deficiency enhanced toxic effects of lead in rats and copper seems to be essential for drug-metabolizing enzymes.[158,159] Vitamins also interact with the toxic effects of metals as vitamin E deficiency decreases lead toxicity.[158] Deficiency in dietary proteins increases lead and cadmium toxicity in rats. Dietary copper and iron deficiencies enhance cadmium toxicity while selenium may protect from mercury toxicity, although the mechanisms of how metals interact with toxic effects have not been established.[158]

Nonnutritional Constituents

In addition to the normal nutrients, a diet contains numerous nonnutritional components, such as nitroso-compounds, environmental contaminants (like polycyclic aromatic hydrocarbons and pesticide residues) and food additives.[53,160-163] The effect of polycyclic hydrocarbons on intestinal drug metabolism has been studied extensively.[164-166] Benzo(a)pyrene causes a marked increase in the intestinal phenacetin metabolism.[164,165] Kuntzman and co-workers found even more pronounced induction of phenacetin metabolism by cigarette smoke exposure in everted intestinal sacs.[164]

Arcos and co-workers found that benzo(*a*)pyrene and 3-methylcholantrene depressed dimethylnitrosamine demethylase activity in the livers of rats.[167] Sternson and Gammans found that nitroso compounds inhibit the oxidation of Type II substrates in the rabbit liver microsomes while they have no influence on Type I substrates [168]

Babish and Stoewsand gave the rats black tea as a 0.5% solution for 13 weeks and they found induction in the aminopyrine *N*-demethylase and *N*-methylaniline *N*-demethylase activities as well as in the *p*-nitroanisole *O*-demethylase activity in the liver.[169] No increase was present, however, in cytochrome P-450 concentration.[169] Pantuck and co-workers studied the effect of vegetables of the Brassicaceae family on intestinal drug metabolism in the rat and found a marked induction in enzyme activities (Table 7).[165] In further studies they also characterized components in these vegetables as having inducing potency (Table 7).

Pantuck and co-workers found that indoles in the Brassicaceae are very potent enzyme inducers in the intestinal mucosa and even in the liver.[98,166] The hydroxylation of benzo(*a*)pyrene was up to 85-fold in the intestine of rats fed Brussels sprouts as compared to controls. Thus these nonnutritional components in the diet may significantly change the fate of drugs in the body and even influence their pharmacokinetic properties by changing the intestinal enzyme levels.

Food Preparation

In previous paragraphs compositional changes in the diet were shown to influence the drug metabolism rate. Even the preparation of food may change the intestinal drug metabolism. Feeding a diet containing charcoal-broiled beef for 4 days decreased half-lives of antipyrine.[98] This diet also decreased the plasma level of orally administered phenacetin without influencing the plasma concentration of the major metabolite of phenacetin, *N*-acetyl-*p*-aminophenol, or the half-life of phenacetin, suggesting enhancement in the phenacetin metabolism in the gastrointestinal tract and/or during its first pass through the liver. This is probably due to the presence of polycyclic aromatic hydrocarbons in the broiled beef diet.[98]

Effect of Drugs on Nutritional Status

Although in previous paragraphs the effects of diet on biotransformation rates have been widely reviewed, it is also possible that extensive drug therapy may change the nutritional demands.

Orally administered antibiotics inhibit β-glucuronidase activity of the microflora in the gastrointestinal tract.[59] Thus, antibiotics may impair the enterohepatic circulation of biliary excreted compounds. On the other hand, when drugs induce monooxygenase systems in the liver the induction causes a rapid deactivation and excretion of other drugs or their toxicity may change. Stimulation of the glucuronate pathway yields increased synthesis and excretion of ascorbate in rats and D-glucarate in man.[59] Increased deactivation of vitamin D_1 hormone (1,25-dihydroxycholecalciferol) may lead to osteomalacia.[172,173] Diphenylhydantoin decreases the absorption of folate in man while there may be increased demand of folate in the enzyme induction.[174,175] The administration of prednisone influences the urinary ascorbic acid excretion.[59] In guinea pigs, first an increase is seen, followed by a decrease due to the depletion of ascorbic acid.

PRINCIPLES IN CARCINOGENICITY

In the carcinogenic transformation in the cells the production of reactive intermediates of chemicals plays a key role according to the chemical carcinogenesis theory.[43,55,57] The genome changes induced by the carcinogenic compounds are counteracted by repair systems in the nuclei (Figure 3). The formation of carcinogenic intermediates often needs metabolic activation with the exception of alkylating and acylating agents per se. Donors of simple alkyl groups such as dialkylnitrosamine and dialkylnitrosamide may be carcinogenic.[176,177] Precarcinogens are activated by mixed-function oxidase enzymes yielding proximate carcinogens and further ultimate carcinogens, according to Miller and Miller.[178] Nucleophilic receptors in the cell act as trapping agents to the ultimate carcinogens to deactivate them.[178] Promoters are not themselves carcinogens, or they will not form carcinogenic metabolites, but they will otherwise promote carcinogenic transformation. Promoters increase the synthesis of phospholipids, RNA, DNA, and protein, and increase the mitotic rate.[53,178] The earliest changes are increases in protease and ornithine decarboxylase activities. Strong electrophilic reactivity is the basic requirement for ultimate chemical carcinogens and for the metabolism of chemicals although generally carcinogens have no overall similarities.[53]

Mutation tests can be used for screening potential electrophilicity. A good correlation has been found between mutagenicity and carcinogenicity in various mutagenicity tests, the discrepancy being only 10%.[179] Electrophilic forms of chemical carcinogens come into contact with DNA in mutagenicity tests, thus having mutagenic activity.[52]

DIETARY FACTORS IN CARCINOGENESIS

General

It has been estimated that 90% of all human cancers are of environmental origin.[12,14,46] Although some of these cancers are due to occupational exposure to carcinogens and to smoking, there still remain 60% of female and 40% of male cancer cases which have been estimated to be caused by nutritional factors or by xenobiotics entering the body as food contaminants.[13,41,46] Numerous compounds present in food are known or suspected carcinogens.[15,51,180] Such carcinogenic food contaminants are mycotoxins that may cause liver cancer and cycasin, which is also possibly carcinogenic to the liver.[51] Nitrites, nitrates, and nitrosamides, have been postulated to be related to gastric cancer, and nitrosamines formed from nitrites and natural amines may cause cancers in various tissues.[181-189] Aflatoxin B_1, N-nitrosamines, and N-nitrosamides are strongly suspected carcinogens causing human cancer; ethionine also is in this group of compounds.[51,190-192] Nutritional deficiencies are known to influence possible carcinogenic transformation in numerous ways, contributing to the transformation of normal cells into neoplastic cells.[15]

The diet may have a double role in promoting cancer formation.[49] First, it is possible that man ingests in the diet substances which work as cancer initiators or promoters. Secondly, nutritional factors might establish conditions increasing organ susceptibility for cancer.

In addition to nutrients the gastrointestinal tract is the entrance for many xenobiotics which may have harmful effects in the body. Although the skin and lungs are acknowledged as passages for foreign compounds to enter the body, the alimentary canal is still by far most frequently exposed to the exchange of molecules of xenobiotics in ratio 1:1000:1000 0000 (skin to lungs to alimentary canal). The composition of the diet also changes tumor incidence as compositional changes may change the metabolic activation of carcinogens. Factors regulating tumor development may influence cellular proliferation or the immunological control of tumor growth. Dietary restriction decreases the incidence of mammary tumor, virus-induced tumors in DBA and C3H mice, spontaneous lung tumors in Swiss and ABC mice, and benzo(a)pyrene-induced skin tumors.[193] Similar effects to those described in mice have been found in rats.[49] Underfeeding may thus prolong the life span and lower tumor incidence.

Table 7
THE EFFECT OF BRASSICACAE VEGETABLES AND THEIR PURIFIED CONSTITUENTS ON INTESTINAL AND HEPATIC BIOTRANSFORMATION RATES IN RATS[99,165,170,171]

Diet/constituent	Phenacetin metabolism	Intestine Ethoxycoumarin O-deethylation	Hexobarbitone hydroxylation	Benzo(a)pyrene hydroxylation	Liver Benzo(a)pyrene hydroxylation
Cabbage	1.91—3.68	9.62—15.78	1.58	11.74—32.92	
Brussels sprouts	2.87—6.59	20.05—42.71	2.18	28.42—85.54	
Indole-3-aceto-nitrile	1.29	4.18	1.04	8.00—15.25	6.33
Indole-3-carbi-nol	1.28	16.13	2.15	22.46—31	56.46
3,3′-Diindolyl-methane	1.28	10.39	3.76	11.25—13.46	15.77
Indole-3-Car-boxaldehyde				1.25	0.95
Ascorbigen				6.50	1.33

Note: Control activity in each experiment is 1 and the data show relative changes in respective units. Rats were on specific diets for 3 to 7 days.

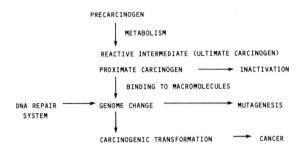

FIGURE 3. The carcinogenic transformation in the cells caused by precarcinogenic compounds via metabolic activation.

Nitroso Compounds
General

Nitroso compounds are composed of a large variety of substances. These compounds and their existence in the food products form a very important question in food safety. Both nitrates and nitrites can be added to food products such as meat, fish, and sausages. However, these compounds as food additives do not form the only source — natural sources also exist.[51,162,194] In some geographic areas water may contain nitrites as well as some vegetables, especially spinach. Although originally the nitrite amounts in the diet may be quite small, nitrate may be reduced to nitrite. Nitrate is a nontoxic compound, actually comparable to sodium chloride. However, due to its potential capacity to be reduced to nitrite, it may form a potential health hazard. Both nitrate and nitrite give a red color to meat products. The bright red color is due to myoglobin and oxymyoglobin. When nontreated meat is heated it turns to grayish brown due to the formation of metmyochromogen and oxidation of fats and sugars. Nitrites form nitrogen oxide which binds to the ferrous part of myoglobin producing nitrosomyoglobin which is a stable, bright red product. However, a far more important factor favoring the use of nitrites in the meat and fish products than the color is the fact that nitrites prevent the growth of numerous bacteria of which the most unwanted is *Clostridium botulinum.*

Although some substitutes have been tested, still nitrates have their advantages in the food industry despite some unwanted effects. Nitrates may be transformed both enzymatically and nonenzymatically to nitrites in food or in the gastrointestinal tract (Figure 4).[51]

Nitrites are toxic mainly due to their effects on the hemoglobin as they oxidize the ferrous iron to ferric form by transferring an electron. Thus the methemoglobin which is formed cannot bind any oxygen and transport it to target tissues. In addition to direct toxic effects, nitrites have other indirect hazardous effects. The *N*-nitroso compounds are formed from nitrites and secondary, tertiary, or quaternary, amines in the acidic environment.[182] The toxicity of *N*-nitroso compounds varies depending on the nature of the compound. Both the doses needed to produce toxic effects and the nature of the toxicity are variable.

Exposure to nitrosamines takes place either through the ingestion of nitroso compounds or through the simultaneous ingestion of nitrosable substances and nitrite.[186,195] Magee and Barnes demonstrated the induction of malignant hepatic tumors in rats by dimethylnitrosamines.[184] Nitrosamines are usually stable compounds being composed either from dialkyl or heterocyclic compounds while nitrosamides are unstable compounds. The acute toxicity varies considerably in experimental animals. For rats, the peroral LD_{50} of dicyclohexylnitrosamine is 5 mg/kg, while the LD_{50} of

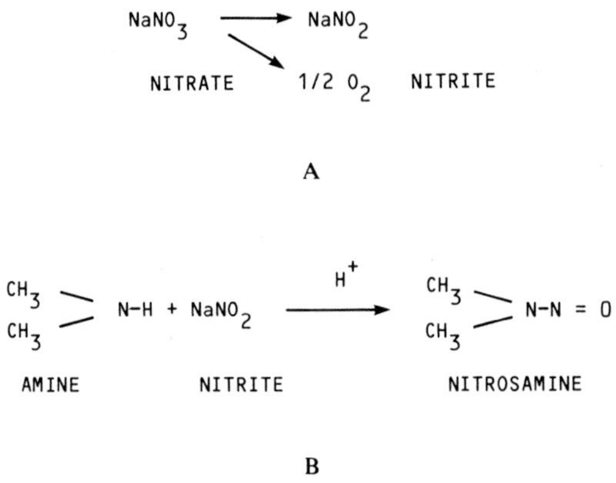

$$NaNO_3 \longrightarrow NaNO_2$$

NITRATE $1/2\ O_2$ NITRITE

A

$$\underset{CH_3}{\overset{CH_3}{>}} N-H\ +\ NaNO_2 \xrightarrow{\ \ H^+\ \ } \underset{CH_3}{\overset{CH_3}{>}} N-N = O$$

AMINE   NITRITE   NITROSAMINE

B

FIGURE 4.   (A) The reduction of nitrate to nitrite. (B) Formation of nitrosamine from amine and nitrite.

N-nitrosoethyl-2-hydroxyethylamine is 7.5 g/kg.[176] Dialkylnitrosamines are selectively hepatotoxic, causing hemorrhagic centrilobular necrosis, as do heterocyclic nitrosamines.

Toxicity of *N*-Nitroso Compounds

The toxicity may appear as carcinogenicity in the liver, gastrointestinal tract, and urinary bladder, as liver necrosis, or as mutagenicity.[196-199] The amines subject to nitrosation originate from various sources such as cigarette smoke, drugs, pesticides, and other contaminants in the diet. Many drugs contain tertiary amines available for nitrosation in the body, including such drugs as oxytetracycline, aminophenazon, disulfiram, and nicetamide. Moreover, even the amino acids from dietary proteins are due to nitrosation.

Amines form, together with nitrites, *N*-nitroso compounds during processing, preparation, and storage of food, and in the stomach. Nitrates can be reduced to nitrites by bacteria.[162] In neutral pH areas as well as in an acidic environment nitrosation is possible, due to microbial processes. In many animal species the relationship between nitrosamines and cancer has been indicated, but in man no actual data exist at the doses present in the diet. The formation of carcinogenic intermediates from some *N*-nitroso compounds needs the mixed-function oxidase enzyme system present in the liver and extrahepatic organs both in man and in animals — thus making man potentially susceptible to health hazards from nitrosamines (Figure 5). Low levels (50 ppm) of dimethylnitrosamines have been reported to cause liver cancer in rats.[184] Over 100 *N*-nitroso compounds have been tested and over 80% were found to be carcinogenic in some species. Because of a wide variation of nitrosamines in the environment it has been suggested that they may account for a significant proportion of human cancers.[195] Some nitroso compounds do not need metabolic activation to produce cancers, e.g., nitrosoureas and nitrosamides, but they produce tumors at the site of administration. Feeding these compounds to experimental animals results in tumors in the stomach. Nitrosamines require metabolic activation preceding induction of tumors in the liver, kidney, lungs, gastrointestinal tract, and bladder. No direct evidence on the relationship between human carcinogenicity and nitroso compounds exists but such a relationship is possible as dimethylnitrosamine has proved to be carcinogenic in all animal species tested. It is not only the presence of nitrates, nitrites, and *N*-nitroso compounds in the diet, but also the formation of nitroso compounds from numerous different

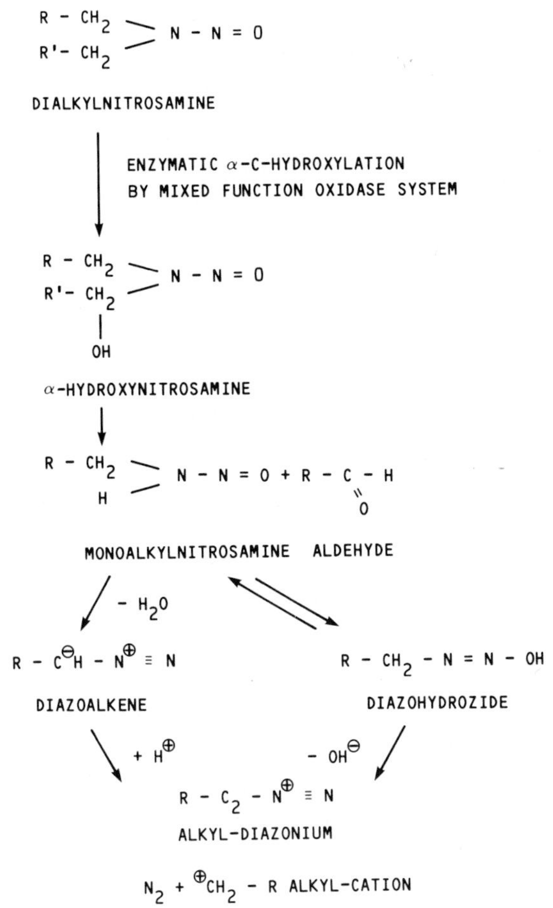

$$
\begin{array}{c}
\left. \begin{array}{l} R - CH_2 \\ R'- CH_2 \end{array} \right\rangle N - N = 0
\end{array}
$$

DIALKYLNITROSAMINE

ENZYMATIC α–C–HYDROXYLATION
BY MIXED FUNCTION OXIDASE SYSTEM

$$
\begin{array}{c}
\left. \begin{array}{l} R - CH_2 \\ R'- CH_2 \end{array} \right\rangle N - N = 0 \\
| \\
OH
\end{array}
$$

α-HYDROXYNITROSAMINE

$$
\left. \begin{array}{l} R - CH_2 \\ H \end{array} \right\rangle N - N = 0 + R - \overset{\displaystyle C}{\underset{\displaystyle \parallel}{}} - H
$$
$$
O
$$

MONOALKYLNITROSAMINE   ALDEHYDE

$- H_2O$

$$R - C^{\ominus}H - N^{\oplus} \equiv N$$

DIAZOALKENE

$$R - CH_2 - N = N - OH$$

DIAZOHYDROZIDE

$+ H^{\oplus}$ $- OH^{\ominus}$

$$R - C_2 - N^{\oplus} \equiv N$$

ALKYL-DIAZONIUM

$$N_2 + {}^{\oplus}CH_2 - R \text{ ALKYL-CATION}$$

FIGURE 5. The formation of active mutagens and proximal carcinogen from dialkylnitrosamines.[200]

sources and the activation of these compounds in the body which regulate the biological effects and fate of nitroso compounds in the body.

In the process of biological carcinogenesis the activation of a specific genetic repressor by carcinogens is a significant event. Magee and Farber studied the in vivo incorporation of labeled dimethylnitrosamine into the liver DNA by identifying 7-methylguanine in acid hydrolysates of the nucleic acids.[201] All mutagens and carcinogens are strong electrophiles (i.e., molecules with electron deficient atoms) to react with nucleophilic sites of cellular constituents (Figure 6). In nitroso compounds alkylation of O^6-position of guanine in DNA leads to the mutagenicity. The sensitivity of each organ to the carcinogenic action of nitroso compounds reflects the ability of each organ to remove the carcinogen-produced O^6-alkylguanine from its DNA.[202] This leads to the substantial repair of the carcinogenic damage induced by dimethylnitrosamine. The repair reflects the enzymatic removal of altered base from DNA. If present in DNA it leads to the induction of irreversible mutation. Dimethylnitrosamine yields chemically reactive methylating intermediates, a methylcarbonium ion which reacts with nucleophilic sites in the nucleic acids and proteins and with water to yield methanol. *N*-Methylnitrosourea does not require metabolic activation but yields some methylating intermediates spontaneously under physiological conditions.[203] Alkylation of

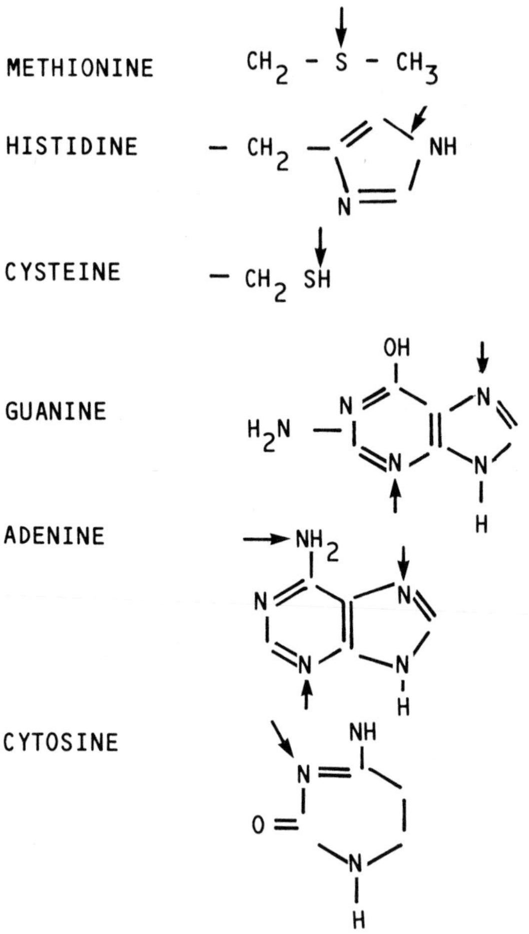

FIGURE 6.   Nucleophilic sites of some common cellular constituents. The electrophiles (mutagens and carcinogens) as the intermediates in the metabolism of nitrosocompounds may attack the nucleophilic sites causing tissue damage (the reactive sites are shown by arrows).

cellular constituents is associated with various biological effects including cytotoxicity, carcinogenesis, and mutagenesis.[177,201] The activity of enzymes removing alkylating bases from DNA varies considerably in different organs leading possibly to differences in organ susceptibility in DNA repair mechanisms. N-Nitroso compounds are extremely potent point mutagens in addition to producing chromosome breaks and aberrations.[204] N-Methyl-N'-nitro-N-nitrosoguanine is the most potent chemical mutagen for bacteria yet discovered.[204] Nitrosamides require no metabolic activation to be mutagenic in microbial systems and they are also mutagenic in *Drosophila*. On the other hand, nitrosamines are mutagenic in *Drosophila* but not in bacteria due to the inability of microbes to metabolize these compounds to active mutagenic forms. When adding an NADPH-dependent drug-metabolizing enzyme system these compounds are mutagenic also in bacteria, indicating the need for metabolic activation which bacteria cannot do themselves. Although mutagenicity of nitroso compounds does not necessarily imply that they are also carcinogenic, many recent studies have shown a correlation between mutagenicity and carcinogenicity according to the somatic mutation concept.[52,199] Montesano and Magee found a correlation between the metabolic conversion of dimethyl- and diethylnitrosamines and the organ distribution of induced tumors in vivo.[205]

Transport of a carcinogen to its target tissue and its potential reactivity at the α-carbon site has an important role in the determination of the carcinogenic activity.[206] N-Nitrosamines are well-known carcinogens[78] and potentially they are important in the etiology of human cancer.[185,187,188,207] The correlation with the partition coefficient in water-hexane and carcinogenicity is transmitted to the biologically active molecules to reach the active site.[207] Initiation in enzymatic oxidation at α-carbon following intermediate steps leads to the formation of diazonium ion and/or carbonium ions. Initial oxidation is rate-limiting, correlating with the reactivity at the α-carbon site.[181]

Dietary Factors in Toxicity of N-Nitroso Compounds

The effect of the high-fat diet on the induction of tumors by N-nitrosodimethylamine, N-nitrosodiethylamine, and N-nitrosodibutylamine, was studied in normal and marginally lipotrope-deficient rats.[194] Lipotrope (choline and methionine) deficiency enhanced hepatocarcinogenesis by both N-nitrosodiethylamine and N-nitrosodibutylamine. Liver cirrhosis, the result of consumption of alcoholic beverages caused, together with malnutrition, liver cancer; this, together with exposure to environmental N-nitroso compounds, enhanced the cancer risk.[194] Dimethylnitrosamine is metabolized by the mixed-function oxidase system yielding demethylation. In animals having protein-free diet the hepatotoxicity of dimethylntrosamine is lowered due to the decreased hepatic metabolism.[176,208] Vitamin A may reduce the incidence of cancer induced by N-nitroso compounds in lungs, skin, bladder, and breast.[51]

The diet may not only contain compounds yielding the production of N-nitroso compounds which themselves may have hazardous effects but diet and its nutritional component also modify the metabolic activation of potentially harmful N-nitroso compounds. This dual role of diet and the versatile nature of different N-nitroso compounds makes it complicated to give a final judgment on N-nitroso compounds in general, but each compound must be judged individually.

Lipids

Lipotrope deficiency frequently causes fatty liver due to choline deficiency. A diet deficient in lipotropes enhances hepatocarcinogenesis by aflatoxin B_1, dimethylnitrosamine, and also the incidence of dimethylhydrazine-induced intestinal tumors.[149,191,209]

When the level of dietary fat increases to 15%, tumor incidence produced by benzo(a)pyrene, methylcholantrene, and dimethylbenzanthracene increases in mice.[210] Tannenbaum and Silverstone showed with equicaloric diets that fat enhances benzo(a)pyrene-induced skin tumors in mice, naturally occurring hepatomas, and reduces the latency of mammary tumors.[193,211-213] The substitution of hydrogenated coconut oil for corn oil reduced the number of hepatomas in rats fed dimethylaminoazobenzene.[214] The tumor-inhibitory fats enable the liver to store riboflavin more efficiently and this leads to the greater activity of detoxifying enzymes as riboflavin is their cofactor. A 35% beef fat enhances the yield of the intestinal tumors induced by azoxymethane in rats.[215] The incidence of colon cancer is also related to the dietary fat intake when comparing the incidence in various nations.[15]

Reddy and co-workers have studied the role of dietary fats in the regulation of the incidence of colon tumors induced by environmental chemicals present in the diet.[216] They fed rats a semipurified diet containing 20% or 5% beef fat from weanlings onward. At 7 weeks they gave 1,2-dimethylhydrazine (150 mg/kg s.c.) or methylazomethanol, one dose, or methylnitrosourea, 2 doses, and had a 35-week observation pe-

Table 8
THE TOXICITY OF CHEMICALS IN
ANIMALS FED LOW-PROTEIN
DIET[74,103,104,197,208,218-222]

Reduced	Enhanced
	Acetaminophen
CCl_4	Dieldrin
	Phenacetin
Dimethylnitrosamine	Lindane
Heptachlor	DDT
Endosulfan	Parathion
	Malathion
Aflatoxin	Strychnine
Polycyclic aromatic hydrocar-bons	Zoxazolamine
	Chlordane
Mutagenity: secondary carcin-ogens	Primary carcinogens

riod. The frequency of colon tumors increased in groups fed 20% fat diet and administered either methylazomethanol or methylnitrosourea. Groups contained 30 rats and the incidence was 60 to 70% in rats fed the high-fat diet compared to the low-fat groups where the tumor incidence was 20%.

Polyunsaturated fats increase the incidence of colon cancers compared to the respective saturated-fat diet.[15] It might be that steroid metabolites would function as carcinogens or procarcinogens.[217] The activity of β-glucuronidase seems to correlate with the amount of bile acid and neutral steroid metabolites in feces.[217] In animals, litocholic acid and taurodeoxycholic acid play a role in the neoplasia formation and enhanced the tumor growth. Thus these bile acids might function as tumor promoters or initiators.[15] In patients with colon cancers, fecal 7α-dehydroxylase activity is higher than in controls, suggesting possibly the production of reactive metabolites from cholesterol, e.g., cholesterol epoxide.

The incidence of breast cancer in many countries has been found to correlate with the high intake of dietary fat and cholesterol.[15] In rats, the incidence of chemically induced breast cancer increases by feeding them high-fat diets, including both saturated and unsaturated fats.[15,44] This may be coupled to enhanced prolactin production in rats. A vegetarian diet has been found to decrease prolactin production by 50%.[15] In studies of the breast fluids of women having a western diet this fluid has been found to contain high amounts of cholesterol and its metabolites. These metabolites might function in vivo as carcinogens or procarcinogens.

Proteins

Table 8 gives a summary of the influence of a low-protein diet on the toxicity of some chemicals. McLean studied the role of protein diets in the toxicity of CCl_4 and acetaminophen in rats.[74] He found that a low-protein diet decreased CCl_4 toxicity but enhanced acetaminophen toxicity, suggesting the role of metabolic activation in producing toxic effects. Protein deficiency decreases hepatic cytochrome P-450 concentration leading to the impairment of the mixed-function oxidase system.[117] This increases the toxicity of those xenobiotics detoxicated by these enzymes and decreases the toxicity of the xenobiotics activated by these enzymes, such as CCl_4 and endosulfan.[197,218-220]

In young male rats fed a low-protein but otherwise complete diet, the resistance to

CCl₄ poisoning seemed elevated as the mortality was decreased and the extent of the liver damage was lowered due to a low mixed-function oxidase activity.[117] The administration of an enzyme-inducing agent like DDT or phenobarbitone returned the toxicity.[218] However, despite the fact that the starvation also decreases the enzyme activities, the toxicity of CCl₄ is elevated during starvation.[218] McLean, and Verschuuren fed a protein-free diet to young male rats for 7 days and found that this diet protects rats from the hepatotoxic effects of dimethylnitrosamine.[208] This probably results from the decreased production rate of methylating metabolites from dimethylnitrosamine by mixed-function oxidase enzymes.[221]

Feeding a 5% casein diet to weanling male rats for 10 days increased threefold the tolerance to heptachlor toxicity caused by the low production rate of toxic heptachlor epoxide.[74] Kato and co-workers demonstrated in young rats that the toxicity of strychnine, pentobarbitone, and zoxazolamine varied inversely with the protein content of the diet.[107] Campbell and Hayes also studied the effect of low-protein diets on the toxicity of xenobiotics in rats.[103] The toxicity of the following compounds was decreased: octamethylpyrophosphoramide, carbon tetrachloride, and heptachlor.[103,117] The toxicity of numerous compounds was increased by a low-protein diet, e.g., chlordane, diazinoson, endrin, lindane, chloroprophan, DDT, diuron, endosulfan, monouron, toxaphene, demeton, carbaryl, parathion, captan, malathion, parathion, and phenacetin.[103] Preston and co-workers found that in rats fed a low- (5%) protein diet the binding of aflatoxin B₁ metabolites to chromatin, DNA, and chromatin protein, was 70% lower than in rats fed a 20% protein diet.[204] In paired rats fed a 20% protein diet the binding was slightly less than in those fed *ad libitum* ⁴ 20% protein diet.[222]

Changing the dietary protein content from 9 to 45% failed to influence the incidence of mammary tumors and polycyclic aromatic hydrocarbon-induced skin tumors in rats.[219] Spontaneous hepatomas in C3H mice were less frequent on a 9% protein diet containing less cysteine and methionine than the average mice diet.[219] High dietary protein levels protect the rat liver against carcinogenesis by 4-dimethylaminoazobenzene. When feeding a protein-free diet for 7 days to rats, a 45% inhibition of liver metabolism of dimethylnitrosamine was found, while the kidney metabolism was unaffected.[219] Thus, one can conclude that a low-protein diet decreases hepatotoxicity of environmental xenobiotics. Very low levels of dietary protein protect the liver from the toxic and carcinogenic chemicals by reducing microsomal drug-metabolizing enzyme activity yielding lowered metabolic production of biologically active intermediates.[218]

Vitamins and Minerals

Vitamin A at high doses may protect the organism against hydrocarbon-induced tumors.[223] The administration of 0.5% vitamin A palmitate to hamsters inhibited the formation of carcinomas of the forestomach and small intestine by dimethylbenzanthracene and benzo(a)pyrene.[13,15] Vitamin A also provides protection against skin tumors working as a lysosomal labilizer of premalignant cells. Vitamin A deficiency, combined with a low-fat diet, may increase the incidence of cervix and stomach cancers. The influence of thiamin (vitamin B₁) is yet to be discovered. Riboflavin (vitamin B₂) inhibits the formation of hepatic tumors induced by dimethylaminoazobenzene.[224] It works as an essential cofactor for detoxification enzymes. Riboflavin deficiency increases the production of liver cancer by N,N-dimethyl-4-aminoazobenzene.[180] Vitamin B₂ deficiency in alcoholics may cause disturbances in the upper gastrointestinal tract and even cancer incidence is elevated.[15] Pyridoxine may work in the xenobiotic metabolism participating in the tryptophan metabolism. Ascorbic acid (vitamin C) reduces sodium nitrite to NOₓ and thus inhibits the nitrosation of secondary and tertiary amines, amides, and ureas. Excessive amounts of copper delay azo dye-induced hepatocarcinogenesis. Liver tumors can be induced by such compounds as 3-methoxy-4-aminoazobenzene and its *N*-methyl derivatives, which formation can be inhibited by 0.5% curpric oxyacetate.[225]

Natural Carcinogens

All known or suspected carcinogens are not the results of man's influence on the environment. About 20 naturally occurring chemical carcinogens exist; most are metabolites of green plants and fungi. A few examples of some of the natural carcinogens and their metabolism in the body will be given (Figure 7). One should bear in mind that most of these compounds do need metabolic activation to yield ultimate carcinogens. Thus, the influence of drug-metabolizing enzymes may be critical in producing carcinogenic products.

Aflatoxins are mycotoxins from *Aspergillus flavus* fungi. The toxicity of aflatoxins varies, that of aflatoxin B_1 being the most toxic.[190,192,226,227] It has been estimated that 10% of aflatoxin B_1 is converted to protein and nucleic acid-bound forms in rat liver where it is, as aflatoxin B_1-2,3-oxide, the ultimate carcinogen (Figure 2B).[51,53]

Cycasin (methylzoxymethanol-β-glucoside) originates from green plants such as cycads.[51,53] Orally, cycasin is highly carcinogenic to the liver and kidney of rats and also induces tumors in other species. Intestinal bacteria contain β-glucosidase, breaking it to methylazomethanol which, at neutral pH, works as an electrophilic intermediate and methylates nucleic acids and proteins as a proximate carcinogen.

Ethionine is an *S*-ethyl analog of methionine and it is formed as a metabolite by several bacteria species.[51,53] When it is fed in the diet to rats, a concentration as low as 0.25% causes hepatocellular carcinoma through ethylation of hepatic nucleic acids. The ultimate carcinogen is the metabolite, *S*-adenosyl ethionine.

Pyrrolizidine alkaloids are also from plants and are known to be highly hepatocarcinogenic causing acute poisoning in humans.[51,53] They contain allylic ester structure for hepatotoxicity and carcinogenicity leading to the formation of pyrrolic ester metabolites which are major toxic metabolites and ultimate carcinogens. Safrole (1-allyl-3,4-methylene dioxybenzene) is found in spices and oils and is also hepatocarcinogenic after metabolic activation.[51,53]

Food Additives

Berenblum has reviewed the carcinogenicity of some additives and chemicals in food.[48] He found that butter yellow (4-dimethylaminoazobenzene) is possibly a liver carcinogen. Tween 60®, a detergent, may be a promoter for skin carcinogenesis. Dulcin may be a liver carcinogen as also may be cyclamate, diethylstilbesterol (also causes cancer in the vagina), lead salts, CCl_4, nitrosamines, cycasin, and aflatoxins. Azo dyes will be reduced to amines in the body. However, none of the dyes presently listed in the U.S. were mutagenic when tested.[228] Butylated hydroxyanisole and butylated hydroxytoluene inhibited the formation of dimethylbenzanthracene-induced forestomach tumors in female mice, mammary tumors in female Sprague-Dawley rats, and renal necrosis and general toxicity in rats.[229,230] In mice, butylated hydroxyanisole reduced lung tumors induced by benzpyrene, dimethylbenzanthracene, urethan, and uracil mustard. Fluorenylacetamide-induced carcinomas were inhibited by butylated hydroxytoluene. Butylated hydroxytoluene also delayed dimethylaminoazobenzene-induced liver tumors and the level of its protein binding.[190] Feeding the antioxidants, butylated hydroxyanisole or ethoxyquin to mice decreased the incidence of lung adenomas induced by diethylnitrosamine or 4-nitroquinoline 1-oxide.[229]

Miscellaneous Factors

Epidemiological studies have shown that inhabitants in countries with a high inci-

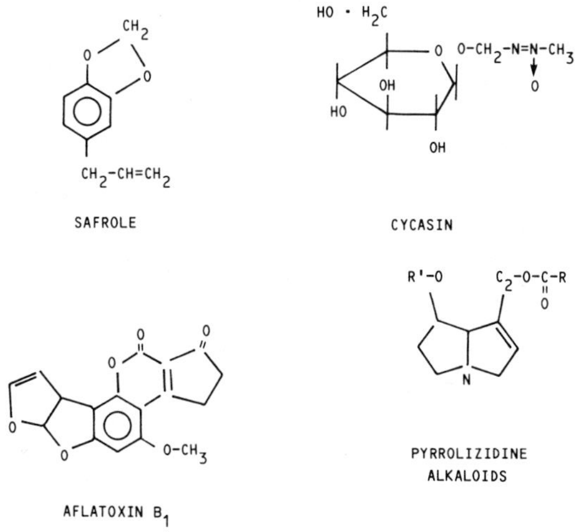

CH_2

SAFROLE

$CH_2-CH=CH_2$

$HO \cdot H_2C$

$O-CH_2-N=N-CH_3$

CYCASIN

AFLATOXIN B$_1$

$O-CH_3$

$R'-O$ $C_2-O-\overset{O}{\underset{\|}{C}}-R$

PYRROLIZIDINE
ALKALOIDS

FIGURE 7.   The molecular structures of naturally occurring carcinogens.

dence of gastric cancer have a low incidence of colon cancer and vice versa.[13] The mechanisms producing gastric cancers are open, although some suggestive proposals have been presented in man.[45] These studies have further shown that populations at a high risk for gastric cancer consume diets low in fat and high in carbohydrate and low in micronutrients.[13,15] It has been proposed that ascorbate would lower the cancer risk by decreasing the nitrosation reactions and by decreasing the reduction of nitrate to nitrite.[45] Gastric cancer correlates negatively with the consumption of raw vegetables and milk. This is based on a study in Japan where among patients with gastric cancer milk drinking was less frequent and consumption of salted foods greater than in controls.[15,45]

In addition to compositional variation in the diet the caloric amounts may also account for cancer formation. Caloric restriction seems to inhibit tumor formation. Low levels or deficiencies of some amino acids may have a therapeutic effect in animal studies. In women, obesity increases the incidence of endometrium and kidney cancers.[13,15]

SAFETY EVALUATION

Recently data have been accumulating about the effects of nutrients and other dietary factors on living organisms. However, despite a few individual studies, very little is known about the interactions of diet with drug metabolism in man. In addition to direct influences on pharmacokinetics of therapeutic drugs, nutrition and diet may be important in other respects. With diet, man ingests a large variety of chemical contaminants and additives. The major goal in the future should involve the development and application of methods for the evaluation of the safety of human food — its nutrients, the optimal concentration and total amount, as well as the methods for the detection of hazardous additives and contaminants in advance.

At present the influences of nutrients on drug metabolism are relatively well known in animals. Still, the biological significance is less well established and in man the possible role of nutrition in the regulation of drug metabolism needs further studies. Possibly even more interesting than drug metabolism, in a strict sense, is the role of nutrition in the regulation of toxic reactions and its possible role in the carcinogenic transformations. These factors makes it of utmost significance to find out means for evaluating the safety of human nutrition. This should include means of estimating the proper caloric intake, adequate nutrition, proper ratio of various nutrients and, moreover, estimation of the safety of intentional food additives and nonintentional contaminants. The estimation of protein, fat, and carbohydrate content is a difficult task as one should, in addition to caloric needs, also take into a consideration other possible effects of nutrients. These factors include the relationship of nutrition to promotion and/or initiation of cancer as seen in previous paragraphs. Although some decisions can be made on the basis of present data, much work is still necessary to obtain final answers in this matter.

A flow-chart for experimental and human evaluation for the safety of nonnutritional contaminants is proposed in Figure 8. These tests can be divided into 3 phases, according to the organisms used. In the first phase, mutagenicity tests should be performed with microbes and human cell cultures. Only negative results would justify further experimentation with animals to establish the toxicological data for the tested compound during the second phase of experiments. In the third phase, such compounds as had no harmful effects in experimental animals might be proposed for human use in a restricted population at the predetermined dose level. Thus, a new additive or a contaminant which cannot be avoided in food processing would be tested preceding its general use. Despite testing, the final decisions on the ultimate toxicity of food contaminants in man are often based on epidemiological findings and confirmed or rejected in further experimental studies, where the metabolic modifications are more easily controlled.

CONCLUSIONS

Numerous dietary factors regulate the rate of drug metabolism; both nutritional deficiencies and excesses may modify the rate. No general conclusion about the effect of nutrients on biotransformation can, however, be drawn, but each enzyme and nutrient must be judged individually. In addition to direct influences of nutrients on the activities of the drug-metabolizing enzymes, nutrients may modify the carcinogenic cellular transformations even in man. Although many factors influence cancer formation, the modification of one factor, diet, may be enough to stop or retard the chain of events leading to the progress of cancer. Although present data are far from definite and preferably only suggestive, one might speculate about an ideal diet with respect to the low cancer risk. This diet should be low in fat, sugar, cholesterol, and salts, while it should contain high concentrations of minerals, micronutrients, vitamins, and bulk materials. The role of dietary protein is vague; on the one hand, proteins supply the body with essential amino acids, and, on the other, a high-protein diet may enhance toxicity and even cancer risk if man is exposed to certain environmental xenobiotics. Naturally the diet should contain as low concentration of environmental xenobiotics as possible. Some food additives such as antioxidants may even be advantageous in the diet, protecting from carcinogenesis induced by foreign compounds. Urgent further studies are necessary before giving final proposals on ''noncarcinogenic'' diets.

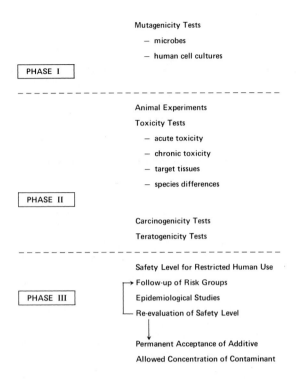

FIGURE 8. The safety evaluation of food additives and contaminants and a proposed schema for the research schema of any chemical in the human diet.

REFERENCES

1. **Basu, T. K. and Dickerson, J. W. T.**, Inter-relationships of nutrition and the metabolism of drugs, *Chem.-Biol. Interact.*, 8, 193—206, 1974.
2. **Dickerson, J. W. T. and Walker, R.**, Nutrition, age and drug metabolism, *Proc. Nutr. Soc.*, 33, 191—202, 1974.
3. **Hartiala, K.**, Metabolism of hormones, drugs and other substances by the gut, *Physiol. Rev.*, 53, 496—534, 1973.
4. **Hietanen, E.**, Dietary factors in drug metabolism, *Acta Pharmacol. Toxicol.*, 41 (Suppl. IV), 30, 1977.
5. **Kato, R.**, Drug metabolism under pathological and abnormal physiological states in animals and man, *Xenobiotica*, 7, 25—92, 1977.
6. **Kato, R. and Gillette, J. R.**, Sex differences in the effects of abnormal physiological states on the metabolism of drugs by rat liver microsomes, *J. Toxicol. Pharmacol. Exp. Ther.*, 150, 285—291, 1965.
7. **McLean, A. E. M.**, Molecules in food that alter drug metabolism, *Proc. Nutr. Soc.*, 33, 197—202, 1974.
8. **Siest, G., Batt, A. M., and Ziegler, J. M.**, Les enzymes du metabolisme des medicamentes, *Lyon Pharm.*, 29, 347—364, 1978.
9. **Vesell, E. S.**, Genetic and environmental factors affecting drug disposition in man, *Clin. Pharmacol. Ther.*, 22, 659—679, 1977.
10. **Williams, R. T.**, Nutrients in drug detoxication reactions, in *Nutrition and Drug Interactions*, Nathcock, J. N. and Coon, J., Eds., Academic Press, New York, 1978, 303—318.
11. **Yoshida, A.**, Interrelationships between the metabolism of xenobiotics and nutrition, *Seikagaku*, 50, 347—352, 1978.

12. **Doll, R.**, *Prevention of Cancer — pointers for Epidemiology,* The Rock Carling Fellowship 1967 — Nuffield Provincial Hospitals Trust 1967, Whitefriars Press Ltd., London, 1967.
13. **Gori, G. B.**, Diet and cancer, *J. Am. Diet. Assoc.,* 71, 375—379, 1977.
14. **Higginson, J.**, *Proc. 8th Can. Cancer Res. Conf.,* 1969, 40—75.
15. **Wynder, E. L.**, The dietary environment and cancer, *J. Am. Diet. Assoc.,* 71, 385—391, 1977.
16. **Campbell, T. C.**, Nutrition and drug-metabolizing enzymes, *Clin. Pharmacol. Ther.,* 22, 699—706, 1977.
17. **Dutton, G. J.**, in *Concepts in Biochemical Pharmacology,* Part II, Brodie, B. B. and Gillette, J. R., Eds., Springer-Verlag, New York, 28, 378, 1971.
18. **Estabrook, R. W., Fouts, J. R., and Mannering, G. J.**, *Microsomes and Drug Oxidations,* Academic Press, New York, 1969.
19. **Lu, A. Y. H.**, Liver microsomal drug metabolizing enzyme system. Functional components and their properties, *Fed. Proc., Fed. Am. Soc. Exp. Biol.,* 35, 2460—2463, 1976.
20. **Parke, D. V.**, *The Biochemistry of Foreign Compounds,* Pergamon Press, New York, 1968.
21. **Vainio, H. and Hietanen, E.**, The role of extrahepatic metabolism in drug disposition and toxicity, in *Concepts in Drug Metabolism,* Testa, B. and Jenner, P., Eds., Marcel Dekker, New York, 1980, 251—284.
22. **Williams, R. T.**, in *Concepts in Biochemical Pharmacology,* Part II, Brodie, B. B. and Gillette, J. R., Eds., Springer-Verlag, New York, 28, 226, 1971.
23. **Jenner, P. and Testa, B.**, Novel pathways in drug metabolism, *Xenobiotica,* 8, 1—25, 1978.
24. **Oesch, F.**, Mammalian epoxide hydrases: inducible enzymes catalysing the inactivation of carcinogenic and cytotoxic metabolites derived from aromatic oleofinic compounds, *Xenobiotica,* 3, 305—340, 1972.
25. **Arias, I. M. and Jakoby, W. B.**, *Glutathione: Metabolism and Function,* Raven Press, New York, 1976.
26. **La Du, B. N., Mandel, H. G., and Way, E. L.**, *Fundamentals of Drug Metabolism and Disposition,* Williams & Wilkins, Baltimore, 1971.
27. **Smith, R. L.**, *The Excretory function of Bile. The Elimination of Drugs and Toxic Substances in Bile,* Chapman and Hall, London, 1973.
28. **Bock, K. W.**, Dual role of glucuronyl- and sulfotransferases converting xenobiotics into reactive or biologically inactive and easily excretable compounds, *Arch. Toxicol.,* 39, 77—85, 1977.
29. **Kinoshita, N. and Gelboin, H. V.**, β-Glucuronidase catalyzed hydrolysis of benzo(a)pyrene-3-glucuronide and binding to DNA, *Science,* 199, 307—309, 1978.
30. **Mulder, G. J., Hinson, J. A., and Gillette, J. R.**, Generation of reactive metabolites of N-hydroxyphenacetin by glucuronidation and sulfation, *Biochem. Pharmacol.,* 26, 189—196, 1977.
31. **Nemoto, N.**, Glucuronidation in the metabolism of benzo(a)pyrene, in *Conjugation Reactions in Drug Biotransformation,* Aitio, A., Ed., Elsevier/North-Holland, Amsterdam, 1978, 17—27.
32. **Berry, C., Allistone, J., and Hallinan, T.**, Phospholipid dependence of UDPglucuronosyltransferase, *Biochim. Biophys. Acta,* 507, 198—206, 1978.
33. **Claude, A.**, *The Harvey Lectures,* Series 43, Academic Press, New York, 1947, 121.
34. **Claude, A.**, *Microsomes and Drug Oxidations,* Academic Press, New York, 1969.
35. **Vainio, H.**, On the Topology and Synthesis of Drug Metabolizing Enzymes in Hepatic Endoplasmic Reticulum, Dissertation, University of Turku, Turku, Finland, 1973.
36. **Seidegård, J., Moron, M. S., Eriksson, L. C., and DePierre, J. W.**, The topology of epoxide hydratase and benzpyrene monooxygenase in the endoplasmic reticulum of rat liver, *Biochim. Biophys. Acta,* 543, 29—40, 1978.
37. **Irjala, K.**, Synthesis of p-aminohippuric, hippuric, and salicyluric acids in experimental animals and man, *Ann. Acad. Sci. Fenn.,* 154, 1—40, Dissertation, University of Turku, Turku, Finland, 1972.
38. **Aitio, A. and Marniemi, J.**, Extrahepatic glucuronide conjugation, in *Extrahepatic Drug Metabolism,* Gram, T. E., Ed., Spectrum Publications, Holliswood, N.Y., 1980, 365—387.
39. **Testa, B. and Jenner, P.**, *Drug Metabolism, Chemical and Biochemical Aspects,* Marcel Dekker, New York, 1976.
40. **Testa, B. and Jenner, P.**, Novel drug metabolites produced by functionalization reactions: chemistry and toxicology, *Drug Metab. Rev.,* 7, 325—369, 1978.
41. **Berg, J. W.**, Can nutrition explain the pattern of international epidemiology of hormone-dependent cancers?, *Cancer Res.,* 35, 3345—3350, 1975.
42. **Castagne, M. and Weisburger, J. H.**, Nutrition et cancer: où est le danger?, *Recherches,* 8, 286—288, 1977.
43. **Heidelberger, C.**, Chemical carcinogenesis, *Annu. Rev. Biochem.,* 44, 79—121, 1975.
44. **Le, M. and Flamant, R.**, Nutrition et cancer du sein: presentation d'une enquête francaise, *Bull. Cancer,* 65, 65—69, 1978.

45. **Weisburger, J. H. and Raineri, R.**, Dietary factors and the etiology of gastric cancer, *Cancer Res,.* 35, 3469, 1975.
46. **Wynder, E. L.**, Nutrition and cancer, *Fed. Proc., Fed. Am. Soc. Exp. Biol.,* 35, 1309—1315, 1976.
47. **Wynder, E. L. and Mabuchi, K.**, Etiological and preventive aspects of human cancer, *Prev. Med.,* 1, 300, 1976.
48. **Berenblum, I.**, Carcinogenesis as a biological problem, North-Holland, Amsterdam, 1974, 1—376.
49. **Clayson, D. B.**, Nutrition and experimental carcinogenesis. A review, *Cancer Res.,* 35, 3292—3300, 1975.
50. **Criciute, L.**, Les substances cancérogènes dans les aliments, *Bull. Cancer,* 65, 53—58, 1978.
51. **Miller, E. C.**, Some current perspectives on chemical carcinogenesis in humans and experimental animals: presidential address, *Cancer Res.,* 38, 1479—1496, 1978.
52. **Miller, E. C. and Miller, J. A.**, The mutagenicity of chemical carcinogens: correlations, problems and interpretations, in *Chemical Mutagens, Principles and Methods for Their Detection,* Holländer, A., Ed., Plenum Press, New York, 1971, 1; 83—119.
53. **Miller, J. A. and Miller, E. C.**, Carcinogens occurring naturally in foods, *Fed. Proc., Fed. Am. Soc. Exp. Biol.,* 35, 1316—1321, 1976.
54. **Burke, M. D., Vadi, H., Jernström, B., and Orrenius, S.**, Metabolism of benzo(a)pyrene with isolated hepatocytes and the formation and degradation of DNA-binding derivatives, *J. Biol. Chem.,* 252, 6424—6431, 1977.
55. **Harbison, R. D.**, Chemical-biological reactions common to teratogenesis and mutagenesis, *Environ. Health Perspectives,* 24, 87—100, 1978.
56. **Thor, H., Moldéus, P., Kristoferson, A., Högberg, J., Reed, D. J., and Orrenius, S.**, Metabolic activation and hepatotoxicity. Metabolism of bromobenzene in isolated hepatocytes, *Arch. Biochem. Biophys.,* 188, 114—121, 1978.
57. **Wiebkin, P., Fry, J. R., and Bridges, J. W.**, Metabolism-mediated cytotoxicity of chemical carcinogens and noncarcinogens, *Biochem. Pharmacol.* 27, 1849—1851, 1978.
58. **Hietanen, E. and Lang, M.**, Control of glucuronide biosynthesis in the gastrointestinal mucosa, in *Conjugation Reactions in Drug Biotransformation,* Aitio, A., Ed., Elsevier/North-Holland, Amsterdam, 1978, 399—408.
59. **Parke, D. V.**, The effects of nutrition and enzyme induction in toxicology, *World Rev. Nutr. Diet.,* 29, 96—114, 1978.
60. **Basu, T. K.**, Effect of nutrition on hepatic microsomal drug metabolizing enzymes in growing rats, Thesis, Guildford, 1971.
61. **Baetjer, A. M. and Rubin, R. J.**, Effect of water and food deprivation on hepatic microsomal metabolism of hexobarbital and aniline, *J. Toxicol. Environ. Health,* 2, 131—138, 1976.
62. **Dixon, R. L., Shultice, W., and Fouts, J. R.**, Factors affecting drug metabolism by liver microsomes. IV. Starvation, *Proc. Soc. Exp. Biol. Med.,* 103, 333—335, 1960.
63. **Kato, R. and Gillette, J. R.**, Effect of starvation on NADPH-dependent enzymes in liver microsomes of male and female rats, *J. Pharmacol. Exp. Ther.,* 150, 279—284, 1965.
64. **Reidenberg, M. M.**, Obesity and fasting — effects on drug metabolism and drug action in man, *Clin. Pharmacol. Exp. Ther.,* 22, 729—734, 1977.
65. **Rogers, C. G.**, Fatty acid composition of liver mitochondria and microsomes in fed and fasted rats, *Nutr. Rep. Int.,* 4, 351—362, 1971.
66. **Hietanen, E. and Vainio, H.**, Interspecies variations in small intestinal and hepatic drug hydroxylation and glucuronidation, *Acta Pharmacol. Toxicol.,* 33, 57—64, 1973.
67. **Marselos, M. and Laitinen, M.**, Starvation and phenobarbital treatment effects on drug hydroxylation and glucuronidation in the rat liver and small intestinal mucosa, *Biochem. Pharmacol.,* 24, 1529—1535, 1975.
68. **Laitinen, M., Hietanen, E., Vainio, H., and Hänninen, O.**, Dietary fats and properties of endoplasmic reticulum. I. Dietary lipid-induced changes in the composition of microsomal membranes in the liver and gastroduodenal mucosa of the rat, *Lipids,* 10, 461—466, 1975.
69. **Joly, J.-G., Hétu, C., Mavier, P., and Villeneuve, J. P.**, Mechanism of induction of hepatic drug-metabolizing enzymes by ethanol. I. Limited role of microsomal phospholipids, *Biochem. Pharmacol.,* 25, 1995—2001, 1976.
70. **Kleemann, W. and McConnell, H. M.**, Interactions of proteins and cholesterol with lipids in bilayer membranes, *Biochim. Biophys. Acta,* 419, 206—222, 1976.
71. **Lang, M.**, Dietary cholesterol caused modification in the structure and function of rat hepatic microsomes, studied by fluorescent probes, *Biochim. Biophys. Acta,* 455, 947—960, 1976.
72. **Marshall, J. W. and McLean, A. E. M.**, The effect of oral phenobarbitone on hepatic microsomal cytochrome P-450 and demethylation activities in rats fed normal and low protein diets, *Biochem. Pharmacol.,* 18, 153—157, 1962.

73. **Marshall, J. W. and McLean, A. E. M.,** A requirement for dietary lipids for induction of cytochrome P-450 by phenobarbitone in rat liver microsomal fraction, *Biochem. J.,* 122, 569—573, 1971.

74. **McLean, A. E. M.,** Diet, DDT, and the toxicity of drugs and chemicals, *Fed. Proc., Fed. Am. Soc. Exp. Biol.,* 36, 1688—1691, 1977.

75. **Norred, W. P. and Wade, A. E.,** Dietary fatty acid-induced alterations of hepatic microsomal drug metabolism, *Biochem. Pharmacol.,* 21, 2887—2897, 1972.

76. **Agradi, E., Spagnuolo, C., and Galli, C.,** Dietary lipids and aniline and benzpyrene hydroxylation in liver microsomes, *Pharmacol. Res. Commun.,* 7, 469—480, 1975.

77. **Century, B.,** Role of the dietary lipid in the ability of phenobarbital to stimulate drug detoxification, *J. Pharmacol. Exp. Ther.,* 185, 185—194, 1973.

78. **Hietanen, E., Hänninen, O., Laitinen, M., and Lang, M.,** Regulation of hepatic drug metabolism by elaidic and linoleic acids in rats, *Enzyme,* 23, 127—134, 1978.

79. **Hietanen, E., Hänninen, O., Laitinen, M., and Lang, M.,** The *in vitro* and *in vivo* changes in drug biotransformation by dietary cholesterol as related to membrane modification, in *Industrial and Environmental Xenobiotics,* Fouts, J. R. and Gut, J., Eds., Excerpta Medica, Amsterdam, 1977, 110—113.

80. **Hietanen, E., Hänninen, O., Laitinen, L., and Lang, M.,** Dietary cholesterol-induced enhancement of hepatic biotransformation rate in male rats, *Pharmacology,* 17, 163—172, 1978.

81. **Hietanen, E. and Laitinen, M.,** Regulation of intestinal UDPglucuronosyltransferase activity by fatty acids in the rat, *Enzyme,* 22, 316—321, 1977.

82. **Hietanen, E. and Laitinen, M.,** Dependence of intestinal biotransformation on dietary cholesterol, *Biochem. Pharmacol.,* 27, 1095—1097, 1978.

83. **Hietanen, E., Laitinen, M., Lang, M., and Vainio, H.,** Inducibility of mucosal drug-metabolizing enzymes of rats fed on a cholesterol rich diet by polychlorinated biphenyl, 3-methylcholanthrene and phenobarbitone, *Pharmacology,* 13, 287—296, 1975.

84. **Hietanen, E., Laitinen, M., Vainio, H., and Hänninen, O.,** Dietary fats and properties of endoplasmic reticulum. II. Dietary lipid-induced changes in the activities of drug metabolizing enzymes in the liver and duodenum of the rat, *Lipids,* 10, 467—472, 1975.

85. **Hopkins, G. J. and West, C. E.,** Effect of dietary fats on pentobarbitone-induced sleeping times and hepatic microsomal cytochrome P-450 in rats, *Lipids,* 11, 736—740, 1976.

86. **Lambert, L. and Wills, E. D.,** The effect of dietary lipid peroxides, sterols and oxidised sterols on cytochrome P-450 and oxidative demethylation in the endoplasmic reticulum, *Biochem. Pharmacol.,* 26, 1417—1421, 1977.

87. **Lambert, L. and Wills, E. D.,** The effect of dietary lipids on 3,4-benzo(a)pyrene metabolism in the hepatic endoplasmic reticulum, *Biochem. Pharmacol.,* 26, 1423—1427, 1977.

88. **Michalek, H., del Carmine, R., and Gatti, G. L.,** Effect of dietary rapeseed oil on hepatic hexobarbital metabolism in mice, *Nutr. Metab.,* 18, 272—282, 1975.

89. **Stier, A.,** Lipid structure and drug metabolizing enzymes, *Biochem. Pharmacol.,* 25, 109—113, 1976.

90. **Strobel, H. W., Lu, A. Y. H., Heidema, J., and Coon, M. J.,** Phosphatidylcholine requirement in the enzymic reduction of hemoprotein P-450 and in fatty acid, hydrocarbon, and drug hydroxylation, *J. Biol. Chem.,* 245, 4851—4854, 1970.

91. **Wade, A. E. and Norred, W. P.,** Effect of dietary lipid on drug-metabolizing enzymes, *Fed. Proc., Fed. Am. Soc. Exp. Biol.,* 35, 2475—2479, 1976.

92. **Wade, A. E., Norred, W. P., and Evans, J. S.,** Lipids in drug detoxication, in *Nutrition and Drug Interactions,* Nathcock, J. N. and Coon, J., Eds., Academic Press, New York, 1978, 475—503.

93. **Wade, A. E., Wu, B., and Caster, W. O.,** Relationship of dietary essential fatty acid consumption to hepatic drug hydroxylation, *Pharmacology,* 7, 305—314, 1972.

94. **Century, B. and Horwitt, M. K.,** A role of dietary lipid in the ability of phenobarbital to stimulate hexobarbital and aminopyrine metabolism, *Fed. Proc., Fed. Am. Soc. Exp. Biol.,* 27, 349, 1968.

95. **Zbinden, G., Brandle, E., and Pfister, M.,** Modification of Adriamycin toxicity in rats fed a high fat diet, *Agents and Actions,* 7, 163—170, 1977.

96. **Lang, M., Koivusaari, U., and Hietanen, E.,** Microsomal drug metabolism and the interaction of three fluorescent probes with microsomes at different temperatures, *Biochim. Biophys. Acta,* 539, 195—208, 1978.

97. **Lang, M., Koivusaari, U., Hietanen, E., and Hänninen, O.,** Use of fluorescent probes in studies of rat liver microsomes: structure and function, in *Conjugation Reactions in Drug Biotransformation,* Aitio, A., Ed., Elsevier/North-Holland, Amsterdam, 1978, 317—326.

98. **Alvares, A., Anderson, K. E., Conney, A. H., and Kappas, A.,** Interaction between nutritional factors and drug biotransformation in man, *Proc. Natl. Acad. Sci. U.S.A.,* 73, 2501—2504, 1976.

99. **Conney, A. H., Pantuck, E. J., Kunzman, R., Kappas, A., Anderson, K. E., and Alvares, A. P.,** Nutrition and chemical biotransformation in man, *Clin. Pharmacol. Ther.,* 22, 707—719, 1977.

100. Fishman, J. and Bradlow, H. L., Effects of malnutrition on the metabolism of sex hormones in man, *Clin. Pharmacol. Ther.*, 22, 721—727, 1977.

101. Kappas, A., Alvares, A. P., Anderson, K. E., Pantuck, E. J., Pantuck, C. B., Chang, R., and Conney, A. H., Effect of charcoal-broiled beef on antipyrine and theophylline metabolism, *Clin. Pharmacol. Ther.*, 23, 445—450, 1978.

102. Pantuck, E. J., Hsiao, K.-C., Conney, A. H., Garland, W. A., Kappas, A., Anderson, K. E., and Alvares, A. P., Effect of charcoal-broiled beef on phenacetin metabolism in man, *Science*, 194, 1055—1057, 1976.

103. Campbell, T. C. and Hayes, J. R., The effect of quantity and quality of dietary protein on drug metabolism, *Fed. Proc., Fed. Am. Soc. Exp. Biol.*, 35, 2470—2474, 1976.

104. Dickerson, J. W. T., Basu, T. K., and Parke, D. V., Protein nutrition and drug metabolizing enzymes in the liver of the growing rat, *Proc. Nutr. Soc.*, 30, 5A, 1971.

105. Eriksson, M., Catz, C., and Yaffe, S. J., Effect of weanling malnutrition upon hepatic drug metabolism, *Biol. Neonat.*, 27, 339—351, 1975.

106. Hospador, M. A., Grosso, L. S., and Manthei, R. W., Influence of age and diet on the induction of microsomal enzymes in the mouse, *Proc. Soc. Exp. Biol. Med.*, 136, 884—888, 1971.

107. Kato, R., Oshima, T., and Tomizawa, S., Toxicity and metabolism of drugs in relation to dietary protein, *Jpn. J. Pharmacol.*, 18, 356—366, 1968.

108. Sachan, D. S. Effects of low and high protein diets on the induction of microcomsal drug-metabolizing enzymes in rat liver, *J. Nutr.*, 105, 1631—1639, 1975.

109. Smith, J. A., Butler, T. C., and Poole, D. T., Effect of protein depletion in guinea pigs on glucuronate conjugation of chloramphenicol by liver microsomes, *Biochem. Pharmacol.*, 22, 981—983, 1973.

110. Wood, G. C. and Woodcock, B. G., Effects of dietary protein deficiency on the conjugation of foreign compounds in rat liver, *J. Pharm. Pharmacol.*, 22, (Suppl.), 60S—63S, 1970.

111. Woodcock, B. G. and Wood, G. C., Effect of protein-free diet on UDPglucuronosyltransferase and sulfontransferase activities in rat liver, *Biochem. Pharmacol.*, 20, 2703—2713, 1971.

112. Basu, T. K., Dickerson, J. W. T., and Parke, D. V., Effect of underfeeding suckling rats on the activity of hepatic microsomal drug metabolizing enzymes, *Biol. Neonat.*, 23, 109—115, 1973.

113. Winick, M., Relation of nutrition to physical and mental development, *Bibl. Nutr. Dieta.*, 18, 114—122, 1973.

114. Winick, M., Brasel, J. A., and Velasco, E., Effects of prenatal nutrition upon pregnancy risk, *Clin. Obstet. Gynecol.*, 16, 184—198, 1973.

115. Winick, M., Brasel, J. A., Velasco, E., and Rosso, P., Effects of early nutrition on growth of the central nervous system, *Infant at Risk*, 10, 29—36, 1974.

116. Marshall, W. J. and McLean, A. E. M., The effect of oral phenobarbitone on hepatic microsomal cytochrome P-450 and demethylation activity in rats fed normal and low protein diets, *Biochem. Pharmacol.*, 18, 153—157, 1969.

117. Kato, R., Oshima, T., and Tomizawa, S., Toxicity and metabolism of drugs in relation to dietary protein, *Jpn. J. Pharmacol.*, 18, 356—366, 1968.

118. Paine, A. J. and McLean, A. E. M., The effect of dietary protein and fat on the activity of aryl hydrocarbon hydroxylase in rat liver, kidney and lung, *Biochem. Pharmacol.*, 22, 2875—2880, 1973.

119. Basu, T. K., Dickerson, W. T., and Parke, D. V., Effect of dietary substitution of sucrose and its constituent monosaccharides on the activity of aromatic hydroxylase and the level of cytochrome P-450 in hepatic microsomes of growing rats, *Nutr. Metab.*, 18, 302—309, 1975.

120. Nash, A. H. and Bender, A. E., The effect of dietary sucrose on the metabolism of pentobarbitone, *Proc. Nutr. Soc.*, 35, 133A, 1976.

121. Becking, G. C., Hepatic drug metabolism in iron-, magnesium- and potassium-deficient rats, *Fed. Proc., Fed. Am. Soc. Exp. Biol.*, 35, 2480—2485, 1976.

122. Becking, G. C. and Morrison, A. B., Hepatic drug metabolism in zinc-deficient rats, *Biochem. Pharmacol.*, 19, 895—902, 1970.

123. Becking, G. C. and Morrison, A. B., Role of dietary magnesium in the metabolism of drugs by NADPH-dependent rat liver microsomal enzymes, *Biochem. Pharmacol.*, 19, 2639—2644, 1970.

124. Kuenzig, W., Tkaczevski, W., Kamm, J. J., Conney, A. H., and Burns, J. J., The effect of ascorbic acid deficiency on extrahepatic microsomal metabolism of drugs and carcinogens in the guinea pig. *J. Pharmacol. Exp. Ther.*, 201, 527—533, 1977.

125. Carpenter, M. P., Role of α-tocopherol in microsomal hydroxylation, *Fed. Proc., Fed. Am. Soc. Exp. Biol.*, 27, 677, 1968.

126. Carpenter, M. P., Vitamin E and microsomal drug hydroxylation, *Ann. N.Y. Acad. Sci.*, 203, 81—92, 1972.

127. Carpenter, M. P. and Howard, C. N., Jr., Vitamin E, steroids and liver microsomal hydroxylations, *Am. J. Clin. Nutr.*, 27, 966—979, 1974.

128. Colby, H. D., Kramer, R. E., Greiner, J. W., Robinson, D. A., Krause, R. F., and Canady, W. J., Hepatic drug metabolism in retinoid-deficient rats, *Biochem. Pharmacol.*, 21, 1644—1646, 1975.

129. Conney, A. H., Bray, G. A., Evans, C., and Burns, J. J., Metabolic interactions between L-ascorbic acid and drugs, *Ann. N. Y., Acad. Sci.,* 92, 115—127, 1961.

130. Horn, L. R., Machlin, L. J., Barker, M. O., and Brin, M., Drug metabolism and hepatic heme proteins in the vitamin E-deficient rats, *Arch. Biochem. Biophys.,* 172, 270—277, 1976.

131. Shargel, L. and Mazel, P., Effect of riboflavin deficiency on phenobarbital and 3-methylcholanthrene induction of microsomal drug metabolizing enzymes of the rat, *Biochem. Pharmacol.,* 22, 2365—2373, 1973.

132. Sikic, B. I., Mimnaugh, E. G., and Gram, T. E., Effects of dietary ascorbic acid supplementation on hepatic drug-metabolizing enzymes in the guinea pig, *Biochem. Pharmacol.,* 26, 2037—2041, 1977.

133. Zannoni, V. C., Ascoribc acid and liver microsomal drug metabolism, *Acta Vitaminol. Enzymol.,* 31, 17—29, 1977.

134. Zannoni, V. G., Flynn, E. J., and Lynch, M., Ascorbic acid and drug metabolism, *Biochem. Pharmacol.,* 22, 2365—2373, 1973.

135. Zannoni, V. G., Sato, P. H., and Rikans, L. E., Ascorbic acid and drug metabolism, in *Nutrition and Drug Interactions,* Nathcock, J. N. and Coon, J., Eds., Academic Press, New York, 1978, 347—370.

136. Degkwitz, E., Luft, D., Pfeiffer, U., and Staudinger, H., Untersuchungen über mikrosomale Enzymaktivitäten (Cumazinhydroxylerung, NADPH-oxydation, Glucose-6-phosphatase und Esterase) und Cytochromgeholte (P-450 und b$_5$) bei normalen, skorbutischen und hungernden Meerschweinden, *Hoppe-Seyler's Z. Physiol. Chem.,* 349, 465—471, 1968.

137. Kato, R., Takanaka, A., and Oshima, T., Effect of vitamin deficiency on the metabolism of drugs and NADPH-linked electron transport system in liver microsomes, *Jpn. J. Pharmacol.,* 19, 25—33, 1969.

138. Leber, H. E., Dekgwitz, E., and Staudinger, H., Untersuchungen zum Einfluss der Ascorbinsäure auf die Aktivität und Gehalt an Hämoproteiden in der Mikrosomenfraktion der Meerschweinchenleber, *Hoppe-Seyler's Z. Physiol. Chem.,* 350, 439—445, 1969.

139. Enkiewitz, M. and Lasker, M., The origin of l-xyloketose (urine pentose), *J. Biol. Chem.,* 110, 443—456, 1935.

140. Harris, C. C., Sporn, M. B., Kaufman, D. G., Smith, J. M., Jackson, F. E., and Saffiotti, U., Histogenesis of squamous metaplasia in the hamster tracheal epithelium caused by vitamin A deficiency or benzo(a)pyrene-ferric oxide, *J. Natl. Cancer Inst.,* 48, 743—746, 1972.

141. Sporn, M. B., Dunlop, N. M., Newton, D. L., and Smith, J. M., Prevention of chemical carcinogenesis by Vitamin A and its synthetic analogs (retinoids), *Fed. Proc., Fed. Am. Soc. Exp. Biol.,* 35, 1332—1338, 1976.

142. Wolbach, S. B. and Howe, P. R., Tissue changes following deprivation of fat-soluble A vitamin, *J. Exp. Med.,* 42, 753—777, 1925.

143. Wong, Y. and Buck, R., An electron microscopic study of metaplasia of the rat tracheal epithelium in vitamin A deficiency, *Lab. Invest.,* 24, 55—66, 1971.

144. Moore, T., Effects of vitamin A deficiency in animals: pharmacology and toxicology of vitamin A, in *The Vitamins,* Vol. 1, 2nd ed., Sebrell, W. H. and Harris, R. S., Eds., Academic Press, New York, 1967, 245—299.

145. Chopra, D. P. and Wilkoff, L. J., Inhibition and reversal of carcinogen-induced lesions in mouse prostate in vitro by all trans-retinoic acid, *Proc. Am. Assoc. Cancer Res.,* 16, 35, 1975.

146. Lasnitzki, I., The influence of A hypervitaminosis on the effect of 20-methylcholantrene on mouse prostate glands grown *in vitro, Br. J. Cancer,* 9, 434—441, 1955.

147. Nettesheim, P., Snyder, C., Williams, M. L., Cone, M. V., and Kim, J. C., Effect of vitamin A on lung tumor induction in rats, *Proc. Am. Assoc. Cancer Res.,* 16, 54, 1975.

148. Cohen, S. M., Wittenberg, J. F., and Bryan, G. T., Effect of hyper- and avitaminosis A on urinary bladder carcinogenicity of N-[4-(5-nitro-2-furyl)-2-thiazolyl] formamide (FANFT), *Fed. Proc., Fed. Am. Soc. Exp. Biol.,* 33, 602, 1974.

149. Rogers, A. E., Herndon, B. J., and Newberne, P. M., Induction by dimethylhydrazine of intestinal carcinoma in normal rats and rats fed high or low levels of vitamin A, *Cancer Res.,* 33, 103—109, 1973.

150. Bjelke, E., Dietary vitamin A and human lung cancer, *Int. J. Cancer,* 15, 561—565, 1975.

151. Genta, V. M., Kaufman, D. G., Harris, C. C., Smith, J. M., Spron, M. B., and Saffiotti, U., Vitamin A deficiency enhances the binding of benzo(a)pyrene to tracheal epithelial DNA, *Nature (London),* 247, 48—49, 1974.

152. Murty, H. S., Caasl, P. I., Brooks, S. K., and Nair, P. D., Biosynthesis of haem in the vitamin E-deficient rat, *J. Biol. Chem.,* 245, 5498—5504, 1970.

153. Dingell, J. V., Joiner, P. D., and Hurwitz, L., Impairment of hepatic drug metabolism in calcium deficiency, *Biochem. Pharmacol.,* 15, 971—976, 1966.

154. **Becking, G. C. and Morrison, A. B.**, Hepatic drug metabolism in zinc-deficient rats, *Biochem. Pharmacol.*, 19, 895—902, 1970.
155. **Hoensch, H., Woo, C. H., and Schmid, R.**, Cytochrome P-450 and drug metabolism in intestinal villous and crypt cells of rats: effect of dietary iron, *Biochem. Biophys. Res. Commun.*, 65, 399—406, 1975.
156. **Hoensch, H., Woo, C. H., Ruffin, S. B., and Schmid, R.**, Oxidative metabolism of foreign compounds in rat small intestine: cellular localization and dependence on dietary iron, *Gastroenterology*, 70, 1063—1070, 1976.
157. **Maines, M. D. and Kappas, A.**, Regulation of cytochrome P-450-dependent microsomal drug-metabolizing enzymes by nickel, cobalt and iron, *Clin. Pharmacol. Ther.*, 22, 780—790, 1977.
158. **Levander, O. A.**, Nutritional factors in relation to heavy metal toxicants, *Fed. Proc., Fed. Am. Soc. Exp. Biol.*, 36, 1683—1687, 1977.
159. **Laitinen, M. and Hietanen, E.**, The copper induced modification of duodenal biotransformation reactions in rats during fat deficiency, *Acta Pharmacol. Toxicol.*, 43, 363—367, 1978.
160. **Bradshaw, L. R. A.**, Factors affecting the introduction and fate of foreign chemicals in food, *Clin. Toxicol.*, 9, 633—646, 1976.
161. **Grasso, P.**, Review of tests for carcinogenicity and their significance to man, *Clin. Toxicol.*, 9, 745—760, 1976.
162. **Issenberg, P.**, Nitrite, nitrosamines and cancer, *Fed. Proc., Fed. Am. Soc. Exp. Biol.*, 35, 1322—1326, 1976.
163. **Vettorazzi, G.**, The safety evaluation of food additives. The dynamics of toxicological decision, *Lebensm. Wiss. Technol.*, 8, 195—201, 1975.
164. **Kuntzman, R., Pantuck, E. J., Kaplan, S. A., and Conney, A. H.**, Phenacetin metabolism: effect of hydrocarbons and cigarette smoking, *Clin. Pharmacol. Ther.*, 22, 757—764, 1977.
165. **Pantuck, E. J., Hsiao, K.-C., Loub, W. D., Wattenberg, L. W., Kuntzman, R., and Conney, A. H.**, Stimulatory effect of vegetables on intestinal drug metabolism in the rat, *J. Pharmacol. Exp. Ther.*, 198, 278—283, 1976.
166. **Wattenberg L. W.**, Dietary modification of intestinal and pulmonary aryl hydrocarbon hydroxylase activity, *Toxicol. Appl. Pharmacol.*, 23, 741—748, 1972.
167. **Arcos, J. C., Bryant, G. M., Venkatesan, N., and Argos, M. F.**, Repression of dimethylnitrosamine demethylase by typical inducers of microsomal mixed function oxidases, *Biochem. Pharmacol.*, 24, 1544—1547, 1975.
168. **Sternson, L. A. and Gammans, R. E.**, Effects of aromatic nitro compounds on oxidative metabolism by cytochrome P-450 dependent enzymes, *J. Med. Chem.*, 19, 174—177, 1976.
169. **Babish, J. G. and Stoewsand, G. S.**, Effect of tea intake on induction of hepatic microsomal enzyme activity in the rabbit, *Nutr. Rep. Int.*, 12, 109—115, 1975.
170. **Pantuck, E. J., Hsiao, K.-C., Kuntzman, R., and Conney, A. H.**, Intestinal metabolism of phenacetin in the rat: effect of charcoal-broiled beef and rat chow, *Science*, 187, 744—745, 1975.
171. **Loub, W. D., Wattenberg, L. W., and Davis, D. W.**, Aryl hydrocarbon hydroxylase induction in rat tissues by naturally occurring indoles of cruxiferous plants, *J. Natl. Cancer Inst.*, 54, 985—988, 1975.
172. **Dent, C. E., Richens, A., Rowe, D. J. F., and Stamp, T. C. B.**, Osteomalacia with long-term anticonvulsant therapy in epilepsy, *Br. Med. J.*, 4, 69—72, 1970.
173. **Lathem, A. N., Milbank, L., Richens, A., and Rowe, D. J. F.**, Liver enzyme induction by anticonvulsant drugs and its relationship to disturbed calcium and folic acid metabolism, *J. Clin. Pharmacol.*, 13, 337—342, 1973.
174. **Gerson, C. D., Hepner, G. W., Brown N., Cohen, N., Hebert, V., and Jonowitz, H. D.**, Inhibition by diphenylhydantoin of folic acid absorption in man, *Gastroenterology*, 63, 246—251, 1972.
175. **Maxwell, J. D., Hunter, J., Stewart, D. A., Ardeman, S., and Williams, R.**, Folate deficiency after anticonvulsant drugs: an effect of hepatic enzymes induction?, *Br. Med. J.*, 1, 297—299, 1972.
176. **Bartsch, H., Margison, G. P., Malaveille, C., Camus, A. M., Brun, G., Margison, J. M., Kolar, G. F., and Wiessler, M.**, Some aspects of metabolic activation of chemical carcinogens in relation to their organ specificity, *Arch. Toxicol.*, 39, 51—63, 1977.
177. **Magee, P. N. and Hultin, T.**, Toxic liver injury and carcinogenesis: methylation of proteins of rat-liver slices by dimethylnitrosamine *in vitro*, *Biochem. J.*, 83, 106—114, 1962.
178. **Miller, E. C. and Miller, J. A.**, Mechanisms of chemical carcinogenesis: nature of proximate carcinogens and interactions with macromolecules, *Pharmacol. Rev.*, 18, 805—838, 1966.
179. **Andrews, A. W., Thibault, L. H., and Lijinsky, W.**, The relationship between mutagenicity and carcinogenicity of some nitrosamines, *Mutat. Res.*, 51, 319—326, 1978.
180. **Poirier, L. A. and Boutwell, R. K.**, Current problems in nutrition and cancer, *Fed. Proc., Fed. Am. Soc. Exp. Biol.*, 35, 1307—1308, 1976.

181. **Chambon, P. and Chambon, R.,** Cancerogenese et environment: les N-nitrosamines, *Lyon Pharm.* 27, 259—265, 1976.

182. **Hashimoto S., Yokokura, T., Kawai, Y., and Mutai, M.,** Dimethylnitrosamine formation in the gastrointestinal tract of rats, *Food Cosmet. Toxicol.,* 14, 553—556, 1976.

183. **Magee, P. N.,** Toxicity of nitrosamines: their possible human health hazards, *Food Cosmet. Toxicol.,* 9, 207—208, 1971.

184. **Magee, P. N. and Barnes, J. M.,** The production of malignant primary hepatic tumors in the rat by feeding dimethylnitrosamine, *Br. J. Cancer,* 10, 114—122, 1956.

185. **Magee, P. N. and Barnes, J. M.,** Carcinogenic nitroso compounds, *Adv. Cancer Res.,* 10, 163—246, 1967.

186. **Olajos, E. J.,** Biological interactions of N-nitroso compounds: a review, *Ecotoxicol. Environ. Safety,* 1, 175—196, 1977.

187. **Scanlan, R. A.,** N-nitrosamines in foods, *Crit. Rev. Food Technol.,* 5, 357—402, 1975.

188. **Swann, P. F.,** The toxicology of nitrate, nitrite and N-nitroso compounds, *J. Sci. Food Agric.,* 26, 1761—1770, 1975.

189. **Swann, P. F.,** Carcinogenic risk from nitrite, nitrate and N-nitrosamines in food, *Proc. R. Soc. Med.,* 70, 113—115, 1977.

190. **Gurtoo, H. L., Dahms, R. P., and Paigan, B.,** Metabolic activation of aflatoxins related to their mutagenicity, *Biochem. Biophys. Res. Commun.,* 81, 965—972, 1978.

191. **Rogers, A. E. and Newberne, P. M.,** Diet and aflatoxin B_1 toxicity in rats, *Toxicol. Appl. Pharmacol.,* 20, 113—121, 1971.

192. **Wogan, G. N., Paglialunga, S., and Newberne, P. M.,** Carcinogenic effects of low dietary levels of aflatoxin B_1 in rats, *Food Cosmet. Toxicol.,* 12, 681—685, 1974.

193. **Tannenbaum, A.,** The dependence of tumor formation on the composition of the calorie-restricted diet as well as on the degree of restriction, *Cancer Res.,* 5, 616—625, 1945.

194. **Rogers, A. E., Sanchez, O., Feinsod, F. M., and Newberne, P. M.,** Dietary enhancement of nitrosamine carcinogenesis, *Cancer Res.,* 34, 96—99, 1974.

195. **Lijinsky, W. and Epstein, S. S.,** Nitrosamines as environmental carcinogens, *Nature(London),* 225, 21, 1970.

196. **Bartsch, H., Camus, A. M., and Malaveille, C.,** Comparative mutagenicity of N-nitrosamines in semi-solid and in a liquid incubation system in the presence of human tissue fractions, *Mutat. Res.,* 37, 149—162, 1976.

197. **McLean, A. E. M., McLean, E. K., and Judah, D.,** Cellular necrosis in the liver induced and modified by drugs, *Int. Rev. Exp. Pathol.,* 4, 127—157, 1965.

198. **Solt, D. B., Medline, A., and Farber, E.,** Rapid emergence of carcinogen-induced hyperplastic lesions in a new model for the sequential analysis of liver carcinogenesis, *Am. J. Pathol.,* 88, 595—618, 1977.

199. **Zeiger, E. and Sheldon, A. T.,** The mutagenicity of heterocyclic N-nitrosamines for Salmonella Typhimurium, *Mutat. Res.,* 57, 1—10, 1978.

200. **Druckrey, H., Preussmann, R., and Ivanlovic, S.,** N-nitroso compounds in organotropic and transplacental carcinogenesis, *Ann. N.Y. Acad. Sci.,* 163, 676—695, 1969.

201. **Magee, P. N. and Farber, E.,** Toxic liver injury and carcinogenesis methylation of rat liver nucleic acids by dimethylnitrosamine *in vitro, Biochem. J.,* 83, 106—114, 1962.

202. **Goth, R. and Rajewsky, M. F.,** Persistence of *O*-6-ethylguanine in rat brain DNA: correlation with nervous system — specific carcinogenesis by ethylnitrosourea, *Proc. Natl. Acad. Sci. U.S.A.,* 71, 639—643, 1975.

203. **Magee, P. N.,** Covalent binding and endogenous incorporation as illustrated by nitroso carcinogens, *J. Toxicol. Environ. Health,* 2, 883—893, 1977.

204. **Natarajan, A. T., Tates, A. D., Van Buul, P. P. W., Meijers, M., and De Vogel, N.,** Cytogenetic effects of mutagens/carcinogens after activation in a microsomal system in vitro. I. Induction of chromosome aberrations and sister chromatid exchanges by diethylnitrosamine (DEN) and dimethylnitrosamine (DMN) in CHO cells in the presence of rat liver microsomes, *Mutat. Res.,* 37, 83—90, 1976.

205. **Montesano, R. M. and Magee, P. N.,** Metabolism of nitrosamines by rat and hamster tissue slices, *in vitro, Proc. Am. Assoc. Cancer Res.,* 12, 14, 1971.

206. **Wishnok, J. S., Archer, M. C., Edelman, A. S., and Rand, W. M.,** Nitrosamine carcinogenicity: A quantitative Hansch-Taft structure-activity relationship, *Chem.-Biol. Interactions,* 20, 43—54, 1978.

207. **Druckrey, H., Preussmann, R., Ivankovic, S., and Schmahl, D.,** Organotrope Carcinogene, Wirkungen bei 65 verschiedenen N-Nitroso-Verbindungen an BD-Ratten, *Z. Krebsforsch.,* 69, 103—201, 1967.

208. **McLean, A. E. M. and Verschuuren, H. G.,** Effects of diet and microsomal enzyme induction on the toxicity of dimethylnitrosamine, *Br. J. Exp. Pathol.,* 50, 22—25, 1969.

209. **Rogers, A. E.**, Dietary effects on carcinogenity of drugs and related compounds, in *Nutrition and Drug Interactions*, Nathcock, J. N. and Coon, J., Eds., Academic Press, New York, 1978, 505—542.

210. **Jakoby, H. P. and Baumann, C. A.**, The effect of fat on tumor formation, *Am. J. Cancer*, 39, 338—342, 1946.

211. **Tannenbaum, A.**, The genesis and growth of tumors. III. Effects of a high-fat diet, *Cancer Res.*, 2, 468—474, 1942.

212. **Silverstone, H. and Tannenbaum, A.**, Influence of thyroid hormone on the formation of induced skin tumors in mice, *Cancer Res.*, 9, 684—688, 1949.

213. **Silverstone, H. and Tannenbaum, A.**, The influence of dietary fat and riboflavin on the formation of spontaneous hepatomas in the mouse, *Cancer Res.*, 11, 442—446, 1951.

214. **Miller, J. A., Kline, B. E., Rusch, H. P., and Baumann, C. A.**, The effect of certain lipids on the carcinogenicity of *p*-dimethylaminoazobenzene, *Cancer Res.*, 4, 756—761, 1944.

215. **Nigro, N. D., Singh, D. U., Campbell, R. L., and Pak, M. S.**, Effect of dietary beef fat on intestinal tumor formation by azoxymethane in rats, *J. Natl. Cancer Inst.*, 54, 439—442, 1975.

216. **Reddy, B. S., Watanabe, K., and Weisburger, J. H.**, Effect of high-fat diet on colon carcinogenesis in F 344 rats treated with 1,2-dimethylhydrazine, methylazoxymethanol acetate, or methylnitrosourea, *Cancer Res.*, 37, 4156—4159, 1977.

217. **Mastromarino, A., Reddy, B. S., and Wynder, E. L.**, Metabolic epidemiology of colon cancer: enzymatic activity of fecal flora, *Am. J. Clin. Nutr.*, 29, 1455, 1976.

218. **McLean, A. E. M. and McLean, E. K.**, The effect of diet and 1,1,1-trichloro-2,2-bis-(*p*-chlorophenyl)-ethane (DDT) on microsomal hydroxylating enzymes and on sensitivity of rats to carbon tetrachloride poisoning, *Biochem. J.*, 100, 564—571, 1966.

219. **Swann, P. P. and McLean, A. E.**, Cellular injury and carcinogenesis. The effect of a protein-free high carbohydrate diet on the metabolism of dimethylnitrosamine, *Biochem. J.*, 124, 283—288, 1972.

220. **Boyd, E. N. and Dubois, I.**, Protein deficiency and tolerated oral doses of Endosulfan, *Arch. Int. Pharmacodyn. Ther.*, 178, 153—165, 1969.

221. **Magee, P. N. and Lee, K. Y.**, Cellular injury and carcinogenesis, *Biochem. J.*, 91, 35—42, 1964.

222. **Preston, R. S., Hayes, J. R., and Campbell, T. C.**, The effect of protein deficiency on the *in vivo* binding of aflatoxin B₁ to rat liver macromolecules, *Life Sci.*, 19, 1191—1198, 1976.

223. **Chu, E. W. and Malmgren, R. A.**, An inhibitory effect of vitamin A on the induction of tumors of forestomach and cervix in the Syrian hamster by carcinogenic polycyclic hydrocarbons, *Cancer Res.*, 25, 884—895, 1965.

224. **Kensler, C. J., Sugiura, K., Young, N. F., Halter, C. R., and Rhoads, C. P.**, Partial protection of rats by riboflavin with casein against liver cancer caused by dimethylaminoazobenzene, *Science*, 93, 308—310, 1941.

225. **Fare, G. and Howell, J. S.**, The effect of dietary copper on rat carcinogenesis by 3-methoxy dyes. I. Tumors induced at various sites by feeding 3-methoxy-4-aminoazobenzene and its *N*-methyl derivatives, *Cancer Res.*, 24, 1279—1284, 1964.

226. **Stoloff, L. and Friedman, L.**, Information bearing on the evaluation of the hazard to man from aflatoxin ingestion, *BAG Bulletin*, 6, 21—32, 1976.

227. **Newberne, P. M. and Rogers, A.**, Rat colon carcinomas associated with aflatoxin and marginal vitamin A, *J. Natl. Cancer Inst.*, 50, 439—448, 1973.

228. **Brown, J. P., Roehm, G. W., and Brown, R. J.**, Mutagenicity testing of certified food colours and related azo, xanthine and triphenylmethane dyes with the Salmonella/microsome system, *Mutat. Res.*, 56, 249—271, 1978.

229. **Wattenberg, L. W.**, Inhibitions of carcinogenic effects of diethylnitrosamine and 4-nitroquinoline-*N*-oxide by antioxidants, *Fed. Proc., Fed. Am. Soc. Exp. Biol.*, 31, 633, 1972.

230. **Wattenberg, L. W.**, Inhibition of carcinogenic and toxic effects of polycyclic hydrocarbons by phenolic antioxidants and ethoxyquin, *J. Natl. Cancer Inst.*, 48, 1425—1430, 1972.

Physical Performance and Behavior

NUTRITION AND WORK PERFORMANCE

V. R. Edgerton and Y. Ohira

INTRODUCTION

Although the search for an optimal diet for optimal performance has been continuing for many years. These studies have been limited in many cases. Too often the practiced diet has been based more on current fads rather than the solidity of the rationale and evidence which proclaims the benefits of a specific diet.

Based on scientifically sound data, one can surmise that there is no one optimal diet; if an individual absorbs the daily recommended proportions of nutrients, then further supplements, for the most part, will not improve work performance capacity. Indeed, excessive supplements can harm an individual's performance as well as general health.

Several nutritional factors have been related to specific types of work performances. These factors are, for the most part, the level of carbohydrate vs. fats and proteins in the diet, which alters the amount of substrate available for a given physical effort, and the capacity to transport oxygen to utilize the available substrates, which is largely dependent on the availability of iron from diet. Consequently, emphasis in this section will be placed on these two factors.

CARBOHYDRATES

It is evident that the level of carbohydrates and fats in a diet affects resting and work metabolism. Krogh and Lindhard[1] found an 11% waste of energy when fat rather than carbohydrates was combusted. It was also evident from this study that the resting postabsorptive respiratory quotient (RQ) which can be modified by the diet dictates to some degree the RQ that will be observed during steady work.[1] The 11% lower efficiency of metabolism of fat compared to carbohydrates is supported by Bierring,[2] who found an 8.3% difference. The calories per oxygen molecule used for combustion of carbohydrates is approximately 5.0 and 4.7 for the combustion of fat. About 10% more energy is utilizable for work from carbohydrates than from fat. Therefore, it can be estimated that a 15% reduction in oxygen requirement for a given amount of work is required if carbohydrates are used exclusively.[3]

Christensen et al.[3] found that subjects working at a rate of 1080 kg·m/min after a high-fat diet could work about 90 min, but work at the same rate was continued for more than 4 hr after a high-carbohydrate diet. On the fat diet, the RQ was 0.745, which means that approximately 30 g of carbohydrates was used. On the carbohydrate diet with an RQ of 0.900 in 90 min, it was calculated that about 180 g was catabolized. It was estimated that a man weighing 72 kg stores about 700 g of glycogen in all tissues,[4] and in 4 hr about 400 g is used.[3] These authors stated that blood glucose fell to 60 mg/100 ml or less when glycogen was depleted.

The experiments of Christensen et al.[3] in 1934 on the relationship of carbohydrates and work performance have been verified by numerous scientists and laboratories in the 1960s through the 1970s. The use of needle muscle biopsies has made it possible for muscle and liver glycogen and other related metabolites to be measured in humans after various diets and exercises.

Hultman and Bergström[5] demonstrated changes in quadriceps femoris muscle glycogen during starvation, during a high-fat and protein diet, and during a high-carbohydrate diet (Figure 1). Figures 2 and 3 demonstrate the effect of starvation, or carbohydrate-free diet followed by a high-carbohydrate diet, on muscle glycogen and the effect of exercise on the muscle glycogen in response to these two diets. It is clear from this study that (1) exercise reduces muscle glycogen; (2) starvation reduces muscle glycogen; (3) a carbohydrate-free diet reduces muscle glycogen; (4) exercise enhances glycogen to greater-than-normal resting values following its depletion by exercise, a carbohydrate-poor diet, or a starvation diet; and (5) the stimulation of glycogen synthesis after exercise is specific to the muscles that were depleted of glycogen.

In 1967 Bergström et al.[6] demonstrated the relationship between diet, muscle glycogen, and work time to exhaustion. The diet and tissue sampling protocol is shown in Figure 4 and the results are shown in Figure 5. Table 1 gives mean values for a number of work-related parameters before, during, and after exercise following a few days of a carbohydrate, a mixed, fast, or a protein diet. In regard to Table 1, it should be noted that the glycogen formation after the mixed diet is not comparable to the protein or carbohydrate diet because glycogen depletion did not precede the mixed diet.

The relationship between the muscle glycogen, diet, and performance in a 30-km cross-country race was demonstrated again by Karlsson and Saltin.[7] The time required to complete the 30-km race after the carbohydrate diet was 135.3 min compared to 143.0 min after a mixed diet.

The population distribution of quadriceps femoris glycogen concentrations in 228 normal subjects is shown in Figure 6.[8] Glycogen values as high as 5.2 g/100 g wet weight have been reported.[9]

Gollnick et al.[10] noted that the muscle fibers of subjects on a normal mixed diet had equal levels of glycogen in high and low ATPase-staining muscle fibers, but more intense glycogen staining was evident in the high ATPase (presumably fast twitch) fibers after a high carbohydrate diet.

Although the relationship between the carbohydrates combusted and the glycogen lost from muscles during exercise at about 75% of the maximal capacity of oxygen consumption ($\dot{V}_{o2}$ max) is very close (Figure 7), blood glucose is an important factor in the length of time that one can work for a prolonged period. Christensen et al.[3] found that blood glucose was lowered during prolonged work and most of the subsequent studies have also found a consistent drop in blood glucose.[4,6,11,12] However, it cannot be stated that the hypoglycemia was the reason for the termination of the exercises. It is not known at what concentration or to the degree that blood glucose level affects performance. A decrease of only 5 to 10 mg/100 mℓ of glucose could be functionally significant at some workloads.

The recovery of normal blood glucose levels after exhaustive exercise is dependent on the diet. Subjects that practically deplete the muscle glycogen stores and are hypoglycemic at the end of an exercise have low glucose levels for more than 60 min after the exercise is completed if they are on a high fat and protein diet. Glucose infusion stimulates the resynthesis of glycogen in the exercised leg.[8,13] During the exercise, blood glucose is lowered more severely and quickly if the subject is on a fat and protein or mixed diet than when on a high-carbohydrate diet (Figure 8). Mean values of blood glucose, pyruvate, lactate, and RQ are shown in Figure 9. However, glucose infusion during exercise[8,13] does not seem to spare a loss of glycogen in muscle (Figure 10).

To summarize the dietary factors that modify blood glucose, it appears that carbohydrate ingestion during or after exercise and the type of diet several days prior to an exercise determine the level of change in blood glucose at a work intensity of about 75 to 85% of $\dot{V}_{o2}$ max which lasts for approximately 1 to 8 hr.

The mechanics involved in the rate of blood glucose and muscle glycogen utilization during prolonged exercise and the return to normal levels after exercise have been investigated. Pruett[14] tested the hypothesis that the exercise-induced hypoglycemia was due to elevated insulin levels which could occur in response to the reported rise in blood glucose in dogs soon after moderate intensity exercise is initiated. However, it was found in normal humans that insulin concentration decreased at a level similar to the drop in blood glucose during exercise intensities of 50 to 70% of $\dot{V}_{o_2}$ max. The resting blood glucose level was similar when the subjects were on a standard diet or a high-fat or high-carbohydrate diet (Table 2). Work at 20%, of $\dot{V}_{o_2}$ max caused a slight but significant drop in blood glucose following a standard or fat diet, but not a car-bohydrate diet.[14] At 50% of $\dot{V}_{o_2}$ max, blood glucose was lowered after all diets to 60% of the preexercise levels (Table 2). Blood glucose levels were similar after work at 50 and 70% of $\dot{V}_{o_2}$ max. It is interesting that in two subjects, the decrease in blood glucose was greater after the standard and carbohydrate diet than after the fat diet.[14] Figures 11 and 12 illustrate the effect of work intensity for up to 6 hr on plasma glucose and insulin after a standard diet. Figures 13 and 14 illustrate the effect of diet and work intensity on blood glucose and insulin levels during prolonged work.

It can be concluded from Pruett's[14] study that plasma insulin cannot account for the changes in blood glucose during exercise. This is not unexpected in light of the evidence that the mechanisms for glucose entry into the muscle seem to be different for insulin and muscle contraction.[15] It also seems that blood glucose alone does not control the plasma insulin levels.

Alteration in muscle glycogen levels during and after exercise is dependent at least in part on the regulation of glycogen synthetase.[16] At rest, 27% of the glycogen syn-thetase is in the I form, whereas 75% is in the I form after muscle glycogen is lowered by exercise.[16] Total glycogen synthetase activity is unchanged by a single bout of exer-cise (Figure 15). The overshoot of glycogen synthesis following exercised-induced gly-cogen is depletion and a high-carbohydrate diet seems to be independent of synthetase activity.[16]

Dietary factors can also affect physical performance due to its effect on liver glyco-gen as well as the effect it exerts via blood glucose and muscle glycogen. Hultman and Nilsson[17] have demonstrated the marked effect of diet on liver glycogen (Figure 16) and the effect of 1 hr of exercise at 75% of $\dot{V}_{o_2}$ max on liver glycogen (Figure 17). During heavy exercise up to 1100 mg/min of glucose was produced by the liver[17] and the blood glucose level was still decreased. These authors estimated that the mean liver carbohydrate used during an hour of exercise was 24 g/kg of liver or a total of 41 g assuming a liver weight of 1.7 kg.

PROTEIN

In a normally fed person, the energy used during exercise is derived totally, for all practical purposes, from carbohydrates and fats. However, this does not necessarily mean that protein intake is unimportant for one to enhance and maintain optimal physical performance. It is apparent that the rate of synthesis of some proteins is greater than the rate of degradation when one is successfully adapting to physical train-ing. Elevated protein levels are indicated, for example, by increases in the citric acid cycle, fatty acid oxidation enzyme activities, and myoglobin (Mb) concentration in skeletal muscle and hemoglobin (Hb) concentration in the blood.

The appropriate question to be answered is, how much dietary protein is optimal for a given tissue to maintain optimal function during growth and maintenance of normal cellular functions. Because the synthesis of many enzymic proteins as men-tioned above exceeds degradation, a greater amount of that protein is assimilated in muscular tissue during the process of adaptation to training. The specific protein that is elevated in a tissue depends on the nature of the physical training. If the training is characterized by high resistance overload, the muscle mass will increase indicating an overall increase of proteins in general. The additional protein will be predominantly myofibrillar. However, if the training is of an endurance nature, the net protein synthesis will be primarily mitochondrial protein. This type of training minimally affects total muscle size[18,19] and, perhaps, the overall total of proteins.

Apparently many people believe (but without scientifically sound support) that the supplementation of a normal diet with protein enhances one's capacity to adapt to a physical training regimen such as weightlifting. There is a scarcity of pertinent and useful information that suggests the desirability of protein supplementation of normal diets in order to enhance physical performance. It was shown in adult female rats that were exercised at a moderate intensity for up to 3 hr daily for 4 weeks that serum total protein, albumin, and globulin decreased.[20] It is highly unlikely that these serum changes would have any effect on physical performance. These serum components were reduced by a 3.8% casein (protein deficient) diet but not a 7.5 or 15.0% casein diet (Table 3). There were four training periods, each for 1 month, on the 5th, 7th, 9th, and 11th to 12th months of age, resulting in elevated DNA, RNA, and nitrogen concentration in the gastrocnemius muscles. Diets of casein concentrations of 3.8, 7.5, and 15.0 for the most part did not affect DNA, RNA, or nitrogen concentration (Table 4).

The quality as well as quantity of dietary protein can affect muscular growth. One of four diets was assigned to 25-day-old male rats for either 4, 8, or 12 weeks. The four diets consisted of 5.2 (C-1), 10.5 (C-2), 21.0% (C-3) casein, or a wheat diet supplemented with soybean meal and fishmeal (SW) which approximately equalled the amount of crude protein as in the 21.0% casein diet but differed in amino acid composition.[21] Weight gains for each subgroup are shown in Table 5. The weight gain after 12 weeks was as follows: SW>C-3>-C-2>C-1. Gastrocnemius weight, protein, RNA, and essential amino acids are shown in Table 6. In general, it can be seen that the quality as well as quantity of dietary protein affects muscle growth as reflected by mass, protein, RNA, and five amino acids. The amino acid response is shown in greater detail in Table 7.

Because adult humans have a positive nitrogen balance during training, it has been recommended by Yamaji[22,23] that 2.0 g/kg of protein of body weight resulted in a greater increase in body weight than a diet containing 1.0 to 1.5 g/kg. He also found that blood Hb and albumin levels initially decreased during training. Also, Teruoka and Saito[24] found a correlation between urinary nitrogen and intensity of work. Protein intake in humans ranging from 75 to 150 g/day had no effect on performance of intermittent work in a variety of environmental conditions.[25]

The qualitative factor of dietary protein has also been explored with respect to mental performance and selected enzyme activities of the cerebrum of rats. A low-protein diet (5% casein) for 6 to 25 weeks beginning with 4- to 5-week-old rats was found to depress some enzymes of the cerebrum and reduce learning performance. This enzymic effect was reversed almost completely by the addition of glutamic acid to the low-protein diet[26] as shown in Tables 8 to 10.

Gontzea et al.[27] presented evidence in a well controlled experiment on 30 normal, hospitalized young men ($\overline{X} = 25$ years of age and 68 kg body weight) which lasted for 28 to 52 days. Figure 18 compares the 24-hr N_2 balance of subjects on a diet of 1 g protein per kilogram body weight or 1.5 g/kg before, during, and after high energy expenditure training on a bicycle ergometer (400 to 900 kg; 8 to 10 kcal/min) several times a day. A negative N_2 balance was observed when the subjects were on a 1 g protein per kilogram diet and exercising but not on a 1.5 g/kg diet. The N_2 imbalance was related to elevated urea excretion and N_2 loss in sweat. Some have said that 40 to 50 g of protein per day for humans is adequate,[28-30] while others suggest that the protein intake should be in proportion to the total energy intake.[31]

LIPIDS

Lipids serve as a major energy source for skeletal muscle and are a more important substrate to the heart than skeletal muscle fibers. Although cholesterol,[32] triglycerides, and free fatty acids (FFA) are metabolized particularly during prolonged work,[33] there is no evidence that the availability of these substrates during exercise can be lowered to a critical level.

Diet can modify the utilization of FFA during exercise. For example, a high-fat low-carbohydrate diet and low-fat low-carbohydrate diet lowers RQ.[34] Glucose ingestion 2 hr before moderate exercise and a low-fat and carbohydrate diet causes RQ to increase during work. However, the links that have been made with changes in performance and diet have been more closely associated with carbohydrate than lipid metabolism.[34] Either a high-carbohydrate or a high-protein diet had no effect on untrained exhausted or trained exhausted run time in rats.[35] These diets did not affect citric acid cycle enzyme activities.

MINERALS

Iron

The effect of iron deficiency anemia has been studied rather intensively in the 1970s. Several major questions are related to the adequacy of iron in one's diet to support normal function. Is work performance affected by iron deficiency and/or anemia? If work performance is affected, what factors are involved? Is Hb concentration the critical component essential for normal function? How important are iron-containing components other than Hb, heme, or nonheme in determining work performance capacity? Data presented in the following tables and figures provide considerable insight into these questions.

Edgerton et al.[36] reported a series of four experiments related to work performance on iron-deficient anemic rats. Sprague-Dawley rats were made anemic with an iron-deficient diet or by injection of phenylhydrazine, a hemolytic agent. On 12 out of 13 occasions in four separate experiments, the performance of rats on an exhaustive endurance or sprint-run test on a motor-driven treadmill was directly related to their Hb concentration and hematocrit. The anemic rats on each occasion ran for a significantly shorter time than their control rats. On one occasion there was a difference in performance capacity after normal Hb levels were established in previously anemic rats. Furthermore, anemic rats that were housed individually in cages equipped with an adjoining activity wheel were voluntarily less active than their controls. Upon repletion to normal Hb levels, the difference in activity between the groups was eliminated. Performance, as gauged by a forced exhaustive run and by voluntary activity, seemed to be more closely related to Hb and packed cell volume (PCV) than Mb or cytochrome levels in skeletal or cardiac muscle.

Experiment 1 — Sixty male rats, 32 days old, were run to exhaustion on a motor-driven treadmill at a rate of 18 m/min. After ranking the rats in ascending order according to running performance, pairs of rats were assigned to one of two experimental groups. The rat with the shortest running time (R) in each pair was alternately assigned to the anemic or control group. The control group's diet was supplemented with 54.0 g of $Fe(NH_4)_2(SO_4)_2 \cdot 6 H_2O$/kg equivalent to 7.69 g Fe per gram diet throughout the 18 weeks of the experiment. The anemic group received no iron supplement until the end of week 10, at which time the period of iron repletion began with an iron supplement of 36.9 g of Fe per kilogram diet. This level of supplementation was changed to 18.5, 9.2, 7.7, and 18.5 g/kg diet at the end of weeks 12, 14, 15, and 17, respectively. During weeks 10 and 18, each rat's capacity to run on a motor-driven treadmill at a rate of 52 m/min was determined and 3 days later they were tested again at a speed of 44 m/min. The rate of running was increased relative to R_1 to accommodate for maturation of the rats by week 10 (Figure 19, Table 11).

Experiment 2 — Sixty male rats, 18 days old, were randomly divided into three groups and housed in plastic cages (27 × 12 × 15 cm). For the first 2.5 weeks of the experiment, the control group's diet was supplemented with 54.0 g of $Fe(NH_4)_2$ $(SO_4)_2 \cdot 6 H_2O$ per kilogram diet (7.69 g Fe per kilogram diet) and moderate anemic rats were unsupplemented. Thereafter, the control group's diet was supplemented with only 1.68 g $Fe(NH_4)_2$ $(SO_4)_6 \cdot H_2O$ per kilogram diet (239 mg Fe per kilogram diet). During the 7.5-week-long depletion phase of the experiment, the moderate anemic group received a single iron dose of 5.40 g/kg diet (769 mg Fe per kilogram diet) so that this group's mean Hb and PCV would be intermediate between control values and third group (severe anemics) whose diet was never supplemented during the depletion phase of the study. After 7 weeks on the respective diets, each rat's capacity to run on a motor-driven treadmill was tested at a rate of 35 m/min (R_1) and 3 days later at 52 m/min (R_2). The iron supplement phase was begun immediately following R_2. At the commencement of the 4-week iron supplement phase (week 8), all three groups were maintained on McCall's[37] diet supplemented with 230 mg Fe per kilogram diet. The same procedures for measuring the two running capacities were repeated at the end of 11 weeks (R_3, R_4) (Figure 20, Table 12).

Experiment 3 — Twenty seven male rats, 18 days old, were divided into three groups of nine which were identified as control, phenylhydrazine, and iron deficient. The diets of the control and phenylhydrazine groups were supplemented with 239 mg Fe per kilogram diet throughout the study. In addition, the diet of the iron-deficient group was supplemented on 3 days (days 8, 9, and 38) with 239 mg Fe per kilogram diet in an effort to keep the mean Hb level close to 9.0 g/100 mℓ. The animals were housed as described in Experiment 2. On day 46, the rats of the phenylhydrazine group were injected subcutaneously with 1.0 mℓ of 1.5% phenylhydrazine. Three separate injections were given at 48-hr intervals. Blood samples were taken from all animals on the day after the final injection; 24 hr later, all rats were run at a rate of 27 m/min to exhaustion. The heart, soleus, and gastrocnemius muscles were frozen for not more than 2 weeks before Mb and cytochrome contents were determined (Figure 21, Table 13).

Experiment 4 — Twenty four male rats, 18 days old, were randomly divided into three groups of eight and housed individually in 12 × 12 × 23 cm cages equipped with an adjacent rotating wheel. The control and phenylhydrazine groups' diets were supplemented with 239 mg Fe per kilogram diet throughout the experiment. The iron-deficient group's diet was not supplemented with iron during the anemic phase of the study (7 weeks), but received 239 mg Fe per kilogram diet for the 2-week repletion phase. Treatment of the phenylhydrazine group consisted of 0.18 mℓ of 2% phenylhydrazine subcutaneously injected on days 26, 29, 48, and 49 of the study, while half of this dosage was administered on days 36 and 39. All rats were exposed to a 5-min training run at 27 m/min on the day before, then forced performance capacity was determined at rates of 27 (R_1) and 35 (R_{2-4}) m/min on experimental days 50, 54, 57, and 61, respectively (Figure 22, Table 14).

The duration of iron deficiency anemia did not appear to be as important a determining factor as the level of anemia in forced performance. As clearly demonstrated in Figures 19 to 22 and Tables 11 to 14, the severity of anemia at the time of the running test was closely related to performance levels. For example, the moderately anemic rats in Experiment 1 and moderately and severely anemic rats in Experiment 2 having 11, 13, and 5 g of Hb per 100 mℓ displayed a 53, 22, and 72% performance decrement, respectively, at 52 m/min. The close relationship of Hb level to work performance was also demonstrated by the quick recovery of performance upon repletion of normal Hb levels (Figure 22 and Table 14). Short-term phenylhydrazine-induced anemia (Experiment 3) yielded performance measures similar to those found with a diet-induced iron-deficient anemia. However, long-term phenylhydrazine injections (Experiment 4) did affect Mb and cytochromes and altered the relationship of Hb to run time (Table 13). This suggested that long-term phenylhydrazine injections did not merely affect the blood but also depleted tissue iron.

At both the faster and slower rates of running, the anemic rats' times were approximately half that of the control rats (Table 11). After iron repletion, the run times were practically identical when tested at the greater speed, but the anemic-repleted rats' run times were significantly less than the controls at the slower speed (12 vs. 9 min). This difference in running capacity at the slower speed, along with the finding that the anemic rats' PCV and Hb reached control levels with some difficulty, suggests that the rats were perhaps adversely affected in subtle measures not manifest in Hb concentration. A marked increase in run time (R_2) 3 days after iron therapy occurred in the phenylhydrazine but not in the iron-deficient group (Table 14). It is doubtful that the Hb change also could account for the increased R_2 over R_1 in the phenylhydrazine group.

Physical work capacity of iron-deficient and anemic rats can return to normal within 3 days of initiation of dietary iron repletion, even though Hb concentration is not completely returned to control levels by this time (Figures 22 and 23 and Table 14). Rakušan[38] reported that the Hb concentration of anemic rats reached near normal values after 3 weeks of feeding a normal diet, while P_{50} values were still higher than normal. This suggests that red blood cell 2,3-diphosphoglycerate (2,3-DPG) levels were still elevated at least 3 weeks after initiation of dietary iron therapy.

Because anemia markedly limits the oxygen-carrying capacity of the blood[38-40] and also lowers the work capacity,[36,41-43] one would expect lactate production at a given work load to be inversely related to the Hb level. For similar reasons, postexercise blood pH after a standard muscular work test was higher after Hb concentration increased in human subjects.

To determine the relationship between Hb levels and physical work capacity, changes in Hb concentration and exhaustive run time before and during 15 days of dietary iron therapy were studied in five anemic rats. In addition, venous blood 2,3-DPG lactate, and pH levels were determined following 10-min treadmill runs (27 m/min) to assess the metabolic reponse to work. By the 3rd day of iron therapy, run times to exhaustion increased to normal levels (Figure 23). In contrast, postexercise 2,3-DPG, lactate, and pH values were not normal until the 8th day of repletion and Hb levels reached control values between the 8th and 15th day. The pH values of Andersen and Staven[44] suggest an even longer time required to return to normal. The overall correlation coefficients between Hb and 2,3-DPG levels and lactate and pH values were -0.76 and -0.91, respectively, while those for all other measures were much lower (Figure 24). The improvement in run time to exhaustion prior to changes in Hb concentration suggests that other iron-dependent factors are capable of improving the work capacity of anemic rats.

The fact that work performance capacity increased to a normal level prior to any significant changes in Hb or 2,3-DPG concentration (Figure 23) suggests that there may be other iron-dependent factors that affect physical performance in iron-deficient anemic rats besides Hb and 2,3-DPG. Both muscle Mb[45] and cytochrome[46] concentrations are related to prolonged running capacity, but the turnover rates of Mb and cytochromes are generally thought to be too slow to change significantly within 3 days.[47] However, even if they did increase, they had no apparent effect on the muscles' metabolism during exercise since blood pH and lactate responses to the standard exercise tests after 3 days of iron therapy were the same as before iron therapy began. However, physical performance capacity as shown by an exhaustive run time was normal after 3 days of dietary iron treatment, as has been observed previously.[36,48]

The lactate production at a given workload was less following improvement in physical work capacity.[49,50] However, the failure of blood lactate and pH values, such as those of Hb and 2,3-DPG, to change in parallel with run times indicates that performance was affected by factors other than those typically associated with the stress of exercise. Furthermore, on the 8th and 15th day after iron repletion began, performance did not differ significantly from the 3rd day, even though it was during this time that postexercise Hb, 2,3-DPG, lactate, and pH values returned to control levels.

It seems that during dietary iron repletion of anemic rats, increased performance and decreased acid-base balance disturbance after a given workload are due to the increased oxygen-carrying capacity and buffering capacity of the blood. However, prior to the normalization of blood parameters, some unknown factors related to iron treatment act immediately to improve the physical performance ability.

Finch et al,[48] evaluated work performance of normal and iron deficient rats. They found that iron deficient anemic rats had impaired work performances even after the anemia was corrected by exchange transfusion. The capacity of the mitochondria from the muscles of iron deficient anemic rats to metabolize pyruvate malate, and succinate was not affected but the capacity to oxidize α-glycerophosphate was. This iron deficient effect was explored further by Finch et al,[51] as shown in Table 16. They found no difference in mean arterial PO_2 before and immediately after a 2-min fast run in iron-deficient but not anemic rats (transfused). The vena caval blood PO_2 and PCO_2 was lower in iron deficient than control rats. Blood lactate was also higher at rest and after exercise. The close relationship of α-glycerophosphate oxidation and work performance was also confirmed in this study (Table 17).

Weanling rats have been used in most studies designed to determine the effects of an iron-deficient diet on work performance and/or selected tissue parameters. In adult rats, neither the actual cytochrome oxidase activity nor Mb concentration was lowered when the rats were placed on an iron-deficient diet.[52] In weanling rats placed on an iron-deficient diet, the normal rate of increase of Mb and cytochrome concentration in muscles is less.[47]

An appropriate question is whether an iron-deficient diet results in a decrease in muscle Mb or cytochrome oxidase in adult animals. The following study was designed to answer this question and to determine the degree that iron-deficient animals can adapt during prolonged periods with inadequate dietary iron.[52]

Male Sprague-Dawley rats (350 to 400 g) were fed McCall's[37] iron-deficient diet. The food for the control rats was supplemented with 19.7 g of $Fe(NH_4)_2(SO_4)_2 \cdot 6 H_2O$ per kilogram diet. The animals assigned to the anemic group were bled from the external jugular vein in order to lower Hb concentrations to 8.0 g/100 mℓ. The volume of blood removed was replaced with 6% dextran. The control group was similarly bled but the blood was returned i.p. After the animals were maintained for the prescribed periods ranging from 3 days to 5 months, work capacity on a treadmill and a treadmill run in which all animals ran for the same period at the same load was administered. The data are present in Table 18.

In general, the data in Table 18 demonstrate that

1. The duration of being iron deficient and moderately anemic from 3 days to 5 months does not affect work capacity.
2. The postexercise blood lactate response is similar over time, also suggesting no significant metabolic adaptation to the iron deficiency anemia for up to 5 months.

3. Blood 2,3-DPG was elevated by the anemia at 5 months but not at 1 month or less.
4. Myoglobin or cytochrome oxidase in muscles that characteristically have either a low oxidative or high oxidative metabolism was not affected by the iron deficiency anemia.

It is often thought that an iron-deficient anemic person will have the expected clinical symptoms of weakness, tiredness, and tachycardia. The following study was designed to determine whether or not the level of voluntary activity was affected in rats by the induction of anemia in adult rats by bleeding.[57] A control group consisted of ten rats in which 6 mℓ of blood was removed retroorbitally and the blood was immediately returned i.p. The anemic group was treated in the same way except that plasma and saline equaling the volume of whole blood removed was returned i.p. All rats were fed McCall's[37] iron-deficient diet but the control rats received an iron supplement (19.7 g $Fe(NH_4)_2(SO_4)_2 \cdot 6H_2O$ per kilogram of diet).

Hemoglobin concentration and voluntary activity over a period of 17 weeks are shown in Figure 25. The relationship of Hb to exhaustive run time is shown in Figure 26. Figure 27 illustrates the percent change in voluntary activity that occurred per gram of Hb change. The effect of anemia on muscular fatigue properties is shown in Figure 28.

These data illustrate the following points:

1. Voluntary activity is dependent on Hb and is seemingly independent of the length of time that the anemia is maintained. An Hb level of less than 12 g seems to be critical in terms of depressing the level of voluntary activity.
2. The severity of the anemia is reflected in the severity of the effect on voluntary activity.
3. The *in situ* gastrocnemius muscle preparation with its blood supply intact is more fatiguable in the anemic than control rats.

The effect of Hb concentration on work performance was also demonstrated by Wranne and Woodson.[58] The Hb level was controlled by transferring whole blood or plasma in normal rats in which the jugular vein had been cannulated. They found that a 10% depression of Hb would cause a 10% decrease in the length of time that rats could run on a treadmill (Figure 29).

Anemia is associated with an elevation in red blood cell 2,3-DPG concentration which decreases the affinity of Hb to O_2; work performance could be affected by this affinity change. This is suggested by data presented in Figure 30 in which 2,3-DPG was reduced by bisulfite so that the P_{50} of the blood was reduced by 13 mm Hg. Work performance was reduced by 9%.[53]

The effect of iron deficiency anemia on work performance in humans has also been studied.[59] The relationship of Hb concentration and work performance on a treadmill is shown in Figure 31. Figure 32 illustrates the workload-heart rate relationships in subjects with varying Hb concentrations. Figure 33 shows the relationship of Hb and the percent effect on heart rate. Figure 34 shows that the lower the Hb the higher the postexercise venous blood lactate in spite of the fact that the more anemic subjects worked for a shorter period and reached a lower workload. Figure 35 shows the relationship of muscle Mb and Hb of subjects of the same population as studied for Figures 31 to 34. Although there is a significant relationship ($r = 0.46$, $P < 0.05$), considerable variation exists between these two variables. Figure 36[60] illustrates a similar effect as shown in Figure 31. Figure 36 shows that the more anemic subjects performed the poorest on the Harvard Step Test which is based on the heart rate response to exercise.

The response of moderately (for 360 days) and severely (for 210 days) iron-deficient and anemic rats to treadmill exercise and their ability to exchange O_2 and CO_2 is shown in Figures 37 to 41.[61] These data are supportive of previous reports, but they also suggest that the rate of O_2 consumption is depressed in an iron-deficient rat at a given submaximal workload (Figures 38,39, and 42).[61] Acute and established anemia (2 weeks) has also been studied with respect to ventilatory and cardiovascular responses (Table 19).[62]

Further insight into the effects of iron deficiency anemia has been gained by determining the effects of iron treatment. The Hb response to i.v. total dose infusion of iron is shown in Figure 43. It illustrates the difference in rate of improvement of Hb as a function of the initial Hb level. Figure 44[63] demonstrates that performance can be improved 4 days after iron dextran (Imferon®) is injected i.v. However, the effect of iron deficiency without anemia on performance is less obvious.

The effect of transfusion on work capacity in humans is shown in Figure 45. This illustrates that work performance is affected immediately and in proportion to the change in Hb.

Iron treatment seems to affect the heart rate response to exercise independently of the Hb effect. Figure 46[64] shows that the heart rate at a given workload is lower in a subject treated with iron dextran than in subjects with the same Hb levels but had not been treated or had received a blood transfusion so that Hb level was the same as in the iron treated subject. Similarly, a non-Hb-related effect has been shown on the rate of O_2 consumption in iron-deficient rats (Figure 42). In humans it was shown that subjects with a low Hb and serum iron have a lower work capacity than subjects with low Hb and high serum iron (Figure 47).

Thirty six healthy female volunteers between the age of 18 and 35 years were divided into four groups to test the effect of training and iron supplements on serum iron and work performance.[65] The groups were

1. Nontrained, placebo supplement
2. Nontrained, iron supplement
3. Trained, placebo supplement
4. Trained, iron supplement.

Training groups trained 20 min a day, 3 days a week for 7 weeks using a bicycle ergometer at a workload equivalent to 70% of $\dot{V}_{o2}$ max obtained in pre-test. Nontrained groups maintained their regular daily activities without any physical training. Iron treatment groups received 18 mg of iron every day and placebo groups received a pill containing identical components but lacking iron (double-blind). All of the subjects were required to maintain their regular diets. Physical training seemed to affect serum iron. Sedentary women placed on a moderate training program had significantly lower serum iron levels than nontrained subjects (Figure 48). In this same study trained subjects that received iron supplementation had improved $\dot{V}_{o2}$ max significantly but trained and unsupplemented subjects did not (Figure 49).

Work productivity has also been tested as it relates to iron deficiency anemia.[66] A significant increase in the amount of tea picked per day was found within a month after iron treatment of moderate to severe iron-deficient workers from Sri Lanka (Figure 50). In addition, when the voluntary activity of iron-deficient anemic subjects that worked daily on a tea estate in Sri Lanka was monitored, it was found that their activity increased significantly within 2 to 3 weeks of initiation of iron treatment (Figure 51). These subjects were compared to placebo treated subjects.

VITAMINS

In 1960, Mayer and Bullen[62] reviewed a sizeable number of reports which support the general view that a number of vitamin deficiencies affect maximal work capacity, but intakes greater than a minimum recommended level do not elevate work capacity above normal levels.[67-71]

ACKNOWLEDGMENTS

We would like to thank D. R. Simpson, B. J. Koziol, and G. W. Gardner for their efforts in the collection and synthesis of much of the data included in this section.

Table 1
STATISTICAL TREATMENT: MEAN VALUES ± STANDARD OF ERROR OF DATA OBTAINED BEFORE, DURING, AND AFTER WORK FOLLOWING THE THREE DIETS[a]

		n	Carbohydrate diet (C)	Mixed diet (M)	Protein-fat diet (P)	C—M[b]	C—P[b]	M—P[b]
Muscle glycogen (g/100 g)	Before work	9	3.31 ± 0.30	1.75 ± 0.15	0.63 ± 0.10	<0.001	<0.001	<0.001
	After work	9	0.43 ± 0.06	0.17 ± 0.05	0.13 ± 0.05	<0.01	<0.01	>0.1
Work time (min)		9	166.5 ± 17.8	113.6 ± 5.3	56.9 ± 1.7	<0.01	<0.001	<0.001
Utilized carbohydrate (g)	During work	9	481.5 ± 47.1	306.4 ± 27.4	85.1 ± 10.1	<0.005	<0.001	<0.001
Oxygen uptake (l/min)		9	3.16 ± 0.14	3.24 ± 0.15	3.17 ± 0.15	>0.1	>0.1	>0.1
Blood pyruvate (mM/l)	At rest	6	0.163 ± 0.011	0.120 ± 0.003	0.092 ± 0.008	<0.05	<0.01	<0.05
	After 30 min work	6	0.238 ± 0.025	0.237 ± 0.011	0.187 ± 0.017	>0.1	<0.05	<0.05
	At end of work	6	0.228 ± 0.038	0.178 ± 0.017	0.185 ± 0.020	>0.1	>0.1	>0.1
Blood lactate (mM/l)	At rest	6	1.73 ± 0.17	1.02 ± 0.16	0.75 ± 0.17	<0.05	<0.01	>0.1
	After 30 min work	6	4.92 ± 0.74	5.22 ± 0.91	2.45 ± 0.18	>0.1	<0.01	<0.01
	At end of work	6	3.61 ± 0.74	2.65 ± 0.53	2.38 ± 0.24	<0.05	<0.05	>0.1
Respiratory quotient	At rest	6	0.943 ± 0.024	0.815 ± 0.004	0.743 ± 0.029	<0.01	<0.01	<0.05
	After 30 min work	6	0.942 ± 0.009	0.915 ± 0.007	0.813 ± 0.009	<0.01	<0.01	<0.01
	At end of work	6	0.918 ± 0.012	0.882 ± 0.020	0.795 ± 0.014	<0.01	<0.01	<0.01
Blood glucose (mg/100 ml)	At rest	6	91.7 ± 5.9	76.8 ± 4.5	84.3 ± 4.0	>0.1	>0.1	>0.1
	After 45 min work	5	77.3 ± 5.4	76.3 ± 8.6	52.6 ± 2.6	>0.1	<0.05	<0.05
	At end of work	6	63.3 ± 2.1	53.8 ± 6.2	50.7 ± 10.8	>0.1	>0.1	>0.1

[a]   Probability calculated on paired t-test of intra-individual differences after the three diets.
[b]   Probabilities of mean differences occurring between the three combinations of diets for each parameter measured.

From Bergström, J., Hermansen, L., Hultman, E., and Saltin, B., *Acta Physiol. Scand.*, 71, 140—150, 1967. With permission.

Table 2
CHANGES IN BLOOD PARAMETERS ASSOCIATED WITH
WORK AND DIET

Diet	Rest	20% of $\dot{V}_{o2}$ Max	50% of $\dot{V}_{o2}$ Max	70% of $\dot{V}_{o2}$ Max
Blood glucose level at end of work (mg/100 ml)				
Standard[a]	96.2 ± 3.8	90.6 ± 3.4	62.0 ± 6.3	62.5 ± 3.2
Prob (n)	<0.3 (7)	<0.02 (7)	<0.001 (7)	<0.001 (8)
High fat	93.5 ± 4.6	94.5 ± 2.4	61.3 ± 3.2	74.4 ± 12.3
Prob (n)	<0.2 (5)	<0.05 (5)	<0.001 (5)	<0.05 (5)
High carbohydrate	102.2 ± 4.5	98.5 ± 4.4	60.6 ± 7.6	62.0 ± 8.8
Prob (n)	<0.7 (5)	<0.8 (5)	<0.001 (5)	<0.01 (5)
Blood glucose level 15 min after work (mg/100 ml)				
Standard		99.8 ± 5.5	69.6 ± 5.4	77.4 ± 5.6
Prob (n)		<0.05 (7)	<0.001 (7)	<0.001 (8)
High fat		106.6 ± 5.9	73.9 ± 3.5	85.2 ± 9.3
Prob (n)		<0.05 (5)	<0.05 (5)	<0.1 (5)
High carbohydrate		109.1 ± 6.7	72.3 ± 6.0	74.1 ± 9.5
Prob (n)		<0.01 (5)	<0.02 (5)	<0.01 (5)
Plasma insulin (IRI) level at end of work (μU/ml)				
Standard	82.9 ± 10.0	81.0 ± 3.4	59.9 ± 6.7	57.5 ± 6.4
Prob (n)	<0.2 (6)	<0.001 (6)	<0.001 (6)	<0.001 (7)
High fat	88.7 ± 6.2	62.2 ± 9.9	55.1 ± 7.7	64.4 ± 11.7
Prob(n)	<0.1 (5)	<0.01 (5)	<0.01 (5)	<0.01 (5)
High carbohydrate	79.9 ± 7.7	87.4 ± 21.3	66.4 ± 8.5	62.1 ± 6.8
Prob (n)	<0.02 (5)	<0.6 (5)	<0.01 (5)	<0.001 (5)
Plasma insulin (IRI) level 15 min after work (μU/ml)				
Standard		92.2 ± 7.5	56.3 ± 6.2	64.7 ± 7.4
Prob (n)		<0.1 (6)	<0.5 (6)	<0.01 (7)
High fat		66.9 ± 7.2	58.2 ± 6.6	74.5 ± 5.7
Prob (n)		<0.6 (5)	<0.7 (5)	<0.9 (5)
High carbohydrate		94.1 ± 21.3	60.9 ± 12.0	63.0 ± 8.4
Prob (n)		<0.8 (5)	<0.4 (5)	<0.01 (5)

[a] Values are expressed as means $\pm$ SEM. The number of subjects that appear in the parentheses follows the probability value.

From Pruett, E. D. R., *J. Appl. Physiol.*, 28, 199—208, 1970. With permission.

Table 3
EFFECT OF EXERCISE, DIETARY PROTEIN LEVEL, AND CONDITIONING ON TOTAL SERUM PROTEINS, ALBUMIN, GLOBULINS, AND ALBUMIN-TO-GLOBULIN (A/G) RATIOS OF ADULT FEMALE RATS[a]

Treatment group	n	Total serum protein (g/100 ml)	Albumin (g/100 ml)	Serum globulin (g/100ml)	A/G ratio (g/100 ml)
No exercise	18	6.57	2.65	3.92	0.68
Exercise	18	6.00[b]	2.30[b]	3.70[b]	0.63[b]
15% casein diet	12	6.44	2.50	3.94	0.65[a,b]
7.5% casein diet	12	6.49	2.67	3.82	0.70[b]
3.75% casein diet	12	5.92[b]	2.25[b]	3.67	0.62
Not conditioned (10.5 months old)	12	6.08	2.45	3.63	0.68
Not conditioned (11.5 months old)	12	6.10	2.48	3.62	0.68
Preconditioned (12.5 months old)	12	6.68[b]	2.51	4.17[b]	0.61[b]

[a]   Means within a column and treatment group are not significantly different (P < 0.05) if followed by the same superscript.

[b]   The mean is significantly different from the others within the column with no footnote.

From Christensen, D. A. and Crampton, E. W., *J. Nutr.*, 86, 369—375, 1965. With permission.

Table 4
EFFECT OF EXERCISE, DIETARY PROTEIN LEVEL AND CONDITIONING ON AMOUNTS OF DNA, RNA AND NITROGEN IN THE LIVER, MUSCLE, AND SKIN OF ADULT FEMALE RATS

Treatment group	n	Liver (mg/liver)				Muscle (mg/both gastrocnemii)				Skin (mg/sample)		
		DNA	RNA	Nitrogen		DNA	RNA	Nitrogen		DNA	RNA	Nitrogen
No exercise	18	22.9	93	262		4.0	27.2	111		10.8	32.6	362
Exercise	18	20.4	81[a]	253		4.5[a]	30.2[a]	124[a]		10.8	34.2	377
15% casein diet	12	21.5	85	274		4.3	29.2	121		10.5	31.9	341
7.5% casein diet	12	21.1	92	267		4.4	29.0	117		10.7	34.4	379
3.75% casein diet	12	22.5	84	231		4.0	27.9	114		11.2	34.0	389
Not conditioned (10.5 months old)	12	20.3	77	244		4.0	27.8	114		10.3	33.1	360
Not conditioned (11.5 months old)	12	20.2	83	230		4.0	27.7	114		10.9	35.3	387
Preconditioned (12.5 months old)	12	24.5[a]	102[a]	297[a]		4.7[a]	30.6[a]	125[a]		11.1	31.5	357

[a] Means within a column and treatment group that are significantly different (P < 0.05) from the other means of that column.

From Christensen, D. A. and Crampton, E. W., *J. Nutr.*, 86, 369—375, 1965. With permission.

Table 5

WEIGHT GAIN (g)[a] OF RATS FED CASEIN AND
SUPPLEMENTED WHEAT (SW) DIETS FOR 4, 8,
AND 12 WEEKS COMPARED WITH THE INITIAL
WEIGHT

Weeks on diet	Diet[b]			
	C_1	C_2	C_3	SW
4	43.8 (300)[c]	115.6 (390)	159.8 (445)	181.8 (510)
8	91.6 (700)	225.8 (970)	307.4 (1103)	304.0 (1120)
12	114.4 (1134)	348.0 (1776)	384.6 (1745)	428.6 (1978)

Note: Each value represents the mean of four rats.

[a] Significantly different for diet, time and diet × time at $P < 0.01$.
[b] C_1, C_2, C_3 represent the diets containing 5.2, 10.5, and 21.0% casein respectively.
[c] The amount of diet (g) consumed is bracketed.

From Giovannetti, P. M. and Stothers, S. C., *Growth*, 39, 1—16, 1975. With permission.

Table 6
GASTROCNEMII WEIGHT, CONCENTRATION AND ACCUMULATION OF RIBONUCLEIC ACID (RNA), PROTEIN AND FREE ESSENTIAL AMINO ACIDS (EAA) OF RATS FED CASEIN OR SUPPLEMENTED WHEAT (SW) DIETS FOR 4, 8, AND 12 WEEKS

Diet[a]	Weeks on diet	mg/g fresh muscle		Per muscle pair				Ratio of protein: RNA
		RNA	Protein	Weight (g)	RNA (mg)	Protein (g)	EAA (mg)	
	0	1.47	167	0.59	0.88	0.10	0.32	113
C_1	4	1.03	185	0.90	0.94	0.17	0.51	179
	8	0.95	202	1.61	1.54	0.32	0.84	213
	12	0.89	209	1.77	1.59	0.37	0.63	232
C_2	4	1.28	188	1.87	2.40	0.35	1.04	147
	8	1.02	204	3.10	3.12	0.63	1.43	200
	12	0.92	201	3.90	3.63	0.78	1.38	218
C_3	4	1.36	192	2.42	3.27	0.46	1.51	141
	8	1.00	216	3.98	4.00	0.86	1.72	216
	12	0.95	215	4.50	4.33	0.97	1.84	226
SW	4	1.31	209	2.61	3.44	0.54	0.76	151
	8	0.91	211	4.29	3.88	0.90	1.25	231
	12	0.83	209	4.58	3.85	0.96	1.11	225
Significance of effects of								
Diet		$P < 0.01$	NS[b]	$P < 0.01$	$P < 0.01$	$P < 0.01$	$P < 0.01$	$P < 0.01$
Time		$P < 0.01$	$P < 0.05$	$P < 0.01$	$P < 0.01$	$P < 0.01$	$P < 0.01$	$P < 0.01$
Diet × time		$P < 0.01$	NS	$P < 0.01$	NS	$P < 0.01$	NS	$P < 0.01$

Note: Each value represents the mean of four rats.

[a] C_1, C_2, and C_3 represent the diets containing 5.2, 10.5, and 21.0% casein respectively.

[b] Not significant.

From Giovannetti, P. M. and Stothers, S. C., *Growth,* 39, 1—16, 1975. With permission.

Table 7

SUMMARY OF NINHYDRIN-REACTING SUBSTANCES FROM RAT GASTROCNEMII AS AFFECTED BY TYPE OF DIET AND LENGTH OF TIME ON DIET

Diet[a]	Weeks on diet	Ninhydrin-reacting substances (μ mol/g fresh muscle)									
		Alanine	Arginine	Aspartic acid	Citrulline	Glutamic acid	Glycine	Histidine	Isoleucine	Leucine	Lysine
	0	3.227	0.293	0.657	0.362	5.722	6.020	0.388	0.168	0.295	2.274
C_1	4	4.690	0.288	0.417	0.339	4.568	1.942	0.405	0.150	0.306	1.566
	8	4.736	0.111	0.367	0.329	3.124	2.108	0.453	0.124	0.212	1.524
	12	4.071	0.104	0.376	0.293	2.048	2.517	0.343	0.131	0.213	0.449
C_2	4	4.413	0.105	0.634	0.239	6.143	2.446	0.350	0.152	0.267	1.417
	8	4.302	0.156	0.530	0.208	3.565	1.932	0.296	0.135	0.214	0.791
	12	3.496	0.103	0.483	0.134	2.150	1.508	0.224	0.170	0.261	0.440
C_3	4	4.352	0.135	0.841	0.240	6.899	1.375	0.326	0.178	0.331	1.287
	8	3.237	0.130	0.462	0.130	2.326	0.978	0.254	0.177	0.268	0.958
	12	2.931	0.126	0.442	0.132	1.938	1.018	0.202	0.158	0.254	0.964
SW	4	2.902	0.154	0.567	0.209	4.192	3.977	0.193	0.147	0.230	0.330
	8	2.513	0.159	0.512	0.141	2.086	2.524	0.185	0.137	0.200	0.519
	12	2.460	0.146	0.491	0.124	1.846	2.113	0.179	0.124	0.208	0.256
Significance of effects of											
Diet		$P < 0.01$	NS	$P < 0.01$	$P < 0.01$	$P < 0.01$	$P < 0.01$	$P < 0.01$	$P < 0.05$	$P < 0.05$	$P < 0.01$
Time		$P < 0.01$	$P < 0.05$	$P < 0.01$	$P < 0.01$	$P < 0.01$	$P < 0.01$	$P < 0.05$	NS	$P < 0.01$	$P < 0.05$
Diet × Time		NS	$P < 0.01$	$P < 0.05$	NS	$P < 0.01$	$P < 0.01$	NS	NS	NS	$P < 0.05$

Note: Each value represents the mean of four rats.

[a] C_1, C_2, and C_3 represent the diets containing 5.2, 10.5, and 21.0% casein respectively.

[b] Not significant.

From Giovannetti, P. M. and Stothers, S. C., *Growth*, 39, 1—16, 1975. With permission.

Table 8
WEIGHT GAIN, WEIGHT OF CEREBRUM, AND THE ACTIVITIES OF CERTAIN CEREBRAL ENZYMES[a] IN RATS FED LOW- AND HIGH-PROTEIN DIETS[b]

Group	Weight gain (g/week) Experiment I, (fed ad libitum for 25 weeks) — First 6 weeks	Total period	Experiment II (pair fed for 6 weeks)	Wt of cerebrum (g) Experiment I	Experiment II	L-Glutamate-NAD-oxidoreductase Experiment I	Experiment II	L-Glutamate-1-carboxy-lyase Experiment I	Experiment II	4-Aminobutyrate-2-oxoglutarate aminotransferase Experiment I	Experiment II
1. 5% casein	2.6 ± 0.4	1.6 ± 0.2	4.5 ± 0.2	1.00 ± 0.04	0.98 ± 0.02	1.46 ± 0.097	1.40 ± 0.110	14 ± 1.1	12 ± 0.7	28 ± 0.3	32 ± 2.8
2. 5% casein (niacin omitted from vitamin mixture)	2.3 ± 0.8	1.2 ± 0.8	5.0 ± 0.2	1.00 ± 0.02	0.98 ± 0.04	1.58 ± 0.051	1.25 ± 0.145	16 ± 1.4	11 ± 0.9	26 ± 2.5	30 ± 1.2
3. 5% casein + niacin	2.6 ± 1.0	2.0 ± 0.8	4.9 ± 0.1	1.02 ± 0.04	1.00 ± 0.03	1.47 ± 0.074	1.55 ± 0.146	17 ± 0.7	12 ± 0.8	29 ± 1.4	32 ± 2.0
4. 5% casein + pyridoxine	3.2 ± 0.8	2.0 ± 0.8	4.7 ± 0.1	1.04 ± 0.04	0.99 ± 0.03	1.46 ± 0.120	1.53 ± 0.090	17 ± 2.7	14 ± 0.1	29 ± 1.0	29 ± 1.7
5. 5% casein + glutamic acid	2.3 ± 1.0	2.5 ± 0.2	3.2 ± 0.2	1.05 ± 0.03	1.04 ± 0.05	1.76 ± 0.145	1.69 ± 0.096	17 ± 1.5	19 ± 1.9	31 ± 1.2	31 ± 1.9
6. 20% casein	5.5 ± 0.5	2.8 ± 0.8	8.2 ± 0.2	1.10 ± 0.03	1.09 ± 0.03	1.86 ± 0.070	1.84 ± 0.140	19 ± 1.0	18 ± 1.6	32 ± 0.1	32 ± 1.2
Groups compared 1 vs. 5						NS[c]	NS[c]	NS[c]	P < 0.01		
1 vs. 6						P < 0.01	P < 0.05	P < 0.01	P < 0.01		

[a] Values are mean enzyme units per gram wet weight of cerebrum (±SEM).

[b] Six animals in each group were used in Experiment 1 and five animals in Experiment II.

[c] Not significant.

From Rajalakshmi, R., Pillai, K. R., and Ramakrishnan, C. V., *J. Neurochem.*, 16, 599—606, 1969. With permission.

Table 9
EFFECT OF GLUTAMIC ACID
SUPPLEMENTATION TO LOW PROTEIN DIET
ON CERTAIN CEREBRAL ENZYMES

	Enzyme units/g cerebral tissue[a]	
	L-Glutamate-NAD-oxidoreductase	L-Glutamate-1-carboxy-lyase
5% casein	1.42 ± 0.082	13 ± 0.60
5% casein + glutamic acid	1.74 ± 0.092	18 ± 0.92
	$P < 0.02$	$P < 0.001$

[a]   Combined means of Experiments I and II ± (SEM); see Table 8.

From Rajalakshmi, R., Pillai, K. R., and Ramakrishnan, C. V., *J. Neurochem.*, 16, 599—606, 1969. With permission.

Table 10
WATER MAZE PERFORMANCE OF RATS FED KODRI
(*PASPALUM SCORBICULATUM L.*) WITH OR
WITHOUT DIFFERENT SUPPLEMENTS[a]

		Mean no. of errors			
Group	Supplement added	Forward trials I	Reversal trials II	Ratio II/I	t and P values[c]
1	None	13±1.5	28±3.1	2.1±0.25	
2	Skim milk powder	16±1.0	19±2.4	1.3±0.39	NS[b]
3	Moth bean	15±1.3	25±4.0	1.6±0.74	NS
4	Peas	15±1.4	20±4.3	1.4±0.58	NS
2,3,4 (combined)		15±0.7	21±0.6	1.4±0.12	P<0.02

[a]   Six animals were used in each group.
[b]   Not significant.
[c]   Relative to group 1.

From Rajalakshmi, R., Pillai, K. R., and Ramakrishnan, C. V., *J. Neurochem.*, 16, 599—606, 1969. With permission.

Table 11
MEAN (± SEM) EXHAUSTIVE RUNNING TIMES OF EXPERIMENT 1

Group	n[b]	Running time (minutes)[a]				
		R$_1$ (18/min)	R$_2$ (52 m/min)	R$_3$ (44 m/min)	R$_4$ (52 m/min)	R$_5$ (44 m/min)
Control	26	108 ± 10	9 ± 1	17 ± 1	10 ± 1	13 ± 1
Anemic	25	118 ± 10	4 ± 0	9 ± 1	9 ± 1	9 ± 1
Probability		NS[c]	P<0.01	P<0.01	NS	P<0.05

[a] R$_1$, R$_2$, R$_3$, R$_4$, and R$_5$ represent the exhaustive run days shown in Figure 19. R$_1$ occurred prior to the induction of anemia. R$_2$ and R$_3$ occurred at the point that Hb and packed cell volume was the most different (about 5g/dl). R$_4$ and R$_5$ represent exhaustive runs after iron therapy.
[b] n = 15 for controls and 17 for anemics in R$_4$ and R$_5$.
[c] Not significant.

From Edgerton, V. R., Bryand, S. L., Gillespie, C. A., and Gardner, G. W., *J. Nutr.*, 102, 381—399, 1972. With permission.

Table 12
MEAN(± SEM) FORCED ENDURANCE AND SPRINT EXHAUSTIVE RUNNING TIMES BEFORE AND AFTER IRON REPLETION OF EXPERIMENT 2

Group	n	Running time (minutes)[a]			
		R$_1$(35 m/min)	R$_2$(52 m/min	R$_3$(35 m/min)	R$_4$(52 m/min)
Controls (C)[b]	15	17.9±1.5	6.4±0.7	11.4±1.8	5.9±0.5
Moderate anemic (M)	15	11.3±2.0	5.0±1.1	9.7±1.4	4.9±0.6
Severely anemic (S)	10	2.1±0.5	1.8±0.7	9.4±2.4	4.1±0.4
Probability		P<0.01	P<0.05	NS[c]	NS
Differences		C > M > S	C > S		

[a] R$_1$, R$_2$, R$_3$, and R$_4$ represent the exhaustive run days shown in Figure 20.
[b] In the control and in the severely anemic groups, a significant performance difference (P<0.05 and P<0.01, respectively) existed before and after iron repletion at 35 m/min (R$_1$ and R$_3$). At 52 m/min only the severely anemic animals differed (P < 0.05) before and after iron.
[c] Not significant.

From Edgerton, V. R., Bryant, S. L., Gillespie, C. A., and Gardner, G. W., *J. Nutr.*, 102, 381—399, 1972. With permission.

Table 13
HEMOGLOBIN, MYOGLOBIN, AND CYTOCHROME
CONCENTRATIONS AND EXHAUSTIVE RUNNING TIME AT A RATE
OF 27 M/MIN OF EXPERIMENT 3 (MEAN ± SEM)

	Control (C)	Phenylhy- drazine (P)	Iron deficient (ID)	Probability	Differences
n	9	9[a]	9[b]		
Hb (g/100 mℓ)	16.2 ± 0.02	7.8 ± 0.02	10.4 ± 0.05	<0.05	C > ID > P
Run time (min)	35 ± 6	6 ± 1	9 ± 4	<0.05	C > P = ID
Gastrocnemius					
Cyt a (mg/g)	0.76 ± 0.07	0.67 ± 0.12	0.63 ± 0.06	>0.05	
Cyt b	0.36 ± 0.04	0.34 ± 0.04	0.29 ± 0.04	>0.05	
Cyt c	0.14 ± 0.01	0.11 ± 0.01	0.06 ± 0.01	<0.05	C > P > ID
Total cyt	1.26 ± 0.12	1.12 ± 0.17	0.97 ± 0.11	<0.05	C > ID
					C = P, ID = P
Heart					
Cyt a	2.78 ± 0.10	2.80 ± 0.13	2.69 ± 0.16	>0.05	
Cyt b	0.85 ± 0.03	0.82 ± 0.04	0.81 ± 0.06	>0.05	
Cyt c	0.58 ± 0.02	0.50 ± 0.02	0.53 ± 0.02	<0.05	C > P
Total cyt	4.21 ± 0.15	4.12 ± 0.19	4.03 ± 0.24	>0.05	C = ID, P = ID
Myoglobin (mg/g)					
Gastrocnemius	0.37 ± 0.02	0.30 ± 0.03	0.28 ± 0.03	>0.05	
Soleus	0.73 ± 0.05	0.51 ± 0.02	0.56 ± 0.07	<0.05	C > P = ID

Note: See Figure 21 for time course of changes in Hb.

[a]   n = 8 for gastrocnemius.
[b]   n = 7 for gastrocnemius.

From Edgerton, V. R., Bryant, S. L., Gillespie, C. A., and Gardner, G. W., *J. Nutr.*, 102, 138—399, 1972. With permission.

Table 14
MEAN EXHAUSTIVE RUNNING TIMES OF EXPERIMENT 4 BEFORE
AND AFTER IRON REPLETION (MIN ± SEM)[a]

		Running time (minutes)[a]			
Group	n	R_1 (27 m/ min)[b]	R_2 (35 m/min)	R_3 (35 m/min)	R_4 (35 m/min)
Controls (C)	8	161 ± 22	105 ± 28	98 ± 28	115 ± 32
Phenylhydrazine (P)	8	22 ± 11	84 ± 28	83 ± 30	90 ± 29
Iron deficient (ID)	8	74 ± 32	90 ± 23	88 ± 24	112 ± 31
Probability		<0.01	>0.05	>0.05	>0.05
Differences		C > ID = P			

[a] R_1 was immediately prior to but on the day iron repletion was begun (between weeks 6 and 7). R_{2-4} were performed every 3rd or 4th day thereafter. Hemoglobin levels are shown in Figure 22.
[b]   The greater running times in this experiment relative to Experiments 1, 2, and 3 are undoubtedly accountable by the fact that only the animals in Experiment 4 were housed in cages equipped with activity wheels while in each of the other cases daily activity was limited by the relatively small cage size.

From Edgerton, V. R., Bryant, S. L., Gillespie, C. A., and Gardner, G. W., *J. Nutr.*, 102, 381—399, 1972. With permission.

Table 15

EFFECTS OF IRON DEFICIENCY ON OXIDATIVE PHOSPHORYLATION IN MITOCHONDRIA FROM SKELETAL MUSCLE, AND HEART MUSCLE

Tissue	State of animal	Pyruvate-Malate[a]					Succinate[a]					α-Glycerophosphate[a]				
		^{33}P: 0	^{33}P esterified	ADP: 0	ADP esterified	RCI	^{33}P: 0	^{33}P esterified	ADP: 0	ADP esterified	RCI	^{33}P: 0	^{33}P esterified	ADP: 0	ADP esterified	RCI
Skeletal muscle	Control	2.9 ±0.2	0.34 ±0.04	2.6 ±0.1	0.30 ±0.02	5.3 ±0.2	1.6 ±0.0	0.25 ±0.03	1.6 ±0.0	0.25 ±0.01	3.0 ±0.1	1.7 ±0.1	0.095 ±0.005	1.4 ±0.0	0.084 ±0.004	1.6 ±0.0
	Iron deficient	2.7 ±0.1	0.16 ±0.02	2.4 ±0.0	0.13 ±0.01	2.8 ±0.2	1.3 ±0.1	0.032 ±0.002	1.3 ±0.1	0.053 ±0.006	1.3 ±0.1	1.5 ±0.1	0.047 ±0.002	1.5 ±0.2	0.055 ±0.006	1.3 ±0.0
	Iron treated[b]	2.6 ±0.1	0.14 ±0.02	2.5 ±0.1	0.15 ±0.02	3.4 ±0.02	1.4 ±0.1	0.040 ±0.003	1.3 ±0.1	0.063 ±0.010	1.7 ±0.2	1.7 ±0.1	0.076 ±0.006	1.4 ±0.1	0.077 ±0.008	1.4 ±0.0
Heart muscle	Control	—	—	2.7 ±0.1	0.48 ±0.03	4.8 ±0.2	—	—	1.5 ±0.0	0.38 ±0.02	2.7 ±0.1	0.9 ±0.1	0.005 ±0.0007	—[c]	—[c]	1.0
	Iron deficient	—	—	2.7 ±0.0	0.45 ±0.05	4.1 ±0.2	—	—	1.6 ±0.1	0.35 ±0.03	2.2 ±0.2	—	—	—	—	—

[a] Activities given above are defined as follows: ^{33}P esterified, μmoles of ^{33}P esterified per minute per mg protein; ADP esterified, μmoles of ADP phosphorylated per minute per mg protein; RCI (Respiratory Control Index) was calculated as the ratio of state 3 rate of oxidation to state 4 rate of oxidation. The data represent averages of data from at least 9 separate experiments ± the standard error of the mean, except for data for heart muscle and brain which represent averages of at least 4 separate experiments.

[b] Studies were performed on iron treated rats 4 days after iron treatment.

[c] No stimulation was observed when ADP was added to assays of heart mitochondria containing α-glycerophosphate as substrate.

From Finch, C. A., Miller, L. R., Inamdar, A. R., Person, R., Seiler, K., and Mackler, B., *J. Clin. Invest.* 58, 447—453, 1976. With permission.

Table 16
BLOOD GASES IN IRON-DEFICIENT AND CONTROL ANIMALS BEFORE AND AFTER A 2-MIN FAST RUN

	Resting		After 2-min. running	
	Control	Iron-deficient	Control	Iron-deficient
Arterial blood[a]				
Hemoglobin before exchange transfusion (g/dℓ)	13.44 ± 0.32	5.52 ± 0.19		
Hemoglobin after exchange transfusion (g/dℓ)	10.13 ± 0.07	9.79 ± 0.07		
PO$_2$ (torr)	72.2 ± 2.6	68.9 ± 1.1	85.7 ± 3.2	85.6 ± 1.8
PCO$_2$ (torr)	36.6 ± 2.1	31.3 ± 1.3	26.4 ± 1.6	21.6 ± 1.4[c]
pH	7.477 ± 0.011	7.443 ± 0.020	7.346 ± 0.13	7.138 ± 0.032[d]
Lactate (mM)	1.07 ± 0.05	1.04 ± 0.13	7.82 ± 0.50	15.3 ± 1.8[c]
Base excess (meq/ℓ)	+ 3.4 ± 0.6	−2.1 ± 1.0[c]	−10.1 ± 1.0	−20.9 ± 1.0[d]
O$_2$ content (mℓ/dℓ)	12.0 ± 0.4	11.8 ± 0.18	11.5 ± 0.5	11.3 ± 0.3
Vena caval blood[b]				
Hemoglobin before exchange transfusion (g/dℓ)	14.80 ± 1.10	5.30 ± 0.30		
Hemoglobin after exchange transfusion (g/dℓ)	9.90 ± 0.10	9.80 ± 0.10		
PO$_2$ (torr)	28.70 ± 1.20	28.40 ± 1.50	17.10 ± 2.50	35.40 ± 3.00[d]
PCO$_2$ (torr)	39.40 ± 0.08	37.10 ± 1.30	47.30 ± 1.80	42.90 ± 1.30
pH	7.46 ± 0.01	7.44 ± 0.01	7.18 ± 0.03	7.00 ± 0.02[d]
Lactate (mM)	0.94 ± 0.05	2.24 ± 0.49[c]	10.90 ± 1.30	13.68 ± 1.93
Base excess (meq/ℓ)	+ 4.00 ± 1.10	+ 1.41 ± 0.64	−10.20 ± 1.19	−20.40 ± 1.16[d]

[a]   Six animals studied in each group.
[b]   Eight animals studied in each group.
[c]   Difference between iron-deficient animals and controls significant to $P<0.05$.
[d]   Difference between iron-deficient animals and controls significant to $P<0.001$.

From Finch, C. A., Gollnick, P. D., Hlastala, M. P., Miller, L. R., Dillman, E., and Mackler, B., *J. Clin. Invest.*, 64, 129—137, 1979. With permission.

Table 17
α-GLYCEROPHOSPHATE OXIDASE ACTIVITY IN CONTROL AND IRON-DEFICIENT RATS SEGREGATED ACCORDING TO RUNNING ABILITY

Animals	No. of animals	Running time (min)	Specific activity[a]	Total activity[b]
Control (CI)	5	>30	0.0032±0.0003	0.60±0.01
Iron-deficient (good runners)	5	>30	0.0025±0.0001[c]	0.45±0.03
Iron-deficient (poor runners)	5	9—19	0.0011±0.0000[d]	0.20±0.00[d]

[a]   Specific activity = μmol α-glycerophosphate oxidized/min/mg protein.
[b]   Total activity = μmol α-glycerophosphate oxidized/min/g tissue.
[c]   Difference between iron-deficient and control animals significant to $P<0.05$.
[d]   Difference between iron-deficient and control animals significant to $P<0.001$.

From Finch, C. A., Gollnick, P. D., Hlastala, M. P., Miller, L. R., Dillman, E., and Mackler, B., *J. Clin. Invest.*, 64, 129—137, 1979. With permission.

Table 18
EFFECT OF A PROLONGED IRON DEFICIENT DIET ON SELECTED PARAMETERS (MEAN ± SEM)[a]

	3 days		2 weeks		4 weeks		5 months	
	Control	Anemic	Control	Anemic	Control	Anemic	Control	Anemic
Hb (g/100ml)	11.3 ± 0.5[i]	6.8 ± 0.6	13.0 ± 1.4[i]	8.1 ± 0.4	11.5 ± 0.5[i]	6.4 ± 0.5	12.8 ± 0.4[i]	7.6 ± 0.4
RT[b] (min)	39.6 ± 3.1[i]	27.1 ± 2.5	34.1 ± 1.4[i]	27.1 ± 1.5	43.5 ± 4.2[i]	30.2 ± 6.9	23.6 ± 1.2[i]	15.8 ± 1.3
LA[c] (mmol/l)	1.85 ± 0.27	3.34 ± 0.59	1.98 ± 0.19[i]	3.27 ± 0.28	1.98 ± 0.07[i]	4.30 ± 0.68	2.57 ± 0.69[i]	5.51 ± 0.99[i]
2,3-DPG[d] (μmol/gHb)	26.7 ± 1.6	23.7 ± 1.0	25.5 ± 0.9	22.9 ± 0.5	26.9 ± 0.7	27.7 ± 1.5	22.2 ± 1.8[i]	27.9 ± 1.5
Plasma Fe (μg/100 ml)	155 ± 14[i]	97 ± 21	167 ± 28[i]	41 ± 11	184 ± 28[i]	38 ± 8	156 ± 12[i]	39 ± 9
Mb[e] (mg/g)								
Heart	4.37 ± 0.28	4.26 ± 0.22	4.22 ± 0.29	4.38 ± 0.16	4.36 ± 0.37	3.93 ± 0.40	6.35 ± 1.00	7.49 ± 0.46
Soleus	2.41 ± 0.23	2.67 ± 0.25	3.09 ± 0.40	2.74 ± 0.10	2.79 ± 0.17	2.82 ± 0.20	4.02 ± 0.24	3.40 ± 0.37
RVL[f]	1.62 ± 0.22	1.65 ± 0.16	1.62 ± 0.12	1.73 ± 0.15	1.39 ± 0.06	1.41 ± 0.08	2.03 ± 0.12	1.72 ± 0.31
WVL[g]	0.84 ± 0.19	1.09 ± 0.68	0.98 ± 0.49	0.68 ± 0.17	0.41 ± 0.06	0.51 ± 0.07	0.90 ± 0.17	0.84 ± 0.19
Cyt ox[h] (k/min)								
Heart	1.36 ± 0.22	1.37 ± 0.22	1.82 ± 0.18	1.75 ± 0.18	1.54 ± 0.07[i]	1.18 ± 0.05	1.01 ± 0.06	1.09 ± 0.05
Soleus	0.36 ± 0.19	0.29 ± 0.21	0.42 ± 0.13	0.44 ± 0.10	0.49 ± 0.05	0.48 ± 0.03	0.58 ± 0.05	0.53 ± 0.06
muscle RVL	0.41 ± 0.18	0.42 ± 0.21	0.65 ± 0.15	0.70 ± 0.09	0.36 ± 0.30	0.43 ± 0.05	0.51 ± 0.08[i]	0.24 ± 0.05

a   Some data taken from Koziol et al.[52]

b   Treadmill exhaustive run time (RT) was a gradual test increasing in workload every 3 min according to Woodson et al.[53]

c   Lactate was determined from blood withdrawn from the external jugular vein within 1 min after 6.0 min run at a rate 20 m/min and a 10% incline.

d   2,3-Diphosphoglycerate.

e   Myoglobin (Mb) was measured according to De Duve.[55]

f   Red vastus lateralis.

g   White vastus lateralis. Muscle samples were taken as described by Gillespie et al.[54]

h   Cytochrome oxidase (cyt ox) was measured with a modification of Smith[56] $k = 2.3(\log OD_{t_2} - \log OD_{t_1})/t_2 - t_1$

i   P <0.05 that the two groups differed on a given parameter.

Table 19

EFFECT OF ACUTE AND ESTABLISHED ANEMIA ON OXYGEN TRANSPORT AND HEMODYNAMIC PARAMETERS

	Subject no.	Supine rest			Standing rest			Maximal exercise		
		Control	Acute anemia	Establ. anemia	Control	Acute anemia	Establ. anemia	Control	Acute anemia	Establ. anemia
$\dot{V}_{21}$, $\text{m}l/\text{min}\cdot\text{kg}$	1	3.57	3.70	3.42	3.68	4.49	4.00	43.8	33.8	31.9
	2	4.03	4.11	3.84	4.51	5.16	4.97	45.5	39.4	35.9
	3	3.90	4.53	4.24	4.61	5.28	5.06	43.0	39.0	26.9
	4	3.14	3.80	2.87	3.46	3.76	3.79	39.9	32.1	27.9
	Mean	3.66	4.04	3.59	4.07	4.67	4.46	43.0	36.1	30.7
$\dot{V}_{E}$, $\text{m}l/\text{min}\cdot\text{kg}$	1	91	83	81	99	102	90	1656	1300	1135
	2	90	84	87	103	168	128	1541	1529	1507
	3	92	89	95	115	128	135	1708	1181	1138
	4	78	94	71	96	94	103	2085		1169
	Mean	88	88	84	103	123	114	1748	1373(982)[a]	1237(716)[a]
$\dot{Q}$, $\text{m}l/\text{min}\cdot\text{kg}$	1	74	118	88	55	79	67	249	254	234
	2	106	152	120	79	89	78	297	308	272
	3	118	156	143	97	100	92	295	354	272
	4	67	137	67	67	87	73	293	325	272
	Mean	91	141	104	74	89	78	284	320(265)	236(238)
HR, beats/min	1	77	82	63	88	102	75	185	185	176
	2	96	112	92	112	143	113	196	195	190
	3	73	104	91	116	124	104	205	192	184
	4	50	80	49	57	77	64	191	185	
	Mean	74	95	73	93	112	89	194	189(178)	183(159)
SV, $\text{m}l/\text{min}\cdot\text{kg}$	1	0.98	1.44	1.39	0.63	0.78	0.90	1.35	1.38	1.34
	2	1.19	1.35	1.31	0.71	0.62	0.69	1.51	1.52	1.44
	3	1.61	1.51	1.57	0.84	0.81	0.89	1.44	2.05	1.48
	4	1.34	1.71	1.36	1.17	1.13	1.13	1.54	1.76	
	Mean	1.28	1.50	1.41	0.84	0.84	0.90	1.46	1.68(1.49)	1.42(1.50)

Measurement										
SOT, mℓ/min·kg	1	14.4	15.9	12.2	11.0	11.2	9.8	51.5	38.8	36.0
	2	20.3	22.0	16.6	15.4	13.6	12.1	62.5	51.4	43.2
	3	21.4	17.9	14.1	17.9	11.8	10.3	59.6	50.6	31.5
	4	11.3	14.6	6.4	11.3	9.8	7.4	55.8	40.6	30.4
	Mean	16.9	17.6	12.3	13.9	11.6	9.9	57.3	45.3(52.7)	35.3(47.1)
SVR, dyn·cm⁻⁵	1	1286	809	1212	1854	1356	1680			
	2	952	633	1137	1355	1142	1742			
	3	895	600	652	952	938	949			
	4	1434	697	1509	1283	1159	1724			
	Mean	1142	685	1128	1361	1149	1524			
PVR, dyn·cm⁻⁵	1	186	135	182	156	149	192			
	2	133	93	118	194	138	168			
	3	179	136	104	152		122			
	4	211	211				193			
	Mean	177	121	154	167		169			
a-vO₂ content diff., vol%	1	4.78	3.13	3.89	6.76	5.71	5.94	17.62	13.32	13.62
	2	3.80	2.71	3.20	5.74	5.82	6.35	15.33	12.79	13.21
	3	3.31	2.91	2.96	4.75	5.29	5.50	14.58	9.89	9.87
	4	4.70	2.77	4.32	5.20	4.33	5.22	13.66	9.87	10.24
	Mean	4.15	2.88	3.60	5.59	5.29	5.86	15.30	11.47(13.7)	11.74(12.8)
$S\bar{v}_{O_2}$, %	1	76	77	73	66	60	59	15	13	10
	2	80	82	78	71	62	59	27	24	17
	3	82	75	71	74	55	51	28	24	14
	4	72	74	56	70	61	49		22	8
	Mean	78	77	70	70	60	55	23	21(31)	12(35)
In vivo Pv_{O_2}, Torr	1	41	44	36	38	37	33	19	19	15
	2	39	40	41	33	29	30	22	21	17
	3	45	43	35	39	32	29	24	22	22
	4	36	38	29	38	30	27		25	15
	Mean	40	41	35	37	32	30	22	22(25)	17(26)

Table 19 (continued)

EFFECT OF ACUTE AND ESTABLISHED ANEMIA ON OXYGEN TRANSPORT AND HEMODYNAMIC PARAMETERS

Subject no.	Supine rest			Standing rest			Maximal exercise		
	Control	Acute anemia	Establ. anemia	Control	Acute anemia	Establ. anemia	Control	Acute anemia	Establ. anemia
Arterial lactate, [b]mM									
1	0.76	1.10	0.84	0.77	0.98	0.84	15.1	13.1	11.9
2	1.40	0.80	1.05	1.05	0.85	0.85	14.6	11.4	11.5
3	0.39	0.40	0.42	0.43	0.48	0.55	11.2	8.0	7.3
4	0.65	0.55	0.71	0.90	0.67	0.60	15.9	9.5	11.6
Mean	0.80	0.71	0.76	0.79	0.75	0.71	14.2	10.5(6.4)	10.6(4.3)

Note: HR = heart rate; SV = stroke volume; SOT = systemic oxygen transport; SVR = systemic vascular resistance; PVR = pulmonary vascular resistance.

[a] Values in parentheses represent values observed (obtained by interpolation) in control subjects as equivalent oxygen consumption. For example, mean maximal cardiac output in control subjects with acute anemia was 320 ml/min·kg at the maximal $\dot{V}_{O_2}$ of 36.1 ml/min·kg; mean cardiac output in control subjects at this $\dot{V}_{O_2}$ was 265 ml/min·kg.

[b] Arterial lactate values listed for maximal exercise were obtained during maximal exercise just prior to cessation. Maximal postexercise lactate values in subjects 2, 3 and 4 were 21.2, 15.4, and 19.1 mM (mean 18.6 mM in the control; 17.0, 8.1, and 11.9 mM (mean 12.3 mM) with acute anemia; and 14.2, 10.0, and 14.5 mM (mean 12.9 mM) with established anemia, respectively.

From Woodson, R. D., Wills, R. E., and Lentant, C., *J. Appl. Physiol.*, 44, 36—43, 1978. With permission.

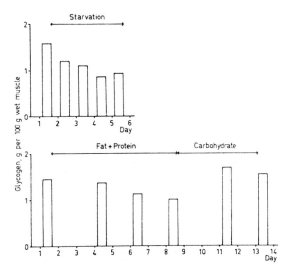

FIGURE 1. Effect of starvation, a high-fat and protein and a high-carbohydrate diet on glycogen in the quadriceps muscle of normal men. (From Hultman, E. and Bergström, J., *Acta Med. Scand.*, 182, 109—117, 1967. With permission.)

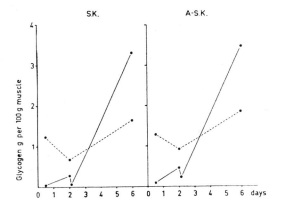

FIGURE 2. Effect of starvation and of a carbohydrate-rich diet on the glycogen concentration in the quadriceps muscles on two normal subjects. One leg (solid line) was exercised before the first biopsy. This was followed by 2 days of starvation, exercise in the same leg, and then a high-carbohydrate diet without exercise. (From Hultman, E. and Bergström, J., *Acta Med. Scand.*, 182, 109—117, 1967. With permission.)

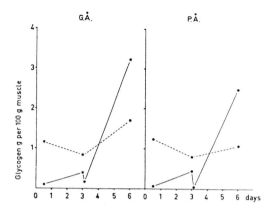

FIGURE 3.   Same condition as in Figure 2 except a high protein-fat diet replaced the period of starvation. (From Hultman, E. and Bergström, J., *Acta Med. Scand.*, 182, 109—117, 1967. With permission.)

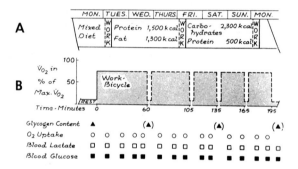

FIGURE 4.   (A) Dietary and work schedule for six subjects for 1 week. (B) Parameter measured at the times indicated. (From Bergström, J., Hermansen, L., Hultman, E., and Saltin, B., *Acta Physiol. Scand.*, 71, 140—150, 1967. With permission.)

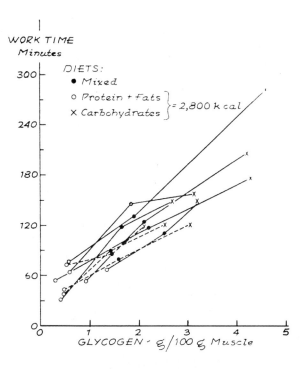

FIGURE 5. Relationship of initial quadriceps femoris muscle glycogen and work time to exhaustion as shown in Figure 4 in normal subjects. The equation for the regression line is $y = 41.6x + 36.8$; $r = 0.92$, $P < 0.001$. Three of the subjects (---) had a carbohydrate diet prior to fat and protein diet. (From Bergström, J., Hermansen, L., Hultman, E., and Saltin, B., *Acta Physiol. Scand.*, 71, 140—150, 1967. With permission.)

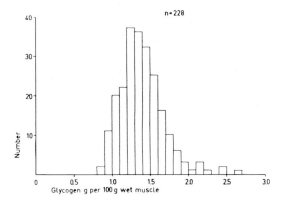

FIGURE 6. Population distributions of quadriceps femoris muscle glycogen of normal male subjects. (From Hultman, E., *Circ. Res.*, 20(Suppl.1), 99—114, 1967. With permission.)

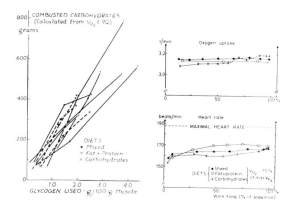

FIGURE 7.   Relationship of the actual glycogen utilized and that estimated from $\dot{V}_{o2}$ and RQ. The upper right shows the rate of O_2 uptake and the lower right illustrates the heart rate response to the exercise. The diets used are indicated in the figure. (From Bergström, J., Hermansen, L., Hultman, E., and Saltin, B., *Acta Physiol. Scand.,* 71, 140—150, 1967. With permission.)

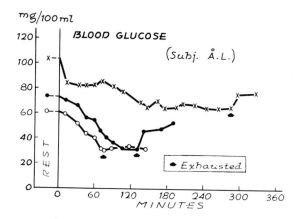

FIGURE 8.   Blood glucose of one subject during bicycle work (approximately 75% $\dot{V}_{o2}$ max) after a carbohydrate (x), mixed (•), and fat and protein (o) diet. (From Bergström, J., Hermansen, L., Hultman, E., and Saltin, B., *Acta Physiol. Scand.,* 71, 140—150, 1967. With permission.)

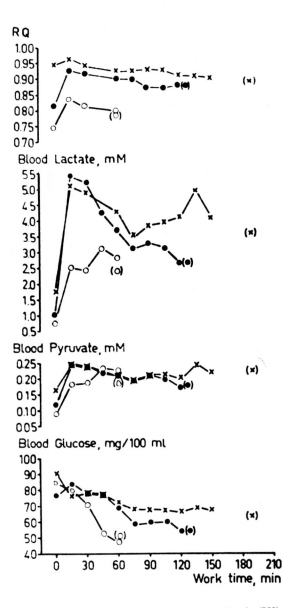

FIGURE 9. Effect of diet and work on a bicycle (75% $\dot{V}_{02}$ max) on mean RQ, blood lactate, pyruvate, and glucose. Symbols are the same as in Figure 8. (From Bergström, J., Hermansen, L., Hultman, E., and Saltin, B., *Acta Physiol. Scand.*, 71, 140—150, 1967. With permission.)

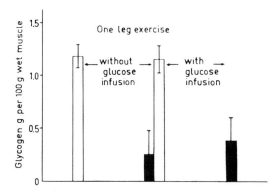

FIGURE 10. Quadriceps femoris muscle glycogen before (open bars) and after (solid bars) exercise with and without glucose infusion with one leg and then the other in six normal subjects (mean ± SD). Glucose was infused in order to maintain blood sugar concentration between 200 and 600 mg/100 ml. (From Hultman, E., *Circ. Res.,* 20(Suppl.1), 99—114, 1967. With permission.)

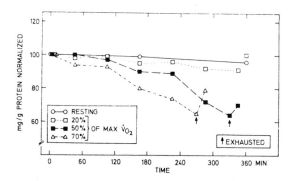

FIGURE 11. Effect of four levels of exercise on blood glucose concentration in five to eight subjects living on a standard diet. (From Pruett, E. D. R., *J. Appl. Physiol.,* 28, 199—208, 1970. With permission.)

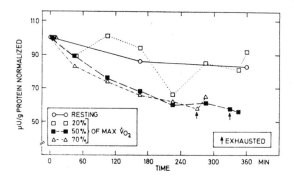

FIGURE 12. Effect of four levels of exercises on plasma immunoreactive insulin levels in five to seven subjects living on a standard diet. (From Pruett, E. D. R., *J. Appl. Physiol.,* 28, 199—208, 1970. With permission.)

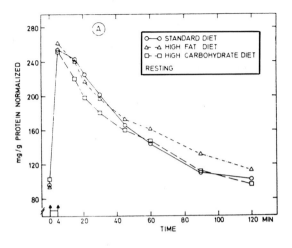

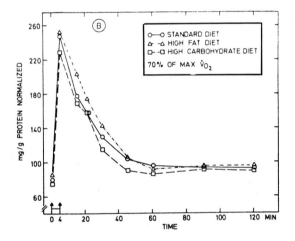

FIGURE 13. Glucose tolerance test at rest (A) and after exercise (B) at 70% of $\dot{V}_{02}$ max in fasting subjects. Mean of seven subjects living on a standard diet, five on high-fat diet, and five on high carbohydrate diet. Glucose (300 mg/ kg body weight) was infused from min 0 to 4 and blood samples drawn at min 5, 15, 22, 30, 45, 60, 90, and 120. (From Pruett, E. D. R., *J. Appl. Physiol.*, 28, 199—208, 1970. With permission.)

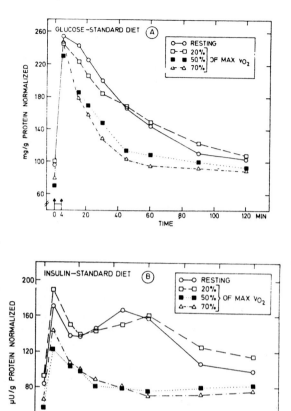

FIGURE 14.   Effect of four work levels on glucose tolerance
(N = 7) and immunoreactive insulin (N = 6) living on a standard
diet. (From Pruett, E. D. R., *J. Appl. Physiol.*, 28, 199—208,
1970. With permission.)

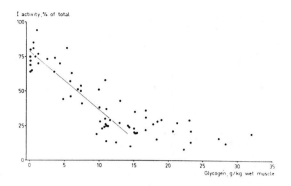

FIGURE 15.   Relationship between glycogen content of
quadriceps femoris muscle and percentage of glycogen synthetase I activity in normal subjects. A range of glycogen
levels were achieved by exercise and carbohydrate diet.
Regression line for values less than the normal mean value
of 14.0 g/kg wet weight is y = −42.2x + 78.8; r = −0.88.
(From Bergström, J., Hultman, E., and Roch-Norlund, A.
E., *Scand. J. Clin. Lab. Invest.,* 29, 231—236, 1972. With
permission.)

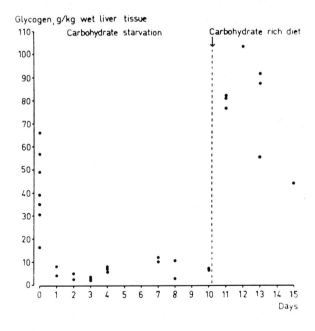

FIGURE 16.   Liver glycogen during long-term carbohydrate
or total starvation followed by refeeding on a carbohydrate-
rich diet. There was total caloric restriction in two subjects.
Others had a caloric intake of 2100 cal/day with less than 5 g
carbohydrate. This diet was followed with a normocaloric, carbohydrate-rich diet containing 400 g of carbohydrate. (From
Hultman, E. and Nilsson, L. H., in *Muscle Metabolism During
Exercise,* Pernow, B. and Saltin, B., Eds., Plenum Press, New
York, 1971, 143—151. With permission.)

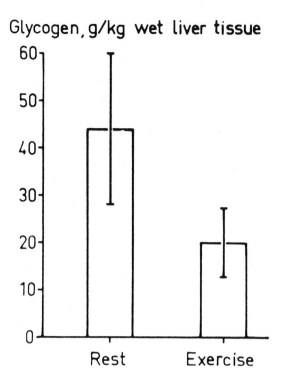

FIGURE 17.   Liver glycogen concentration at rest in the morning after an overnight fast (N = 33) and 1 hr after exercise (n = 14) at 75% of $\dot{V}_{o2}$ max (Mean ± SD): glycogen concentration decreased after exercise (P<0.001). (From Hultman, E. and Nilsson, L. H., in *Muscle Metabolism During Exercise,* Pernon, B. and Saltin, B., Plenum Press, New York, 1971, 143—152. With Permission.)

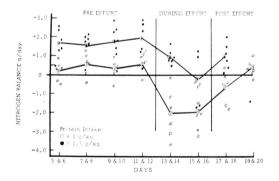

FIGURE 18.   Influence of exercise which consisted of six to seven times daily for 20-min periods. Effort was 400 to 900 kgm/min. (From Gontzea, I., Sutzescu, P., and Dumitrache, S., *Nutr. Rep. Int.,* 10, 35—43, 1974. With permission.)

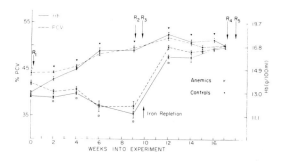

FIGURE 19.   Mean Hb and PCV of rats at various stages
of iron depletion and repletion. Bars represent the standard
errors. Significant differences, P < 0.05, are indicated by ▼
(HB) and □ (PCV), and exhaustive runs are indicated by
arrows R_1 to R_5. See Table 11 for actual running time.
(From Edgerton, V. R., Bryant, S. L., Gillespie, C. A., and
Gardner, G. W., *J. Nutr.,* 102, 381—399, 1972. With permission.)

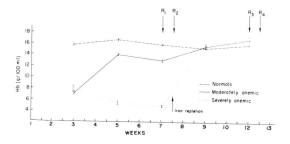

FIGURE 20.   Mean Hb ± SEM of rats at various stages
of iron depletion and repletion. At the end of week 5, the
mean Hb concentrations of each group were significantly
different (P < 0.001). At the end of 9 weeks, there were no
differences. At 3.5 weeks, the iron-deficient diet was supplemented with 760 mg Fe per kilogram diet for 1 day for
the moderate anemic group. At the end of 7 weeks and for
the remainder of the experiment, supplement was 240 mg
Fe per kilogram for all groups. See Table 12 for running
time. (From Edgerton, V. R., Bryant, S. L., Gillespie, C.
A., and Gardner, G. W., *J. Nutr.,* 102, 381—399, 1972.
With permission.)

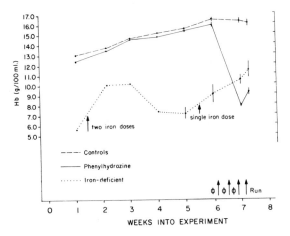

FIGURE 21.   Demonstration of the effect of phenylhydrazine and an iron-deficient diet on mean Hb. Arrows indicate initiation of phenylhydrazine (φ) and exhaustive run
(see Table 13). All standard errors for values prior to week
6 (not shown) are less than those indicated on the graph.
(From Edgerton, V. R., Bryant, S. L., Gillespie, C. A., and
Gardner, G. W., *J. Nutr.*, 102, 381—399, 1972. With permission.)

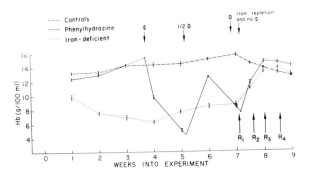

FIGURE 22.   Mean Hb levels ± SEM of control, phenylhydrazine-induced and diet-induced anemic rats at various stages
of the experiment are shown. φ represents 0.18 ml of 2% phenylhydrazine injected i.p. and 1/2 φ is half that dose. Hb of all
three groups differed significantly (P < 0.05) between weeks 4
and 6. At 8 and 8.5 weeks, the Hb of the phenylhydrazine
group was significantly greater than the iron-deficient group
and the controls (P < 0.05), respectively. No significant difference existed on the final Hb determination (9 weeks). See Table
14 for running times. (From Edgerton, V. R., Bryant, S. L.,
Gillespie, C. A., and Gardner, G. W., *J. Nutr.*, 102, 381—399,
1972. With permission.)

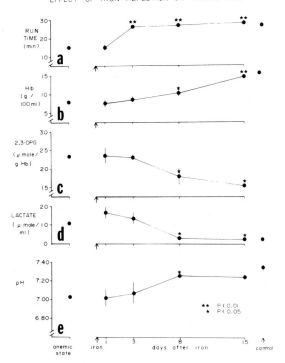

FIGURE 23. The changes in run time to exhaustion (a), Hb (b), 2,3-DPG (c), venous blood lactate (d), and venous whole blood pH (e) 3 min after a 10-min standard treadmill run, before and during dietary iron repletion in anemic rats. The control values were obtained from the standard exercise test administered to normal rats. The mean values and SEM are shown. Correlated t-tests were performed between the anemic state and 1, 3, 8, and 15 days after iron repletion. Significant differences from the anemic state are indicated in the figures.

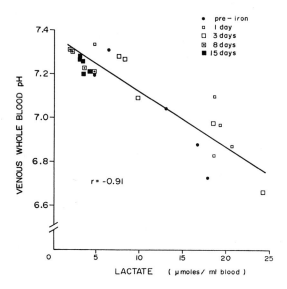

RELATIONSHIP BETWEEN BLOOD LACTATE AND

pH DURING IRON TREATMENT

FIGURE 24. The relationship between venous whole blood pH and venous blood lactate values 3 min after a 10 min treadmill run at 27 m/min, 15% grade, before and during dietary iron repletion in anemic rats. pH = −0.025 (lactate) + 7.366, significant at P < 0.001.

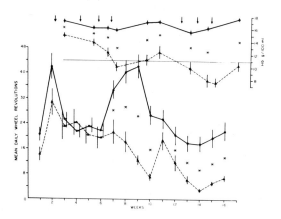

FIGURE 25. The two top lines (anemic [---], control [   ]) represent Hb concentration (mean ± SEM). Arrows indicate days at which blood was withdrawn. Voluntary activity (wheel revolutions) per day averaged weekly is shown by the two lower lines. *P < 0.05 by unpaired t-test between these two groups. (From Edgerton, V. R., Diamond, L. B., and Olson, J., *J. Nutr.,* 107, 1595—1601, 1977. With permission.

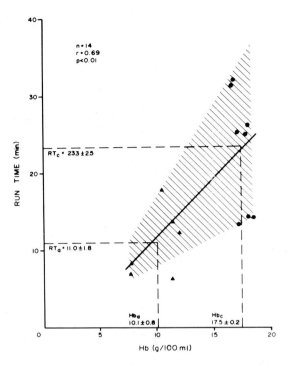

FIGURE 26. The relationship of exhaustive run time (RT) and Hb is illustrated. RT and Hb (mean ± SEM) for control (c or •) and anemic rats (a or ▲) are shown numerically and plotted. The cross-hatched area is to emphasize the apparent increasing criticalness of Hb as a determining factor on RT with decreasing Hb concentrations of whole blood. RT = 1.5 (Hb) −3.4 (From Edgerton, V. R., Diamond, L. B., and Olson, J., *J. Nutr.*, 107, 1595—1601, 1977.

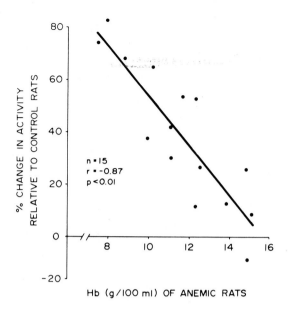

FIGURE 27.   The relationship between Hb and percent differences in voluntary activity is shown. Percent change in activity $= -9.56$ (Hb) $+ 149.59$. (From Edgerton, V. R., Diamond, L. B., and Olson, J., *J. Nutr.*, 107, 1595—1601, 1977. With permission.)

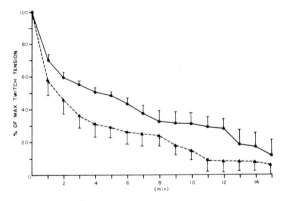

FIGURE 28.   Mean (±SEM) unfused twitch tension, expressed as the percent to the maximum level, in the in situ gastrocnemius during repetitive stimulation (7 per second). The overall mean tension was greater in the control than the anemic group (P<0.05 by unpaired t-test). (●—●) control, n = 5; ▲-----▲ anemic, n = 4. (From Edgerton, V. R., Diamond, L. B., and Olson, J., *J. Nutr.*, 107, 1595—1601, 1977. With permission.)

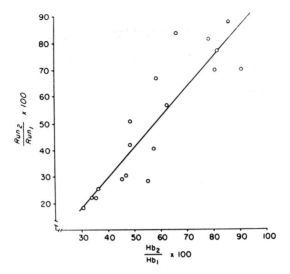

FIGURE 29. Work performance in relation to Hb. Rats were run on a treadmill increasing the workload in increments by increasing speed and slope. The rats were run 24 hr before (Hb_1, Run_1) and 0.5 to 2 hr after (Hb_2, Run_2) acute induction of anemia accomplished by exchange transfusion using plasma. $y = 1.13x -16$ ($r = 0.90$, $P < 0.001$). (From Wranne, B. and Woodson, R. D., *J. Appl. Physiol.*, 34, 732—735, 1973. With permission.)

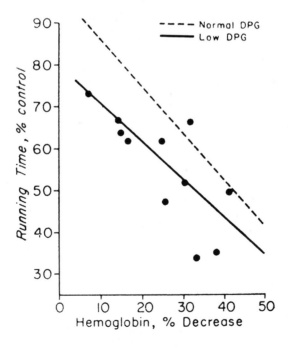

FIGURE 30. Relation between change in Hb and performance of rats on a treadmill. The dashed line represents data reported in Reference 58. The solid line is the least squares regression of the points shown when the 2, 3-diphosphoglycerate of red blood cells is depressed so that P_{50} (P_{O_2} at which half saturation of Hb with O_2 is achieved) is decreased from 36 to 23 mm Hg. (From Woodson, R. D., Wranne, B., and Ditter, J. C., *J. Clin. Invest.*, 52, 2717—2724, 1973. With permission.)

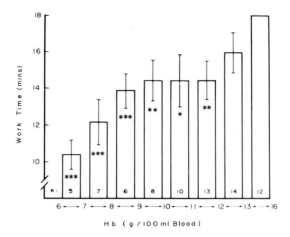

FIGURE 31.   Maximum treadmill work time in different Hb groups. Means (±SEM) were compared using an unpaired t-test between the highest Hb group and each of the lower Hb groups (P<0.05*, P<0.01**, P<0.001***). Female tea pluckers in Sri Lanka performed a standard multistage treadmill test in which they walked for 3 min up a 10% grade at 1.59 km/hr. The speed was then increased to 3.18 km/hr for 3 min and to 4.77 km/hr for 3 min, both at the 10% grade. After that, the grade was changed to 14 and then 18% and, if possible, the top workload was 3 min at 6.36 km/hr and 20% grade. The test was discontinued if any of the following conditions occurred: (1) the subjects completed the maximum exercise time on the treadmill (18 min); (2) the subjects attained the target heart rate (95% of maximum as predicted for age; (3) S-T segment depression was observed; (4) local muscle fatigue made walking impossible; (5) the subjects had severe respiratory distress; or (6) the subjects became dizzy and disoriented. (From Gardner, G. W., Edgerton, V. R., Senewiratne, B., Barnard, R. J., and Ohira, Y., *Am. J. Clin. Nutr.*, 30, 910—917, 1977. With permission.)

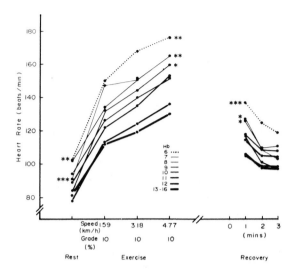

FIGURE 32. Heart rate response at rest and three work-loads and during 3 min of recovery as it related to the Hb level of the subjects. Significance of the differences of the group with a Hb of > 13.0 g/100 mℓ is compared with each of the lower Hb groups (P<0.05*, P<0.01**, P<0.001*** by unpaired t-test). (From Gardner, G. W., Edgerton, V. R., Senewiratne, B., Barnard, R. J., and Ohira, Y., *Am. J. Clin. Nutr.,* 30, 910—917, 1977. With permission.)

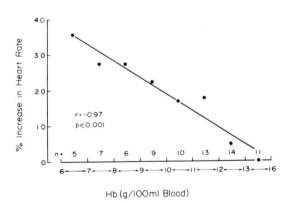

FIGURE 33. Percentage increase of mean heart rate (HR), relative to the subjects with a Hb > 13.0 g/100 mℓ of blood, for each Hb group at a workload of 4.77 km/hr at 10% grade. Δ in HR = −4.7 × Hb + 66.1. (From Gardner, G. W., Edgerton, V. R., Senewiratne, B., Barnard, R. J., and Ohira, Y., *Am. Clin. Nutr.,* 30, 910—917, 1977. With permission.)

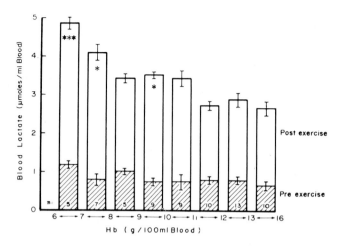

FIGURE 34.   Mean (±SEM) pre- and postexercise venous blood lactate levels. (*) = $p < 0.05$ and (***) = $p < 0.001$ were the results of unpaired t-tests between the highest hemoglobin (Hb) group and each of the lower Hb groups. The n represents the number of subjects. (From Gardner, G. W., Edgerton, V. R., Senewiratne, B., Barnard, R. J., and Ohira, Y., *Am. J. Clin. Nutr.*, 30, 910—917, 1977. With permission.)

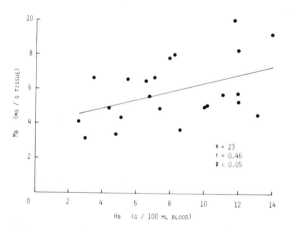

FIGURE 35.   Relationship between resting blood Hb and Mb content in human vastus lateralis muscle obtained by needle biopsy. Mb = $0.24 \times$ Hb + 3.91.

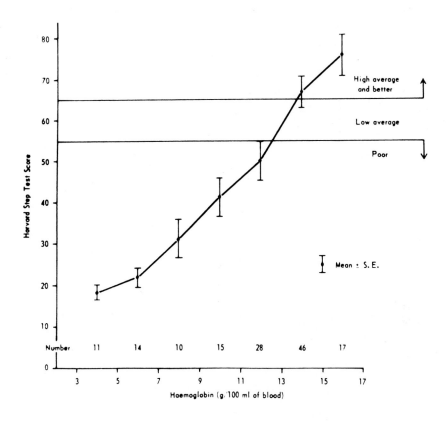

FIGURE 36. Harvard step test score in Guatemalan agricultural laborers with different Hb concentrations. (From Viteri, F. E. and Torún, B., *Clin. Haematol.*, 3, 609—626, 1974. With permission.)

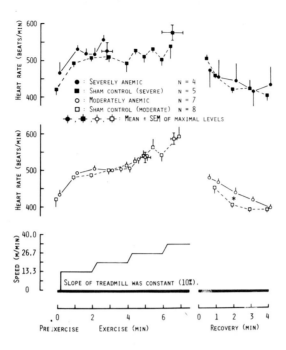

FIGURE 37.   Mean (±SEM) heart rate at submaximal and maximal workloads and during recovery for four groups. Significant differences between each sham control group and their respective anemic group are indicated by * = p < 0.05. Mean run time to exhaustion was significantly less in both severely (p < 0.01) and moderately (p < 0.001) anemic groups than their control groups. Mean maximal heart rate was taken irrespective of the time during the treadmill run at which the maximum occurred.

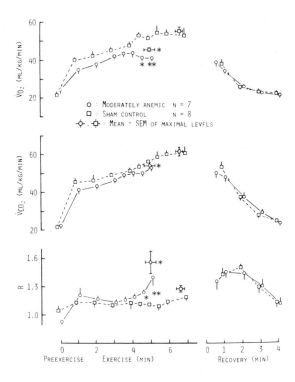

FIGURE 38. Mean (±SEM) oxygen consumption ($\dot{V}_{O_2}$), carbon dioxide production ($\dot{V}_{CO_2}$) and respiratory exchange ratio (R) at submaximal and maximal workloads and during recovery for moderately anemic rats. Significant differences between sham control and anemic groups are indicated by (*) = $p < 0.05$ and (**) = $p < 0.01$. Mean maximal $\dot{V}_{O_2}$, $\dot{V}_{CO_2}$ and R were taken irrespective of the time during the treadmill running at which the maximum occurred.

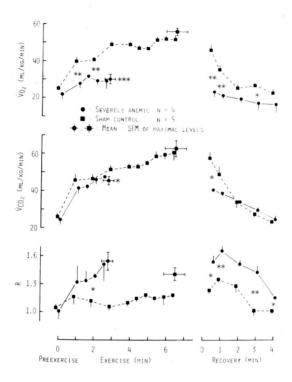

FIGURE 39.   Mean (±SEM) oxygen consumption ($\dot{V}_{O_2}$), carbon dioxide production ($\dot{V}_{CO_2}$) and respiratory exchange ratio (R) at submaximal and maximal workloads and during recovery for severely anemic rats. Significant differences between sham control and anemic groups are indicated by (*) = $p < 0.05$, (**) = $p < 0.01$ and (***) = $p < 0.001$. Mean maximal $\dot{V}_{O_2}$, $\dot{V}_{CO_2}$, and R were taken irrespective of the time during the treadmill running at which the maximum occurred.

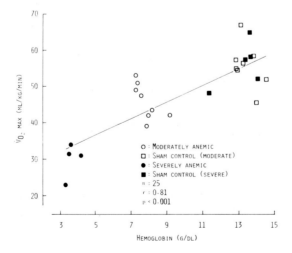

FIGURE 40.   Relationship between hemoglobin (Hb) and maximal oxygen consumption ($\dot{V}_{O_2}$ max). $\dot{V}_{O_2}$ max = 2.26 (Hb) + 25.38. Correlation coefficients for the moderately anemic and severely anemic rats were 0.52 ($p < 0.05$) and 0.95 ($p < 0.001$), respectively, and 0.81 when combined.[61]

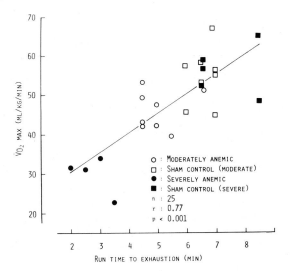

FIGURE 41. Relationship between run time to exhaustion (RT) and maximal oxygen consumption ($\dot{V}_{O_2}$ max). $\dot{V}_{O_2}$ max = 4.91 (RT) + 20.51. Correlation coefficients for the moderately anemic and severely anemic groups were 0.54 (p < 0.05) and 0.86 (p < 0.01), respectively, and 0.77 when combined.[61]

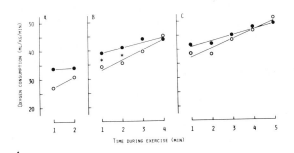

FIGURE 42. The comparison of oxygen consumption ($\dot{V}_{O_2}$) during exercise between the rats with higher (•) and lower (o) plasma iron levels but with equal, or similar Hg levels. B-⊙: $\dot{V}_{O_2}$ = 1.71(WL) + 37.55 (r = 0.94, p < 0.05), B-o : $\dot{V}_{O_2}$ = 3.67(WL) + 29.35 (r = 0.96, p < 0.05), C-• : $\dot{V}_{O_2}$ = 2.08(WL) + 38.70 (r = 0.98, p < 0.01) and C-o : $\dot{V}_{O_2}$ = 3.30(WL) + 33.60 (r = 0.97, p < 0.01). The WL represents the time during exercise. * = p < 0.05 by paired t-tests between • and O at each workload. A : Hb = 3.6 (•) and 3.5 g/dℓ (O), Fe = 61 (•) and 23 (O); B : Hb = 7.6 ± 0.1 (Mean ± SEM, •) and 7.6 ± 0.2 g/dℓ (O), Fe = 157 ± 11 (•) and 85 ± 20 ug/dℓ (O); C : Hb = 13.4 ± 0.2 (•) and 13.4 ± 0.3 g/dℓ (O), Fe = 232 ± 16 (•) and 163 ± 12 μg/dℓ (O).

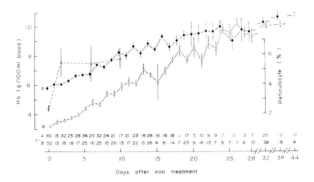

FIGURE 43.   The time course of change (Mean ± SEM) in Hb levels and reticulocyte counts (open triangle) after Imferon ® infusion i.v. Solid circles represent subjects with initial Hb levels greater than 4.0 g/100 mℓ of blood and open circles with Hb less than or equal to 4.0 g/100 mℓ. In both groups, Hb concentration increased significantly (p < 0.05 by paired t-tests) 1 day after iron treatment. Reticulocyte counts increased within 3 days after iron treatment (p < 0.05). Numbers of subjects for reticulocyte counts on day 0, 1 to 3, 4 to 7, and ≥ 8 were 55, 7, 10, and 24, respectively.

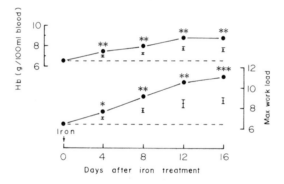

FIGURE 44.   Changes in Hb at rest and maximum workload reached following iron treatment in Sri Lankans (vertical bars represent SE of mean difference). Significant differences were determined by a paired t-test between the values before and each day after treatment. The work intensity of workloads 6, 8, 10, and 12 were 2.40 at 17, 4.41 at 14, 5.19 to 19, and 6.42 km/hr at 20%, respectively. (P< 0.05*, P< 0.01,** and P< 0.001***.) (From Edgerton, V. R., Gardner, G. W., Senewiratne, B., Barnard, R. J., and Ohira, Y., unpublished observations, 1977.)

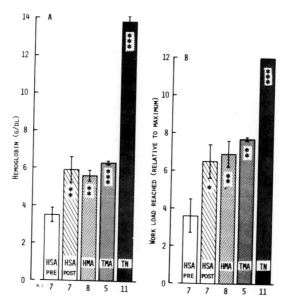

FIGURE 45. Hemoglobin (A) and maximal workload reached (B, expressed in relative numbers, see Table 2) are shown prior to and 1 day after transfusion of 570 mℓ of whole blood (mean ± SEM). The n represents the number of subjects in each case. HSA: Hospital severely anemic (pre- and post-transfusion), HMA: Hospital moderately anemic, TMA: Tea estate moderately anemic, and TN: Tea estate normal subjects. The * = $p < 0.05$, ** = $p < 0.01$ and *** = $p < 0.001$ were obtained by paired or unpaired t-tests between pre-transfusion and each group. Only TN group had significantly higher values than HSA post both in Hb and maximal workload tolerated ($p < 0.001$ by unpaired t-test).

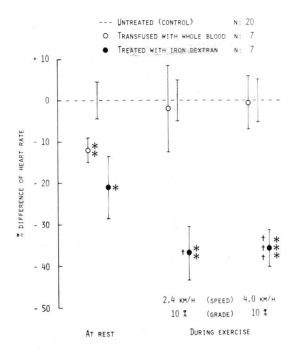

FIGURE 46.   Effects of whole blood transfusion and iron dextran infusion in iron-deficient anemic subjects on heart rates at rest and during exercise. The heart rates in the transfused subjects and the iron-treated subjects were compared with the values in the untreated control subjects. Mean ± SEM are shown. The * = p < 0.05, ** = p < 0.01, and *** = p < 0.001 were obtained by unpaired t-tests between the mean value in the untreated control group and individual values in the transfused and iron-treated subjects. The † = p<0.05 and were obtained by unpaired t-tests between the transfused and iron treated subjects. All of the groups had the same Hb levels. Note that even though their Hb levels were the same, heart rates in the iron-treated subjects were significantly lower than those in the subjects who received no treatment or were transfused with whole blood. (From Ohira, Y., Edgerton, V. R., Gardner, G. W., Senewiratne, B., and Simpson, D. R., *Nutr. Rep. Int.*, 18, 647—651, 1978. With permission)

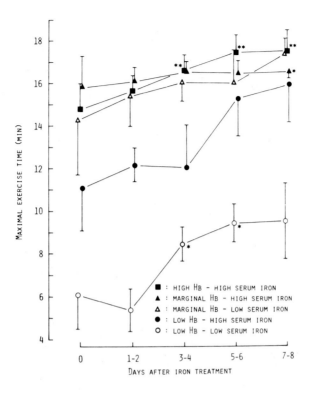

FIGURE 47. Changes in mean maximal work capacity in response to iron treatment (± SEM). * = p < 0.05 and ** = p < 0.01 by paired t-tests between, before, and each day after treatment. Initial work time in the low Hb - low serum iron group was significantly less than the high Hb - high iron, marginal Hb - high iron (p < 0.01) and marginal Hb - low iron groups (p < 0.05).

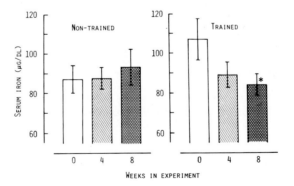

FIGURE 48. Changes in serum iron levels in response to physical training. Mean ± SEM. Both trained groups and both non-trained groups were combined. The * = p < 0.05 is the result of a paired t-test between pre- and post-treatments. (From Ohira, Y., Ph.D. dissertation, University of Southern California, 1980.)

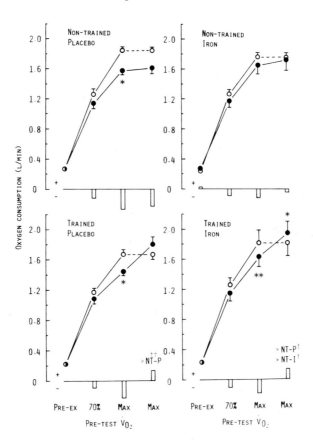

FIGURE 49.   Changes in oxygen consumption (pre-exercise, at 70% of $\dot{V}_{o2}$ max and $\dot{V}_{o2}$ max in pre-test, and maximal levels in both tests). Mean ± SEM. O = pre-test and $\bullet$ = post-test. The maximal levels connected with broken lines were obtained at the same, or lower, or higher work load than for $\dot{V}_{o2}$ max. Thus, broken lines show that exercise was not always continued. $*$ = $p < 0.05$ and $**$ = $p < 0.01$ among pre- and post-tests. The bars represent the mean differences between pre- and post-tests. Statistical significances in the magnitude of these changes between each group are shown by $\dagger$ = $p < 0.05$ and $\dagger\dagger$ = $p < 0.01$. (From Ohira, Y., Ph.D. dissertation, University of Southern California, 1980.)

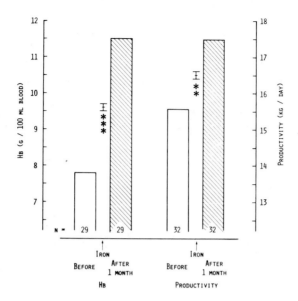

FIGURE 50.   Changes in Hb and daily productivity (tea picked) in response to daily oral iron treatment in subjects whose initial Hb levels were less than 9 g/dℓ. The ** = p < 0.01, *** = p < 0.001, and vertical bars. Mean ± SEMD were obtained from paired t-tests between the values before and 1 month after iron treatment. The N represents the number of subjects.

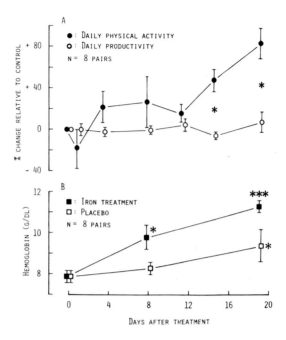

FIGURE 51.   **(A)** Percent changes (Mean ± SEM) in daily physical activity and productivity (tea picked) compared to the pre-treatment recordings in response to oral iron treatment. The percent changes of experimental group relative to placebo group which were matched by initial Hb levels were examined. The * = p < 0.05 was obtained by paired t-tests between the activity levels before and each day after treatment. **(B)** Changes in Hb levels (Mean ± SEM) in response to iron or placebo treatment. The * = p < 0.05, ** = p < 0.01 and *** = p < 0.001 were obtained by paired t-tests between day 0 (pre-treatment) and each day after treatment. (From Edgerton, V. R., Gardner, G. W., Ohira, Y., Gunawardena, K. A., and Senewiratne, B., *Br. Med. J.*, 2, 1546—1549, 1980.)

REFERENCES

1. **Krogh, A. and Lindhard, J.**, The relative value of fat and carbohydrate as sources of muscular energy. With appendices on the correlation between standard metabolism and the respiratory quotient during rest and work, *Biochem. J.*, 14, 290—363, 1920.
2. **Bierring, E.**, The respiratory quotient and the efficiency of moderate exercise (measured in the initial stage and in the steady state during postabsorptive conditions). With special reference to the influence of diet, *Arbeitsphysiologie*, 5, 17—48, 1932.
3. **Christensen, E. H., Krogh, A., and Lindhard, J.**, Investigations on heavy muscular work, *League Nations Bull. Health Organ.*, 3, 388—417, 1934.
4. **Hedman, R.**, The available glycogen in man and the connection between rate of oxygen intake and carbohydrate usage, *Acta Physiol. Scand.*, 405, 305—321, 1957.
5. **Hultman, E. and Bergström, J.**, Muscle glycogen synthesis in relation to diet studied in normal subjects, *Acta Med. Scand.*, 182, 109—117, 1967.
6. **Bergström, J., Hermansen, L., Hultman, E., and Saltin, B.**, Diet, muscle glycogen and physical performance, *Acta Physiol. Scand.*, 71, 140—150, 1967.
7. **Karlsson, J. and Saltin, B.**, Diet, muscle glycogen, and endurance performance, *J. Appl. Physiol.*, 31, 203—206, 1971.

8. Hultman, E., Physiological role of muscle glycogen in man, with special reference to exercise, *Circ. Res.*, 20 (Suppl. 1), 99—114, 1967.

9. Taylor, A. W., The effects of different feeding regimens and endurance exercise programs on carbohydrate and lipid metabolism, in *Proc. 1st Int. Congr. Nutrition and the Athlete*, University of Leningrad Press, Leningrad, 1976.

10. Gollnick, P. D., Piehl, K., Saubert, C. W., IV, Armstrong, R. B., and Saltin, B., Diet, exercise, and glycogen changes in human muscle fibers, *J. Appl. Physiol.*, 33, 421—425, 1972.

11. Houston, M. E., Reid, P. A., and Green, H. J., Carbohydrate ingestion during prolonged running performance, *Nutr. Rep. Int.*, 9, 377—381, 1974.

12. Ehrenstein, W., Emans, C., and Muller-Limmroth, W., Glycogen reduction in working muscle during 8-hour bicycle work and its inhibition by moderate elevation of the blood glucose level, *Pflügers Arch.*, 320, 233—246, 1970.

13. Ahlborg, B., Bergström, J., Ekelund, L.-G., and Hultman, E., Muscle glycogen and muscle electrolytes during prolonged physical exercise, *Acta Physiol. Scand.*, 70, 129—142, 1967.

14. Pruett, E. D. R., Glucose and insulin during prolonged work stress in men living on different diets, *J. Appl. Physiol.*, 28, 199—208, 1970.

15. Holloszy, J. O. and Narahara, H. T., Studies of tissue permeability. X. Changes in permeability to 3-methylglucose associated with contraction of isolated frog muscle, *J. Biol. Chem.*, 240, 3493—3500, 1965.

16. Bergström, J., Hultman, E., and Roch-Norlund, A. E., Muscle glycogen synthetase in normal subjects. Basal values, effect of glycogen depletion by exercise and of a carbohydrate-rich diet following exercise, *Scand. J. Clin. Lab. Invest.*, 29, 231—236, 1972.

17. Hultman, E. and Nilsson, L. H., Liver glycogen in man. Effect of different diets and muscular exercise, in *Muscle Metabolism During Exercise*, Pernow, B. and Saltin, B., Eds., Plenum Press, New York, 1971, 143—151.

18. Edgerton, V. R., Neuromuscular adaptation to power and endurance work, *Can. J. Appl. Sport Sci.*, 1, 49—58, 1976.

19. Edgerton, V. R., Exercise and the growth and development of muscle tissue, in *Physical Activity: Human Growth and Development*, Rarick, G. L., Ed., Academic Press, New York, 1971, chap. 1.

20. Christensen, D. A. and Crampton, E. W., Effects of exercise and diet on nitrogenous constituents in several tissues of adult rats, *J. Nutr.*, 86, 369—375, 1965.

21. Giovannetti, P. M. and Stothers, S. C., Influence of diet and age on ribonucleic acid, protein and free amino acid levels of rat skeletal muscle, *Growth*, 39, 1—16, 1975.

22. Yamaji, R., Studies on protein metabolism during muscular exercise, I. Nitrogen metabolism in training for heavy muscular exercise, *J. Phys. Soc. Jpn.*, 13, 476—482, 1951.

23. Yamaji, R., Studies on protein metabolism during muscular exercise. II. Changes of blood properties during training for heavy muscular exercise, *J. Phys. Soc. Jpn.*, 13, 483—489, 1951.

24. Teruoka, G. and Saito, K. H., The protein demand in workers, *Chem. Abstr.*, 51, 18172, 1957.

25. Pitts, G. C., Consolazio, F. C., and Johnson, R. E., Dietary protein and physical fitness in temperature and hot environments, *J. Nutr.*, 27, 497—508, 1944.

26. Rajalakshmi, R., Pillai, K. R., and Ramakrishnan, C. V., Effects of different supplements to low protein and poor quality protein diets on performance and brain enzymes in the albino rat, *J. Neurochem.*, 16, 599—606, 1969.

27. Gontzea, I., Sutzescu, P., and Dumitrache, S., The influence of muscular activity on nitrogen balance and on the need of man for proteins, *Nutr. Rep. Int.* 10, 35—43, 1974.

28. Cathcart, E. P. and Burnett, W. A., The influence of muscle work on metabolism in varying conditions of diet, *Proc. R. Soc. London*, 99, 405—426, 1926.

29. Garry, R. C., The static effort and the excretion of uric acid, *J. Physiol.*, 62, 364—372, 1927.

30. Keys, A., Physical performance in relation to diet, *Fed. Proc. Fed. Am. Soc. Exp. Biol.*, 2, 164—187, 1943.

31. Crampton, E. W., Nutrient-to-calorie ratios in applied nutrition, *J. Nutr.*, 82, 353—365, 1964.

32. Malinow, M. R., McLaughlin, P., Perley, A., Laastuen, L., and Van Hook, E., Hepatic and adrenal degradation of cholestrol during rest and muscular activity, *J. Appl. Physiol.*, 29, 323—327, 1970.

33. Issekutz, B., Jr., Shaw, W. A. S., and Issekutz, T. B., Effect of lactate on the FFA and glycerol turnover in resting and exercising dogs, *J. Appl. Physiol.*, 39, 349—353, 1975.

34. Issekutz, B., Jr., Birkhead, N. C., and Rodahl K., Effect of diet on work metabolism, *J. Nutr.*, 79, 109—115, 1963.

35. Dohm, G. L., Huston, R. L., Askew, E. W., and Fleshood, H. L., Effects of exercise, training, and diet on muscle citric acid cycle enzyme activity, *Can. J. Biochem.*, 51, 849—854, 1973.

36. Edgerton, V. R., Bryant, S. L., Gillespie, C. A., and Gardner, G. W., Iron deficiency anemia and physical performance and activity of rats, *J. Nutr.*, 102, 381—399, 1972.

37. McCall, M. G., Newman, G. E., O'Brien, J. R. P., Valberg, L. S., and Witts, L. J., Studies in iron metabolism. I. The experimental production of iron deficiency in the growing rat, *Br. J. Nutr.,* 16, 297—304, 1962.

38. Rakušan, K., Oxygen affinity of blood in rats during chronic anemia and after its correction, *Respir. Physiol.,* 17, 263—267, 1973.

39. Eaton, J. W. and Brewer, G. J., The relationship between red cell 2,3-diphosphoglycerate and levels of hemoglobin in the human, *Biochemistry,* 61, 756—760, 1968.

40. Sproule, B. J., Mitchell, J. H., and Miller, W. F., Cardiopulmonary physiological responses to heavy exercise in patients with anemia, *J. Clin. Invest.,* 39, 378—388, 1960.

41. Davies, C. T. M., Chukweumeka, A. C., and Van Haaren, J. P. M., Iron-deficiency anaemia: its effect on maximum aerobic power and responses to exercise in African males aged 17—40 years, *Clin. Sci.,* 44, 555—562, 1973.

42. Woodson, R., Wranne, B., and Detter, J., Effect of erythrocyte 2,3-DPG and hemoglobin concentration on O_2 delivery and work performance, *Clin. Res.,* 20, 628, 1972.

43. Vellar, O. D. and Hermansen, L., Physical performance and hematological parameters. With special reference to hemoglobin and maximal oxygen uptake, *Acta Med. Scand., Suppl.,* 522, 1—40, 1971.

44. Andersen, H. T. and Stavem, P., Iron deficiency anaemia and the acid-base variations of exercise, *Nutr. Metab.,* 14, 129—135, 1972.

45. Pattengale, P. K. and Holloszy, J. O., Augmentation of skeletal muscle myoglobin by a program of treadmill running, *Am. J. Physiol.,* 213, 783—785, 1967.

46. Barnard, R. J. and Peter, J. B., Effect of exercise on skeletal muscle. III. Cytochrome changes, *J. Appl. Physiol.,* 31, 904—908, 1971.

47. Dallman, P. R. and Schwartz, H. C., Myoglobin and cytochrome response during repair of iron deficiency in the rat, *J. Clin. Invest.,* 44, 1631—1638, 1965.

48. Finch, C. A., Miller, L. R., Inamdar, A. R., Person, R., Seiler, K., and Mackler, B., Iron deficiency in the rat. Physiological and biochemical studies of muscle dysfunction, *J. Clin. Invest.,* 58, 447—453, 1976.

49. Ekblom, B., Effect of physical training on oxygen transport system in man, *Acta Physiol. Scand., Suppl.,* 328, 1—45, 1969.

50. Saltin, B., Hartley, L. H., Kilbom, Å., and Åstrand, I., Physical training in sedentary middle-aged and older men. II Oxygen uptake, heart rate, and blood lactate concentration at submaximal and maximal exercise, *Scand. J. Clin. Lab. Invest.,* 24, 323—334, 1969.

51. Finch, C. A., Gollnick, P. D., Hlastala, M. P., Miller, L. R., Dillman, E., and Mackler, B., Lactic acidosis as a result of iron deficiency, *J. Clin. Invest.,* 64, 129—137, 1979.

52. Koziol, B. J., Ohira, Y., Simpson, D. R., and Edgerton, V. R., Biochemical skeletal muscle and hematological profiles of moderate and severely iron deficient and anemic adult rats, *J. Nutr.,* 108, 1306—1314, 1978.

53. Woodson, R. D., Wranne, B., and Detter, J. C., Effect of increased blood oxygen affinity on work performance of rats, *J. Clin. Invest.,* 52, 2717—2724, 1973.

54. Gillespie, C. A., Simpson, D. R., and Edgerton, V. R., High glycogen content of red as opposed to white skeletal muscle fibers of guinea pigs, *J. Histochem. Cytochem.,* 18, 552—558, 1970.

55. de Duve, C., A spectrophotometric method for the simultaneous determination of myoglobin and hemoglobin in extracts of human muscle, *Acta Chem. Scand.,* 2, 264—289, 1948.

56. Smith, L. B., Spectrophotometric assay of cytochrome c oxidase, in *Methods of Biochemical Analysis,* Glick, D., Ed., Interscience, New York, 1975.

57. Edgerton, V. R., Diamond, L. B., and Olson, J., Voluntary activity, cardiovascular and muscular responses to anemia in rats, *J. Nutr.,* 107, 1595—1601, 1977.

58. Wranne, B. and Woodson, R. D., A graded treadmill test for rats: maximal work performance in normal and anemic animals, *J. Appl. Physiol.,* 34, 732—735, 1973.

59. Gardner, G. W., Edgerton, V. R., Senewiratne, B., Barnard, R. J., and Ohira, Y., Physical work capacity and metabolic stress in subjects with iron deficiency anemia, *Am. J. Clin. Nutr.,* 30, 910—917, 1977.

60. Viteri, F. E. and Torún, B., Anaemia and physical work capacity, *Clin. Haematol.,* 3, 609—626, 1974.

61. Ohira, Y., Koziol, B. J., Edgerton, V. R., and Brooks, G. A., Oxygen consumption and work capacity in iron deficient anemic rats, *J. Nutr.,* in press.

62. Woodson, R. D., Wills, R. E., and Lenfant, C., Effect of acute and established anemia on O_2 transport at rest, submaximal and maximal work, *J. Appl. Physiol.,* 44, 36—43, 1978.

63. Ohira, Y., Edgerton, V. R., Gardner, G. W., Senewiratne, B., Barnard, R. J., and Simpson, D. R., Work capacity, heart rate and blood lactate responses to iron treatment, *Br. J. Haematol.,* 41, 365—372, 1979.

64. Ohira, Y., Edgerton, V. R., Gardner, G. W., Senewiratne, B., and Simpson, D. R., Non-hemoglobin related effects on heart rate in iron deficiency anemia, *Nutr. Rep. Int.,* 18, 647—651, 1978.

65. Ohira, Y., Hematological responses and work capacity after iron supplementation in sedentary and trained women, Ph.D. Dissertation, University of Southern California, 1980.

66. Edgerton, V. R., Gardner, G. W., Ohira, Y., Gunawardena, K. A., and Senewiratne, B., Iron-deficiency anaemia and its effect on worker productivity and activity patterns, *Br. Med. J.,* 2, 1546—1549, 1980.

67. Mayer, J. and Bullen, B., Nutrition and athletic performance, *Physiol. Rev.,* 40, 369—397, 1960.

68. Shephard, R. J., Campbell, R., Pimm, P., Stuart, D., and Wright, G. R., Vitamin E. Exercise, and the recovery from physical activity, *Eur. J. Appl. Physiol.,* 33, 119—126, 1974.

69. Simonson, E., Enzer, N., Baer, A., and Braun, R., The influence of vitamin B (complex) surplus on the capacity for muscular and mental work, *J. Indust. Hyg. Toxicol.,* 24, 83—90, 1942.

70. Keys, A., Henschel, A. F., Mickelsen, O., and Brozek, J. M., The performance of normal young men on controlled thiamine intakes, *J. Nutr.,* 26, 399—415, 1943.

71. Montoye, H. J., Spata, P. J., Pinckney, V., and Barron, L., Effects of vitamin B_{12} supplementation on physical fitness and growth of young boys, *J. Appl. Physiol.,* 7, 589—592, 1955.

NUTRITIONAL FACTORS AND PHYSICAL PERFORMANCE IN MAN

Ivan M. Sharman

HISTORICAL INTRODUCTION

Ever since his creation man has had to perform physical exercise. During the early period of his existence upon earth such exercise may well have been confined to meeting his most pressing needs for survival, viz., the obtaining of sufficient food to satisfy his pangs of hunger. Anything edible would have been consumed, of course, without regard to nutritional values. Gradually, however, man would have become aware that certain foods were more desirable than others because of their taste and smell and also because of the sense of satisfaction that they provided when eaten. Primitive man is known to have endowed food with various attributes such as fears, hopes, and friendly and unfriendly feelings. Such was the primitive belief that eating the heart or flesh of strong or agressive animals would confer courage and strength, whereas eating the flesh of timid and weak animals would undermine man's most valued attributes.[1]

Minimum nutritional requirements were, no doubt, met by man in those early days through use of the natural vegetation in his particular area, and by the slaughter for food of those animals he was able to catch. Later, the tilling of the ground led to the sowing and harvesting of crops. Such tilling required much physical activity on the part of man. The invention of the plough substantially reduced man's physical efforts in the field as did also the harnessing of animals for draught purposes.

After his essential needs for existence had been met, the advent of spare time enabled man to develop the idea of recreation. Physical exercise for recreative purposes, viz., the various forms of athletics, gradually emerged. Such forms of exercise are known to have been in existence for thousands of years, and it is from this sphere of activity that some of the earliest information about the nutritional needs for physical performance can be gleaned.

Organized athletics are said to have appeared in history when the first Olympic games were held in Greece in 776 BC. These games continued to be held every four years for over a thousand years. However, according to Harris, there is evidence that the first Olympics were not really the beginning of organized sports as references to athletic events are included in the Homeric poems, thereby indicating an origin some five centuries earlier.[2]

In those far off days of the first Olympic games there are records that the athlete was concerned with what he ate.[3] For example, Charmis of Sparta, who was victor at the games held in 668 BC, is known to have trained on a special diet of dried figs. Tradition indicates that as a sprinter he found the extra sugar in fruit helpful.[2] Pausanius, the classical writer of the second century AD says that the first athlete to train on a diet mainly of meat was Dromeus of Stymphalus, a long-distance runner, in about 480 BC. However, Harris considers that this innovation is probably more correctly attributed to Eurymenes of Samos, a heavyweight competitor of the previous century.[2] A curiosity about this tradition is that he is said to have been advised so to do by his trainer who was Pythagoras, the mathematician and philosopher, who is generally supposed to have been a vegetarian. Harris says that the temptation to eat large quantities of meat must have been particularly strong for competitors in the fighting events of the games as in these events sheer body-weight counted for so much.

It is probable that the only meat eaten in the normal course of events would have been that consumed at religious festivals. So, the idea that athletes might perform better with more meat was plausible especially when it was realized that muscles are made up of proteins. It was logical to expect that the ingestion of large quantities of protein would encourage muscle growth and so, performance. However, it has now been known for well over a century that there is in fact no evidence to support the view that extra protein is beneficial.[4] Even so, it is still held in some quarters that large amounts of meat are a desirable asset for the athlete. A recent survey of Olympic athletes has shown that their intakes of protein do in fact vary from 60 to 300 g daily.[5]

During the centuries that have followed the first Olympic games, experience, traditions, the fads and fancies of trainers, and the whims of individual competitors have all influenced the items that have been proposed for inclusion in the diet of athletes.

DEVELOPMENT OF NUTRITION AS A SCIENCE

During the present century as nutrition developed into a science, it is surprising, even disappointing, that in general, nothing has been firmly proved regarding the suitability of any particular type of diet for athletes.[6] If a diet is to be suitable for athletes, or indeed for anyone having to carry out physical performance, it must contain adequate quantities of protein, fats, and carbohydrate together with the necessary amounts of vitamins and minerals. Furthermore, it must be sufficient to meet the high energy requirements for those undertaking physical work. This is especially true for athletes participating in long distance endurance events. On the other hand, it should not be so excessive that it causes obesity, if this were possible, by those undergoing a vigorous training program though weight lifters and wrestlers may sometimes want to put on weight intentionally.

Despite what has been said above, our understanding of the science of nutrition has opened the door to the idea of supercharging the body with the nutrients believed to be of special importance for those carrying out physical activity of any kind.[6] It is hoped, thereby, to raise performance levels above that possible on a normal diet. One of the more imaginative attempts in this direction has been the suggestion that the queen bee substance, or royal jelly, should be included in an athlete's diet.[7]

Many of the more bizarre nutritional beliefs of coaches echo Greek, Roman, or even older tribal advice. For example, a current best-seller attributes a number of exceptional properties for athletic nutrition to honey. While eating honey may be a pleasant way of consuming carbohydrates, there is no evidence to show that honey is inherently superior to other carbohydrate foods from a physiological point of view.[7] The composition of both the queen bee substance and of honey has been detailed by Steyn.[8]

On the other hand, scientific trials have been reported in which serious attempts have been made to ascertain whether extra amounts of vitamins can improve athletic and physical performance. There have also been extensive tests, carried out mainly in Scandinavia, to see whether additional quantities of carbohydrates can be ingested to meet the higher energy requirements of those participating in long distance athletic events. The details of these trials, and the effectiveness, if any, of the proposed additions to the normal diet in aiding performance will now be considered.

ROLE OF VITAMINS IN PHYSICAL PERFORMANCE

The recommended intakes of each of the vitamins are essential to all athletes and others undertaking physical work.[9,10] Such vitamins are needed for general health and development irrespective of physical exercise.

When they occur, severe vitamin deficiencies are known to impair work performance. However, as it is sometimes difficult to recognize borderline deficiency states, a favorable effect of vitamin supplementation on performance may be observed. This is, of course, nothing more than a therapeutic effect of correcting the symptoms of deficiency.

Many workers have attempted to see whether the ingestion of vitamins additional to the accepted daily intakes, can be helpful in meeting the additional stress imposed by strenuous exercise. Furthermore, there are sometimes good scientific reasons for believing that extra quantities of vitamins may be needed, e.g., it is known that a deficiency of vitamin E in various animals causes the muscles to become dystrophic and it could be argued that when muscles are under stress an increased demand for this vitamin is made which is not provided by a normal diet.

WATER SOLUBLE VITAMINS

B Vitamins

Simonsen et al. have examined the influence of extra B vitamins on the performance of a dozen healthy subjects engaged in different types of muscular work.[11] No beneficial effects on total output or efficiency were found although in 8 of the 12 subjects flicker-fusion frequency increased, a finding usually regarded as an indication of decreased fatigue of the central nervous system. Keys and Henschel who carried out a series of tests on pretrained army men receiving adequate diets supplemented with five B vitamins and ascorbic acid, found no beneficial effects on endurance, recovery from exertion, resistance to fatigue, or muscular strength and dexterity.[12] However, in a series of carefully controlled experiments Harper et al. found that mixed vitamin supplementation did increase the vital capacity of a group of students.[13]

Some individual members of the group of B vitamins have been examined separately for their possible ergogenic or work-producing effects. The three best known members of the complex, thiamin, riboflavin, and niacin (nicotinic acid), are all involved in carbohydrate metabolism. Thiamin, for example, is connected with decarboxylation and carboxylation of pyruvic acid, one of the intermediary degradation products of carbohydrate breakdown. Bourne, who injected rats with thiamin or thiamin ascorbate, found that they ran on a treadmill longer than untreated rats before becoming fatigued.[14] Vytchikova has suggested that the thiamin content of athletes' rations should be increased above the usual daily intake of 1.5 to 2 mg on the basis of the fact that following vigorous exercise, the levels of both thiamin and pyruvic acid in the blood were found to be raised.[15] Vytchikova found that by supplementing the diet of some athletes with 10 to 20 mg thiamin, the levels of pyruvic acid in their blood were reduced to values similar to those found in manual workers engaged in only moderate exercise. It also improved reaction time before and after training.

Experiments with animals have shown that the rate of thiamin utilization depends upon the amount of carbohydrate metabolized, and epidemiological studies in man also suggest that thiamin requirements are closely allied to carbohydrate intake. However, little accuracy is lost if they are related to the total energy intake, and it is now general practice to express requirements for thiamin per 1000 kcal (4.2 MJ) ingested. Increased physical activity raises thiamine requirements because of the greater energy involved; but when expressed per 1000 kcal the requirement for the vitamin is constant and does not vary. The level needed to saturate the tissues varies between 0.3 and 0.35 mg thiamin/1000 kcal and any excess will be excreted. To allow for variations between individuals an intake of 0.4 mg/1000 kcal has been recommended.[9] Any excess above this level of intake will be excreted, so no benefit can be expected by the provision of extra quantities. This means that thiamin is ruled out as an ergogenic aid so long as the needs for carbohydrate metabolism are met.

A similar conclusion is reached when riboflavin and niacin are considered. Daily intakes of 0.44 mg riboflavin/1000 kcal and 6.6 mg nicotinic acid equivalents/1000 kcal have been recommended.[9] No further increases are deemed necessary apart from the related increase resulting from the larger amounts of energy needed for energetic exercise.

Other B vitamins, e.g., pyridoxin and possibly pantothenic acid and biotin, are concerned with aspects of metabolism. The requirements for these vitamins may be increased when metabolism is speeded up as in muscular exercise.[14] Confirmation of such higher requirements are not, however, forthcoming. When vitamin B_{12} was used to supplement the diet of boys aged 12 to 17 no improvement was observed on the Harvard Step Test Score, half-mile running time, height, weight, or a combination of age, height, and weight (Wetzel Grid) when all the boys were considered.[16] Some claims that pangamic acid (vitamin B_{15}) may aid physical performance have been reported.[17] Such claims, however, have not been confirmed. In general, it may be said that the B vitamins do not appear to be useful in aiding physical performance when added in amounts above those normally required.

Vitamin C

A number of observations have been made that suggest that vitamin C may have a connection with the ability of the body to perform physical work. One of the earliest of such observations was that outbreaks of scurvy often occurred during those periods when sailors were subjected to severe physical stress. Thus, Lind, in his famous treatise published in the eighteenth century, pointed out that outbreaks of the disease occurred during or immediately following periods of rough weather and, therefore, heavy manual work.[17]

One of the difficulties in assessing whether extra vitamin C will improve physical performance is the evaluation of the amount of the vitamin normally required. Various recommendations have been made for daily intake. It is known that 5 to 10 mg will prevent scurvy, but that higher levels, 20 mg or more, are needed for wound healing.[18] Levels of 30 mg in the U.K. and 60 mg in the U.S. have been suggested. Some authors have proposed that levels ranging from 100 to 300 mg are necessary for optimal physical efficiency, and still higher intakes have been suggested for what has become known as megatherapy. Thus, daily intakes of 1 g of the vitamin and even more have been used for treating the common cold.[19] With such wide variations in intake it can be easily understood that the investigator has difficulty in answering the question of whether additional amounts of the vitamin will aid physical performance. We can conclude, however, that the amount of the vitamin needed to prevent scurvy may be insufficient to maintain physical fitness and the potential for fulfilling maximum performance.

Despite the difficulties outlined above, several authors have attempted to ascertain whether supplementing a normal diet with vitamin C will improve physical performance. Thus, Margaria et al. gave an additional 250 mg to an athlete and two nonathletes. In a double blind trial in which either the vitamin or a placebo was given 90 min before a variety of tests of performance, no significant effect of the vitamin was observed.[20] Gey et al., in a much larger trial with nearly 300 male Air Force officers, investigated the effect of a daily dose of 1000 mg ascorbic acid on endurance performance and the rate, severity, and duration of athletic injury.[21] Each officer ran a 12-min field test at the beginning of a 12-week training period, was given the ascorbic acid or comparable placebo tablets daily, and was retested at the end of the training period. The results showed that any differences between those on the vitamin C supplement and on the placebos were negligible.

In another trial the effect of 2 g ascorbic acid per day on the performance of 20 trained and 20 untrained young males on a treadmill was investigated over a 5-day period. The results obtained were compared with those found after a similar period during which the subjects were given placebo tablets. Again, no significant differences were observed.[22] More recently, Bender and Nash have reviewed the literature on vitamin C and physical performance and have reported the details of their own investigations.[23] In view of the uncertainty that additional vitamin C might be beneficial in physical activity these authors made prolonged observations of athletes using their normal performance in regular competitive running as a criterion of improvement. They suggest that as far as the athletes themselves are concerned, unless a noticeable improvement in field performance can be observed, any changes measured in the laboratory would have little practical importance. They gave daily supplements of 250 mg vitamin C either the pure compound or the equivalent amount in orange juice. Both long and short distance athletes were investigated and the trials extended over two seasons. Besides field performances, work efficiency was measured by the Harvard Step Test. Oxygen consumption and pulse rate in some laboratory subjects were also measured and one experiment was repeated with doses up to 1 g vitamin C. The results of all these experiments showed that the addition to the regular diet of these athletes of vitamin C in tablet form or as orange juice had no beneficial effect on their competitive athletic performance or on their work efficiency and physical fitness index.

It must be concluded from the results of the trials described above that vitamin C cannot be regarded as an ergogenic aid. Therefore, little, if any, advantage can be expected by giving supplements of this vitamin so long as adequate amounts are provided in the diet to meet the requirements of normal metabolic processes.

FAT SOLUBLE VITAMINS

Vitamin E

As already mentioned in the introduction to this section, there are some good reasons for believing that additional quantities of vitamin E might aid physical performance. This vitamin has attracted special interest with regard to assisting performance for three main reasons, the first of which is the fact that in many species of animal a deficiency of the vitamin causes muscles to become dystrophic. It is tempting, therefore, to assume that when muscles are under stress their demand for vitamin E may be increased and may not be met by the amounts available in a normal diet. It is not suggested that a deficiency of the vitamin would cause dystrophy in the human, but it could result in lower muscular performance than might have been possible had the intakes of the vitamin been greater.

A second reason is that convincing evidence has been obtained with experimental animals that their resistance to hypoxia and hyperoxia can be influenced by their vitamin E status.[24,25] This finding may be linked with the ability of the vitamin to act as an antioxidant, as has been established in a number of investigations both in vivo and in vitro. Once again, there is a temptation to suggest that since a deficiency of vitamin E can cause an increased susceptibility to hypoxia, an increased intake of the vitamin might serve as a shield against those stresses that are inevitably imposed during all-out muscular performance.

A possible reason for thinking that vitamin E might benefit athletic performance originates from the alleged value of the vitamin in the treatment of those human diseases involving defects of the heart and circulation.[26,27] Although it is not claimed that the vitamin, even in large doses, can effect a permanent cure, it could be presumed that if it is able to ameliorate the conditions of circulatory strain, then it would act similarly under the stress of extreme exertion.

A number of claims have been made that vitamin E can improve physical performance. The claim of Percival in 1951 appears to be one of the earliest.[28] He examined a group of young sportsmen by a variety of tests including distance running, jumping, step tests, and push ups and concluded that supplementation with vitamin E improved their physical performance. Vitamin E has also been given to racehorses and improved performances reported.[29,30] In 1960, Prokop investigated the short-term effects of dosing with vitamin E on the performance of a standard exercise task by human volunteers.[31] He found that vitamin E increased the speed of recovery after the exercise and that the "oxygen debt" incurred was reduced. However, because of the small dose given, the apparently considerable benefit derived from ingestion of a placebo and the failure to make any due allowance for a possible training effect during the course of the study make his findings equivocal.

The relationship between athletic performance and the energy-yielding quality of wheat germ oil containing vitamin E has been extensively investigated by Cureton. In a series of experiments extending over many years he found significant improvement in endurance and various cardiorespiratory measurements.[32,33] Some of the beneficial effects of wheat germ oil have been attributed to octocosanol — a long straight chain primary alcohol — rather than to vitamn E. However, in two long-term studies by Consolazio et al. the effects of octacosanol and wheat germ oil on the performance of swimming rats was investigated; comparisons made during these studies indicated that the performance of the rats receiving these substances did not differ significantly from those of a control group.[34]

Moreover, the findings of Thomas with vitamin E contradict those of Cureton and Prokop.[35] They investigated 30 young male students; 15 were given 450 IU of α-tocopheryl acetate daily for 5 weeks and then placebos for an additional 5 weeks. The remaining 15 students received placebos first, and then vitamin E. At the commencement of the trial and at 5 and 10 weeks later, measurements were made of anthropometric status, reclining pulse-rate, resting respiratory rate, speed sit-ups, vertical jump, and pulse and respiratory rates immediately after activity. No significant differences were found between the dosed and undosed subjects during either test period. Thomas also reported that no changes were seen in temperature, in disposition, or in general feeling of well-being. The investigations of Consolazio also showed no beneficial effects of supplementation with vitamin E.[34]

It is, however, a reasonable comment to say that the findings of Thomas and Consolazio cannot be compared fairly with those of Cureton because, at least in some experiments, Cureton obtained greater effects with wheat germ oil than with pure vitamin E. With the intention of definitely ascertaining whether or not vitamin E per se might be used as an ergogenic aid, Sharman et al. carried out a trial with two matched groups of thirteen boarding-schoolboy swimmers.[36] Each boy received either 400 mg of α-tocopheryl acetate or a placebo daily during a 6-week training period. Evaluation of the possible effect of vitamin E was conducted with a battery of tests, including measurements of muscular development, heart and lung efficiency, and muscle fitness and coordination. The tests were administered at the beginning and end of an experimental period of 6 weeks. As might be expected, training was found to improve both physiological function and performance in both groups but there was no further improvement in the group given vitamin E. Therefore, it was concluded from this trial that vitamin E is of no value as an ergogenic aid. A similar conclusion was reached by Shephard and colleagues when they compared the perfmance of male swimmers given three capsules daily each containing 400 IU of d-α-tocopheryl acid succinate with those given only a placebo.[37]

After the publication of the work by Sharman et al., it was suggested that a positive effect might have been obtained with vitamin E had highly trained swimmers been investigated so that any effect of training was obviated.[36] Some years later, an opportunity occurred for them to test an elite group of competition swimmers including a number of Olympic competitors.[38] The use of such a highly motivated squad of swimmers ensured a precise control over the quantity and quality of the training undertaken, and also that their recreational activity was generally limited, if only by lack of spare time, to swimming. In this further trial two experimental groups of eight young male and seven young female swimmers each were daily given either 400 mg of α-tocopheryl acetate or placebos in addition to their usual diet during the 6-week period of swimming training. An evaluation of the experimental treatments was again made from tests of anthropometric status, cardiorespiratory efficiency, and motor fitness and performance. These tests were administered at the beginning and end of the experimental period. No significant differences between the two groups were observed resulting from the treatment with vitamin E. The slight improvements in cardiorespiratory efficiency, as shown by the submaximal and maximal work tests, and the marked improvements in muscular endurance, as indicated by the motor fitness tests, were common to both groups and, so, were a training effect, despite the fact that it had been expected that the effects of vitamin E would be eliminated. Therefore, from the results of this further trial there are no grounds for considering vitamin E as an ergogenic aid to performance. This neutral effect of vitamin E supplementation has since been confirmed by Talbot and Jamieson.[39]

Other Fat Soluble Vitamins

The recommended daily intakes of each of the other fat soluble vitamins besides vitamin E, viz., vitamins A, D, and K have been published.[9,10] Amounts in excess of those recommended are not known to improve performance in any way. Therefore, provided the recommended amounts are available in the daily diet no apparent advantage will be gained by giving more.

SOURCES OF MUSCULAR ENERGY

The energy necessary for every muscle contraction comes ultimately from dietary sources; in other words, by the combustion of food. Baldwin has said that living organisms are like machines and must conform to the law of conservation of energy; they must pay for all their activities in the currency of metabolism.[40] In the case of muscles, the immediate source of energy is ATP (adenosine triphosphate). This compound is capable of splitting into ADP (adenosine diphosphate) and phosphoric acid and when it does, it provides the actual power for muscle contraction. As muscles contain only small quantities of ATP, it is necessary that this compound be continuously resynthesized. This can be achieved by the recombination of its breakdown products, the energy necessary for the process being provided by another energy-yielding reaction in the cell, viz., the splitting of creatine phosphate. This additional phosphagen, as it has been called, also has to be constantly replaced since it is present only in small quantities. There are two primary sources of energy for the resynthesis of the phosphagens: the combustion of food, which can be measured by the consumption of oxygen, and the process known as glycolysis, that is, the breakdown of glycogen with the formation of lactic acid. Since the latter process is reversible, an input of energy from food combustion will cause a resynthesis of glycogen from the lactic acid. Therefore, in all, five biochemical reactions have to be considered. Three of them, phosphagen splitting, food combustion, and glycolysis are energy providing; whereas the other two, phosphagen resynthesis and glycogen reconstitution are energy absorbing.[41]

Carbohydrate and fat are the main nutrients in the diet that supply energy to the muscles of the body; protein, as we have seen plays a nonessential role.[4] The relative amounts of fat and carbohydrate used during physical exercise will depend on the composition of the diet, the intensity of work performed, the extent of the exercise, and the fitness of the subject concerned.[42] Since studies have indicated that fat is mobilized from the body's reserve depots and that it is transported to the muscles and combusted in the cell during exercise, the alleged importance of carbohydrates for prolonged exercise was challenged. However, a number of Scandinavian investigators have shown decisively that carbohydrates play an essential role in the building up of glycogen stores. By developing the needle biopsy technique, it has been possible to collect muscle specimens for the direct determination of glycogen.[43-45]

The technique consists of making an incision in the skin under local anesthesia, and then inserting the needle into the deeper part of the quadriceps femoris muscle. The lateral portion of the muscle group is most frequently used. This contains no big vessels or nerves and is large enough for repeated sampling. The amount of tissue material that can be obtained in a single biopsy varies between 10 and 50 mg wet weight. The time between insertion of the needle and removal of the specimen is about 2 to 5 sec. By making use of a bicycle ergometer modified so that only one leg is exercised it has been possible to investigate specimens from both exercised and resting legs. From such studies it has been possible to show that with prolonged heavy exercise the glycogen content of the working muscle is reduced from an average normal value of 15 g/kg muscle to almost zero when the subject is exhausted.[46] During prolonged exercise, when the relative work load is over 75% of the subject's maximal oxygen uptake, there is a high and constant rate of carbohydrate combustion and this is equally applicable whether the concentration of glycogen in the muscle is high or low. The importance of carbohydrate as a fuel during heavy exercise is therefore confirmed.

In another trial, well-trained and untrained subjects were worked to complete exhaustion on a bicycle ergometer with work loads averaging 77% of their individual maximal aerobic power.[47] Determinations of the glycogen used by working muscles and of combusted carbohydrate were performed at fixed intervals from the commencement of work to exhaustion. The glycogen was estimated by similar techniques, i.e., by taking biopsy specimens of the lateral portion of the quadriceps femoris muscles. At a combustion rate of about 3 g carbohydrate per minute and at average values for glycogen in resting muscle of 1.6 g/100 g wet muscle, the effective work time was about 85 min for the untrained and 90 min for the trained subjects. At the termination of the exhaustive exercise, the glycogen content averaged 0.06 g in the untrained and 0.12 g/100 g wet muscle in the trained subjects. A close relationship between utilized glycogen and combusted carbohydrate was found so that it seems highly probable that at high relative work loads it is primarily the magnitude of the glycogen stores that limits the capacity for strenuous work to be prolonged.[47]

DIETARY MANIPULATION IN PREPARATION FOR COMPETITION

In this section consideration will be given to the question whether use can be made of the above conclusion, viz., that the capacity for strenuous work depends on the magnitude of glycogen stores, in preparation for competitions involving physical prowess. It shall be determined whether glycogen stores can be increased by dietary manipulation and if so, how effective such regimes are. The desirability of such procedures will also be briefly considered.

When the glycogen stores of healthy subjects are exhausted by heavy exercise it has been shown that the glycogen content of the muscles can be altered in individual subjects by varying the subsequent diet. Thus, when a diet consisting mainly of fat and protein was given, e.g., one consisting of bacon, eggs, meat, butter, and vegetable oils together with small amounts of lettuce and tomato, the glycogen content remained low at about 6 g per kg of muscle.[48,49] However, when a high carbohydrate diet was given, e.g., one consisting of bread, potatoes, spaghetti, sugar, with some fruit and juices, the glycogen content rose to levels as high as 47 g / kg muscle. These results led Åstrand to recommend that athletes should first exhaust their stores of muscle glycogen by fairly heavy work, remain on a high protein-fat diet for a short period of 1 or 2 days, and then consume a high carbohydrate diet for the remaining 4 days or so before a competition.[50] This would therefore appear to be an effective way of building up an extra high content of glycogen in the muscles and one that will be effective for improving athletic performance.

In a further trial, Karlsson et al. have demonstrated that, besides a beneficial effect on the rate of running, an increase in muscle glycogen can increase endurance as well. Ten physical education students ran a race, once after a normal mixed diet and once after a special diet designed to increase muscle glycogen levels.[51] Some of the students were only slightly trained whereas others were regular competitors in cross-country running. The subjects twice ran a distance of 30 km (about 19 miles), once after the normal diet and once after the high carbohydrate diet. There was an interval of 3 weeks between the two runs. The first run was a regular race involving over 1000 competitors. The second race was run only by the subjects in the study. For the first 3 days of the week of the race six subjects ate a diet without carbohydrates. For the next 3 days a minimum of 2500 kcal per day came from dietary carbohydrate and no heavy exercise was allowed during this period. The remaining four subjects kept to the normal mixed diet before the first race. All subjects reversed their diets before the second race. To motivate runners in the second race a reward of five dollars was offered for every 4 km maintained at a pace similar to the pace run in the first race. A total of $40 could therefore be received if a contestant performed as well in the second race as in the first.

Biopsy specimens were obtained from the quadriceps muscle before and after both races. In those subjects eating the high carbohydrate diet before the race muscle glycogen amounted to 32 g/kg muscle compared with 18 g in subjects eating the mixed diet, although one subject had a high glycogen content, 36 g/kg muscle, even though he was eating the mixed diet. Glycogen values after the race were found to have decreased to 19 g/kg muscle in subjects eating the mixed diet. None of the subjects receiving the high carbohydrate diet had particularly low glycogen levels after their race but glycogen was almost depleted in six subjects who had consumed the mixed diet. The best performance by each runner occurred after eating the high carbohydrate diet. Observations of running time differences and of abilities to keep a good pace indicated that higher initial levels of muscle glycogen resulted in better performance. As glycogen levels approached low values there was a marked reduction in running speed. It was found that 3 to 5 g/kg muscle was the critical lower limit for the maintenance of a rapid and continuous pace of exercise.

It was calculated that about 350 g of glycogen was utilized in the race. Respiratory quotients were found to be between 0.90 and 0.95. Karlsson and colleagues observed that although enhanced muscle glycogen stores did not have a direct effect on the speed that each subject attained at the beginning of the prolonged period of heavy exercise, or on the pace which was set, the high initial level of muscle glycogen was an important prerogative for maintaining the pace for the duration of the race.

This further trial seems to decisively demonstrate that prior depletion of glycogen reserves by a low carbohydrate diet followed by a very high carbohydrate diet for 3 or 4 days immediately before long-term physical exercise results in a building up of muscle glycogen reserves which are of real benefit to the athlete. It is understood that a number of long distance and marathon runners are now using this dietary regimen and are finding it beneficial. However, it is unlikely that the sprinter will derive any benefit from adopting this dietary procedure.

One adverse comment on the regimen described above for increasing stores of muscle glycogen is that glycogen retains water in both liver and muscle tissues and tends to increase body weight. However, when the regimen includes an initial few days on a high protein diet there is a reduction in body weight and this will partly offset the subsequent increase in weight following the ingestion of the high carbohydrate diet. Thus, Heeley et al. noted an average fall in weight of 1.4 kg in their subjects after 4 days on a high-protein diet.[52] Another comment on the use of this regimen is the fact that it is neither known how frequently it can be repeated with the same beneficial effects, nor whether the procedure is entirely innocuous. As a first step to providing an answer to this last question Heeley and colleagues examined six healthy young men before and after being given a high-protein diet for 4 days.[52] They examined blood specimens collected at the beginning and ending of the experimental period. Urine specimens were collected for the 24-hr period immediately preceding and during the last 24 hr on the special high-protein diet. The blood and urine specimens were analyzed for a variety of elements and compounds. Significant differences were observed in a number of the indexes examined in the blood. Thus, there were significant average rises in urea from 4.65 to 8.13 mmol/ℓ, in cholesterol from 4.66 to 5.52 mmol/ℓ, in total phosphorus from 2.87 to 3.16 mmol/ℓ, in phosphatides from 2230 to 2440 mg/ℓ, and in osmolarity from 282 to 293 mosmol/ℓ. There were significant falls in triodothyronine levels from 83 to 31% and in glucose from 4.90 to 4.53 mmol/ℓ. Significant changes were also observed in urine. Thus, average rises in urea from 22.5 to 38.7 g/24 hr and in cyclic AMP from 15.7 to 31.5 μmol/24 hr were found. There was also a significant rise in chromium from 6.01 to 11.68 μg/24 hr. A significant average fall in uric acid from 2.89 to 0.62 mmol/24 hr was also noted. The implications of these various differences however, remain to be understood.

Dangers of carbohydrate loading in older long distance runners have been cited by Mirkin and Spring.[53a] These authors reported the case of a 40-year-old man who had started running 10 years previously because he had a high serum cholesterol level. He had attained some proficiency in distance running. He had run a marathon event in less than 2 hr and 50 min and was training on 18.6 to 24.8 km a week with one long run and two runs of moderate length. He raced four or five times a year generally at 6.2 to 12.4 km. He weighed 67.8 kg and at the time had a serum cholesterol level of 240 mg. Four weeks before a marathon in which he was due to participate, he ran 6.2 km in 59 minutes with little effort. Seven, six and five days before the marathon he changed to a diet of cheese, meat and turkey; and on days four, three and two he added as much bread as he could eat. At one sitting he consumed almost two loaves. On day three he felt a dull pain in the left side of his chest and on day two the pain became more severe and constant. He did not take part in the race and an electrocardiogram showed flattening and inversion of the T wave, and S-T segment depression. He immediately changed to one small meal daily whereupon the pain subsided after five days. This case raises serious questions not only about carbohydrate loading in older distance runners but also about the wisdom of eating large meals at night by those susceptible to infarction.

For further details of the regimen for building up muscle glycogen stores by high carbohydrate diets the reader is referred to the paper by Saltin and Hermansen.[53] A more recent review of the use of such diets as an aid to preparation for competition has been provided by Hultman, and details of energy metabolism in skeletal muscle fibers with exercise are given in the paper by Saltin.[54,55]

GLUCOSE SYRUP AND PHYSICAL PERFORMANCE

Allied with the last section, where consideration was given to the use of high carbohydrate diets for building up glycogen reserves, is the use of glucose drinks for aiding long distance athletes and others having to carry out prolonged physical work. Such drinks may consist of a simple solution of glucose in water, but usually of glucose syrup prepared by the hydrolysis of starch. A number of commercial preparations also contain small quantities of mineral salts with the intention of replacing such salts lost in sweat. A number of trials have shown beneficial results of the use of such drinks either before or during the performance of physical activities.[56-63]

Thus, the effects of ingestion of an experimental glucose syrup drink, containing 46% w/v glucose syrup and mineral salts, were studied in physical education students during vigorous exercises of differing intensities and duration.[56] The glucose syrup ingestion followed three routines: (1) one intake of 150 mℓ consumed 15 or 45 min before exercise, (2) one intake of 150 mℓ consumed 30 or 45 min before exercise followed by three intakes of 50 mℓ at 30 min intervals, and (3) one intake of 150 mℓ consumed 20 min before exercise followed by three intakes of 50 mℓ at 45 min intervals. All conditions were compared to similar conditions with a placebo and with no exercise. Glucose syrup ingestion caused a significant rise in exercise blood-glucose levels with a time-lag and magnitude specific to each individual subject. The elevation of blood glucose caused by the glucose syrup ingestion was maintained during both moderate and severe exercise of various types and also during the hour following exercise. Concurrent with the elevation of blood glucose, there was an improvement in the performance of both submaximal and maximal exercise, in terms of increased work done and decreased heart rate during the work.

In another investigation male racing cyclists each cycled to exhaustion on four occasions on an Ergowheels® ergometer adjusted to approximate their racing load, 65 to 70% of each individual's maximum physical work capacity.[57] On each occasion the prolonged maintenance of physical power output was assessed on one of the following dietary treatments: T_1 (glucose syrup); T_2 ("normal" diet — canned rice pudding, canned fruit salad, and sucrose); T_3 (low-energy drink with electrolytes as in T_1); T_4 (no dietary supplement). Subjects ate their normal diet before each test. In T_1 and T_2 the energy expended was replaced every 20 min; in T_3 a volume of drink equal to that used in T_1 was given. In all treatments, an additional 150 mℓ of an electrolyte solution, approximating the concentration of sweat, was given every 20 min. Exhaustion was defined as the inability of the subject to voluntarily maintain the power output required. The mean work times, in minutes, to exhaustion were T_1, 216; T_2, 201; T_3, 180; T_4, 148. The differences between any two pairs of mean work times were all statistically significant. Therefore, those subjects who had the glucose syrup worked longer than when they had any of the other treatments. Mean blood-glucose levels, mg/100 mℓ, at 120 minutes were T_1, 72; T_2, 82; T_3, 66; and T_4, 55. However, when the subjects took the glucose syrup before exhaustion, the mean blood-glucose levels rose to 96 mg/100 mℓ. These results are an advance on earlier work in that for the maintenance of physical work, they differentiate between a high-energy diet in the form of a glucose syrup drink, and the diet which includes fat and protein normally used by cyclists. Therefore, when cycling under the conditions of this trial the most efficient work of longest duration is performed before exhaustion occurs when a glucose drink has been taken.

The possible beneficial effects of glucose syrup to improve the performance and prevent accidents among factory workers has also been investigated. In a preliminary trial among foundrymen it was found that low-carbohydrate availability appeared to be associated with accident incidence.[58] There were more morning than afternoon accidents, and more occurred before than after the morning break. In a second study, over a 3-day period, factory workers were given three different dietary treatments, each in addition to their normal diet; (1) two 250 mℓ portions of glucose syrup, each of 1486 kJ energy value, in the first session; (2) a low-energy drink in identical volumes, each of energy value less than 20 kJ; and (3) no treatment.[58] Dietary surveys were made and respiratory quotients were measured. The normal respiratory quotient pattern was similar to that of the first study; the respiratory quotients revealed a boost in available carbohydrate with the glucose syrup supplement in comparison with the normal diet. In a further study lasting over 18 weeks, male forge workers, acting as their own controls, each working morning were given supplements of either 500 mℓ glucose syrup of energy value 710 kcal and containing added salts, or 500 mℓ of a low-energy fluid of less than 9.6 kcal but including the salts.[59] Treatments were reversed after 4, 8, and 13 weeks. Reported accidents and body weights before and after experiment were recorded and random determinations made of blood glucose and respiratory quotient. Accidents among the men on the glucose syrup treatment were significantly fewer than those on the low-energy treatment. The differences were more apparent in the morning than in the afternoon work sessions. Changes in body weights were found insignificant. The authors of this study point out that because of the problems in carrying out the program in the environment of forge hot-shops, the relations between the measures of metabolism and accident incidence must be treated with caution. However, the work did suggest that there may be a relationship between a reduction in factory accidents and the intake of glucose syrup. Details of the dietary intakes of these forge workers at different times of the day have been published.[60] The energy contributions from fat, protein, carbohydrate, and alcohol were also computed.

Glucose syrup ingestion has also been shown to be beneficial in aiding recovery from physical work exhaustion. During the first 10 min after they became exhausted, cyclists were given 250 mℓ glucose syrup with added salts (1486 kJ energy value), a normal diet for racing cyclists — canned rice pudding with added sucrose (1486 kJ energy value), or 250 mℓ of a low-energy fluid with added salts ($<$ 20 kJ energy value).[61] The subjects recommended work at the same load 40 min after exhaustion performed on an Ergowheel®, as in the first part of the trial. The amount of work done after recovery was greatest after ingestion of the glucose syrup drink and lowest on the low-energy drink; the 'normal' diet giving an intermediate result. Therefore, recovery from exhaustion due to reduced carbohydrate availability is more rapidly achieved with a dietary supplement of a glucose syrup drink than with a normal diet or low-energy drink. In keeping with Christensen and Hansen,[42] Brooke and Green believe that the basis of this improved recovery does not lie solely in the fuel-for-muscle metabolism, although the effects may be seen in the blood sugar concentrations.

More recently further trials have shown the beneficial effects of glucose syrup on the performance of male racing cyclists.[62] Thus, after preliminary road trials, laboratory loads of power output were selected which would bring the subjects to exhaustion in about 4 hr, thereby simulating a road race over one hundred miles. This experimental work load elicited 67% of the maximum oxygen intake of the cyclists. Four dietary treatments were randomly distributed over subjects and trials according to a replicated Latin square design. These treatments, which were presented every 20 min during work, were (1) glucose syrup drink with added salts, (2) a normal race diet of canned rice pudding with added sucrose to be isocaloric with (1), (3) a very low energy isovolumetric drink with similar salts to (1), and (4) no food. By calculating energy expenditure from oxygen uptake, the energy utilized was matched by the energy value of the treatment. Both of the high energy diets delayed the onset of exhaustion, providing more combusted carbohydrate as shown by elevated RQ and blood glucose levels. More efficient work was performed when the glucose syrup drink was taken in comparison to the other diets. It was concluded that the raised blood glucose levels with the high energy treatments contributed carbohydrate as fuel for the active skeletal muscles. It was also concluded that, when resulting from glucose syrup ingestion, this raised blood glucose level may benefit neural function in the physical work performance.

In fasting subjects, the onset of exercise results in a transient decrease in the concentration of glucose in the blood sufficient for hypoglycemic symptoms to occur. On the other hand, the ingestion of glucose syrup prior to exercise results in an increase in the blood glucose concentration during physical work and improved performance.[57] In an attempt to eliminate the reported initial exercise hypoglycemia, an experiment was conducted with adult male subjects to assess the most appropriate time for the prework ingestion of glucose syrup.[63] After a 30 min rest period, subjects exercised on a leg ergometer at 150 W for 20 min, a work schedule that induced a heart rate of 140 to 150 beats per min. After habituation and an initial trial with no feeding, a drink of 300 mℓ glucose syrup was given at 0, 10, 20, or 30 min before exercise in a design balanced for treatments to subjects over the trials. Trials per subject were one week apart. Capillary blood was sampled every 5 min during rest and exercise and analyzed by the glucose oxidase method. With no feeding, the transient hypoglycemia previously reported was observed. It was, however, fully alleviated by ingestion of glucose syrup at the commencement of exercise. But as the time of ingestion before exercise was lengthened, there was an earlier increase in the peak blood glucose concentration, followed by a subsequent decrease as exercise progressed towards lower values observed in the subjects not given glucose syrup. It is therefore concluded that intelligent use of glucose syrup demands evaluation of the behavioral needs and appropriate timing of ingestion.

TIMING OF MEALS IN RELATION TO PHYSICAL EXERCISE

Another aspect of the subject of nutrition in relation to physical performance, and one that is of practical concern to the would-be athlete or other person contemplating extensive physical exercise, is the time interval that should be allowed after a meal before participating in the exercise. Or, to put it another way, since the time of the particular contest or physical activity may have been predetermined, how long before the event should the last meal be taken?

There is no precise answer to this question, but large bulky meals should certainly be avoided shortly before exercise. This is especially true for the athlete competing in an endurance event or in hot climatic conditions. During the period immediately following the ingestion of food, blood is directed mainly to the alimentary tract to aid the process of digestion and a reduced amount is therefore available for muscular activity. This may be partly responsible for the feeling of lethargy that often follows the ingestion of a large meal. Should exercise be attempted under these conditions, cramp or intestinal stasis with a delay in gastric emptying may result, and if the practice is continued, nausea, abdominal pain, and even vomiting and diarrhea may ensue. Therefore it is recommended that a period of 2 hr or more should elapse after a heavy meal before participation in any form of strenuous exercise.

The details of the content of the pregame meal has been given attention by a number of authors. It is usually recommended that it should be made up of foods that can be easily digested and rapidly absorbed. Items that are likely to cause flatulence should be excluded. The latter can be disturbing to the athlete and detrimental to peak performance. The following foods should therefore be avoided: beans, peas and other legumes, sauerkraut and other cabbage preparations. This is particularly important prior to competition.

It is usually suggested that a sportsman's main meal should be taken in the evening after the cessation of the day's physical activities. The same advice is probably applicable to others who have to undergo extensive physical exertion during the day. A substantial breakfast may be taken but luncheon should be light and easily digested for the reasons mentioned above. In view of the fact that the majority of sporting activities usually take place in the afternoon, care should be exercised to see that luncheon is taken at least 1 hr or preferably two before physical work is begun.

SUMMARY AND CONCLUSIONS

The athlete, or any other person contemplating physical exercise, requires a good well-balanced diet. This should be palatable and supply all nutrients in adequate amounts to meet the recommended daily requirements. In general, there is little evidence to suggest that quantities in excess of those recommended for the normal subject are required by those undertaking physical performance, so long as these quantities are sufficient to meet the extra demands for energy. Nevertheless, some modifications may be beneficial in certain cases.

Supplementing an adequate normal diet with extra vitamins does not appear to aid physical performance, though there may be a small increase in the requirement of the B vitamins to metabolize additional carbohydrate given to provide extra energy. The claims made that supplements of vitamin E are an ergogenic aid have generally been disproved.

The ingestion of a very high carbohydrate diet after a brief period on a high protein diet to exhaust existing stores of muscle glycogen, leads to the building up of stores of glycogen in excess of those originally present. Such increased stores are of real use to the long distance or marathon runner though they are unlikely to benefit the sprinter. The same applies to others expecting to have to undertake prolonged physical work. Details are included for implementing this dietary regime.

The beneficial effects of glucose syrup as an aid to preparation for competition, for refreshment during exercise, and for aiding recovery after exertion, are considered in detail. The provision of glucose syrup drinks in factories may help performance and prevent accidents.

The timing of meals before athletic events or other physical exercise is considered. At least 2 hr should elapse after a meal before training or participation in a sports contest. Consideration is also given to the content of the pregame meal.

REFERENCES

1. McCollum, E. V., A history of nutrition, Houghton Mifflin, Boston, 1957, 2.
2. Harris, H. A., Nutrition and physical performance: the diet of Greek athletes, *Proc. Nutr. Soc.*, 25, 87-90, 1966.
3. Harris, H. A., *Greek Athletes and Athletics,* Hutchinson, London, 1964, 171—173.
4. Pettenkofer, M. and Voit, C., Untersuchungen über den Stoffrerbranch des normalen Uenschen, *Z. Biol. (Munich),* 2, 459—573, 1866.
5. Steel, J. E., A nutritional study of Australian Olympic athletes, *Med. J. Aust.,* 2, 119—123, 1970.
6. Sharman, I. M., Nutrition and athletic performance, *Br. Nutr. Found. Bull.,* No. 8, 36—43, 1973.
7. Mayer, J. and Bullen, B., Nutrition and athletics, in *Proc. 6th Int. Congr. Nutr.,* Mills, C. F. and Passmore, R., Eds., Livingstone, Edinburgh, 1964, 27—39.

8. **Steyn, D. G., Honey,** in *Molecular Structure and Function of Food Carbohydrate,* Birch, G. G. and Green, L. F., Eds., Applied Science Publishers, London, 1973, 81—106.

9. Department of Health and Social Security, Recommended intakes of nutrients for the United Kingdom, Reports on Public Health and Medical Subjects, No. 120, Her Majesty's Stationery Office, London, 1969, 4—33.

10. National Academy of Sciences, Recommended Dietary Allowances, 8th ed., National Academy of Sciences, Washington, D. C., 1974, 50—81.

11. **Simonson, E., Enzer, N., Baer, A., and Braun, R.,** The influence of vitamin B (complex) on the capacity for muscular and mental work, *J. Ind. Hyg.,* 24, 83—90, 1942.

12. **Keys, A. and Henschel, A. F.,** Vitamin supplementation of U.S. Army rations in relation to fatigue and the ability to do muscular work, *J. Nutr.,* 23, 259—269, 1942.

13. **Harper, A. A., Mackay, I. F. S., Raper, H. S., and Camm, G. L.,** Vitamins and physical fitness, *Br. Med. J.,* 1, 243—245, 1943.

14. **Bourne, G. H.,** Vitamins and muscular exercise, *Br. J. Nutr.,* 2, 261—263, 1948—49.

15. **Vytchikova, M. A.,** Increasing the vitamin B_1 content in the rations of athletes, *Chem. Abstr.,* 52, 14787, 1958.

16. **Montoye, H. J., Spata, P. J., Pinckney, V., and Barron, L.,** Effects of vitamin B_{12} supplementation on physical fitness and growth of young boys, *J. Appl. Physiol.,* 7, 589—592, 1955.

17. **Lind, J.,** *Lind's Treatise on Scurvy,* Stewart, C. P. and Guthrie, D., Eds., University Press, Edinburgh, 1953, 69.

18. Medical Research Council, Accessory Food Factor Committee Report No. 280, Vitamin C requirements of human adults, Her Majesty's Stationery Office, London, 1953.

19. **Pauling, L.,** *Vitamin C and the Common Cold,* Freeman, San Francisco, 1970, 39—52 and 83—88.

20. **Margaria, R., Aghemo, P., and Revelli, E.,** The effect of some drugs on the maximal capacity of athletic performance in man, *Int. Z. Angew. Physiol. Einschl. Arbeitsphysiol.,* 20, 281—287, 1964.

21. **Gey, G. O., Cooper, K. H., and Bottenberg, R. A.,** Effect of ascorbic acid on endurance performance and athletic injury, *JAMA,* 211, 105, 1970.

22. **Bailey, D. A., Carron, A. V., Teece, R. G., and Wehner, H.,** Effect of vitamin C supplementation upon the physiological response to exercise in trained and untrained subjects, *Int. J. Vitam. Nutr. Res.,* 40, 435—441, 1970.

23. **Bender, A. E. and Nash, A. H.,** Vitamin C and physical performance, *Plant Foods for Man,* 1, 217—231, 1975.

24. **Hove, E. L., Hickman, K., and Harris, P. L.,** The effect of tocopherol and of fat on the resistance of rats to anoxic anoxia, *Arch. Biochem.,* 8, 395—404, 1945.

25. **Taylor, D. W.,** Effects of vitamin E deficiency on oxygen toxicity in the rat, *J. Physiol.,* 121, 47P—48P, 1953.

26. **Shute, W. E. and Shute, E. V.,** Alpha-tocopherol in cardiovascular disease, *Summary,* 2, 3—58, 1950.

27. **Shute, W. E.,** A critique of 'classical' treatment of coronary artery disease, *Summary,* 3, 77—82, 1951.

28. **Percival, L.,** Vitamin E in athletic efficiency (preliminary report), *Summary,* 3, 55—64, 1951.

29. **Darlington, F. G. and Chassels, J. B.,** A study on the breeding and racing of thoroughbred horses given large doses of alpha tocopherol, *Summary,* 8, 1—20, 1956.

30. **Darlington, F. G. and Chassels, J. B.,** A further study of breeding and racing of thoroughbred horses given large doses of alpha tocopherol, *Summary,* 8, 55—82, 1956.

31. **Prokop, L.,** Die Wirkung von natürlichem Vitamin E auf Sauerstoffverbrauch und Sauerstoffschuld, *Sportärztl. Praxis,* 1, 19—23, 1960.

32. **Cureton, T. K.,** Effect of wheat germ oil and vitamin E on normal human subjects in physical training programs, *Am. J. Physiol.,* 179, 628, 1954.

33. **Cureton, T. K.,** The physiological effects of wheat germ oil and related substances as ergogenic aids, *Br. J. Sports Med.,* 7, 31—33, 1973.

34. **Consolazio, C. F., le Matoush, R. O., Nelson, R. A., Isaac, G. J., and Hursh, L. M.,** Effect of octacosanol, wheat germ oil, and vitamin E on performance of swimming rats, *J. Appl. Physiol.,* 19, 265—567, 1964.

35. **Thomas, P.,** The Effects of Vitamin E on Some Aspects of Athletic Efficiency, Ph.D. thesis, University of Southern California, Los Angeles, 1957.

36. **Sharman, I. M., Down, M. G., and Sen, R. N.,** The effects of vitamin E and training on physiological function and athletic performance in adolescent swimmers, *Br. J. Nutr.,* 26, 265—276, 1971.

37. **Shephard, R. J., Campbell, R., Pimm, P., Stuart, D., and Wright, G. R.,** Vitamin E, exercise, and the recovery from physical activity, *Eur. J. Appl. Physiol. Occup. Physiol.,* 33, 119—126, 1974.

38. **Sharman, I. M., Down, M. G., and Norgan, N. G.,** The effect of vitamin E on physiological function and athletic performance of trained swimmers, *J. Sports Med. Phys. Fit.,* 16, 215—225, 1976.

39. Talbot, D. and Jamieson, J., An examination of the effect of vitamin E on the performance of highly trained swimmers, *Can. J. Appl. Sports Sci.*, 2, 67—69, 1977.

40. Baldwin, E., *Dynamic Aspects of Biochemistry*, 4th ed., Cambridge University Press, London, 1963, 57.

41. Margaria, R., The sources of muscular energy, *Sci. Am.*, 226, 84—91, 1972.

42. Christensen, E. H. and Hansen, O., Zur Methodik der Respiratorischen Quotient - Bestimingen in Ruhe und bei Arbeit, *Skand. Arch. Physiol.*, 81, 137—151, 1939.

43. Bergström, J., Muscle electrolytes in man determined by neutron activation analysis on needle biopsy specimens. A study on normal subjects, kidney patients and patients with chronic diarrhoea, *Scand. J. Clin. Lab. Invest.*, 14 (Suppl. 68), 7—110, 1962.

44. Hultman, E., Muscle glycogen in man determined in needle biopsy specimens. Method and normal values, *Scand. J. Clin. Lab. Invest.*, 19, 209—217, 1967.

45. Harris, R. C., Hultman, E., and Nordesjö, L.-O., Glycogen, glycolytic intermediates and high-energy phosphates determined in biopsy samples of musculus quadriceps femoris of man at rest. Methods and variance of values, *Scand. J. Clin. Lab. Invest.*, 33, 109—120, 1974.

46. Saltin, B. and Hermansen, L., Glycogen stores and prolonged severe exercise, *Symp. Swed. Nutr. Found.*, 5, 32—46, 1967.

47. Hermansen, L., Hultman, E., and Saltin, B., Muscle glycogen during prolonged severe exercise, *Acta Physiol. Scand.*, 71, 129—139, 1967.

48. Bergström, J., Hermansen, L., Hultman, E. and Saltin, B., Diet, muscle glycogen and physical performance, *Acta Physiol. Scand.*, 71, 140—150, 1967.

49. Hultman, E. and Bergström, J., Muscle glycogen synthesis in relation to diet studied in normal subjects, *Acta Med. Scand.*, 182, 109—117, 1967.

50. Astrand, P.-O., Diet and athletic performance, *Fed. Proc.*, 26, 1772—1777, 1967.

51. Karlsson, J. and Saltin, B., Diet, muscle glycogen and endurance performance, *J. Appl. Physiol.*, 31, 203—206, 1971.

52. Heeley, D. M., Sharman, I. M., and Cooper, D. F., Variations in the compostion of blood and urine following the ingestion of a high-protein diet, *Proc. Nutr. Soc.*, 34, 69A, 1975.

53. Saltin, B. and Hermansen, L., Glycogen stores and prolonged severe exercise, in *Nutrition and Physical Activity*, Blix, G., Ed., Almquist & Wiksells, Uppsala, 1967, 32.

53a. Mirkin, G. and Spring, S., Carbohydrate loading: a dangerous practice, *JAMA*, 223, 1511—1512, 1973.

54. Hultman, E., Dietary manipulations as an aid to preparation for competition, in *XXth World Congress in Sports Medicine, Congress Proceedings 1974*, Congress Secretariat, Carlton 3053, Australia, 1974, 239—265.

55. Saltin, B., Energy metabolism in skeletal muscle fibres of man with exercise, in *XXth World Congress in Sports Medicine, Congress Proceedings 1974*, Congress Secretariat, Carlton 3053, Australia, 1974, 266—267.

56. Green, L. F. and Thomas, V., Some effects of glucose syrup ingestion during vigorous exercises of differing intensities and duration, *Proc. Nutr. Soc.*, 31, 5A—6A, 1972.

57. Brooke, J. D., Davies, G. J., and Green, L. F., Nutrition during severe prolonged exercise in trained cyclists, *Proc. Nutr. Soc.*, 31, 93A—94A, 1972.

58. Brooke, J. D., Toogood, S., Green, L. F., and Bagley, R., Dietary pattern of carbohydrate provision and accident incidence in foundrymen, *Proc. Nutr. Soc.*, 32, 44A—45A, 1973.

59. Brooke, J. D., Toogood, S., Green, L. F., and Bagley, R., Factory accidents and carbohydrate supplements, *Proc. Nutr. Soc.*, 32, 94A—95A, 1973.

60. Brooke, J. D. and Green, L. F., A survey of some forge workers, *Proc. Nutr. Soc.*, 33, 97A—98A, 1974.

61. Brooke, J. D. and Green, L. F., Carbohydrate availability in human recovery from physical work exhaustion, *Proc. Nutr. Soc.*, 33, 12A—13A, 1974.

62. Brooke, J. D., Davies, G. J., and Green, L. F., The effects of normal and glucose syrup work diets on the performance of racing cyclists, *J. Sports Med. Phys. Fit.*, 15, 257—265, 1975.

63. Brooke, J. D., Llewelyn, K., and Green, L. F., Time of glucose syrup ingestion to alleviate initial exercise hypoglycaemia, *Proc. Nutr. Soc.*, 35, 136A—137A, 1976.

NUTRITION AND BEHAVIOR: ANIMALS (OTHER THAN PRIMATES)

S. Fraňková

I. INTRODUCTION

The study of behavioral responses to the quantity and quality of ingested food has been marked by periods of increased interest alternating with a declined interest. To some extent, these trends reflect the progress made in nutritional science. The discovery of vitamins stimulated an avid interest in the study of the behavioral effects of deficiency or excess of vitamins. Knowledge of the etiology of kwashiorkor initiated, among other things, intensive research into the effect of early protein deprivation on the behavior of experimental animals. While during the first half of this century the theoretical and analytical approach to nutrition was typical, behavioral research during the latter half is characterized by a remarkable upswing of interest in the solution of practical and complex nutritional problems, such as the consequences of early protein-calorie malnutrition.

Recently, attempts have been made to formulate a synthetic approach to nutrition, study its role in relation to the external factors affecting the individual, and determine its limits. An increasing number of studies attempt to explain the mechanisms underlying nutrition-induced behavioral changes and to discover the interaction between physiological and psychological variables.

There are many reasons for the use of animal laboratory models in investigation of the behavioral responses to nutrition. The nutritional status of the currently used laboratory animals may be precisely defined; the requirements of most vital substances are relatively well known, and construction of experimental diets is without problems. Their behavioral responses can be observed under controlled external conditions. Moreover, the use of rodents allows the performance of long-term experiments for study of the effects of nutritional intervention on consecutive generations. Studies on relatively large homogeneous samples make possible statistical analysis of the results.

Laboratory experiments help solve many problems of interest to human psychologists. The animal becomes a model for the study of mental development and long-term behavioral responses to early nutritional impacts. Starvation has been used as a basal drive in motivational studies and learning experiments. The practical questions of current interest include, for example, enhancement of physical and mental performance and better resistance to stress. Although nutrition cannot fully compete with psychopharmacology, it is important to realize there are findings which show that certain food constituents exert excitatory or inhibitory effects on the central nervous system (CNS). Nutritional therapy, especially that involving reduced food intake, has a serious impact on behavior. Finally, human psychologists are interested in the possibility of discovering potential nutritional bases for some abnormal states.

The value of an individual finding and its degree of generalization is limited by the conditions under which it is obtained. Methodical factors in behavioral research are of great importance because spontaneous behavior is extremely sensitive to changes in the environment; it reflects both the actual functional status of the CNS and responses to nonnutritional stimuli which may be erroneously interpreted as results of a changed nutritional variable.

Nutritional research employs methods developed for the study of various psychological phenomena. There is no procedure specific for the field of nutrition. A survey of the commonly used techniques is presented in Table 1. For many years measurement

Table 1
SURVEY OF BEHAVIORAL TESTS COMMONLY USED IN NUTRITIONAL STUDIES

Technique	Description	Criteria	Ref.
Locomotor activity			
Revolving drum, wheel activity cages	Long-term cycles of total body movements; animal lives in the device or the revolving drum is attached to the cage; activity measured automatically	Number of revolutions, sum of all movements; activity expressed as one number	1, 2
Open field activity	Short-term record of spontaneous activity, especially exploration; the box is usually larger than the living cage and is illuminated, with the floor divided into squares; activity recorded by the observer or by means of photocells, capacitance system, etc.; originally used to test the "emotionality"	Horizontal exploration: number of traversed squares; vertical exploration: frequency of rearing reactions; defecation: number of boluses	3, 4
Learning			
Maze learning	Space of the box divided into alleys and blind arms, usually of the type Y or T; animal placed in the starting box and must find the way to the goal; running is motivated by food, water, or an aversive stimulus (shock, cold water)	Speed of running, number of correct responses or errors, entries of the blind arms, speed of running, selection of route	1, 2
Hebb-Williams maze	Widely used method; food box (the goal) is always in the same location; barriers dividing the space vary and the animal must find a new route every day		5
Problem box	Box or cage which the animal enters or leaves after solving certain task; used as a test of discrimination; most commonly used modification is the Lashley jumping test		6
Classical conditioning	Unconditioned stimulus (UCS) (shocks, water, food) elicits the unconditioned response (UCR) connected with originally indifferent stimulus [conditioned stimulus (CS)—sound, light],	Latent periods of responses, number of responses necessary to meet the criterium of conditioned	1, 7

Table 1 (continued)
SURVEY OF BEHAVIORAL TESTS COMMONLY USED
IN NUTRITIONAL STUDIES

Technique	Description	Criteria	Ref.
	which is presented before or simultaneously with the UCS; originally developed in Pavlovian laboratories; animal learns to react in the presence of CS	response, number of responses performed during the presentation of CS	
Shuttle box (one-way or two-way)	Animal must run from one part of the box, where it receives shocks from the grid, to the other part of the box, which is temporarily safe; shocks are preceded by CS		
Instrumental (operant) learning	Situation involving a mechanism which can be operated by the animal (usually a lever); by means of lever pressing, it can regulate the reinforcement; original methods: Skinner box; modification: Sidman avoidance learning (lever pressing delays the shocks from the grid)		8, 9
"Emotionality" Defecation	Usually measured in the open field box, in which no other stimuli are presented; animal reacts to the novelty	Number of boluses	
Startle response	Duration of freezing induced by an intensive stimulus (sound)	Duration of freezing, defecation, startle reaction	10
Conditioned emotional response (CER)	Conditioned response to the aversive stimulus is elaborated; the animal is later exposed to the same environment without the CS or UCS		

of total activity and performance in a maze predominated. Behavior was simply expressed as a sum of movements in the running wheel or activity cage or as a number of correct responses. These data were objective and of great value when taken as a first approximation, but the simplified view on animal behavior prevented more detailed analysis of the consequence of a given nutritional impact. Only recently has more attention been paid to more complex forms of behavior; a wider scale of activities of the animal and interaction with other individuals of the same species have been recorded.

In the interpretation of experimental data it is necessary to consider motivational factors involved in the test situation. In some procedures food reward means unequal motivation for the deprived as opposed to satiated animals. Another factor is the animal's motor ability. Various extreme nutritional situations may result in gross motor impairment that prevents the animal from exhibiting any response.

Designs of experimental diets are another source of methodological problems. A decreased or increased amount of one dietary compound (vitamin, amino acid, or mineral) may result in dysbalance which, in turn, may manifest itself in behavioral changes. An extreme dose of specific dietary component may have toxic effects. Lastly, drastic intervention in the diet should preferably be avoided for ethical reasons if and where a lesser deviation from the optimal composition is capable of eliciting behavioral response.

The commonly used experimental animals are rats, mice, dogs, guinea pigs, and pigs. In comparative studies care should be given to the widely differing nutritional requirements of individual animal species. Developmental studies[11] indicate that the rate of brain growth differs from species to species. In some species the highest rate of brain growth occurs in the prenatal period, while in others it takes place in the postnatal period. This may modify the long-term effects of diet on behavior. Other methodological problems will be considered in the respective parts of this contribution.

II. CALORIC VALUE OF FOOD

Intake of food with calorie value which does not satisfy the physiological requirements of the individual affects the function of different organs and body weight rapidly decreases. The adult brain is predominantly protected against the consequences of altered food supply, and its weight and composition change very little.[12-14] On the other hand, even a short-term deprivation elicits behavioral changes in the animal.

A. Acute Effects of Short-term Calorie Deprivation

Psychologists and nutritionists sometimes differ in their approaches to starvation as an experimental variable. For the former, starvation is considered an essential and easily measurable drive and is, therefore, a suitable tool for studies of motivation and learning. For the latter, starvation represents a state of deficiency during which a lack of vital substances induces alteration in various physiological functions.

Ample literature exists on the effect of starvation on spontaneous activity of adult animals (for detailed reviews of earlier studies see References 1, 2, 15, and 16). Most experimental studies[17-23] showed the enhancement of the total locomotor activity in starved rats. Locomotor activity usually achieves peak values on the fourth or fifth day after removal of the food, declining rapidly thereafter. Refeeding restores the pretreatment activity level. A significant relationship was found between weight deficit and wheel running.[23,24] Several studies reported an opposite effect of starvation on activity. The discrepancies in the findings of various authors stimulated more profound analysis of experimental conditions. It appeared that the course, intensity, and trend of behavioral changes was determined by numerous factors, of which the most important appear to be

1. The type of measuring equipment. Locomotor activity was recorded by means of various techniques (see Table 1) which, in fact, registered different behavioral manifestations. Olewine et al.[25] showed reduced food intake to be associated with a decrease of total random movements, but with an increase of voluntary wheel activity. Activity expressed as a total number of all movements of the body and

measured over a prolonged period in a familiar environment should be distinguished from that tested during a short-term observation in a novel, exploratory activity-promoting situation. It was observed[26] that exploratory activity of the hungry animal in a new environment increased.

2. Environmental stimulation. Campbell and Sheffield[18] observed that food-deprived animals displayed an extremely increased sensitivity to external stimuli; the animals reacted with an enhanced activity to any change in the experimental situation. According to Adlerstein and Fehrer,[27] exploratory activity of the hungry animal in an environment with the lack of variety of the stimulation (such as Y maze) is low. They predicted that in the complex maze, exploratory activity would be higher. Their assumption was confirmed by Fehrer[19] who found the increased exploration of hungry rats in novel situations provided more stimuli. Other studies[12,28,29] confirmed that a novel environment stimulated the activity of food-deprived rats when compared with familiar conditions. Woods and Bolles[30] distinguished three categories of behavior: object exploration, nonobject exploration, and nonexploratory behavior. They observed food-deprived rats to explore more than the satiated rats, but whereas starvation stimulated the nonobject exploration, object exploration declined.

3. Age of the animal. It was shown[31] that differences existed in the response to food deprivation in rats aged 23, 38, 54, and 100 days. After 24 hr of deprivation, 23-day-old rats quadrupled their activity and lost approximately 18% of their initial body weight. On the other hand, adult rats showed no increase in their activity level and lost only 9% of their initial body weight. In young rats there is a larger ratio of skin surface to body mass and higher metabolic and activity levels.

4. Species difference. The rat is the laboratory animal most often used in deprivational studies. However, there are interspecies differences in behavioral responses to starvation. In a comparison of the activities of deprived chicks, guinea pigs, hamsters, and rabbits in stabilimeter-type cages and running wheels, it appeared that each species showed consistent activity patterns for each condition. However, these patterns were very different and sometimes opposite for various species and activity devices.[32]

5. Previous nutritional history. The reaction to starvation depends on the life history of the individual, i.e., on the experienced food and water deprivation.[33-37] Observations suggest that experience with deprivation may have a long-term effect persisting even after Ss have recovered under free-feeding conditions.[38,39]

B. Effects of Semistarvation

Moderately reduced feeding does not elicit an explicitly unfavorable effect, especially in adult animals. Better discrimination and learning in instrumental or escape situations and shorter running time in the maze were reported in early psychological studies.[40,41] However, the reward used in these experiments is questionable. If food is the reward, there is an obvious explanation for a better performance in the semistarved animals. The results of experiments using a water maze should also be considered with reservations, as the stimulus intensity may be different for normal and calorie-deprived rats. The deprived animals lose weight and body fat stores, become cold earlier, and are more exhausted by swimming.

C. Water Deprivation

There is ample evidence[39,42,43] of the interaction between solid food and water intake. Behavioral effects of food and water deprivations are not always identical.[44-47] When rats are allowed to explore and/or to drink and eat, thirsty animals tend to drink first and eat later.[48] Thirst appears to be a stronger motive initially than either hunger or exploration, but is sooner satiated. Hunger is initially weaker than either thirst or the tendency to explore and is slow to be satiated, causing hungry rats to explore initially. After the reduction of exploration, the animal starts to eat.

D. Food Restriction in Early Life and Long-Term Effects of Undernutrition

As opposed to the reversible effect of calorie deprivation in adult animals, lack of food during the suckling or even prenatal period may disturb neural and behavioral development and result in long-term behavioral abnormalities.

Rat pups deprived of food for 24 hr between the fifth and sixth days of life exhibited marked reduction in spontaneous motor activity. The recorded values did not reach the level found in normal pups until the 28th day of life.[49] The effect of 48 hr of hunger and thirst induced in 15-day-old rat pups was evident even when the rats became adults. When tested for the speed of elaboration of conditioned responses on the 90th day of life and retention of the memory trace over 3 months, the previously deprived rats were inferior in all criteria to the control group.[50]

The lasting calorie reduction in infancy, although permitting most animals to survive and grow, may result in retarded neuromuscular development and functional changes in the CNS. Several techniques were developed for the study of calorie undernutrition. The most common are

1.   Variation of the litter size. Litter size is one of the factors determining the quantity of food for individual pups. When 15 to 20 rat pups are nursed by one dam, they grow slowly; show signs of undernutrition; and, despite ad libitum feeding after weaning, they never reach the weight of animals nursed in small litters. The physical and behavioral development of rats from large litters is often compared (without use of a control group of medium size) with the development of animals reared in litters of three to four pups which grow faster and are actually overfed.[51-54]

2.   Restricted feeding of pregnant or lactating dams. Chow and Lee,[55] Lee and Chow[56] and Altman et al.[51] developed and used in numerous experiments a method in which rat dams were fed approximately 50% of the amount of food consumed by control females fed ad libitum. Irreversible changes were found in various metabolic characteristics and neuromuscular development.

3.   Intermittent separation of pups from their mothers. Pups separated daily for given periods of time from the dam are unable to compensate for this deficit by increased suckling during the remainder of the day and develop symptoms of physical handicap.[58-61] This procedure grossly interferes with the natural psychological environment. It leads not only to a reduction of nursing care, but also to physical and social deprivation. Moreover, both the mother and control pups may be disturbed through manipulation of the litter. It is difficult to keep the handling of experimental and control groups absolutely identical; therefore, this method, although valuable in biochemical and physiological research, does not appear to be especially suitable for behavioral experiments in which more precise control of psychological variables is required.

The disturbed development of CNS and behavioral consequences due to early calorie deprivation were demonstrated by many authors. There is good agreement in the findings reported by different laboratories. Undernourished pups exhibit retarded development of electric activity of the brain and evoked potentials. Latency of evoked potentials is prolonged, wave amplitudes are lower, and the capacity to respond to stimulation reduced.[62] The offspring of calorie-restricted dams show a delayed development of various reflexes,[63] poor motor coordination as measured in swimming tests,[61] retarded development, and reduced motor and exploratory activities.[63-65] A low level of exploratory activity was also observed in pups reared in large litters as compared with pups from small[66] or medium-sized litters.[67]

Some behavioral disturbances persevere long after the initiation of nutritional rehabilitation. Exploratory activity of rats undernourished early in life continues to be depressed in adulthood.[54,67,68]

Reduced learning performance was observed in various situations involving food as reward, such as escape from a water maze or an electrified grid.[69-73] Undernourished rats also showed stronger passive avoidance behavior than controls[74] and a lower threshold of response to electric shock.[75] Rats undernourished early in life respond with elevated "emotionality" as measured by defecation, startle response, or vocalization in different testing situations.[54,74,76]

Early calorie deprivation can modify feeding behavior in adults. Rats from large litters hoarded more food and were more successful in competition for food[54] or water.[77] Hoarding was maximized when nutritional deprivation was started before weaning, but not 12 days after weaning.[78] According to Seitz,[54] the rats deprived early were more sexually active and vicious, but recent studies[79] have not confirmed these findings and have shown retarded development of sexual behavior. In social interactions the undernourished rats were found to be more aggressive[80] and more socially active than controls.[77]

E. Overnutrition

In recent years obesity in children has been receiving growing attention because of accumulated evidence that overfeeding during the critical developmental periods (i.e., the prepubertal period of postnatal growth) may initiate the onset of cardiovascular disorders, carbohydrate intolerance, or obesity during later life.[81,82] Overfeeding during the preweaning period leads to an increased number of adipose cells and results in hyperplastic obesity.[83]

There is one way to induce overnutrition in experimental animals during the suckling period, i.e., by reducing the number of pups in the litter. Animals reared in small litters were long used as antagonists of undernourished pups. During the period of rapid growth they displayed higher exploratory activity[66] and various biochemical indices of accelerated development. However, further studies demonstrated that in adulthood the animals overnourished early in life were not superior to normally fed animals of medium-sized litters, and in some behavioral tests they behaved similarly to previously undernourished rats. In avoidance learning, the best performance was found in animals from medium-sized litters.[69,71]

III. BASAL CALORIC NUTRIENTS AND BEHAVIOR

In nutritional research two distinct approaches to the study of behavioral effects of isolated nutrients exist. The first lies in the elimination (or drastic reduction) of a substance from food, or, conversely, feeding in excess. In this way, extreme nutritional conditions are created which may also occur in human nutrition under some circumstances.

The second approach is based on the testing of the effect of one nutrient of a limited quantity in food while maintaining all nutrients within relatively physiological limits not causing deficiencies, gross metabolic disorders, symptoms of poisoning, marked mortality, or other pathological conditions. This method has been widely used in the study of behavioral effects of dietary protein, fats, and carbohydrates.

A. Proteins

Many studies have confirmed the effect of protein level on spontaneous activity of adult animals (see References 16 and 84). The early findings gave contradictory results. Abderhalden and Wertheimer[85] reported increased spontaneous activity in rats fed diets with high volumes of meat. Hitchcock[86] found elevated activity in the revolving drum in those rats fed a diet consisting of 12% vegetable protein, but only after general emaciation of the animals by inadequate diet.

Later studies[87.88] were more consistent, revealing an inverse relationship between amount of dietary protein and intensity of spontaneous activity in adult rats. Fifty percent of dietary protein markedly inhibited activity level.[89] Lát and Faltová[90] tested exploratory activity in a new environment in groups of rats fed diets with different protein-carbohydrate ratios but a constant amount of fat. Exploratory activity increased with decreasing protein and increasing carbohydrates and vice versa. Further studies[91-96] confirmed their results.

Learning performance was studied under various testing conditions. A low-protein vegetable diet deteriorated the capacity of rats to learn.[97] Short-term experiments failed to show marked interaction between the amount of dietary protein and performance in learning.[88.89]

Andriasov[99] studied conditioned avoidance responses in freely moving rats. He compared the effects of diet with 3.8, 18, and 36% of calories as protein. Decreased protein levels resulted in the weakening of inhibitory cortical processes and in the predominance of excitatory processes. In contrast, the high protein diet exerted an inhibitory effect on conditioned reflexes in the long-term feeding and finally resulted in pathological symptoms of experimental neurosis.

Decrease of dietary protein to 3 cal % disturbed the conditioned responses of dogs.[100] A diet with a medium protein content, i.e., 23.8 cal % proved to have an optimum effect on the discriminatory capacity of rats.[90] Studies[101] on the susceptibility of rats to convulsions showed the animals on a medium-protein diet to be most resistant to seizures.

B. Amino Acids

Under natural conditions where there is free choice of foods, an animal can meet its biological requirements through adequate intake of individual amino acids. Animals are able to distinguish food containing a balanced mixture of amino acids from that with a dysbalanced amino acid ratio. Rats refused to eat food from which some amino acids were eliminated, tending to prefer even a protein-free diet over an imbalanced diet, despite the fact that the former produced gradually severe malnutrition.[102.103]

Dietary amino acid dysbalance disturbs various physiological functions and elicits disorders in the CNS. Excess of some amino acids grossly interferes with growth;[104] excess of others may induce cerebral lesions[105] or mental retardation. Their potential effect on behavior, performance, and intelligence is discussed below.

Before interpreting the results of behavioral research, careful attention should be given to experimental variables, especially the following:

1. The age at which intervention was initiated.
2. The duration of experimental feeding.
3. The isomer of the amino acid used.
4. The type of behavioral test — e.g., whether food was used for motivation (in animals with loss of appetite) or whether motor ability was preserved to enable the animal to perform the task.
5. The constancy of psychological conditions during early life, i.e. uniform litter size, adequate maternal care, etc.

1. Methionine

Both deficiency and excess of methionine manifests itself in behavioral changes. Weisz et al.[106] tested conditioned reflex activity in methionine-deficient animals and found rapid extinction of previously fixed conditioned reflexes. In another experiment[100] rats were given a low-protein diet which disturbed conditioned responses. After the dietary methionine was increased, the level of conditioned responses increased, but without positively affecting discriminatory ability.

The adverse effect of methionine excess has been demonstrated in many studies. A higher dose of L-methionine disturbed the social behavior of mice.[107,108] Beaton et al.[109] studied the effect of methionine and its metabolites, including cysteine. Methionine reduced the percentage of efficient responses in Sidman avoidance learning. Behavioral abnormalities manifested themselves through inadequate reactions to external stimuli and premature response to stimulation. According to Beaton et al.,[109] the methyl group was not responsible for this effect and betaine, a metabolite of methionine, and methionine in combination with serine had only weak initial effects. Homocysteine might be the most active metabolic product of methionine. Patients with homocysteinuria displayed symptoms resembling schizophrenia and mental retardation.

The effect of methionine on CNS activity also manifested itself by electroencephalographic changes during sleep. L-Methionine, L-methionine with L-histidine, and L-methionine with nicotinamide led to a significant decrease of rapid eye movement (REM) sleep, while betaine, L-serine, L-histidine, L-methionine, and L-serine did not affect the REM phase of sleep and L-cysteine alone had a lesser effect than methionine.

2. Phenylalanine

Phenylalanine has become one of the most studied amino acids since the 1960s, when massive feeding of phenylalanine (Phe) was found to induce symptoms analogous to genetically determined phenylketonuria (PKU) in children.

PKU-like conditions are induced by L-Phe given in food or injected in doses exceeding metabolic requirements and resulting in serotonine depletion through the inhibition of tryptophan hydroxylase, which increases Phe by inhibiting phenylalanine hydroxylase.[110] Because mental retardation and psychic alterations are typical symptoms of PKU, similar symptoms have been sought for in animals. (For a review see Reference 111.)

Animals treated with Phe after weaning or later were less able to learn water maze or in operant conditioning tasks.[112-115] This effect was reversible; administration of a normal diet eliminated learning deficit after 20 days or more.[116]

The effect of Phe feeding after weaning on spontaneous activity has not been established unequivocally. Different dynamics of habituation of exploratory activity were found in Phe-treated rats as compared with control rats. The Phe-treated rats exhibited an abrupt decrease of activity in habituation tests, interpreted as a decreased capacity to maintain arousal and lesser ability to show exploratory behavior.[110]

Phe administered either neonatally or in the diet of pregnant dams elicits massive behavioral changes. Reduced learning capacity and inadequate behavior was observed in classical avoidance learning, Sidman avoidance learning, and shuttle box; it results in increased conditioned emotional reactions, lower exploratory activity, and higher defecation score.[117-120]

The time factor appears to play a significant role in the extent and reversibility of behavioral changes.[121,122] Thus, as in other nutritional interventions, treatment during the early developmental periods elicits mental disturbances because of its direct interaction with the developing CNS, although the precise correlation between mental deficiency and structural or metabolic changes has not been accurately determined.[123]

The reduced DNA synthesis and lower brain weight in the course of Phe treatment give evidence of abnormal brain development.[124,125] Low brain weight may be caused by a subnormal lipid content.

The metabolic disorders during PKU are supposedly the primary factor responsible for mental retardation. However, the adequacy of animal models for PKU-like conditions has often been discussed.[110,115] For example, some biochemical alterations do not correspond to those seen in humans. One of the crucial problems is the reversibility of changes. Whereas in humans mental retardation is irreparable, the disturbances in learning performance in animals have been found by many authors to be only temporary. The controversial findings may be due to some extent to methodological factors, sensitivity of methods, duration of exposure to Phe, and selection of controls. Many designs use pair-fed animals as controls. However, the reduced food intake during the period of growth produces behavioral abnormalities whereby the differences between Phe-treated and control groups are diminished. If Phe is given during the suckling period, litter size is often reduced to prevent undernutrition of PKU pups of mothers with reduced lactating ability. It should be remembered that litter size is an important psychological factor modifying behavioral development.[66,67]

Many studies use *p*-chlorophenylalanine instead of Phe to induce PKU-like states.[125-129] However, the observed effects often differ from those of Phe. Apart from this, *p*-chlorophenylalanine does not occur as a normal food component and therefore belongs to the field of psychopharmacology rather than nutrition.

3. Tryptophan

Some species exhibit reduced motor activity when given large doses of tryptophan.[130,131] Modigh[132] found that the inhibition of activity appeared only at doses greater than 800 mg per kilogram body weight.

A much argued point is whether tryptophan alone or some of its metabolic products directly influence the CNS. L-Tryptophan is metabolized by different pathways both in peripheral tissues and in the CNS. Two of them are 5-Ht (serotonin) and tryptamine. Findings on inhibitory effects on animal locomotor activity, which describe a sedative and antidepressant effect of tryptophan, agree with those in humans.[133,134] According to Modigh,[132] this effect is not mediated by any of its metabolic products, but by the amino acid itself; he supposes that L-tryptophan loading by a saturating transport mechanism induces deficiency of the other amino acids essential for the maintenance of spontaneous motor activity.

Tryptophan is the precursor of nicotinic acid. Efremov et al.[135] found that combined deficiency of nicotinic acid and tryptophan results in changes in the higher nervous functions of dogs.

4. Lysine

Behavioral changes in rats on lysine-deficient diets were described in the early psychological literature. Lysine deprivation enhanced activity in the running wheel.[136] The lysine-deficient rats required a longer period of time to master the problem box; they made more errors during learning, but the time required to run across the maze was shorter.[137,138] In the elevated maze they took a longer length of time to reach the goal, there were more errors and a higher number of trials were needed to meet the criterion of correct performance.[139] Conditioned reflex activity in deficient animals was also impaired; these changes appeared before weight loss.[106]

Symptoms such as increased motor activity and poorer learning ability resemble those of rats subject to acute calorie deprivation. When lysine-deficient and calorie-deprived rats of equal weight were compared, no differences in their learning performance were revealed.[140] The behavioral changes may merely reflect deprivation or other factors acting on the organism. Lysine is assumed to be the growth-limiting factor[141] and is of essential importance, especially in the initial phases of ontogenesis. Despite the fact that a lysine-deprived pregnant dam is capable of supplying the developing fetus with lysine, the birth weight of pups is slightly retarded; however, as early as 21 days after birth the prenatally deficient group shows drastically reduced body weights.[141]

The effect of excess dietary lysine on animal behavior has not been demonstrated. Lysine excess is known to inhibit weight increments in chickens, but an adverse effect of lysine on growth was observed after only 6% supplementation if administered from weaning.[142]

5. Glutamic Acid

Biochemical research has demonstrated the importance of glutamic acid (GA) in the nervous system, especially in the brain, where it plays an essential role in carbohydrate and protein metabolism.[143] The young brain is permeable to GA even though the transfer of free GA from blood to brain is limited.[144,145]

Initial observations of the influence of GA on the intellectual functions of normal or mentally retarded individuals have indicated that it has a favorable effect on cognitive processes (see References 146 and 147 for a review).

Behavioral studies on experimental animals proceeded parallel to human research. Positive findings on the possibility of promoting learning in problem box situations and mazes of various types[148-150] were followed by a large number of negative results regardless of the type of learning situations[151-153] (for a review see Reference 16). This has by no means put an end to the question of the behavioral effects of GA. Phillips[149] described elevated activity of GA-treated animals in the running wheel. More recently, Winczle and Vogel[154] studied the interaction between GA and exploration in an activity cage. A basal diet was supplemented with GA in doses of 50, 200, or 400 mg per kilogram body weight. Diets were administered to rats between the ages of 30 to 90 days. Activity in the running wheel, operant conditioning, and extinction of bar-pressing responses were recorded. The effect was related to dose: the lowest dose had no essential effect on behavior; 200 mg/kg proved to be an optimum dose, resulting in elevated activity, the lowest number of responses required to master bar pressing, and the fastest extinction. The largest dose (400 mg/kg) had an adverse effect both on learning and activity; these animals were also hyperemotional, with aggressive tendencies.

Braksh[155] studied conditioned alimentary responses in dogs. Supplementation with GA of a normal diet did not influence conditioned activity; however, after administration of a low-protein diet which disturbed the higher nervous functions, GA had a normalizing effect.

From numerous studies it appears that GA has an effect on animal behavior; however, methodological questions, as well as the specificity of the effect of GA, remain open. Interpretation of findings, especially of increased spontaneous activity, is based primarily on the adrenergic effect of GA.[143] GA stimulates the release of epinephrine, which in turn may lead to stimulation of mental and physical activity. It was previously shown that adrenergic states facilitated performance in simple situations such as bar pressing, but disturbed performance in more complex situations which included discrimination.

6. Monosodium Glutamate

Some researchers use the salt of GA, monosodium glutamate (MSG) instead of GA itself, apparently because it produces no gastric disorders in patients and because of its easier application.[146] However, it appears that the effects of MSG differ markedly from those of GA.[156,157] Unlike GA, which decreased epileptic activity, MSG increased it, eliciting both clinical symptoms and changes in electroencephalograms (EEG). Favorable effects of MSG on the intellect of mentally retarded patients were not established.

Berry et al.[158] studied biochemical and behavioral effects of MSG applied in doses of 4 mg per kilogram body weight during the first 10 days of life. From the 50th day on, learning in a water maze was tested. The treated group showed lower swimming speed and made more errors than the control group. The groups did not differ from one another in simple tasks, but the treated animals were markedly inferior in tasks requiring more complex discrimination.

Several experiments[159-161] gave evidence of the toxic effect of MSG on pups of various animal species; they showed that MSG causes neuroanatomical lesions, primarily in the retina and hypothalamus. The mortality rate of MSG pups was high. The toxic effect of MSG was mitigated when added to diet rather than given parenterally. MSG supplementation of 40% of the basal diet suppressed food intake and body and brain weight. A lower dose (20% supplementation) had a less marked effect. Weight of the adrenal glands significantly increased.[162]

7. Cysteine

Earlier papers[137] reported reduced learning performance, a longer period of time required to reach the goal, more errors, and a higher number of responses to meet the criterion of adequate performance in cysteine-deficient rats. Cysteine supplementation failed to affect their behavior.[98]

Recent studies have been concerned with the long-term effects of excess cysteine during the early periods of postnatal development. Feeding with cysteine induces damage in various part of the brain, e.g., the dorsal hippocampus, amygdala, thalamus, and cerebral cortex.[163] Sharpe et al.[164] studied the long-term effect of a single dose of 1.2 to 1.3 mg L-cysteine per kilogram body weight in 4-day-old mice. The experimental group had a high mortality — 75% of the pups died before weaning. The surviving pups displayed no impaired growth or loss of motor capacity, but demonstrated behavorial abnormalities which persisted into adulthood.

L-Cysteine induces lesions, primarily in the limbic structures of the brain. Behavioral symptoms resemble the disorders seen in animals with hippocampal lesions. For example, hippocampectomized animals do not exhibit typical spontaneous alteration in the T-maze, make more errors in learning, lack habituation, and display persistence or fixation of reactions. It is assumed that neonatal injection of L-cysteine prevents a normal maturation of the inhibitory hippocampal system.[164]

8. Histidine

Experiments with histidine showed dysbalance of dietary amino acids to induce aversion to administered food. Simson and Booth[165] demonstrated that a single intragastric administration of a mixture containing amino acids in the same proportions found in a fully adequate dietary protein followed by presentation of odorized food increased preference for food with this odor; on the other hand, the same mixture with the elimination of histidine resulted in conditioned aversion to odors added to this diet. The conditioned aversion was extremely strong.[166]

9. Other Amino Acids

The behavioral effects of the other amino acids are not well known. An excitatory effect on CNS neurons was found with aspartate; some amino acids caused brain lesions when administered in large doses to infant mice.[163] Mice treated with tyrosine from birth until the seventh or eighth week of life showed subnormal performance in learning situations for a short period of time after they were transferred to a normal diet.[121]

C. Long-term Effect of Early Protein Deprivation and Protein-calorie Malnutrition

Feeding of a diet with extremely low dietary protein drastically disturbs development of the CNS and behavior when administered early in life. Conditions both of extreme forms of protein deprivation (see in human kwashiorkor) and milder forms of protein deficiency have been modeled in experimental animals. Feeding a low-protein diet leads to the loss of appetite and, therefore, to reduced food intake, resulting in complex manifestation of protein-calorie malnutrition (PCM). In humans, various types of early PCM represent some of the most urgent problems of contemporary nutritional science.[167] Many workers[168-176] have reviewed the physiological and mental symptoms of PCM in animals and humans.

The interference of acute PCM with the normal development of the brain has been evidenced by biochemical and electrophysiological findings. Deviations in the development of EEGs were observed in dogs malnourished from the early postnatal periods; the maximum differences appeared between weeks 8 and 13 of life. PCM animals displayed slow, rhythmic activity of low amplitude with sharp, multifocal spikes.[177] Disturbances in EEGs were also found in PCM pigs.[178]

Administration of a low-protein diet (12% casein or less) to the lactating female after giving birth leads to rapid weight loss and reduced milk secretion. At first the pups are calorie deprived; when spontaneously transferred to solid food, they gradually also develop symptoms of protein deficiency, resulting in the picture of combined protein-calorie malnutrition.

In PCM infant rats, slower growth and retarded development of exploratory activity was found in the preweaning period,[179] together with quantitative and qualitative differences in interactions with littermates and the mother.[180,181] Young rats transferred to a diet containing 5% protein displayed irritability and resistance to handling.[182]

Behavioral abnormalities in malnourished dogs were described in detail by Platt and Stewart.[183] Their PCM puppies showed unusual postures and, when forced into activity, responded with agitation, running in circles, seizures, and defecation.

Behavioral abnormalities in pups originating during the suckling period may reflect (to a degree) alteration in the maternal behavior of the lactating female suffering from acute PCM. Abnormal behavior of mother toward infants and less active contacts were observed both in dogs and rats.[184,185] Abnormal behavioral manifestations can also be observed in other malnourished species. For example, wing flapping, turning around in circles, and rapid head bobbing near the wall of the cage were recorded in malnourished pigeons.[186]

Many behavioral disorders persevere after the termination of protein deprivation. Thus, rats displayed a reduced level of open field exploratory activity.[179,187] Their reactions in various social situations also differ from those of normal animals. While the exploratory activity of normally fed rats is enhanced by the presence of an animal of the same species,[188,189] young PCM rats show inhibition of exploration in this situation.[180] A striking feature is their aggressiveness, observed even toward a larger, normally fed animal.[190,191]

Abnormalities in sexual behavior in the presence of a female were observed and lower exploratory (sniffing) activity in an environment previously scented by a female in estrus were observed in adult, nutritionally rehabilitated male rats.[192]

There are controversies concerning learning performance of young PCM animals. Cowley and Griesel[193,194] showed that rats maintained for a prolonged period of time on a diet with a moderately lowered level of protein were not consistently inferior in learning ability if cold water was used for motivation. Poorer responses were recorded in rehabilitated PCM rats in a learning set with a food reward.[195] Fraňková and Barnes[196] studied conditioned avoidance responses in adult rats after realimentation. The rats learned to jump on a vertically placed screen to avoid the shocks from the electrified grid, signalled by an acoustic stimulus. The previously PCM rats did not differ from controls either in the speed of learning or in mean latencies of conditioned responses. However, in the course of learning, the excitement of the PCM rats gradually increased and manifested itself in panic reactions, restlessness, stereotype jumps on the screen (Figure 1), and the inability to inhibit learned response. Similar behavioral patterns in avoidance learning were seen in realimented pigs.[197]

Experiments demonstrating the effects of PCM on animal learning suggest that learning capacity ("intelligence") is not damaged by early protein deprivation. Changes in learning, if any, are the result of motivational disturbances, increased fear of novel environment, or higher "emotionality." The experimental animal exhibits exaggerated response to unusual or aversive stimuli.[198] When motivation (in a bar-pressing situation) was adjusted to a constant level for both the young PCM and normal rats, no difference in response was found in a visual discrimination test,[199] and fear-motivated panic responses in the course of avoidance learning were prevented when these animals were first acclimated to the experimental conditions.[200]

Long-term effects of PCM which affect the preweaning period have been evidenced by numerous studies. On the other hand, PCM initiated after weaning supposedly has mild, transient behavioral effects, if any. However, a detailed study[201] demonstrated that if the PCM was severe enough and extended over the period of sexual maturation, it resulted in long-term behavioral disturbances.

D. Fats

Interest in the behavioral effects of fats was stimulated by the extensive research of the role of dietary fat in various metabolic disorders and obesity. Early studies were concerned primarily with the effect of fats on working capacity. According to Hajdu,[202] a diet with a well-balanced fat/carbohydrate ratio ensures optimal growth and working performance. Other authors[203-205] observed better physical performance and an elevated activity in various situations with such a diet, especially when compared with a fat-free diet.

The study of Smith and Conger[89] was the first to contain detailed experimental data on the behavioral effect of dietary fat. Spontaneous activity in a revolving drum remained at a normal level up to 56 cal % of fats, while 72 cal % inhibited activity. Other workers[93,95,206] reported an elevation of spontaneous activity with increasing fat level. Fraňková[206] tested open field exploratory activity in rats. Groups of normal adult males were transferred to diets with the following fat/carbohydrate ratios: 75:10, 35:50, and 10:75. After 5 weeks of dietary treatment the group on the high-fat diet displayed increased exploratory activity as compared with the other groups. A high activity level persisted throughout the administration of the high-fat diet (19 weeks). The high-fat diet also normalized the activity level of the rats undernourished at an early age.[67] Comparison of isocaloric diets with high levels of fats, carbohydrates, or proteins revealed that the maximum exploratory activity was elicited by a high-fat diet; a carbohydrate diet had a lesser, but also excitatory effect, while the high-protein diet inhibited exploratory activity.[95,96]

Less attention has been paid to the interaction between dietary fat and learning.

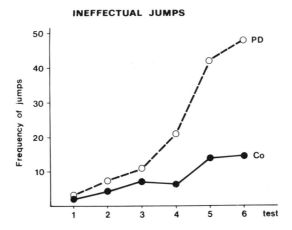

FIGURE 1. Mean number of spontaneous jumps on the screen during avoidance conditioning in adult male rats protein-calorie malnourished from birth to the 49th day of life. PD, the experimental group; CO, controls. (Data from Fraňková, S. and Barnes, R. H., *J. Nutr.*, 96, 477—484, 1968.)

Razenkov[207] showed that, similar to the effect on activity, a high-fat diet promoted conditioned reflex activity in dogs; a lesser effect was elicited by carbohydrates, and a high level of dietary protein inhibited conditioned reflexes. These results were confirmed in experiments with rats.[208]

The effect of administration of a fat-free diet during gestation on the development and learning ability of the progeny was studied by Caldwell and Churchill.[209] Pregnant dams were maintained on a fat-free diet throughout the gestation period. The offspring had lower birth weights. The weight later became normalized, but the experimental group was inferior in learning at 50 days of life as compared with the controls (Figure 2).

When taking into account findings on the enhancing effect of fats on the susceptibility to convulsions,[210-212] it can be assumed that fats have an excitatory effect on CNS activity.

1. Fatty Acids and Behavior

Behavioral effects of individual fatty acids have not been studied systematically, although the composition of fat may be responsible for some observed behavioral changes. Fraňková[213] studied the influence of high-fat diets with a prevalence of either unsaturated fatty acids (sunflower oil) or saturated fatty acids (mutton suet) on the exploratory activity of adult rats. Both diets increased the activity, as had been observed previously.[206,208] Fats were later replaced by mixtures of either unsaturated or saturated fatty acids. The activity levels of animals with unsaturated fats in their diets declined to the levels recorded in control groups maintained on a commercial diet. A high level of saturated fatty acids drastically suppressed spontaneous activity and growth of animals was markedly decreased, suggesting the possibility of a toxic effect of an excess saturated fatty acids.

In the short-term acute experiment, the effect of arachidonic fatty acid was studied on mice. Intraperitoneal administration of 100 or 200 mg per kilogram body weight inhibited activity. Reduction of activity was so severe that it was possible even to inhibit the antagonistic effect of d-amphetamine.[214]

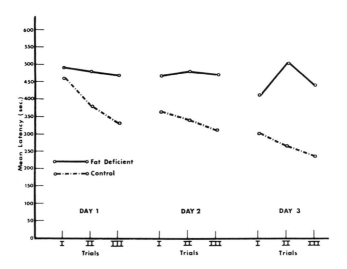

FIGURE 2.   Mean response latency in the Lashley III maze in the progeny of rats fed either lipid-free or control diet throughout the gestation period. (From Caldwell, D. F. and Churchill, J. A., *Psychol. Rep.*, 19, 99—102, 1966. With permission.)

E. Carbohydrates

The influence of dietary carbohydrates on activity and learning become evident when compared with those of proteins or fats. Carbohydrates attracted attention primarily in relation to preference for certain dietary compounds. Faltová and Lát,[42] Lát and Faltová,[90] and Lát[216] tested interindividual differences in preference for carbohydrates, fats, and proteins. In male rats, intensity of exploratory activity was established; then self-selection of dietary compounds (SSDC) was tested. Rats with low levels of exploratory activity tended to select a high amount of protein, while rats with high values of exploration preferred carbohydrates (Figure 3).

Many studies[216,217] have shown a high preference for carbohydrates by various animal species (for a review see Reference 2). When no other factors interfere, rats prefer carbohydrates of higher concentration to those of lower ones.[218-220] This preference also depends on the type of diet administered. High protein-low carbohydrate diets result in a high bar-pressing rate (sucrose reward), while the administration of low protein-high carbohydrate diet leads to a low rate of bar pressing when a 32% sucrose reward on a fixed-interval (1 min) schedule was employed.[94] Nutritional conditions also influence preference for sucrose given in lower concentrations.[221] These findings are of importance for the interpretation of the effect on learning performance of diets with different levels of protein or carbohydrate. Using sugar- or carbohydrate-containing food as reinforcement induces the factor of unequal motivation.

IV. VITAMINS

Deficiency of one or more vitamins in the diet manifests itself very quickly through behavioral changes. Elevation of total motor activity is often the earliest symptom of vitamin deficiency. Severe or protracted vitamin deprivation may elicit massive neurological disorders which make the performance of animals in behavioral tests based on motor responses impossible. Excesses of some vitamins, especially in the diets of pregnant dams, has a teratogenic effect and results in abnormal development of the CNS.

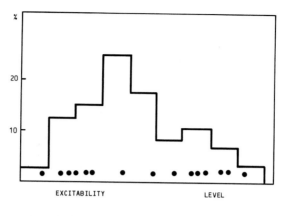

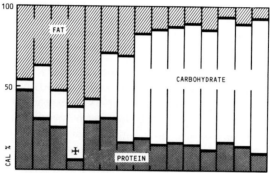

FIGURE 3. (Top) Frequency distribution of individual levels of excitability measured by means of the sum of exploratory (rearing) reaction in the habituation period. Black circles are the 15 rats of 59 chosen for the SSDC experiment. (Bottom) average intake of margarine, starch, and casein (cal %) in 15 male rats represented by 15 columns and arranged in the same order as in the upper graph, i.e., from less excitable rats (left side) to highly excitable ones (right side). Rat 13 died on day 70 of SSDC experiment. Average values were calculated from the period in which rats regularly gained weight and showed good regulation. (From Lằt, J., in *The Chemical Senses and Nutrition*, Kare, M. K. and Maller, O., Eds., Johns Hopkins Press, Baltimore, 1967, 169—180. With permission.)

In interpretation of the results it is necessary to consider the motor ability of the animal to respond to the stimulation and the mode of reinforcement used, because of the potential suppression of appetite by vitamin deficiency. In many of the older studies, adequate nutritional control was lacking and there was no precise control over other nutritional and nonnutritional variables.

A. B-complex Vitamins

Early experiments[224-227] using B-complex vitamins were not able to differentiate among the effects of individual vitamins; therefore, it was not possible to determine whether the effects observed were caused by a deficiency of all vitamins or of only one (apparently thiamine). Because they are closely related to both the peripheral and central nervous systems, B-complex vitamins have marked behavioral effects. Early psychological studies[224-227] described various behavioral disorders accompanying deficiency. Deficiency of B-complex vitamins manifests itself firstly by an elevation of locomotor activity[222] (for reviews see References 16 and 84); the activity gradually falls.[223]

The deficiency of B-complex vitamins adversely affected maze learning.[224-226] Behavioral disturbances were more profound in animals already exposed to deprivation during the suckling period.[227] Abnormalities induced by vitamin deficiency persevere. As long as 3 months after termination of deprivation, poor performance of rats in the water maze was observed.[228-230] Disorders of conditioned reflex activity were found in dogs.[231]

Food preference tests[232] in deficient rats revealed that they chose to hoard normal, nondeficient diets. A distinct preference for new foods in those rats deficient of vitamins (including those of the B-complex) was demonstrated by Rodgers and Rozin[233] and Rozin and Rodgers.[234]

There is evidence on the adverse effect of B-complex deficiency on sexual behavior. In the terminal stage or deficiency there is reduced sexual activity;[235] in young rats the development of copulatory behavior is delayed.[236]

1. Thiamine

Anorexia is the earliest symptom of thiamine deficiency; motor and neurological disturbances develop later (for details see Brožek and Grande.[237]) Thiamine deficiency manifests itself first by an increase in total activity; this gradually decreases with advancing polyneuritis.[238,239] No difference in short-term open field activity was found.[240] Thiamine-deficient rats were inferior in learning when food was used as reward.[241-243] However, objections that anorexia during deficiency lowered reinforcing properties of food and therefore decreased the motivation to learn was disproved by late studies which tested the rate of learning in a water maze.[229,230] In the studies of Poe et al.,[229,230] the deficiency was induced during gestation and extended through the nursing period and weaning. Young deprived rats showed retarded development of conditioned eyelid responses.[244] Soviet authors[245,246] revealed disturbances in conditioned reflex activity in thiamine-deficient dogs.

Observations on the spontaneous behavior of rats showed that the deficient animals were overreactive in conflict situations and displayed rigidity of learned response and behavior irrelevant in respect to external stimuli. They reacted with sudden attacks and biting.[247] In social situations, thiamine deficiency did not influence the aggressiveness of mice (which is relatively high in normal animals) unless the mice were physically so weak that they were unable to respond to the partner.[248]

The effect of thiamine was studied extensively with respect to food preference and self selection of dietary compounds. Richter et al.[249] previously reported that thiamine-deprived rats preferred food containing thiamine. If a diet containing thiamine was associated with a specific flavor and the flavor of the food was later altered, the thiamine-deficient rats preferred the food flavor originally associated with thiamine.[250,251] Recent studies[233,252,253] indicate the relationship between deficiency and the ability to choose thiamine is not simple and little is known about the mechanism of preference. It is not clear whether an animal is able to adequately regulate the spontaneous intake of thiamine with respect to its physiological requirements, whether the ability to select thiamine (if any) is innate or learned.

The thiamine-deficient rats invariantly prefer novel diet over the familiar one even when it is deficient in thiamine while the familiar one is supplemented with thiamine.[233] Given a choice from diets where only one contained thiamine, the deficient rats often developed a strong preference for the thiamine- containing diet. They selected their food systematically and tended to choose one type of the diet to constitute one meal.[252] On the other hand, Rozin et al.[253] found no preference for thiamine if it was given in water rather than administered in solid food despite the fact that the physiological effects were identical in both cases.

Fewer studies have dealt with the effect of elevated doses of thiamine on behavior. Thiamine supplementation of a normal diet improved the speed of escape from water if supplementation was initiated during the gestational period.[254] Supplementation was initiated on the 35th day of life was ineffective.[255] Havliček[256] observed that 35 mg/kg i.v. of thiamine normalized higher nervous activity in dogs. The effect of a higher dose of thiamine (and also of riboflavine, pyridoxine, and some minerals) on susceptibility to seizures was described by Patton et al.[257] The frequency of seizures dropped to a very low level within a few days, indicating that these substances may promote the utilization of dietary compounds.

On the other hand, an excess of thamine may also have an adverse effect. Disturbances of reproduction were found in thiamine-supplemented females; it was possible to repair the damage through an increased pyridoxine level.[258]

2. Riboflavine

The behavioral consequences of riboflavine deficiency in animals have not been studied in detail, apparently because mental disorders related to riboflavine deficiency in humans have not been confirmed.[259] Besides, behavioral manifestations in animals are masked by neurological symptoms resulting from myelin degeneration.[260]

Early experiments on riboflavine-deprived rats demonstrated that, like the deficiency of other vitamins, the lack of dietary riboflavine resulted in elevation of total motor activity[239] and poorer learning in both the dry maze[224] and the water maze.[262] The younger the animal, the more profound were the symptoms of deficiency.

The deleterious effect of riboflavine deficiency on conditioned responses was reported by Efremov et al.[263] Improvement of higher nervous activity after refeeding lasted for a long period of time, but the normalization was never complete.

3. Nicotinic Acid (Niacin)

Despite the wide symptomatology of niacin deficiency in man,[259,264] studies of the behavioral responses in animals to lack of this vitamin have not been conducted in detail to date.

The Soviet authors Efremov et al.[135] studied the effect of niacin on conditioned reflex activity in dogs. They found changes in EEG and reduction of excitability of the cerebral cortex. Apart from the disturbance of conditioned reflex activity, the dogs showed neurotic behavior and refused to eat. This can be attributed to the dysbalance of dietary amino acids rather than to vitamin deficiency. Subsequent therapy failed to restore the functions of the CNS.

Nikolov et al.[265] observed that a low dose of vitamin supplementation promoted excitatory processes while a high dose had the opposite effect. Improvement of salivary conditioned reflexes and establishment of positive conditioned reflexes were also described.[266]

4. Pyridoxine (Vitamin B_6)

Interest in the behavioral effects of pyridoxine has been stimulated by biochemical studies which demonstrated the importance of pyridoxine in the metabolism of amino acids, gamma aminobutyric acid (GABA), nucleic acids, proteins, lipids, etc. Interaction between the symptoms of protein-calorie malnutrition and of vitamin B_6 has also been considered.[267] Requirement for pyridoxine is relative and depends on other dietary components. Its requirement increases with increased protein level. Winczle and Vogel[154] called attention to the relationship between pyridoxine and glutamic acid.

Increased doses of pyridoxine may result in the depletion of glutamic acid. Hoff et al.[268] studied the relationship of growth and behavior to the vitamin content. It appeared that there was no equal optimum level for both growth and spontaneous activity. While activity reached its peak at 3 μg per 10 g of diet, maximum growth was recorded after 20 μg.

Results of experiments on animals transferred to a vitamin B$_6$ deficient diet after weaning or later in life have not been universal. Reduction of dietary protein did not influence learning in a water maze.[269,270] In learning lever pressing to avoid electric shock or to obtain water after deprivation, deficient animals were inferior to controls.[271] Conditioned reflex activity was also disturbed in deficient dogs.[272,273] In a biochemical study by Bhagavan and Coursin,[274] postweaning pyridoxine deficiency resulted in significantly reduced brain weight, but the number and size of brain cells of the deprived rats did not differ from the controls. Behavioral deficit was reversed by pyridoxine therapy.[275,276]

Severe consequences were demonstrated after pre- and neonatal pyridoxine deficiency. Interaction between the symptoms of protein-calorie malnutrition and the level of vitamin B$_6$ has also been considered.[267] Requirements for pyridoxine is relative and depends on other dietary components; they increase with increased protein level.

The susceptibility of pyridoxine-deficient rats and mice to convulsions has been widely studied. Both audiogenic stimuli and electric shocks increased the incidence of seizures in vitamin B$_6$-deprived rats.[279-281] Dakshinamurti et al.[282] reported that the "majority of rats exhibited a peculiar tendency to hide in the corners of the cage." This behavioral pattern was absent in both controls and pair-fed (calorie-restricted) animals. The susceptibility to seizures in vitamin-deficient rats appears, to a certain extent, to be genetically determined.[279]

The deficient rats showed disorders in development and characteristics of EEG, with high-voltage waves (up to 300 to 400 μV) and spike discharges in motor and auditory cortex under nembutal anesthesia; control rats showed spindles rather than spikes in their EEG. The difference was evident in the character of cortical-auditory evoked potentials, especially in rats with distinct symptoms of deficiency; the evoked potentials had longer latencies.[282]

Pre- and neonatal pyridoxine deficiency was found to affect neuromotor development. Alton-Mackey and Walker[283] administered to rats diets with 0, 25, 50, 75, 100, or 400% of the recommended pyridoxine allowance. Both the development of reflexes and the onset of some behavioral patterns such as rearing, grooming, or startle response were markedly delayed in groups maintained on a low-pyridoxine level. The startle response was much more intense than in controls. The pups of pyridoxine-deficient mothers were undernourished, as the milk secretion in these dams decreased. The 100 or 400% groups did not differ in most criteria, although acceleration of development was observed in some indices in the latter group.

The therapeutic effect of elevated pyridoxine intake has been studied primarily in humans.[284] Pyridoxine was found to be effective in treatment of certain behavioral disorders in rats which were calorie or protein deprived during the early postnatal periods. An intraperitoneal dose of 40 mg/kg body weight injected between the 40th and 50th day of life normalized spontaneous behavior in the course of avoidance learning.[285]

5. Biotin

There are controversies among findings on the neurological symptomatology of biotin-deficient animals. Nielsen and Elvehjem[286] recorded locomotor abnormalities, paralysis and spasticity of varying degrees. On the other hand, Lazere et al.[287] observed no neuromuscular disturbances. Interestingly, biotin-deficient rats were more sensitive to handling.

Stewart et al.[288] tested learning capacity in biotin-deficient rats using conditioned avoidance and escape reactions. They reported an impaired learning in the experimental group; however, neuromuscular disturbances could not have been responsible for this effect because there was no difference between the experimental and control groups in unconditioned avoidance reaction to electric shocks. This finding supported their hypothesis that motor syndrome does not induce a degree of muscular weakness strong enough to prevent an animal from exhibiting an avoidance reaction unless an extreme state of deficiency is induced.

6. Pantothenic Acid

Little attention has been given thus far to the behavioral consequences of experimental pantothenic acid deficiency or excess. Gantt et al.[272] observed in dogs disturbance of conditioned reflex activity which was not associated with obvious neurological changes. Vitamin supplementation rapidly restored the conditioned reflexes. Weiss and Danford[289] combined vitamin deficiency with starvation and found enhanced sensitivity to cold which manifested itself in a higher rate of bar pressing in order to obtain heat.

7. Folic Acid

There is evidence that folic acid deficiency has an adverse effect, primarily on the nervous system of the developing fetus. Animal studies have shown that maternal folic acid deficiency results in a high occurrence of hydrocephali and abnormalities of the CNS in the progeny.[290] Delayed maturation of electric activity of the brain was observed in both rats and infants fed maternal milk containing low serum folate levels.[291,292]

Maze learning of those rats exposed to deficiency after weaning was not impaired, but animals subjected to deficiency during both the prenatal and suckling periods exhibited disorders in learning performance.[270] Efremov[293] reported lower values of conditioned reflexes in deficient dogs.

8. Cyanocobalamin (Vitamin B_{12})

Deficiency of vitamin B_{12} in the diet of a pregnant mother elicits congenital defects and structural changes in the nervous system. Pups of deficient mothers develop hydrocephalus (for a review see Reference 237). If there are any detectable behavioral effects, it is not known if they are caused by deficiency of the vitamin (its structure being complex) or to what extent some of its components, such as cobalt, play a role.

B. Vitamin C

Interest in vitamin C in human psychology has been stimulated by experimental studies which demonstrated enhanced working capacity and better economy of work after vitamin C supplementation.[294-296] On the other hand, reduced performance in various tests of mental functions, psychomotor performance, and physical fitness, as well as changes in personality, were observed during deficiency states.[297]

The only animal species known to be dependent on dietary vitamin C intake are humans, monkeys, and guinea pigs; however, other animal species are able to metabolize it. Experiments on subprimates are rare. Recently, Adlard et al.[298] studied the behavioral effect of vitamin C deficiency on guinea pigs. Performance in a T-maze after 2 months of vitamin depletion was not significantly altered, although the content of ascorbic acid measured in brain, brain stem, liver, and adrenal glands was distinctly lower in the deficient group.

C. Vitamin A

Vitamin A deficiency in pups results in growth retardation, disorders of motor co-ordination, and paralysis, usually of the hind legs. The rapid development of symptoms is accounted for by the inability to store this vitamin in the body. However, the deficiency can be rapidly compensated for by the administration of retinoic acid.[299]

Experimental studies of vitamin A deficiency on behavior produced rather controversial results. Moore and Mathias[242] reported impairment of maze learning. The difference in the rate of learning in the maze between the deficient and control groups was later found to be insignificant; however, the former group required a longer period of time to run from the start to the goal box.[300,301] Behavioral disorders could be related to conditions accompanying xerophthalmia and general emaciation of the animal. Studies of conditioned reflexes indicated that in deprived animals a longer period of time was required to learn a task and differentiation between two acoustic stimuli was poor. Vitamin A-deficient rats also exhibited reduced locomotor activity.[303] Another common symptom of vitamin A deficiency is the loss of normal taste preference.[304] Bernard and Halpern[305] tested spontaneous preference for NaCl and quinine sulfate (QSO$_4$) in rats. Normal rats tend to prefer NaCl and refuse QSO$_4$. At the onset of the experiment, vitamin A-deficient rats also refused QSO$_4$, but their aversion gradually weakened. It appeared that the loss of discriminatory capacity coincided with the onset of growth disturbance. While Duncan[304] supposed the mechanism of disorder was of central origin and linked to general debility, Bernard and Halpern[305] suggested that structural and functional changes at the periphery were involved in the behavioral taste deficit.

Hypervitaminosis during pregnancy has a teratogenic effect on the developing embryo and fetus: it disturbs the development of the CNS and produces anencephalus, anophthalmia, microphthalmia, and spina bifida.[306-309]

D. Vitamin D

Both deficiency and excess of vitamin D result in behavioral abnormalities. Rats maintained on a diet composed predominantly of corn exhibited signs of deficiency accompanied by decreasing spontaneous activity.[310]

Observation of the effect of vitamin D deficiency on learning are inconsistent. Inferior learning and relearning of the maze[311] may be a sign of neuromuscular pathology. Wilder[312] found no learning deficit in the maze when the reward was a normal or rachitogenic diet. Rachitic rats exhibit a preference for normal diet. This preference develops gradually and is evident only after 40 days on a rachitogenic diet.[313]

Excess of vitamin D may have serious mental consequences. Reed et al.[314] found an increased concentration of calcium in various tissues of dogs treated with irradiated ergosterol. His finding of an increased calcium concentration in the brain indicates that impaired CNS may be related to mental deficiency. More recently, evidence has been accumulated indicating that hypercalcemia in infancy is often associated with mental retardation (for a review see Reference 315).

E. Vitamin E (α-Tocopherol)

Vitamin E deficiency is manifested by anorexia, muscular debility, and paralysis and in advanced stages by the inability to maintain an upright position. Progressive behavioral changes occur (for a review see Reference 316). Wiesner and Bacharach[317] described changes in the sexual behavior of rats. Behavioral changes may be related to the level of brain biogenic amines. A decreased value of brain norepinephrine was found in vitamin E-deficient rats.[318] Administration of vitamin E resulted in elevation of the brain norepinephrine level. The therapeutic effect of dietary supplementation with vitamin E has not been convincingly established.[319] Rosen et al.[320] supplemented the diets of animals with weights maintained at 85% of the initial weight throughout the experiment with 50 or 100 mg of vitamin E. The 100 mg-supplemented rats performed better in instrumental learning and extinguishing as compared with controls; however, a food reward was used to motivate learning.

V. MINERALS

In the nutritional sciences attention has been paid to minerals because of the increasing evidence of their role in a large number of physiological processes in the mammalian body. They are important for the activity of the nervous system through their effect on the regulation of excitability, activation of enzymatic systems, and maintenance of the nervous structure (for a comprehensive review see Reference 237).

The behavioral effects of some minerals have been subjected to detailed investigation. The role, if any, of some seems to be obscure. An obvious problem is the complexity of interaction of individual minerals. A limited or excessive administration of one mineral may upset the balance of the requirements of other minerals. For example, higher doses of calcium can elicit symptoms of zinc deficiency[321-324] and so on.

In evaluating the effect on the behavior of laboratory animals, it is necessary to distinguish the specific effect of a particular mineral on nervous system functions from the nonspecific response to complex metabolic processes and energetic and (when providing the mineral in excess) toxic effects which lead to serious impairment of the activity of the CNS as a whole. Therefore, it is important to accept the results of older papers with caution. On the other hand, as seen in vitamins, there are many dysbalances which do not show up clinically, yet may quickly modify behavior.

A. Sodium and Potassium

Many studies are concerned with the balance between sodium and potassium in relation to brain activity. Decreased susceptibility to seizures is associated with reduced sodium content (for a review see Reference 325). There is much information available on the effect of dietary NaCl and KCl on mental activity. Salt deprivation causes nervous dysfunction both in conditions of acute restriction and chronic deprivation. Hypochloremia manifests itself by restlessness, tremors, anxiety, etc.[326] Rats fed a low-NaCl diet with water as an unconditioned stimulus elaborated conditioned reflexes less easily.[327] In an experiment in which conditioned reflexes were established and dietary NaCl then replaced by KCl, conditioned reflex activity deteriorated.[328] A positive effect of a decreased amount of NaCl on conditioned reflex activity was found in hypertensive dogs.[329]

Prenatal restriction of sodium in the maternal diet resulted in retarded motor development in the offspring despite the feeding of a diet with a normal amount of NaCl during the nursing period.[330]

Faltová and Lât[42] and Lât and Faltová[331,332] studied the interaction between spontaneous selection of NaCl and KCl in relation to selection of other nutrients. Rats which preferred protein and spontaneously selected high amounts of casein also selected high amounts of KCl. Conversely, animals with a pronounced preference for carbohydrate spontaneously selected large quantities of NaCl. A group of rats transferred from a high-carbohydrate diet to a high-protein diet rapidly lowered their intake of NaCl and increased their KCl intake.

Many experimental studies have dealt with the ability of animals to distinguish minerals in their diets. Most species, including rats, have been found to regulate sodium intake by apppropriate alimentary behavior.[333] Adrenalectomized rats or animals fed a low-sodium diet develop a distinct preference for sodium.[334]

Potassium-deficient rats show a "specific hunger" for potassium.[335] However, spontaneous regulation of potassium intake is far from simple. Potassium-depleted rats prefer NaCl to KCl when given free choice of both minerals. Adam and Dawborn[336] tested the selection of NaCl, KCl, CaCl₂, and quinine sulfate, offering a choice between water and one mineral. A clear preference for NaCl was demonstrated, but no preference for either KCl or CaCl₂ was established. Other authors[334,337] reported similar results.

Potassium depletion results in the aversion for the diet associated with the depletion and in a distinct preference for a novel diet, irrespective of whether or not it contains KCl or NaCl,[338] while the nondeficient rats display preference for a familiar diet to a novel one.[339-340] The preference of potassium-depleted rats for a novel diet is similar to that reported for thiamine deficiency.[234]

B. Calcium

The effect of calcium on the nervous system is well known. Calcium is considered a sedative substance (for a review see Reference 341). Calcium salts alter the spontaneous electric activity of the brain of cats, rats, and rabbits and decrease alpha rhythm and the voltage of slow waves,[342] indicating an inhibitory effect on the brain.[342] Decreased calcium level results in elevated excitability. Rats receiving a low amount of calcium and a high quantity of phosphorus develop tetanus (for a review see Reference 237).

Behavioral manifestations of calcium are not uniform. Rats fed a low-calcium diet showed higher retention of learned tasks in the maze.[343] Overton[344] reported similar results. He found that the brain calcium level can be affected by dietary intake. A significant elevation in the brain calcium level was accompanied by significantly decreased retention of previous maze learning. Lawson and Gulick,[345] using the same diet as Overton, failed to reproduce these results. No difference between the experimental and control groups was found either in the concentration of calcium in the brain or in visual discrimination. The brain level of calcium in rats was found to be extremely variable, with the tissue of the CNS considerably resistant to even drastic changes in the calcium concentration in the blood.[346]

Hughes and Wood-Gush[347] reported interesting behavioral manifestations in calcium-deficient chickens. The deficient birds showed elevated locomotor and pecking activity. They were restless and constantly moved from one part of the cage to another. Their pecking activity was high, but of a stereotyped nature directed toward walls or ceiling or performed as "air pecking." The level of circulating parathyroid hormone increased simultaneously. However, administration of the hormone alone did not alter behavior.

C. Magnesium

Interactions between magnesium and functions of the nervous system have been extensively studied in various species. Mild reduction in magnesium exerted a depressive effect on the nervous system; prolonged hypomagnesia resulted in increased nervous excitability, tremor, and seizures[348] (for a detailed review see Reference 237). An increased level of magnesium was also found to have an adverse effect on nervous functions.[237]

Behavioral symptoms were observed in magnesium-deficient animals. Decreased spontaneous activity had previously been recorded in deprived rats.[239] In a more recent study, Dalley et al.[349] studied the influence of a magnesium-deficient diet on escape and avoidance learning of growing rats in a lever-pressing situation with shocks as reinforcement. Transfer to a magnesium-deficient diet resulted in the decline of avoidance responses (Figure 4). Escape response to shock was not affected, suggesting that

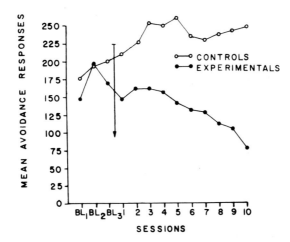

FIGURE 4.   Effect of magnesium deficiency on avoidance responses in rats. Mean avoidance responses for each daily session for control (n = 5) and experimental (n = 5) rats. BL₁, BL₂, and BL₃ are the pretreatment sessions. The arrow denotes the institution of magnesium-deficient diet. (From Dalley, M. B., Mahoney, A., and Cheney, C., *Nutr. Rep. Int.*, 11, 507—515, 1975. With permission.)

motor functions were not seriously impaired. Interesting changes of spontaneous behavior were observed. Animals frequently responded to sound and other sudden stimuli with a startle reaction. These stimuli also elicited tremor and seizures. After 5 days of deficiency, the following marked emotional changes appeared during the presentation of conditioned stimulus: vocalization; tremors; and, occasionally, freezing until the onset of shock. The symptoms were only slowly reversible by the administration of normal diet.

D. Zinc

Dietary zinc deficiency manifests itself very quickly. In young animals the deficiency results in growth disorders, in females impairment of the estrus cycle appears, and in more severe cases reproduction is damaged. Zinc deficiency is responsible for a variety of malformations in pups even if the deficiency is of a short duration.[350] In 47% of pups of deficient mothers, brain malformations were found, including numerous cases of hydrocephalus, hydranencephalus, etc.[350] Prenatal zinc deficiency results in a reduction in brain size of the fetus and the newborn animal.[351]

Dams maintained on a zinc-deficient diet throughout gestation and lactation exhibited disturbance of maternal behavior. Complete absence of typical maternal activities such as nest building, cleaning of pups, retrieval, and consumption of the placenta were recorded.[352,353]

Similar symptoms also occur in animals exposed to post-natal deficiency. Typical symptoms include slow movements and lethargy[354] reminiscent of the apathy seen in kwashiorkor. Exploratory activity in the open field was lower than that of the supplemented group[355] (Figure 5). Poor learning performance was observed in the one-way avoidance test, water maze, and Tolman-Honzik elevated maze.[355,356]

These results give convincing evidence on the behavioral consequences of zinc deficiency. However, attention should be given to methodological problems. For example, some observations have been made on small samples of animals because of the high mortality rate of pups of zinc-deficient mothers. Because a diet low in zinc elicits an-

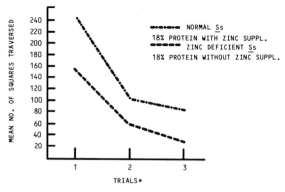

FIGURE 5.   Mean number of squares traversed for each of three daily 5-min test periods on the open field test for subjects receiving either a zinc-supplemented (*N* = 12) or nonsupplemented (*N* = 12) soy protein diet for 48 days commencing at time of weaning. (From Caldwell, D. F., Oberleas, D., Clancy J. J., and Prasad, A. S., *Proc. Soc. Exp. Biol. Med.*, 133, 1417—1421, 1970. With permission.)

orexia and therefore inhibits growth, pair-fed animals are used as controls. Calorie deprivation has been found to impair behavior and, therefore, to mask the real difference between the normal and zinc-deprived individual.

Zinc deficiency often accompanies protein-calorie malnutrition. In PCM animals and especially children it is not known whether the lack of protein or of zinc is responsible for the apathy observed. Zinc is necessary for the utilization of dietary protein and has an important role in the growth of the brain via nucleic acid and protein synthesis.[357-359]

E. Iron

Iron deficiency is often associated with protein-calorie malnutrition, especially in children (for a review see Reference 360).

Iron requirements increase primarily during the period of most rapid growth. The deficiency of a pregnant dam is transmitted to the offspring.[361-364] Even in the absence of major malformations in neonates, survival is reduced.[364] Scarpelli[365] studied the effect of maternal deficiency on behavior of the offspring. A deficient diet was fed during the prenatal period, but the pups were fostered by a normal dam. Although the newborn weight was lower in the deficient group than in controls, the difference gradually disappeared. No effect was found on learning tested at 42 days in a maze. Bernhardt[366] and, more recently, Edgerton et al.[367] recorded during iron deficiency a lower level of spontaneous motor activity which was normalized after iron supplementation.

F. Phosphorus

So far, phosphorus has received little attention in experimental studies on animals, and results of human studies are inconsistent[368,369] (for a review see Reference 370). Neither maze learning nor performance in multiple-choice tests was influenced by phosphorus level.[366]

G. Copper

Copper deficiency can exert its behavioral effect in different ways. As showed in guinea pigs[371] and lambs,[372] copper has an important influence on myelin formation. Maternal deficiency results in congenital malformations.[350] A copper-deficient diet administered from weaning to age 70 days led to a decreased copper concentration in the brain, spinal cord, and other organs, combined with a decrease in food intake and retarded growth.[373]

Schlesinger and Lieff[281] studied susceptibility to seizures in mice of different strains. Four weeks of dietary treatment did not influence susceptibility to audiogenic stimuli.

Roshchina[329] reviewed the work of Soviet authors. They showed a shift in copper in various organs of the body during changes in the functional state of the CNS (for example, in the course of conditioned reflex formation). In rats, an increased level of copper in the brain and declined levels in the liver and kidney were recorded during electroconvulsive siezures. Raitses and Tradadyuk[374] studied the effect of an increased level of copper on higher nervous activity. The conditioned motor reflexes of dogs were established, and the diet was then supplemented with copper in doses from 0.2 to 0.5 mg per kilogram body weight. Conditioned reflex activity gradually declined. First, the intensity of responses decreased and the balance between excitatory and inhibitory processes was impaired, followed later by a complete inhibition of conditioned reflexes after high doses of copper.

H. Manganese

The symptoms of manganese deficiency in humans have not been reliably confirmed. In birds and rodents experimental deficiency retarded growth and induced structural and chemical abnormalities of the bones and disturbance of fat metabolism, etc. Deficiency in the maternal diet elicits congenital abnormalities[350] and seizures in the offspring.[375] Prolonged manganese deprivation disturbs maternal behavior. The dams often desert their young and do not feed them.[576] Maternal deficiency also manifests itself in loss of balance and coordinated movement in rats[377] and pigs.[378,379]

Elevated manganese intake has toxic effects that have been observed, for example, in miners who inhaled manganese dust over a long time period. There are few behavioral studies on animals. Soviet physiologists showed symptoms of manganese intoxication including functional changes in the CNS; impaired differentiation; disturbance of inhibitory processes; and, later, paradoxical and ultraparadoxical phases in conditioned reflex activity. Restoration of normal activity in dogs lasted for 2 to 3 months after the termination of intoxication.[380] Inhibition of higher nervous activity was also observed in rabbits and cats (reviewed by Roshchina[329]).

I. Other Minerals

Some minerals not discussed in this chapter may elicit mental symptoms as a result of major deviations in the metabolism and activity of different organs. Thus, behavior may reflect changes in the activity of endocrine organs and circulatory system, severe bone malformations, and disturbances which make the motor activity of the animal impossible.

The symptoms of iodine deficiency and excess have been investigated in detail in humans, but not in animals. Gantt and Fleishmann[381] found that the ability to develop conditioned reflexes was impaired in dogs.

Cadmium was studied in relation to hypertension. Injection of cadmium elicited hypertension.[382] Galoyan[383] observed that injections of cadmium inhibited both conditioned and unconditioned reflexes in rats. He observed morphological changes in the hypothalamopituitary system simultaneous with the changes in higher nervous activity.

The influence of cobalt materializes primarily via its relationship to cyanocobalamine (vitamin B_{12}).

It is evident that behavioral studies on the effect of minerals on laboratory animals are far from being complete.

REFERENCES

1. **Kreezer, G. L.,** Technics for the investigation of behavioral phenomena in the rat, in *The Rat in Laboratory Investigation,* Farris, E. J. and Griffith, J. Q., Jr., Eds., J. B. Lippincott, Philadelphia, 1942, 203—277.

2. **Munn, N. J.,** *Handbook of Psychological Research on the Rat,* Houghton Mifflin, Boston, 1950.

3. **Hall, C. S.,** Emotional behavior in the rat. I. Defecation and urination as measures of individual differences in emotionality, *J. Comp. Psychol.,* 18, 385—403, 1934.

4. **Lát, J. and Gollová-Hémon, E.,** Permanent effects of nutritional and endocrinological intervention in early ontogeny on the level of nonspecific excitability and on lability (emotionality), *Ann. N.Y. Acad. Sci.,* 159, 710—720, 1969.

5. **Hebb, D. O. and Williams, K.,** A method of rating animal intelligence, *J. Gen. Psychol.,* 34, 59—65, 1946.

6. **Lashley, K. S.,** The mechanism of vision. XV. Preliminary studies of the rat's capacity for detail vision, *J. Gen. Psychol.,* 18, 123—193, 1938.

7. **Hinde, R. A.,** *Animal Behavior: A Synthesis of Ethology and Comparative Psychology,* 2nd ed., McGraw-Hill, New York, 1966, 568—584.

8. **Skinner, B. F.,** *The Behavior of Organisms: An Experimental Analysis,* Appleton-Century-Crofts, New York, 1938; as cited in Hinde, R. A., *Animal Behavior: A Synthesis of Ethology and Comparative Psychology,* McGraw-Hill, New York, 1966, 568—584.

9. **Sidman, M.,** *Scientific Research. Evaluating Experimental Data in Psychology,* Basic Books, New York, 1960.

10. **Leaf, R. C. and Muller, S. A.,** Simple method for CER conditioning and measurements, *Psychol. Rep.,* 17, 211, 1965.

11. **Dobbing, J.,** The effect of undernutrition on myelination in the central nervous system, *Biol. Neonat.,* 9, 132—147, 1965/1966.

12. **Donaldson, H. H.,** A comparison of the albino rat with man in respect of the growth of the brain and of the spinal cord, *J. Comp. Neurol.,* 18, 345, 1908.

13. **Donaldson, H. H.,** The effect of underfeeding on the percentage of water, on the ether-alcohol extract and on modulation in the central nervous system of the albino rat, *J. Comp. Neurol. Psychiatr.,* 21, 139, 1911.

14. **Dobbing, J.,** Effects of experimental undernutrition on development of the nervous system, in *Malnutrition, Learning and Behavior,* Scrimshaw, N. E. and Gordon, J. E., Eds., MIT Press, Cambridge, 1968, 181—202.

15. **Vaes, G.,** L'influence des malnutritions sur le comportement. I. Comportement général, apprentisage et intelligence, *Encephale,* 49, 30—73, 1960.

16. **Brožek, J. and Vaes, G.,** Experimental investigations on the effects of dietary deficiencies on animal and human behavior, *Vitam. Horm.,* (N.Y), 19, 43—94, 1961.

17. **Richter, C. P.,** A behavioristic study of the activity of the rat, *Comp. Psychol. Monogr.,* 1, 1—55, 1922.

18. **Campbell, B. A. and Sheffield, F. D.,** Relation of random activity to food deprivation, *J. Comp. Physiol. Psychol.,* 46, 320—322, 1953.

19. **Fehrer, E.,** The effects of hunger and familiarity of locale on exploration, *J. Comp. Physiol. Psychol.,* 49, 549—552, 1956.

20. **Treichler, F. R. and Hall, J. F.,** The relationship between deprivation weight loss and several measures of activity, *J. Comp. Physiol. Psychol.,* 55, 346—349, 1962.

21. **Moskowitz, M. J.,** Running-wheel activity in the white rat as a function of combined food and water deprivation, *J. Comp. Physiol. Psychol.,* 52, 621—625, 1959.

22. **Richards, W. J. and Leslie, G. R.,** Food and water deprivation as influences on exploration, *J. Comp. Physiol. Psychol.,* 55, 834—837, 1962.

23. **Duda, J. J. and Bolles, R. C.,** Effects of prior deprivation, current deprivation and weight loss on the activity of the hungry rat, *J. Comp. Physiol. Psychol.,* 56, 569—571, 1963.

24. **Treichler, F. R. and Collins, C. W.,** Comparison of cyclic and continuous deprivation effects on wheel running, *J. Comp. Physiol. Psychol.,* 60, 447—448, 1965.

25. **Olewine, D. A., Barrows, C. H., Jr., and Shock, N. W.,** Effect of reduced dietary intake on random and voluntary activity in male rats, *J. Gerontol.,* 19, 230—233, 1964.

26. **Bolles, R. C. and DeLorge, J.,** Exploration in Dashiell maze as a function of prior deprivation, current deprivation and sex, *Can. J. Psychol.,* 16, 221—227, 1962.

27. **Adlerstein, A. and Fehrer, E.,** The effect of food deprivation on exploratory behavior in a complex maze, *J. Comp. Physiol. Psychol.,* 48, 250—254, 1955.

28. **Zimbardo, P. G. and Millier, N. E.,** Facilitation of exploration by hunger in rats, *J. Comp. Physiol. Psychol.,* 51, 43—46, 1958.

29. **Hughes, R. N.,** Food deprivation and locomotor activity in the white rat, *Anim. Behav.,* 13, 30—32, 1965.

30. **Woods, P. J. and Bolles, R. C.,** Effects of current hunger and prior eating habits on exploratory behavior. A study with rats, *J. Comp. Physiol. Psychol.,* 59, 141—143, 1965.

31. **Campbell, B. A., Teghtsoonian, R., and Williams, R. A.,** Activity, weight loss, and survival time of food-deprived rats as a function of age, *J. Comp. Physiol. Psychol.,* 54, 216—219, 1961.

32. **Campbell, B. A., Smith, N. F., Misanin, J. R., and Jaynes, J.,** Species differences in activity during hunger and thirst, *J. Comp. Physiol. Psychol.,* 61, 123—127, 1966.

33. **Sheffield, F. D. and Campbell, B. A.,** The role of experience in the "spontaneous" activity of hunger rats, *J. Comp. Physiol. Psychol.,* 47, 97—100, 1954.

34. **Ghentt, L.,** Some effects of deprivation on eating and drinking behavior, *J. Comp. Physiol. Psychol.,* 50, 172—176, 1957.

35. **Capaldi, E. J. and Robinson, D. E.,** Performance and consummatory behavior in the runway and maze as a function of cyclic deprivation, *J. Comp. Physiol. Psychol.,* 53, 159—164, 1960.

36. **Bolles, R. D.,** The readiness to eat and drink: the effect of deprivation condition, *J. Comp. Physiol. Psychol.,* 55, 230—234, 1962.

37. **Fallon, D.,** Effects of cyclic deprivation upon consummatory behavior: the role of deprivation history, *J. Comp. Physiol. Psychol.,* 60, 283—287, 1965.

38. **Dufort, R. H. and Blick, K. A.,** Adjustment of the rat to a 23-hour water deprivation schedule, *J. Comp. Physiol. Psychol.,* 55, 649—651, 1962.

39. **Verplanck, W. S. and Hayes, J. R.,** Eating and drinking as a function of maintenance schedule, *J. Comp. Physiol. Psychol.,* 46, 327—333, 1953.

40. **Dodson, J. D.,** Relative values of reward and punishment in habit formation, *Psychobiology,* 1, 231—276, 1917.

41. **Tolman, E. C., Honzik, C. H., and Robinson, E. W.,** The effect of degrees of hunger upon the order of elimination of long and short blinds, *Univ. Calif. Berkeley Publ. Psychol.,* 4, 189—202, 1930.

42. **Faltová, E. and Lát, J.,** The activity of the feeding center. II. Regulation of proteins, electrolytes and water intake, *Cesk. Fysiol.,* 3, 225—234, 1954.

43. **Bolles, R. C.,** The interaction of hunger and thirst in the rat, *J. Comp. Physiol. Psychol.,* 54, 580—584, 1961.

44. **Petrinovich, L. and Bolles, R.,** Deprivation states and behavioral attributes, *J. Comp. Physiol. Psychol.,* 47, 450—453, 1954.

45. **Campbell, B. A. and Cicala, G. A.,** Studies of water deprivation in rats as a function of age, *J. Comp. Physiol. Psychol.,* 55, 763—768, 1962.

46. **Campbell, B. A.,** Theory and research on the effect of water deprivation on random activity in the rat, in *Thirst,* Wayner, M. J., Ed., Pergamon Press, Oxford, 1964, 317—394.

47. **Fallon, D., Thompson, D. M., and Schild, M. E.,** Concurrent food- and water-reinforced responding under food, water and food and water deprivation, *Psychol. Rep.,* 16, 1305—1311, 1965.

48. **Zimbardo, P. G. and Montgomery, K. C.,** The relative strengths of consummatory response in hunger, thirst and exploratory drive, *J. Comp. Physiol. Psychol.,* 50, 504—508, 1957.

49. **Mysliveček, J. and Rokyta, R.,** Conditioned and "spontaneous" behaviour after elimination of the neocortex during the early postnatal period, in *Central and Peripheral Mechanism of Motor Functions,* Guttman, E. and Hnik, P., Eds., Československá Akademie Věd, Prague, 1963, 183—190.

50. **Nováková, V.,** Effect of starvation and thirst in early ontogeny on higher nervous activity of adult rats, *Act. Nerv. Super.,* 8, 36—38, 1966.

51. **Kennedy, G. C.,** The development with age of hypothalamic restraint upon the appetite of the rat, *J. Endocrinol.,* 16, 9, 1957.

52. **McCance, R. A.,** The bearing of early nutrition on later development, in *Proc. 6th Int. Congr. Nutrition,* Mills, C. F. and Passmore, R., Eds., Livingstone, E. and S., Edinburgh, 1964, 74—81.

53. **Widdowson, E. M. and McCance, R. A.,** Some effects of accelerating growth. I. General somatic development, *Proc. R. Soc. London Ser. B,* 1. 152, 188—206, 1960.

54. **Seitz, P. F. D.,** The effects of infantile experience upon adult behavior in animal subjects. I. Effects of litter size during infancy upon adult behavior in the rat, *Am. J. Psychiatr.,* 110, 916—927, 1954.

55. **Chow, B. F. and Lee, C. J.,** Effect of dietary restriction of pregnant rats on body weight gain of the offspring, *J. Nutr.,* 82, 10—18, 1964.

56. **Lee, C. J. and Chow, B. F.,** Protein metabolism in the offspring of underfed mother rats, *J. Nutr.,* 87, 439—443, 1965.

57. **Altman, J., Das, G. D., Sudarshan, K., and Anderson, J. B.,** The influence of nutrition on neural and behavioral development. II. Growth of the body and brain in infant rats using different techniques of undernutrition, *Dev. Psychobiol.,* 4, 55—70, 1971.

58. Culley, W. J., Mertz, E. T., Lineburger, R. O., and Gotts, R. E., Effect of early undernutrition on brain composition of adult rats, *Fed. Proc. Fed. Am. Soc. Exp. Biol.,* 26, 519, 1967.
59. Cheng, M., Rozin, P., and Teitelbaum, P., Starvation retards development of food and water regulations, *J. Comp. Physiol. Psychol.,* 70, 206—218, 1971.
60. Howard, E. and Granoff, D. M., Effect of neonatal food restriction in mice on brain growth, DNA and cholesterol, and an adult delayed response learning, *J. Nutr.,* 95, 111—121, 1968.
61. Salas, M. and Cintra, L., Nutritional influences upon somatosensory evoked responses during development in the rat, *Physiol. Behav.,* 10, 1019—1022, 1973.
62. Mysliveček, J., Fox, M. W. and Záhlava, J., Maturation retardée de l'activité bioélectrique corticale provoquée par malnutrition, *J. Physiol.* (Paris), 58, 572—573, 1966.
63. Smart, J. L. and Dobbing, J., Vulnerability of developing brain. II. Effects of early nutritional deprivation on reflex ontogeny and development of behaviour in the rat, *Brain Res.,* 28, 85—91, 1971.
64. Simonson, M., Sherwin, R. W., Anilane, J. K., Yu, W. Y., and Chow, B. F., Neuromotor development in progeny of underfed mother rats, *J. Nutr.,* 98(7), 18—24, 1969.
65. Altman, J., Sudarshan, K., Das, G. D., McCormick, N., and Barnes, D., The influence of nutrition on neural and behavioral development. III. Development of some motor, particularly locomotor patterns during infancy, *Dev. Psychobiol.,* 4(2), 97—114, 1971.
66. Lát, J., Widdowson, E. M., and McCance, R. A., Some effects of accelerating growth. III. Behaviour and nervous activity, *Proc. R. Soc. London Ser. B,* 153, 347—356, 1961.
67. Franková, S., Nutritional and psychological factors in the development of spontaneous behaviour in the rat, in *Malnutrition, Learning and Behavior,* Scrimshaw, N. E. and Gordon, J. E., Eds., MIT Press, Cambridge, 1968, 312—322.
68. Franková, S., Nutritional and environmental determinants of rat behaviour, Proc. 8th Int. Congr. Nutrition, Prague, 1969, *Excerpta Med. Int. Congr. Ser.,* 213, 236—239, 1970.
69. Franková, S. Behavioral responses of rats to early overnutrition, *Nutr. Metab.,* 12, 228—239, 1970.
70. Simonson, M. and Chow, B. F., Maze studies on progeny of underfed mother rats, *J. Nutr.,* 100, 685—690, 1970.
71. DiBenedetta, C. and Cioffi, L. A., Early nutrition, brain glycoproteins and behaviour in rats, *Bibl. Nutr. Dieta,* 17, 69—82, 1972.
72. Leathwood, P., Bush, M., Bernet, C., and Mauron, J., Effect of early malnutrition on swiss white mice: avoidance learning after rearing in large litters, *Life Sci.,* 14, 157, 1974.
73. Smart, J. L. and Dobbing, J., Vulnerability of developing brain. IV. Passive avoidance behavior in young rats following maternal undernutrition, *Dev. Psychobiol.,* 5, 129—136, 1972.
74. Lynch, A., Passive avoidance behavior and response thresholds in adult male rats after postnatal undernutrition, *Physiol. Behav.,* 16, 27—32, 1976.
75. Smart, J. L., Whatson, T. S., and Dobbing, J., Thresholds of response to electric shock in previously undernourished rats, *Br. J. Nutr.,* 34, 511—516, 1975.
76. Seminginovský, B., Mysliveček, J., Springer, V., and Rokyta, R., Testing of emotionality in animals with different level of nutrition, *Act. Nerv. Super.,* 11, 282—283, 1969.
77. Whatson, T. S., Smart, J. L., and Dobbing, J., Dominance relationship among previously undernourished and well fed male rats, *Physiol. Behav.,* 14, 425—429, 1975.
78. Hunt, J. McV., The effects of infant feeding-frustration upon hoarding in the albino rat, *J. Abnorm. Soc. Psychol.,* 36, 338—360, 1941.
79. Larsson, K., Carlsson, S. G., Sourander, P., Forsström, B., Hansen, J., Henriksson, B., and Lindquist, A., Delayed onset of sexual activity of male rats subjected to pre- and postnatal malnutrition, *Physiol. Behav.,* 13, 307—312, 1974.
80. Whatson, T. S., Smart, J. L., and Dobbing, J., Social interactions among adult male rats after early undernutrition, *Br. J. Nutr.,* 32, 413—419, 1974.
81. Mayer, J. and Thomas, D. W., Regulation of food intake and obesity, *Science,* 156, 328, 1967.
82. Wohl, M. G., Obesity, in *Modern Nutrition in Health and Disease,* Wohl, M. G. and Goodhart, R. S., Eds., Lea & Febiger, Philadelphia, 1968, 971—983.
83. Czajka-Narins, D. M. and Hirch, J., Supplementary feeding during the preweaning period, *Biol. Neonat.,* 25, 176, 1976.
84. Reed, J. D., Spontaneous activity of animals: a review of the literature since 1929, *Psychol. Bull.,* 44, 393—412, 1947.
85. Abderhalden, E. and Wertheimer, E., Ernährung und Zellfunktionen. V. Das psychische Verhalten verschieden ernährter Ratten, *Pfluegers Arch. Gesamte Physiol.,* 216, 396—404, 1927.
86. Hitchcock, F. A., The effects of low protein and protein-free diets or starvation and voluntary activity of the albino rat, *Am. J. Physiol.,* 84, 410—416, 1928.
87. Slonaker, J. R., The effect of different percentage of protein in the diet on six generations of rats, *Biol. Sci.,* 6, 257—321, 1939.

88. **Bernhardt, K. S.**, Protein deficiency and learning in the rat, *J. Comp. Psychol.,* 22, 269—272, 1936.
89. **Smith, E. A. and Conger, R. M.**, Spontaneous activity in relation to diet in the albino rat, *Am. J. Physiol.,* 142, 663—665, 1944.
90. **Lát, J. and Faltová, E.**, Influence of nutrition on higher nervous activity. I. Influe nce of various ratios of animal proteins on higher nervous activity of rats, *Cesk. Fysiol.,* 4, 171—180, 1955.
91. **Watson, R. H. J.**, Modifications of the effects of drugs on behaviour by the nutritional state, in *Animal Behaviour and Drug Action,* Steinberg, H., de Reuck, A. V. S., and Knight, J., Eds., J. A. Churchill, London, 1964, 249—256.
92. **Beaton, J. R., Feleki, V., Stevenson, J. A. F.**, Activity and patterns of rats fed a low-protein diet and the effects of subsequent food deprivation, *Can. J. Physiol. Pharmacol.,* 42, 705—718, 1964.
93. **Collier, G., Squibb, R. L., and Jackson, F.**, Activity as function of the diet. I. Spontaneous activity, *Psychonomic. Sci. Sect. Anim. Physiol. Psychol.,* 3, 173—174, 1965.
94. **Collier, G., Squibb, R. L., and Jackson, F.**, Activity as a function of diet. II. Instrumental activity, *Psychonomic Sci. Sect. Anim. Physiol. Psychol.,* 3, 175—176, 1965.
95. **Collier, G. and Squibb, R. L.**, Diet and activity, *J. Comp. Physiol. Psychol.,* 64, 409—413, 1967.
96. **Franková, S.**, Influence of diet with a different ratio of fat, carbohydrate and protein on the behaviour of ageing rats, *Cesk. Psychol.,* 10, 111—112, 1966.
97. **T'ang, Y., Ch'in, K., and Tsang, Y. H.**, The effect of a vegetarian diet on the learning ability of albino rats, *Contrib. Nat. Res. Inst. Psychol. Acad. Sinica,* 1, 1—16, 1934; *Psychol. Abstr.,* No. 4052, 1934.
98. **Pilgrim, F. J., Zabarenko, L. M., and Patton, R. A.**, The role of amino acid supplementation and dietary protein level in serial learning performance of rats, *J. Comp. Psychol.,* 44, 25—35, 1951.
99. **Andriasov, A. N.**, Vliyanie razlichnogo soderzhaniya belka v pishche na uslovnoreflektornuyu deyatelnost krys, *Zh. Vyssh. Nervn. Deyat. im. I.P. Pavlova,* 2, 113—125, 1952.
100. **Alekseeva, I. A. and Kaplanskaya-Raiskaya, S. I.**, Vliyanie metionina na vysshuyu nervnuyu deyatelnost krys pri belkovom golodaniyu, *Vopr. Pitan.,* 19(1), 44—48, 1960.
101. **Faltová, E., Poupa, O., and Servít, Z.**, Influence of the ration between proteins and carbohydrates in the diet on the susceptibility to seizures in mice, *Cesk. Fysiol.,* 4, 10—13, 1955.
102. **Sanahuja, J. C. and Harper, A. E.**, Effect of amino acid imbalance on food intake and preference, *Am. J. Physiol.,* 202, 165—170, 1962.
103. **Leung, P. M. B., Rogers, Q. L., and Harper, A. E.**, Effect of amino acid imbalancy on dietary choice in the rat, *J. Nutr.,* 95, 483—492, 1968.
104. **Murumatsu, K., Odagiri, H., Morishita, S., and Takeuchi, H.**, Effect of excess levels of individual amino acids on growth of rats fed casein diets, *J. Nutr.,* 101, 117—1126, 1971.
105. **Olney, J. W., Ho, O. L., and Rhee, V.**, Cytotoxic effects of acidic and sulphur containing amino acids on the infant mouse central nervous system, *Exp. Brain Res.,* 14, 61—76, 1931.
106. **Weisz, B., Sos, J., Gati, T., Harmos, D., and Rigo, J.**, *Vopr. Pit.,* 15, 15—21, 1956; as cited in Brožek, J., and Vaes, G., Experimental investigations on the effects of dietary deficiencies on animal and human behaviour *Vitam. Horm.* (N.Y.), 19, 43—94, 1961.
107. **Carranza, J., Ortega, B., and Ludlow, A.**, Group dispersion in mice produced by chronic administration of alfa-amphetamine, 7th Congr. Coll. Int. Neuropsychopharmacologicum, *Psychopharmacol.,* 26, (suppl. 1972), Abstr. 54, 1972.
108. **Beaton, J. M., Smythies, J. R., Bridgers, W. F., McClain, L. D., Pegram, G., and Bradley, R. J.**, A study of behavioral disruption of mice induced by L-methionine and related compounds, *Psychopharmacologia,* 36, 101, 1974.
109. **Beaton, J. M., Smythies, J. R., and Bradley, R. J.**, The behavioral effects of L-methionine and related compounds in rats and mice, *Biol. Psychiatr.,* 10, 45—52, 1975.
110. **Hole, K.**, Arousal deficit in L-phenylalanine fed rats, *Dev. Psychobiol.,* 5, 149—156, 1972.
111. **Karrer, R. and Cahilly, G.**, Experimental attempt to produce phenylketonuria in animals. A clinical review, *Psychol. Bull.,* 64, 52—64, 1965.
112. **Hwa, L. W. and Waisman, H. A.**, Experimental phenylketonuria in rats, *Proc. Soc. Exp. Biol. Med.,* 108, 332—335, 1961.
113. **Louttit, R. T.** Effect of phenylalanine and isocarboxazid feeding on brain serotonin and learning behavior in the rat, *J. Comp. Physiol. Psychol.,* 55, 425—428, 1962.
114. **McFarland, J. N., Peacock, L. J., and Watson, J. A.**, Mental retardation and activity level in rats and children, *Am. J. Ment. Defic.,* 71, 376—380, 1966.
115. **Polidora, V. J., Cunningham, R. F., and Waisman, H. A.**, Dosage parameters of a behavioral deficit associated with phenylketonuria in rats, *J. Comp. Physiol. Psychol.,* 61, 436—441, 1966.
116. **Polidora, V. J., Cunningham, R. F., and Waisman, H. A.**, Phenylketonuria in rats: reversibility of behavioral deficit, *Science,* 151 (3707), 219—221, 1966.
117. **Hess, M., Paulsen, E. C., Muller, S. A., and Carlton, P. L.**, A comparison of behavioral tests for measuring the effects of phenylketonuria in rats, *Life Sci.,* 5, 927—937, 1966.

118. **Shalock, R. L., Brown, W. J., Copenhauer, J. H., and Gunter, R.**, Model phenylketonuria in the albino rat: behavioral, biochemical and neuroanatomical effects, *J. Comp. Physiol. Psychol.*, 89, 655—666, 1975.

119. **Leaf, R. C., Carlton, P. L., and Hess, S. M.**, Behavioral deficit in the rat induced by feeding phenylalanine, *Nature*, 208 (5014), 1021—1022, 1965.

120. **Thompson, W. R. and Kano, K.**, Effects on rat offspring of maternal phenylalanine diet during pregnancy, *J. Psychiatr. Res.*, 3, 91—98, 1965.

121. **Woolley, D. W. and Van der Hoeven, T.**, Serotonin deficiency in infancy as one cause of mental defect in phenylketonuria, *Science*, 144, 883—884, 1964.

122. **Lo, G. S., Lee, S., Cruz, N. L. and Longenecker, J. G.**, Temporary induction of phenylketonurial-like characteristics in infant rats: effect on brain protein synthesis, *Nutr. Rep. Int.*, 2, 59—72, 1970.

123. **Reed, P. B., White, M. N., and Longenecker, J. B.**, Temporary induction of phenylketonuria-like characteristics in infant rats: effect on brain DNA synthesis, *Nutr. Rep. Int.*, 2, 73—85, 1970.

124. **Shah, S. N., Peterson, N. A., and McKean, C. M.**, Impaired myelin formation in experimental hyperphenylalaninaemia, *J. Neurochem.*, 19, 479—485, 1972.

125. **Tenen, S. S.**, The effect of *p*-chlorophenylalanine, a serotonin depletor, on avoidance acquisition, pain sensitivity and related behavior in the rat, *Psychopharmacologia*, 10, 204—219, 1967.

126. **McFarlain, R. A. and Bloom, J. M.**, The effects of *para*-chlorophenylalanine on brain serotonin, food intake and U-maze behavior, *Psychopharmacologia*, 27, 85—92, 1972.

127. **Fibiger, H. C., Mertz, P. H., and Campbell, B. A.**, The effect of *para*-chlorophenylalanine in aversion thresholds and reactivity to foot shock, *Physiol. Behav.*, 8, 259—263, 1972.

128. **Hole, K.**, Behavior and brain growth in rats treated with *p*-chlorophenylalanine in first weeks of life, *Dev. Psychobiol.*, 5, 157—173, 1972.

129. **Adlard, B. P. F. and Smart, J. L.**, Some aspects of the behavior of young and adult rats treated with *p*-chlorophenylalanine in infancy, *Dev. Psychobiol.*, 7, 135—144, 1974.

130. **Ashcroft, W. C., Eccleston, D., and Crasford, T. B. B.**, 5-Hydroxyindole metabolism in rat brain. A study of intermediate metabolism using the technique of tryptophan loading. 1, *J. Nuerochem.*, 12, 483—492, 1965.

131. **Brown, B. B.**, CNS drug action and interaction in mice, *Arch. Int. Pharmacodyn. Ther.*, 128, 391—414, 1960.

132. **Modigh, K.**, Effects of L-tryptophan on motor activity in mice, *Psychopharmacologia*, 30, 123—134, 1973.

133. **Wyatt, R. J., Engelman, K., Kupfer, D. J., Frams, D. H., Sjoerdsma, A., and Snyder, F.**, Effects of L-tryptophan (a natural sedative) on human sleep, *Lancet*, 2, 842—846, 1970.

134. **Coppen, A., Shaw, D. M., Herzberg, B., and Maggs, R.**, Tryptophan in the treatment of depression, *Lancet*, 2, 1178—1180, 1967.

135. **Efremov, V. V., Makarychev, A. I., and Tikhomirova, A. N.**, Vliyanie PP-avitaminoza na uslovno-reflektornuyu deyatelnost sobak, *Vopr. Pit.*, 3, 10—15, 1954.

136. **Bevan, W., Lewis, G. T., Bloom, W. L., and Abess, A. T.**, Spontaneous activity in rats fed an amino acid deficient diet, *J. Physiol.*, 163, 104—110, 1950.

137. **Anderson, J. E. and Smith, A. H.**, The effect of quantitative and qualitative stunting on maze learning in the white rat, *J. Comp. Psychol.*, 6, 337—359, 1926.

138. **Anderson, J. E. and Smith, A. H.**, Relation of performance to age and nutritive condition in the white rat, *J. Comp. Psychol.*, 13, 409—446, 1932.

139. **Riess, B. F. and Block, R. J.**, The effect of amino acid deficiency on the behaviour of the white rat: lysine and cystine deficiency, *J. Psychol.*, 14, 101—113, 1942.

140. **Bevan, W. and Frieman, O. I.**, Some effects of an amino acid deficiency upon the performance of albino rats in a simple maze, *J. Genet. Psychol.*, 80, 75—82, 1952.

141. **Stapleton, P. and Hill, D. C.**, Plasma amino acid levels and offspring viability of rats fed a diet low in lysine during pregnancy and lactation, *Nutr. Rep. Int.*, 6, 199—207, 1972.

142. **Acheampong-Mensah, D. K. and Hill, D. C.**, Effect of excess dietary lysine on the weaning rat, *Nutr. Rep. Int.*, 2, 9—17, 1970.

143. **Weil-Malherbe, H.**, Significance of glutamic acid for the metabolism of nervous tissue, *Physiol. Rev.*, 30, 549—568, 1950.

144. **Himwich, W. A., Peterson, J. C., and Allen, M. L.**, Hematoencephalic exchange as a function of age, *Neurology*, 7, 705—710, 1957.

145. **McLaughlan, J. M., Noel, F. J., Botting, M. G., and Knipfel, J. E.**, Blood and brain levels of glutamic acid in young rats given monosodium glutamate, *Nutr. Rep. Int.*, 1, 131—138, 1970.

146. **Vogel, W.**, The therapeutic effect of L-glutamite, *Gerontologist*, 6, 51—53, 1966.

147. **Vogel, W., Broverman, D. M., Draguns, J. G., and Klaiber, E. L.**, The role of glutamic acid in cognitive behaviors, *Psychol. Bull.*, 65, 367—382, 1966.

148. **Zimmermann, T. T. and Ross, S.**, Effect of glutamic acid and other amino-acids on maze learning in the rat, *AMA Arch. Neurol. Psychiatry,* 51, 446—451, 1944.

149. **Phillips, H. J.**, Activity of rats on free, normal, and excess glutamic acid diets, *Fed. Proc. Fed. Am. Soc. Exp. Biol.,* 13, 112, 1954.

150. **Hughes, K. R. and Zubek, J. P.**, Effect of glutamic acid on the learning ability of bright and dull rats. I. Administration during infancy, *Can. J. Psychol.,* 10, 132—138, 1956.

151. **Helm-Zeller, H.**, Über die Wirkung von Glutaminsäure auf das Antriebs und Lernverhalten bei Ratten, *Z. Psychol.,* 159, 54—84, 1956.

152. **Adamo, N. J. and Ratner, A.**, Monosodium glutamate: lack of effects on brain and reproductive function in rats, *Science,* 169, 673—674, 1970.

153. **Oser, B. L., Carson, S., Vogin, E. E., and Cox, G. E.**, Oral and subcutaneous administration of monosodium glutamate to infant rodents and dogs, *Nature,* 229, 411—413, 1971.

154. **Winczle, J. P. and Vogel, W.**, The effects of glutamic acid upon operant conditioning in rats, *J. Genet. Psychol.,* 115, 97—105, 1969.

155. **Braksh, T. A.**, Vliyanie L-glutaminovoi kisloty na vysshuyu nervnuyu deyatelnost i nekotorie pokazateli belkovogo obmena u sobak, *Vopr. Pit.,* 16(2), 20, 1957.

156. **Pond, D. A. and Pond, M. H.**, Glutamic acid and its salts in epilepsy, *J. Ment. Sci.,* 97, 663—673, 1951.

157. **Himwich, W. A.**, Absorption of L-glutamic acid, *Science,* 120, 351—352, 1954.

158. **Berry, H. K., Butcher, R. E., Elliot, L. A., and Brunner, R.L.**, The effect of monosodium glutamate on the early biochemical and behavioral development of the rat, *Dev. Psychobiol.,* 7, 165—173, 1974.

159. **Freedman, J. K. and Potts, A. M.**, Repression of glutaminase I in the rat retina by administration of sodium L-glutamate, *Invest. Ophtalmol.,* 1, 118—121, 1962.

160. **Arees, E. M. and Mayer, J.**, Monosodium glutamate-induced brain lesions: electron microscopic examination, *Science,* 170, 549—550, 1970.

161. **Olney, J. S.**, Brain lesions, obesity and other disturbances in mice treated with monosodium glutamate, *Science,* 164, 719—721, 1969.

162. **Wen, C. P., Hayes, K. C., and Gershoff, S. N.**, Effects of dietary supplementation of monosodium glutamate on infant monkeys, weanling rats and suckling mice, *Am. J. Clin. Nutr.,* 26, 803—813, 1973.

163. **Olney, J. W. and Ho, O. L.**, Brain damage in infant mice following oral intake of glutamate, aspartate or cysteine, *Nature,* 227, 609, 1970.

164. **Sharpe, L. G., Olney, J. W., Ohlendorf, C., Lyss, A., Zimmerman, M., and Gale, B.**, Brain damage and associated behavioral deficits following the administration of L-cysteine to infant rats, *Pharmacol. Biochem. Behav.,* 3, 291—298, 1975.

165. **Booth, D. A. and Simson, P. C.** Food preferences acquired by association with variations in amino acid nutrition, *Q. J. Exp. Psychol.,* 23, 135—145, 1971.

166. **Simson, P. C. and Booth, D. A.**, Olfactory conditioning by association with histidine-free or balanced amino acid loads in rats, *Q. J. Exp. Psychol.,* 25, 354—359, 1973.

167. **Latham, M. C.**, Protein-calorie malnutrition in children and its relation to psychological development and behavior, *Psychol. Rev.,* 54, 541—565, 1974.

168. **Trowell, H. C., Davies, J. N. P., and Dean, R. F. A.**, *Kwashiorkor,* E. Arnold, London, 1954.

169. **Scrimshaw, N. E. and Gordon, J. E.**, Eds., *Malnutrition, Learning and Behavior,* MIT Press, Cambridge, 1968.

170. **Manocha, S. L.**, *Malnutrition and Retarded Development,* Charles C Thomas, Springfield, Ill., 1972.

171. **Kallen, D. J.**, Ed., Nutrition, Development and Social Behavior, Department of Health, Education, and Welfare Publ. No. (NIH) 73—242, U.S. Government Printing Office, Washington, D.C., 1972.

172. **Read, M. S.**, Malnutrition, hunger and behavior. I. Malnutrition and learning, *J. Am. Diet. Assoc.,* 63, 378—385, 1973.

173. **Read, M. S.**, Malnutrition, hunger and behavior. II. Hunger, school programs and behavior, *J. Am. Diet. Assoc.,* 63, 386—391, 1973.

174. **Cravioto, J., Hambraeus, L., and Vahlquist, B.**, Eds., *Early Malnutrition and Mental Development,* Swedish Nutrition Foundation Symposia XII, Almqvist and Wiksell, Uppsala, Sweden, 1974.

175. **Prescott, J. W., Read, M. S., and Coursin, D. B.**, Eds., *Brain Function and Malnutrition,* John Wiley & Sons, New York, 1975.

176. **Franková, S.**, *Starvation and Behavior. Progress in Food and Nutrition Science, Proc. Federation of Nutritional Scientists,* Vol. 2, Pergamon Press, Oxford, 1977, 323—331.

177. **Pampiglione, G.**, *Development of Cerebral Function in the Dog,* Butterworths, London, 1963.

178. **Platt, B. S., Pampiglione, G., and Stewart, R. J. C.**, Experimental protein-calorie deficiency: clinical, electroencephalographic and neuropathological changes in pigs, *Dev. Med. Child Neurol.,* 7, 9—26, 1965.

179. **Fraňková, S. and Barnes, R. H.** Influence of malnutrition in early life on exploratory behavior of rats, *J. Nutr.,* 96, 477—484, 1968.

180. **Fraňková, S.,** Effect of protein-calorie malnutrition on the development of social behavior in rat, *Dev. Psychobiol.,* 6, 33—43, 1973.

181. **Levitsky, D. A., Massaro, T. F., and Barnes, R. H.** Maternal malnutrition and the neonatal environment, *Fed. Proc. Fed. Am. Soc. Exp. Biol.,* 34, 1583—1586, 1975.

182. **Kirsch, R. E., Saunders, S. J., and Brock, J. F.,** Animal models and human protein-calorie malnutrition, *Am. J. Clin. Nutr.,* 21, 1225—1228, 1968.

183. **Platt, B. S. and Stewart, R. J. C.,** Effect of protein-calorie deficiency on dogs. I. Reproduction, growth and behavior, *Dev. Med. Child Neurol.,* 10, 3—24, 1968.

184. **Fraňková, S.,** Relationship between nutrition during lactation and maternal behaviour of rats, *Act. Nerv. Super.,* 13, 1—8, 1971.

185. **Fraňková, S.,** Effects of protein deficiency in early life and during lactation on maternal behaviour, *Baroda J. Nutr.,* 1, 21—28, 1974.

186. **Brown, W. G., Mostofsky, D. I., and Warren, S. A.,** Protein deficiency and performance of pigeons on a multiple schedule of reinforcement, *Dev. Psychobiol.,* 7, 1—6, 1974.

187. **Guthrie, H. A.,** Severe undernutrition in early infancy and behavior in rehabilitated albino rat, *Physiol. Behav.,* 3, 619—624, 1968.

188. **Simmel, E. C. and McGee, D. P.,** Social facilitation of exploratory behavior in rats: effects of increased exposure to novel stimuli, *Psychol. Rep.,* 18, 587—590, 1966.

189. **Hughes, R. N.,** Social facilitation of locomotion and exploration in rats, *Br. J. Psychol.,* 60, 385—388, 1969.

190. **Levitsky, D. A. and Barnes, R. H.,** Nutritional and environmental interactions in the behavioral development of the rat: long term effects, *Science,* 176, 68—70, 1972.

191. **Tikal, K., Benešová, O., and Fraňková, S.,** The effects of pyrithioxine and pyridoxine in rats with early protein or calorie malnutrition. I. Effect on social interaction and avoidance acquisition in adult rats, *Act. Nerv. Super.,* 15, 22—24, 1973.

192. **Hliňák, Z. and Fraňková, S.,** Sexual behavior of male rats rehabilitated after early protein calorie malnutrition, *Physiol. Bohemoslov.,* 26, 1—7, 1977.

193. **Cowley, J. J. and Griesel, R. D.,** Some effects of a low protein diet on a first filial generation of white rats, *J. Genet. Psychol.,* 96, 187—201, 1959.

194. **Cowley, J. J. and Griesel, R. D.,** Pre- and post-natal effects of a low-protein diet on the behavior of the white rat, *Psychol. Afr.,* 9, 216—225, 1962.

195. **Baird, A., Widdowson, E. M., and Cowley, J. J.** Effects of calorie and protein deficiencies early in life on the subsequent learning ability of rats, *Br. J. Nutr.,* 25, 391—403, 1971.

196. **Fraňková, S. and Barnes, R. H.** Effect of malnutrition in early life on avoidance conditioning and behavior in rat, *J. Nutr.,* 96, 485—493, 1968.

197. **Barnes, R. H., Moore, U. A., and Pond, W. G.,** Behavioral abnormalities in young adult pigs caused by malnutrition in early life, *J. Nutr.,* 100, 149—155, 1970.

198. **Levitsky, D. A. and Barnes, R. H.,** Effect of early malnutrition on the reaction of adult rats to aversive stimuli, *Nature,* 225, 468—469, 1970.

199. **Levitsky, D. A. and Barnes, R. H.,** Malnutrition and the biology of experience, in *Proc. 9th Int. Congr. Nutrition,* Vol. 2, S. Karger, Basel, 1975, 330—334.

200. **Fraňková, S.,** Interaction between the familiarity with the environment, avoidance learning and behavior of early malnourished rats, *Act. Nerv. Super.,* 15, 207—216, 1973.

201. **Fraňková, S.,** Long-term behavioural effects of postweaning protein deficiency in rat, *Baroda J. Nutr.,* 2, 85—93, 1971.

202. **Hajdu, I.,** Über den Einfluss körperlicher Arbeit auf das Wachstum und Arbeitsvermögen weisser Ratten, den Glykogen — und Fettgehalt ihrer Leber und ihres Muskels, das Gericht ihrer Nebennieren bei unterschiedlicher Kohlenhydrat — und fetthaltiger Diät, *Pfluegers Arch. Gesamte Physiol. Menschen Tiere,* 245, 556, 1942.

203. **Scheer, B. F., Codie, J. F., and Deuel, H. J., Jr.,** The effect of fat level of the diet on general nutrition. III. Weight loss, mortality and recovery in young adult rats maintained on restricted calories, *J. Nutr.,* 33, 641, 1947.

204. **Samuels, L. T., Gilmore, O., Reinecke, R. M.,** The effect of previous diet on the ability of animals to do work during subsequent fasting, *J. Nutr.,* 36, 639, 1948.

205. **Deuel, H. J., Meserve, E. R., Straub, E., Hendrick, C., and Scheer, B. T.,** The effect of fat level of the diet on general nutrition. I. Growth, reproduction and physical capacity of rats receiving diets containing various levels of cottonseed oil or margarine fat ad lib., *J. Nutr.,* 33, 569, 1947.

206. **Fraňková, S.** Relationship between dietary fat intake and higher nervous activity in rats, *Act. Nerv. Super.,* 4, 471—475, 1962.

207. **Razenkov, I. P.,** *Kachestvo Pitaniya i Funktsii Organizma,* Meditsina, Moscow, 1946.

208. Franková, S., Influence of a changed dietary pattern on the behaviour of rats with a different excitability of the CNS, *Cesk. Psychol.,* 10, 13—25, 1966.

209. Caldwell, D. F. and Churchill, J. A., Learning impairment in rats administered a lipid free diet during pregnancy, *Psychol. Rep.,* 19, 99—102, 1966.

210. Davenport, V. D. and Davenport, H. W., The relation between starvation, metabolic acidosis and convulsive seizures in rats, *J. Nutr.,* 36, 139, 1948.

211. Lee, Y. Ch.P., Jardetzky, O., King, J. T., and Visscher, M. B., Effect of dietary factors on incidence of "spontaneous" and induced convulsions in C_3H male mice, *Proc. Soc. Exp. Biol. Med.,* 95, 204, 1957.

212. Swank, R. L. and Engel, R., Production of convulsions in hamsters by high butterfat intake, *Nature,* 181, 1214—1215, 1958.

213. Franková, S., Influence of fat of different composition on exploratory and conditioned reflex activity of rats, *Act. Nerv. Super.,* 5, 366—372, 1963.

214. Laborit, H., Thuret, F., and Laurent, J., Action de l'acide arachidonique sur l'activité locomotorice de la souris, *Agressologie,* 14, 381—385, 1973.

215. Lát, J., Nutrition, learning and adaptive capacity, in *The Chemical Senses and Nutrition,* Kare, M. R. and Maller, O., Eds., Johns Hopkins Press, Baltimore, 1967, 169—180.

216. Jacobs, H. L., Some physiological, metabolic and sensory components in the appetite for glucose, *Am. J. Physiol.,* 203, 1043—1054, 1932.

217. Hutt, P. J., Rate of bar pressing as a function of quality and quantity of food reward, *J. Comp. Physiol. Psychol.,* 47, 235, 1954.

218. Collier, G. H. and Myers, L., The loci of reinforcement, *J. Exp. Psychol.,* 61, 57—76, 1961.

219. Collier, G. H. and Willis, F., Deprivation and reinforcement, *J. Exp. Psychol.,* 62, 377—384, 1961.

220. Wagner, M. W., The effect of age, weight and experience on relative sugar preference in the albino rat, *Psychonomic Sci.,* 2, 243—244, 1965.

221. Titlebaum, L. F. and Mayer, J., Alteration of relative preference for sugar and saccharine caused by ventromedial hypothalamic lesions, *Experientia,* 19, 539, 1963.

222. Bloomfield, A. D. and Tainer, M. L., The effects of vitamin B deprivation on spontaneous activity of the rat, *J. Lab. Clin. Med.,* 28, 1680—1690, 1943.

223. Jackway, I., Voluntary activity in the rat as related to the intake of whole yeast, *J. Comp. Psychol.,* 26, 157—162, 1938.

224. Maurer, S. and Tsai, L. S., Vitamin deficiency in nursing young rats and learning ability, *Science,* 70, 456—458, 1929.

225. Maurer, S. and Tsai, L. S., Vitamin B deficiency and learning ability, *J. Comp. Psychol.,* 11, 51—62, 1937.

226. Fritz, M. F., Maze performance of the white rat in relation to unfavourable salt mixture and vitamin B deficiency, *J. Comp. Psychol.,* 13, 365—390, 1932.

227. Bernhardt, K. S. and Herbert, R., A further study of vitamin B deficiency and learning with rats, *J. Comp. Psychol.,* 24, 263—267, 1937.

228. Poe, E., Poe, C. F., and Muenzinger, K. F., The effect of vitamin deficiency upon the acquisition and retention of the maze habit in the white rat, I. The vitamin B-complex, *J. Comp. Psychol.,* 22, 69—78, 1936.

229. Poe, E., Poe, C. F., and Muenzinger, K. F., The effect of vitamin deficiency upon the acquisition and retention of the maze habit in the white rat. III. Vitamin B, *J. Comp. Psychol.,* 23, 67—76, 1937.

230. Poe, E., Poe, C. F., and Muenzinger, K. F., The effect of vitamin deficiency upon the acquisition and retention of the maze habit in the white rat. IV. Vitamin B-complex, B_1 and B_2 (G), *J. Comp. Psychol.,* 27, 211—214, 1939.

231. Gantt, W. H., Effect of B-complex vitamin in conditioned reflexes in dogs, *Am. J. Clin. Nutr.,* 5, 121—124, 1957.

232. Gross, N. B. and Cohn, V. H., The effect of vitamin B deficiency on the hoarding behavior of rats, *Am. J. Psychol.,* 67, 124—128, 1954.

233. Rodgers, W. and Rozin, P., Novel food preferences in thiamine-deficient rats, *J. Comp. Physiol. Psychol.,* 61, 1—4, 1966.

234. Rozin, P. and Rodgers, W., Novel diet preferences in vitamin deficient rats and rats recovered from vitamin deficiencies, *J. Comp. Physiol. Psychol.,* 63, 421—428, 1967.

235. Evans, H. M., *J. Nutr.,* 1, 1—21, 1928; as cited in Brožek, J. and Vaes, G., Experimental investigations on the effects of dietary deficiencies on animal and human behavior, *Vit. Horm.* (N.Y.), 19, 43—94, 1961.

236. Stone, C. P., *J. Comp. Psychol.,* 5, 177—201, 1925; as cited in Brožek, J. and Vaes, G., Experimental investigations on the effects of dietary deficiencies on animal and human behavior, *Vit. Horm.* (N.Y.), 19, 43—94, 1961.

237. Brožek, J. and Grande, F., Abnormalities of neural function in the presence of inadequate nutrition, in *Handbook of Physiology,* Sect. 1, Vol. 3, Field, J., Ed., American Physiological Society, Washington, D.C., 1960, 1891—1910.

238. Guerrant, N. B. and Dutcher, R. A., The influence of exercise on the growing rat in the presence of vitamin B₁, *J. Nutr.,* 20, 589—598, 1940.

239. Wald, G. and Jackson, B., Activity and nutritional deprivation, *Proc. Natl Acad. Sci., U.S.A.,* 30, 255—263, 1944.

240. Knopfelmacher, F., Khairy, M., Russell, R. W., and Yudkin, J., Q., *J. Exp. Psychol.,* 8, 54—65, 1956; as cited in Brožek, J. and Vaes, G., Experimental investigations on the effects of dietary deficiencies on animal and human behavior, *Vit. Horm.,* (N.Y.), 19, 43—94, 1961.

241. Maurer, S., The effect of early depletion of vitamin B₂ upon performance in rats, *J. Comp. Psychol.,* 20, 385—387, 1935.

242. Moore, H. and Mathias, E., The effect of vitamin A and B deficiency on the maze-learning ability of the white rat, *J. Comp. Psychol.,* 19, 487—496, 1935.

243. Stevens, H., Avitaminosis B (B₁), maze performance and certain aspects of brain biochemistry, *J. Comp. Psychol.,* 24, 441—458, 1937.

244. Biel, W. C. and Wickens, D. D., The effect of vitamin B₁ deficiency on the conditioning of eyelid responses in the rat, *J. Comp. Psychol.,* 32, 329—340, 1941.

245. Aptekar, S. G., Sostoyanie uslovnoreflektornoy deyatelnosti kak pokazatel thiaminovoy nedostatoch, *Vopr. Pit.,* 15, 21—28, 1956.

246. Shekun, L. A., B₁-avitaminos v opytach na sobakach, *Vopr. Pit.,* 16, 29—33, 1957.

247. Khairy, M., Russell, R. W., and Yudkin, J., Some effects of thaimine deficiency and reduced caloric intake on avoidance training and on reactions to conflict, *Q. J. Exp. Psychol.,* 9, 190—205, 1957.

248. Beeman, E. A. and Allee, W. O., Some effects of thiamine on the winning of social contacts in mice, *Physiol. Zool.,* 18, 195—221, 1945.

249. Richter, C. P., Holt, L. E., and Barelare, B., Jr., Vitamin B craving in rats, *Science,* 86, 354, 1937.

250. Harris, L. J., Clay, J., Hargreaves, F. J., and Ward, A., Appetite and choice of diet, the ability of the vitamin B deficient rat to discriminate between diets containing and lacking the vitamin, *Proc. R. Soc.,* 113, 161—190, 1933.

251. Scott, E. M. and Verney, E. L., Self-selection of diet. VI. The nature of appetites for B vitamins, *J. Nutr.,* 34, 471—480, 1947.

252. Rozin, P., Adaptive food sampling patterns in vitamin deficient rats, *J. Comp. Physiol. Psychol.,* 69, 126—132, 1969.

253. Rozin, P., Wells, C., and Mayer, J., Specific hunger for thiamine: vitamin in water versus vitamin in foods, *J. Comp. Physiol. Psychol.,* 57, 78—84, 1964.

254. O'Neill, P. H., The effect of subsequent maze learning ability of graded amounts of vitamin B₁ in the diet or very young rats, *J. Genet. Psychol.,* 74, 85—95, 1949.

255. Marx, M. H., Maze learning as a function of added thiamine, *J. Comp. Physiol. Psychol.,* 41, 364—371, 1948.

256. Havlíček, V., Über den Einfluss von Vitamin B₁ auf die höhere Nerventätigkeit, *Physiol. Bohemoslov.,* 6, 492, 1957.

257. Patton, R. A., Karn, H. W., and King, C. G., Studies on the nutritional basis of abnormal behavior in albino rats. I. The effect of vitamin B₁ and vitamin B-complex deficiency on convulsive seizures, *J. Comp. Psychol.,* 32, 543—550, 1941.

258. Richards, M. B., Imbalance of vitamin B factors. Pyridoxine deficiency caused by addition of aneurin and chalk, *Br. Med. J.,* 1, 433, 1945.

259. Castellanos, G., Nutritional Factors Related to Neurological and Mental Disorders, paper presented before the International Brain Research Organization (UNESCO) World Health Organization Workshop on Nutritional Influences on Function of the Brain, Ibadan, Nigeria, February 2—March 3, 1973.

260. Zimmerman, H. M., Assoc. Res. Nerv. Ment. Dis. Proc., 22, 49, 1943; as cited in Castellanos, G., Nutritional Factors Related to Neurological and Mental Disorders, paper presented before the International (UNESCO) World Health Organization Workshop on Nutritional Influences on Function of the Brain, Ibadan, Nigeria, 1973.

261. Reed, J. D., Spontaneous activity of animals. A review of the literature since 1929, *Psychol. Bull.,* 44, 393—412, 1947.

262. Muenzinger, K. F., Poe, E., and Poe, C. F., The effect of vitamin deficiency upon the acquisition and the maze habit in the white rat. II. Vitamin B₂ (G), *J. Comp. Psychol.,* 23, 59—66, 1937.

263. Efremov, V. V., Makarychev, A. I., Maslennikova, E. M., and Tikhomirova, A. N., Vliyaniya ariboflavinoza na vysshuyu nervnuyu deyatelnost i troficheski funktsii organizma, *Vopr. Pit.,* 16, 37—44, 1957.

264. Eiduson, S., Geller, E., Yuwiller, A., Eiduson, B. T., *Biochemistry and Behavior,* Van Nostrand, Princeton, N.J., 1964.

265. Nikolov, N. A., Gheorghiyeva, E. I., Vassileva, A. V., and Dimitrova, N. V., The influence of the nicotinic acid on the function of the brain cortex in men, *Folia Med.* (Plovdiv), 1(4), 233, 1959.

266. Maksimovich, Y. B., K mekhanizmu vliyaniya nikotinovoi kisloty na vysshyu nervnuyu deyatelnost, in *Proc. 10th Sci. Conf. Institute of Nutrition, Moscow,* Abstr., Institute of Nutrition, Moscow, 1956, 135—137.

267. Dakshinamurti, K. and Stephens, M. C., Pyridoxine deficiency in the neonatal rat, *J. Neurochem.,* 16, 1515—1522, 1969.

268. Hoff, L. A., Peacock, L. J., Meadows, J. S., and Caster, W. O., The vitamin B_6 requirement of the rat as estimated with weight gain and general activity measurements, *Physiol. Behav.,* 3, 301—303, 1968.

269. Smith, D. E. and Pett, L. B., Learning ability of rats cured of rat pellagra, *Psychol. Bull.,* 30, 518—519, 1939.

270. Porter, P. B., Griffin, A. C., and Stone, C. P., Behavioral assessment of glutamic acid metabolism with observations on pyridoxine and folic acid deficiencies, *J. Comp. Physiol. Psychol.,* 44, 543—550, 1951.

271. Sloane, H. N. and Chow, B. F., Vitamin B_6 deficiency and the initial acquisition of behavior, *J. Nutr.,* 83, 379—384, 1964.

272. Gantt, W. H., Chow, B. F., and Simonson, M., Effect of pyridoxine and pantothenic acid deficiency on conditioned relfexes, *Am. J. Clin. Nutr.,* 7, 411—415, 1959.

273. Kosenko, S. A., Znachenie vitamina B_6 v normalnoy deyatelnosti kory bolshikh polusharii golovnogo mozga, *Zh. Vyssh. Nerv. Deytal. im. I. P. Pavlova,* 10(2), 291, 1960.

274. Bhagavan, H. N. and Coursin, D. B., Effect of pyridoxine deficiency on nucleic acid and protein contents of brain and liver in rats, *Int. J. Vit. Nutr. Res.,* 41, 419—423, 1971.

275. Stewart, C. N., Bhagavan, H. N., and Coursin, D. B., Avoidance and escape learning in vitamin B_6-deficient rats, *Fed. Proc. Fed. Am. Soc. Exp., Biol.,* 25, 670, 1966.

276. Stewart, C. N., Bhagavan, H. N., and Coursin, D. B., Position and reversal learning in biotin and pyridoxine deficient rats, *Fed. Proc. Fed. Am. Soc. Exp. Biol.,* 26, 444; abstr. No. 882, 1967.

277. Stephens, M. C., Havliček, V., and Dakshinamurti, K., Pyridoxine deficiency and development of the central nervous system in the rat, *J. Neurochem.,* 18, 2407—2416, 1971.

278. Lyon, J. B., Williams, H. L., and Arnold, E, A., The pyridoxine deficiency state in two strains of inbred mice, *J. Nutr.,* 66, 261—275, 1958.

279. Schlesinger, K. and Schreiber, R. A., Interaction of drugs and pyridoxine deficiency on central nervous system excitability, *Ann. N.Y. Acad. Sci.,* 166, 281—287, 1969.

280. Coleman, D. L. and Schlesinger, K., Effects of pyridoxine deficiency on audiogenic seizure susceptibility in inbred mice, *Proc. Soc. Exp. Biol. Med.,* 119, 264—266, 1965.

281. Schlesinger, K. and Lieff, B., Levels of pyridoxine and susceptibility to electroconvulsive and audiogenic seizures, *Psychopharmacologia,* 42, 27—32, 1975.

282. Dakshinamurti, K., Stephens, M. C., and Bhuvaneswaran, C., Commun. 2nd Meet. International Society of Neurochemistry, Milan, Abstr., 1969, 143.

283. Alton-Mackey, M. G. and Walker, B. L., Graded levels of pyridoxine in the rat diet during gestation and the physical and neuromotor development of offspring, *Am. J. Clin. Nutr.,* 26, 420—428, 1973.

284. Coursin, D. B., Vitamin B_6 and brain function in animals and man. In: Vitamin B_6 in metabolism of the nervous system, *Ann. N.Y. Acad. Sci.,* 166, 7—15, 1969.

285. Tikal, K., Benešová, O., and Franková, S., The effect of pyridoxine and pyrithioxine on individual behavior, social interactions, and learning in rats malnourished in early postnatal life, *Psychopharmacologia,* 46, 325—332, 1976.

286. Nielsen, E. and Elvehjem, C. A., Cure of paralysis in rats with biotin concentrates and crystalline biotin, *J. Biol Chem.,* 144, 405, 1942.

287. Lazere, B., Thomson, J. D., and Hines, H. M., Studies on muscle and nerve in biotin-deficient rats, *Proc. Soc. Exp. Biol. Med.,* 53, 81, 1943.

288. Stewart, C. N., Bhagavan, H. N., Coursin, D. B., and Dakshinamurti, K., Effect of biotin deficiency on escape and avoidance learning in rats, *J. Nutr.,* 88, 427—433, 1966.

289. Weiss, B. and Danford, M. D., Reward Value of Heat and Low Temperatures During Inanition and Pantothenic Acid Deprivation, Rep. No. 56—72, School of Aviation Medicine, U. S. Air Force, Randolph Air Force Base, Texas, 1956.

290. Stenpak, J. G., Etiology of antenatal hydrocephalus by folic acid deficiency in the albino rat, *Anat. Rec.,* 151, 287, 1967.

291. Arakawa, T., Mizuno, T., Honda, Y., Tamura, T., Sakai, K., Tatsumi, S., Chiba, F., and Coursin, D. B., Brain function of infants fed on milk from mothers with low serum folate levels, *Tohoku, J. Exp. Med.,* 97, 391, 1969.

292. **Arakawa, T., Mizuno, T., Honda, Y., Tamura, T., Watanabe, A., Konatushiro, M., Takagi, T., Iinuma, K., and Yamaguchi, N.,** Longitudinal study on maturation pattern of EEG brain waves of infants fed on milk from mothers with low serum folate levels, *Tohoku, J. Exp. Med.,* 102, 81, 1970.

293. **Efremov, V. V.,** Vitaminy i funktsii tsentralnoi nervnoi sistemy, in *Pitaniya i Vysshaya Nervnaya Deyatelnost,* Andriasov, A. N. and Braksh, T., Eds., Meditsina, Leningrad, 1966, 79—117.

294. **Farmer, C. J.,** Some aspects of vitamin C metabolism, *Fed. Proc. Fed. Am. Soc. Exp. Biol.,* 3, 179, 1944.

295. **Hoitink, A. W. J. H.,** Researches on the influence of vitamin C administration on human organism, in particular in connection with the working capacity, *Acta Brev. Neerl. Physiol.,* 14, 62, 1946.

296. **Hoogerwerf, A. and Hoiting, A. W. J. H.,** The influence of vitamin C administration on the mechanical efficiency of the human organism, *Int. Z. Angew. Physiol. Einschl. Arbeitsphysiol.,* 20, 164—172, 1963.

297. **Kinsman, R. A. and Hood, J.,** Some behavioral effects of ascorbic acid deficiency, *Am. J. Clin. Nutr.,* 24, 455—464, 1971.

298. **Adlard, B. P. F., Moon, S., and Smart, J. L.,** Discrimination learning in ascorbic acid-deficient guinea pigs, *Nature,* 247(5440), 398, 1974.

299. **Rogers, W. E., Jr. and Bieri, J. G.,** Vitamin A deficiency in the rat prior to weaning, *Proc. Soc. Exp. Biol. Med.,* 132, 622—624, 1969.

300. **Maurer, A.,** The effect of acute vitamin A depletion upon performance in rats, *J. Comp. Psychol.,* 20, 389—391, 1935.

301. **Bernhardt, K. S.,** Vitamin A deficiency and learning in the rat, *J. Comp. Psychol.,* 22, 277—278, 1936.

302. **Mamish, P. M.,** in *Vitaminy,* Vol. 4, Akademiya Nauk USSR, Institut Biokhemii, Kiev, 1959; as cited in Efremov, V. V., Vitaminy i funktsii tsentralnoi nervnoi sistemy, in *Pitaniya i Vysshaya Nervnaya Deyatelnost,* Andriasov, A. N. and Braksh, T., Eds., Meditsina, Leningrad, 1966, 79—117.

303. **Guerrant, N. B., Dutcher, R. A., and Chornock, F.,** The influence of exercise on the growing rat in the presence and absence of vitamin A, *J. Nutr.,* 17, 473—484, 1939.

304. **Duncan, C. J.,** The taste bud membrane and role of vitamin A acid, *Int. Z. Vitaminforsch.,* 34, 410, 1964.

305. **Bernard, R. and Halpern, B. P.,** Taste changes in vitamin A deficiency, *J. Gen. Physiol.,* 52, 444—464, 1968.

306. **Cohlan, S. Q.,** Congenital anomalies in the rat produced by excessive intake of vitamin A during pregnancy, *Pediatrics,* 13, 556—567, 1954.

307. **Giroud, A. and Martinet, M.,** Hypervitaminose A et anomalies chez le foetus de rat, *Rev. Int. Vit.,* 26, 10—18, 1955.

308. **Kalter, H. and Warkany, J.,** Experimental production of congenital malformations in strains of inbred mice by maternal treatment with hypervitaminosis A., *Am. J. Pathol.,* 38, 1—21, 1961.

309. **Langman, J. and Welch, G. W.,** Effect of vitamin A on development of the central nervous system, *J. Comp. Neurol.,* 128, 1—16, 1966.

310. **Richter, C. P. and Rice, K. U.,** Effects produced by vitamin D on energy, appetite and oestrus cycles of rats kept on an exclusive diet of yellow corn, *Am. J. Physiol.,* 139, 693—699, 1943.

311. **Frank, M.,** The effect of a ricket producing diet on the learning ability of white rats, *J. Comp. Psychol.,* 13, 87—105, 1932.

312. **Wilder, C. E.,** Selection of rachitic and antirachitic diets in the rat, *J. Comp. Psychol.,* 24, 547—577, 1937.

313. **Gross, N. B., Fisher, A. H., and Cohn, V. H.,** *J. Comp. Physiol. Psychol.,* 48, 451—455, 1955; as cited in Brožek, J. and Vaes, G., Experimental investigations on the effects of dietary deficiencies on animal and human behaviour, *Vit. Horm.*(N.Y.), 19, 43—94, 1961.

314. **Reed, C. I., Dillman, E. A., Thacker, E. A., and Klein, R. I.,** The calcification of tissues by excessive doses of irradiated ergosterol, *J. Nutr.,* 6, 371, 1933.

315. **Seelig, M. S.,** Vitamin D and cardiovascular, renal and brain damage in infancy and childhood, *Ann. N.Y. Acad. Sci.,* 147, 537—583, 1969.

316. **Mason, E.,** in *Structure and Function of the Muscle,* Vol. 3, Bourne, G. H., Ed., Academic Press, New York, 1960, 171—207.

317. **Wiesner, B. P. and Bacharach, A. L.,** *Nature,* 140, 972—973, 1937; as cited in Brožek, and Vaes, G., Experimental investigations on the effects of dietary deficiencies on animal and human behaviour, *Vit. Horm.*(N.Y.), 19, 43—94, 1961.

318. **Burkard, W. P., Goy, K. F., Weiser, H., and Schweiter, U.,** Decrease of norepinephrine in brain and heart of vitamin E deficient rats, *Experientia,* 24, 807, 1968.

319. **Consolazio, C. F., Matoush, L. O., Nelson, R. A., Issag, G. J., and Hursh, L. M.,** Effect of octacoxanol, wheat germ oil, and vitamin E on performance of swimming rats, *J. Appl. Physiol.,* 19, 265, 1964.

320. **Rosen, A. J., Cohen, M. E., and Pieken, L.,** DL-alpha Tocopherol acetate and instrumental conditioning in the rat, *Nutr. Rep. Int.,* 6, 181—186, 1972.

321. **Forbes, R. M. and Yohe, M.,** Zinc requirement and balance studies with rat, *J. Nutr.,* 70, 53, 1960.

322. **Hoekstra, W. G.,** Recent observation on mineral interrelationships, *Fed. Proc. Fed. Am. Soc. Exp. Biol.,* 23, 1068—1076, 1964.

323. **Likuski, H. J. A. and Forbes, R. M.,** Mineral utilization in the rat. IV. Effects of calcium and phytic acid on the utilization of dietary zinc, *J. Nutr.,* 85, 230—234, 1965.

324. **Spencer, H., Vankinscott, V., Lewin, I., and Samachson, J.,** Zinc-65 metabolism during low and high calcium intake in man, *J. Nutr.,* 86, 169—177, 1965.

325. **Keynes, R. D. and Lewis, P. R.,** Electrolytes and nerve function, in *Neurochemistry,* Elliott, K. A. C., Page, I. H., and Quastel, J. H., Eds., Charles C Thomas, Springfield, Ill., 1955, 440—457.

326. **Saphir, W.,** *JAMA,* 129, 510, 1945; as cited in Brožek, J. and Grande, F., Abnormalities of neural function in the presence of inadequate nutrition, in *Handbook of Physiology,* Sect. 1, Vol. 3, Field, J., Ed., American Physiological Society, Washington, D.C., 1960, 1891—1910.

327. **Nováková, V., Šterc, J., and Faltin, J.,** The role of sodium chloride in the excitability of the CNS of the rat, *Physiol. Bohemoslov.,* 12, 317, 1963.

328. **Šterc, J., Nováková, V., and Faltin, J.,** Veränderungen der Hirntätigkeit von Ratten bei Substitution von Natriumchlorid durch Kaliumchlorid in der Nahrung, *Acta Biol. Med. Ger.,* 14, 146—157, 1965.

329. **Roshchina, L. F.,** Mineralnye veshchestva i central naya nervnaya sistema, in *Pitaniya i Vysshaya Nervnaya Deyatelnost,* Andriasov, A. N. and Braksh, T., Eds., Meditsina, Leningrad, 1966, 118—143.

330. **Goeller, J. C.,** Effect of Dietary Sodium Restriction During Pregnancy upon the Physical Development of the Offspring, M. Sc. thesis, University of Guelph, Ontario, Canada, 1971; as cited in Alton-MacKey, M. G. and Walker, B. L., Graded levels of pyridoxine in the rat diet during gestation and the physical and neuromotor development of offspring, *Am. J. Clin. Nutr.,* 26, 420—428, 1973.

331. **Lát, J. and Faltová, E.,** On the activity of the feeding center. I. Regulation of water and solid food intake, *Cesk. Fysiol.,* 3, 132—142, 1954.

332. **Lát, J.,** Nutrition, learning and adaptive capacity, in *The Chemical Senses and Nutrition,* Kare M. R. and Maller, O., Eds., Johns Hopkins Press, Baltimore, 1967, 169—180.

333. **Smith, M. H., Holman, G. L., and Fortune, K. H.** Sodium need and sodium consumption, *J. Comp. Physiol. Psychol.,* 65, 33—37, 1968.

334. **Zucker, I.,** Short-term salt preference of potassium-deprived rats, *Am. J. Physiol.,* 208, 1071—1074, 1965.

335. **Milner, P. and Zucker, I.,** Specific hunger for potassium in the rat, *Psychonomic Sci.,* 2, 17—18, 1965.

336. **Adam, W. R. and Dawborn, J. K.,** Effect of potassium depletion on mineral appetite in the rat, *J. Comp. Physiol. Psychol.,* 78, 51—58, 1972.

337. **Blake, W. P. and Jurf, A. N.,** Increased voluntary Na intake in K deprived rats, *Commun. Behav. Biol. A.,* 1, 1—7, 1968.

338. **Adam, W. R.,** Novel diet preferences in potassium-deficient rats, *J. Comp. Physiol. Psychol.,* 84, 286—288, 1973.

339. **Barnett, S. A.,** Experiment in "neophobia" in wild and laboratory rats, *Br. J. Psychol.,* 49, 195—201, 1958.

340. **Rzóska, J.,** Bait shyness: a study in rat behavior, *Br. J. Anim. Behav.,* 1, 128—135, 1953.

341. **Aschkenasy-Lelu, P.,** Le retentissement de la nutrition sur les phenomènes psychiques. I. Alimentation et conduite, *Encephale,* 4, 341—379, 1951.

342. **Komendantova, M. B.,** *Pharmakol. Toksikol.,* 2, 99, 1960; as cited in Roshchina, L. F., Mineralnye veshchestva i centralnaya nervnaya sistema, in *Pitaniya i Vysshaya Nervnaya Deyatelnost,* Andriasov, A. N. and Braksh, T., Eds., Meditsina, Leningrad, 1966, 118—143.

343. **Morgan, C. T.,** *Psychol. Rev.,* 54, 335—341, 1947; as cited in Brožek, J. and Vaes, G., Experimental investigations on the effects of dietary deficiencies on animal and human behaviour, *Vit. Horm.* (N.Y.), 19, 43—94, 1961.

344. **Overton, R. K.,** An effect of high- and low-calcium diets on the maze performance of rats, *J. Comp. Physiol. Psychol.,* 51, 697—700, 1958.

345. **Lawson, R. B. and Gulick, W. L.,** The efficacy of modification of brain calcium through dietary manipulation, *Psychol. Rev.,* 15, 191—196, 1965.

346. **Rubin, M. A., Hoff, H. E., Winkler, A. W., and Smith, P. K.,** Intravenous potassium, calcium and magnesium and the cortical electrogram of the cat, *J. Neurophysiol.,* 6, 23—28, 1943.

347. **Hughes, B. O. and Wood-Gush, D. G. M.,** An increase in activity of domestic fowls produced by nutritional deficiency, *Anim. Behav.,* 21, 10—17, 1973.

348. **Harriman, A. E.,** Seizing by magnesium-deprived mongolian gerbils given open field tests, *J. Gen. Psychol.,* 90, 221—229, 1974.

349. **Dalley, M. B., Mahoney, A., and Cheney, C.,** Magnesium deficiency effects on discriminated avoidance in rats, *Nutr. Rep. Int.,* 11, 507—515, 1975.

350. **Hurley, L. S.,** Zinc deficiency in the developing rat, *Am. J. Clin. Nutr.,* 22, 1332—1339, 1969.

351. **Halas, E. S., Hanlon, M. J., and Sandstead, H. H.,** Intrauterine nutrition and aggression, *Nature,* 257, 221—222, 1975.

352. **Apgar, J.,** Effects of zinc deficiency on parturition in the rat, *Am. J. Physiol.,* 216, 160, 1968.

353. **Caldwell, D. F. and Oberleas, D.,** Effects of protein and zinc nutrition on behavior in the rat, in *Perinatal Factors Affecting Human Development,* Pan American Health Organization Scientific Publ. No. 185, 1—8, 1969.

354. **Ronaghy, H., Fox, M. R. S., Garn, S. M., Israel, H., Harp, A., Moe, P. G., and Halsted, J. A.,** *Am. J. Clin. Nutr.,* 22, 1279, 1969; as cited in Caldwell, D. F., Oberleas, D., Clancy, J. J., and Prasad, A. S., Behavioral impairment in adult rats following acute zinc deficiency, *Proc. Soc. Exp. Biol. Med.,* 133, 1417—1421, 1970.

355. **Caldwell, D. F., Oberleas, D., Clancy, J. J., and Prasad, A. S.,** Behavioral impairment in adult rats following acute zinc deficiency, *Proc. Soc. Exp. Biol. Med.,* 133, 1417—1421, 1970.

356. **Lokken, P. M., Halas, E. S., and Sandstead, H. H.,** Influence of zinc deficiency on behavior, *Proc. Soc. Exp. Biol. Med.,* 144, 680—682, 1973.

357. **Sandstead, H. H., Burk, R. F., Booth, G. H., and Darby, W. J.,** Current concepts on trace minerals, *Med. Clin. North Am.,* 54, 1509—1531, 1970.

358. **Terhune, M. W. and Sandstead, H. H.,** *Science,* 177, 68, 1972; as cited in Lokken, P. M., Halas, E. S., and Sandstead, H. H., Influence of zinc deficiency on behavior, *Proc. Soc. Exp. Biol. Med.,* 144, 680—682, 1973.

359. **Sandstead, H. H., Gillespie, D. D., and Brady, R. N.,** *Pediatr. Res.,* 6, 119, 1972; as cited in Lokken, P. M., Halas, E. S., and Sandstead, H. H., Influence of zinc deficiency on behaviour, *Proc. Soc. Exp. Biol. Med.,* 144, 680—682, 1973.

360. **Read, M. S.,** Anemia and behavior, *Mod. Probl. Pediatr.,* 14, 189—202, 1974.

361. **Alt, H. L.,** Iron deficiency in pregnant rats: its effect on the young, *Am. J. Dis. Child.,* 56, 975—984, 1938.

362. **Lintzel, W., Rechenberger, J., and Schirer, E.,** Über den Eisenstoffwechsel des Neugeborenen und des Säuglings, *Z. Gesamte Exp. Med.,* 113, 591—612, 1944.

363. **Nylander, G.,** On the placental transfer of iron. An experimental study in the rat, *Acta Physiol. Scand. Suppl.,* 29 (107), 1—105, 1953.

364. **O'Dell, B. L., Hardwick, B. C., and Reynolds, G.,** Mineral deficiencies of milk and congenital malformations in the rat, *J. Nutr.,* 73, 151—157, 1961.

365. **Scarpelli, E. M.,** Maternal nutritional deficiency and intelligence of the offspring (thiamine and iron), *J. Comp. Physiol. Psychol.,* 52, 536—539, 1959.

366. **Bernhardt, K. S.,** Phosphorus and iron deficiencies and learning in the rat, *J. Comp. Psychol.,* 22, 273, 1936.

367. **Edgerton, V. R., Bryant S. L., Gillespie, C. A., and Gardner, G. W.,** Iron deficiency anemia and physiological performance and activity of rats, *J. Nutr.,* 102, 381—400, 1972.

368. **Powers, H. D.,** Biochemistry in relation to intelligence, *Science,* 73, 316—317, 1937.

369. **Rich, G. J.,** Intelligence and body chemistry, *Science,* 74, 21—22, 1931.

370. **Aschkenasy-Lelu, P.,** Le retentissement de la nutrition sur les phénomènes psychiques. II. Nutrition et psychisme, *Encephale,* 1, 45—88, 1952.

371. **Everson, G. J., Shrader, R. E., and Wang, T.,** Chemical and morphological changes in brains of copper deficient guinea pigs, *J. Nutr.,* 96, 115, 1968.

372. **Underwood, E. J.,** *Trace Elements in Human and Animal Nutrition,* 3rd ed., Academic Press, New York, 1971, 208—244.

373. **Warren, P. J.,** The effect of a copper-deficient diet on the concentration of copper in the nervous system and other tissues of the rat, *Br. J. Nutr.,* 16, 167—173, 1962.

374. **Raitses, V. S. and Tradadyuk, A. A.,** *Phisiol. Ukr. Zh.,* 3, 319, 1963; as cited in Roshchina, L. F., Mineralnye veshchestva i centralnaya nervnaya sisrema, in *Pitaniya i Vysshaya Nervnaya Deyatelnost,* Andriasov, A. N. and Braksh, T., Eds., Meditsina, Leningrad, 1966, 118—143.

375. **Hurley, L. S., Woolley, D. E., Rosenthal, F., and Timiras, P. S.,** Influence of manganese on susceptibility of rats to convulsions, *Am. J. Physiol.,* 204, 493, 1963.

376. **Orent, E. R. and McCollum, E. V.,** Effects of deprivation of manganese in the rat, *J. Biol. Chem.,* 92, 651—678, 1931.

377. **Shils, M. E. and McCollum, E. V.,** Further studies on the symptoms of manganese deficiency in the rat and mouse, *J. Nutr.,* 26, 1—19, 1943.

378. **Keith, T. B., Miller, R. C., Thorp, W. T. S., and McCarty, M. A.,** *J. Anim. Sci.,* 1, 120, 1942; as cited in Brožek, J. and Grande, F., Abnormalities of neural function in the presence of inadequate nutrition, in *Handbook of Physiology,* Sect. 1, Vol. 3, Field, J., Ed., American Physiological Society, Washington, D.C., 1960, 1891—1910.

379. **Plumlee, M. P., Thrasher, D. M., Beeson, W. M., Andrews, F. N., and Parker, H. E.**, *J. Anim. Sci.*, 15, 352, 1956; as cited in Brožek, J. and Grande, F., Abnormalities of neural function in the presence of inadequate nutrition, in *Handbook of Physiology*, Sect. 1, Vol. 3, Field, J., Ed., American Physiological Society, Washington, D.C., 1960, 1891—1910.

380. **Makarchenko, A. F.**, *Vopr. Fiziol.*, 9, 33, 1954; as cited in Roshchina, L. F.- Mineralnye veshchestva i centralnaya nervnaya sistema in, *Pitaniya i Vysshaya Nervnaya Deyatelnost*, Andriasov, A. N. and Braksh, T., Eds., Meditsina, Leningrad, 1966, 118—143.

381. **Ganitt, W. H. and Fleishmann, W.**, Am. J. Psychiatr., 104, 673, 1948; as cited in Brožek, J. and Grande, F., Abnormalities of neural function in the presence of inadequate nutrition, in *Handbook of Physiology*, Sect. 1 Vol. 3, Field, J., Ed., American Physiological Society, Washington, D.C., 1960, 1891—1910.

382. **Schroeder, H. A., Kroll, S. S., Little, J. W., Livingston, P. O., and Meyers, M. A. C.**, Hypertension in rats by injection of cadmium, *Arch. Environ. Health,* 13, 788, 1966.

383. **Galoyan, A. A.**, *Probl. Endokrinol. Gormonoter.,* 11, 46, 1960; as cited in Roshchina, L. F., Mineralnye veshchestva i centralnaya nervnaya sistema, in *Pitaniya i Vysshaya Nervnaya Deyatelnost*, Andriasov, A. N. and Braksh, T., Eds., Meditsina, Leningrad, 1966, 118—143.

Adaptation and Resistance to
Environmental Stress

NUTRITION IN COLD ENVIRONMENTS

O. Héroux

Recommended daily allowances of nutrients (Table 1) are intended to ensure the maintenance of good nutrition in essentially healthy, normally active persons under current conditions of living and usual environmental stresses.[1]

A comfortable ambient temperature of 20 to 25°C (68 to 77°F) probably applies to most living conditions in temperate climates. Most individuals are protected against the effect of cold by warm clothes, central heating, and heated means of transportation. Yet it cannot be assumed that everyone is insulated from environmental exposure, and when there is prolonged exposure to cold, nutrient allowances may need adjustments.

There is evidence[2] that, all other factors being equal, the energy cost of work is slightly greater (approximately 5%) in a mean temperature below 14°C than in a warm environment. In addition, there is a relatively small (2 to 5%) increased energy expenditure associated with carrying the extra weight of cold weather clothing and footgear. Such clothing also slightly increases energy expenditure by its "hobbling" effect. If the body is inadequately clothed, body cooling will occur and calorie needs will increase because of the increased metabolic rate associated with shivering and other involuntary or voluntary movements. Also, there is a tendency to increase activity in the cold. Assumedly, this situation often occurs in the Arctic.

Under normal conditions, food intake increases in cold environments. It is generally believed that a greater consumption of a well-balanced diet, which satisfies the recommended allowances, will provide all the additional nutrients in the right amount and right proportion under conditions of elevated metabolism.

However, many suspect that under cold conditions the daily nutrient requirement may be quite different than the recommended allowance established for temperate climates. Some nutrients may be needed in greater quantity or in different proportions.

Table 1
NUTRITIONAL STANDARDS: MAN (70-kg ADULT MALE)[1,2]

Nutrient	Daily recommended allowance	Daily average intake	Toxic intake
Calories (kcal)	2600		
Protein (g)	70		
Fat (g)	—		
Carbohydrate (g)	100		
Water (liters)	1.5		
Amino acids (mg/day)			
L-Tryptophane	250		
L-Histidine	—		
L-Threonine	500		
L-Methionine	200		
L-Cystine	810		
L-Arginine	—		
L-Lysine	800		
L-Isoleucine	700		
L-Valine	800		
L-Leucine	1100		
L-Phenylalanine	300		
L-Tyrosine	1100		

Table 1 (continued)
NUTRITIONAL STANDARDS: MAN (70-kg ADULT MALE)[1],[2]

Nutrient	Daily recommended allowance	Daily average intake	Toxic intake
Vitamins			
A (IU)	5000	7500	500,000
D (IU)	400	100–400	1000–2000
E (IU)	30	2–66	56,000
C (mg)	70	21	–
B_1 (thiamine) (mg)	1.4	–	1,400
B_2 (riboflavin) (mg)	1.7	–	8,000 (rat)
B_6 (pyridoxine) (mg)	2.0	2.2–2.9	200
Nicotinic acid (mg)	20.0	16–33	20,000
H (biotin) (μg)	–	250–300	20,000 (mouse)
Pantothenic acid (mg)	5–10	10–15	100,000
Choline (mg)	250–600	500–1000	?
B_{12} (μg)	6.0	2–31	?
Minerals			
Calcium (mg)	800	200–1500	?
Magnesium (mg)	600[3]	300	None
Sodium (g)	–	2.3–6.9	1.2–1.5 (infant)
Potassium (g)	0.8–1.3	2.5–4.5	?
Phosphorus (mg)	800	200–1500	?
Iron (mg)	10	15.6	
Iodine (μg)	50.75	150	?
Copper (mg)	2.0	2–5	?
Fluoride (ppm)	–	–	?
Zinc (mg)	10–15	10–15	?
Cobalt (mg)			
Manganese (mg)			
Selenium (ppm)	?	?	5[4]
Molybdenum (ppm)			
Cadmium (μg)		200–400[5]	

REFERENCES

1. *Recommended Dietary Allowances,* 8th rev. ed., National Academy of Sciences, Washington, D.C., 1974.
2. **Altman, P. L. and Dittmer, D. S.,** Eds., *Metabolism,* Federation of American Societies for Experimental Biology, Bethesda, Md., 1968.
3. **Seelig, M. S.,** *Am. J. Clin. Nutr.,* 14, 342, 1964.
4. **Krehl, W. A.,** *Nutr. Today,* 5(4), 26, 1970.
5. **Gurdarshan, S. et al.,** *Am. J. Physiol.,* 219, 577, 1970.

As will be seen in the following review of the literature, many attempts have been made to increase cold tolerance in men as well as in animals, mostly in rats, either by raising the calorie content of the diet, varying the proportion of protein, fat, and carbohydrate, using lipids of different qualities, or supplementing the diets with large amounts of vitamins.

The greater calorie requirement in cold environments is now well recognized; in fact, the Canadian Army provides its troops with daily rations containing 3500 cal in temperate climates and 4720 cal in the Arctic. However, no definite conclusions have been reached concerning quality of protein, lipid or carbohydrate, vitamin, or mineral supplementation despite the fact that some experimental evidence, as will be seen later on, supports the idea that certain nutrients may be needed in greater quantity or in different proportions under conditions of elevated metabolism.

Nutrient deficiency has also been considered. Many experiments, on rats in particular, have indicated that in specific avitaminosis the animal body is more susceptible to climatic stress than when in a condition of adequate nutrition.[3] It has been revealed recently[4] that in the well-fed Canadian population living in temperate climates, there exists in one fourth of the population a low or nonexistent liver reserve of vitamin A.

Recently, it was found in our laboratory that rats fed a diet containing a suboptimal amount of Mg^{++}, which otherwise satisfied the daily requirements recommended by the National Academy of Sciences[7] (Table 2), became increasingly sensitive to cold with age. The degree of cold resistance of rats fed the same diet but containing a sufficient amount of Mg^{++} did not change with age.[8] Therefore, evidence exists that cold tolerance can be decreased by vitamin or trace mineral deficiencies, or, as will be seen later, can be increased by supplementation of certain vitamins. However, the concept that cold environments modify nutrient requirements or that dietary modification can alleviate the impact of cold stress is still questioned by physiologists and nutritionists.

Table 2
NUTRITIONAL STANDARDS FOR RATS

Nutrient	Daily requirement
Protein (g %)	20.0
Fat (g %)	5.0
Carbohydrate (g %)	—
Amino acids	
L-Tryptophane (g %)	0.15
L-Histidine (g %)	0.30
L-Threonine (g %)	0.50
L-Methionine (g %)	0.60
L-Cystine (g %)	0.20
L-Arginine (g %)	0.75
L-Lysine (g %)	0.90
L-Isoleucine (g %)	0.50
L-Valine (g %)	0.70
L-Leucine (g %)	0.80
L-Phenylalanine (g %)	0.90
L-Tyrosine (g %)	—
Fatty acids	
Linoleic acid (g %)	0.2—0.7
Vitamins (%)	
A (IU)	200.0
D (IU)	—
E (mg)	6.0
C (mg)	—
B_1 (mg)	0.12
B_2 (mg)	0.25
B_6 (mg)	0.12
B_{12} (mg)	0.0005
p-Amino benzoic acid (ml)	—
Niacin (ml)	1.00
Ca-pantothenate (ml)	0.800
K (menadione) (ml)	0.01
H (biotin) (μg)	—
Folic acid (μg)	—
Inositol (mg)	—
Choline (mg)	75.0

Table 2 (continued)
NUTRITIONAL STANDARDS FOR RATS

Nutrient	Daily requirement
Minerals (%)	
Calcium (mg)	600.0
Magnesium (mg)	40.0
Sodium (mg)	50.0
Potassium (mg)	180.0
Iron (mg)	2.5
Phosphorus (mg)	500.0
Zinc (mg)	1.2
Copper (mg)	0.5
Iodine (mg)	0.015
Cobalt (mg)	—
Selenium (mg)	4.0
Manganese (mg)	5.0

NUTRIENT REQUIREMENTS IN COLD ENVIRONMENTS

Calories

Johnson and Kark observed that fully acclimatized troops living under a wide range of climatic conditions voluntarily consumed more calories in cold regions than in warm regions.[9] On the basis of this data, Keys has calculated that the caloric intake varies with temperature according to the formula cal/man/day = 4660 − 15.9 T, where T is the temperature in degrees Fahrenheit. This finding has been confirmed by Swain et al.[10] in a survey of the voluntary food consumption by a garrison of soldiers stationed at Fort Churchill, Manitoba.

The relation of diet to survival and food intake in normal and cold environments has been extensively investigated by Stevenson.[11] In animals chronically exposed to cold temperature, increased food intake is well known.[12] Johnson and Kark[9] attribute the temperature-calorie relationship to (a) a greater calorie expenditure for a given task in the colder climates because of the hobbling effect of Arctic clothing and equipment, and (b) the need for more heat in cold climates to maintain thermal equilibrium.

It has been claimed that if more calories are needed in the cold, their distribution between protein, carbohydrate, and fat does not have to change. Johnson and Kark,[9] Swain et al.,[10] and Milan et al.[13] all found that the percentage of calories in protein, carbohydrate, and fat does not change with environmental temperature in normal voluntary nutrition.

Proteins

Many observations indicate that protein metabolism is altered by cold exposure. When fasting rats are exposed to −5°C for 6 hr[14] there is a marked decrease in plasma proline, followed by decreases in methionine, threonine, arginine, and lysine. In contrast, the plasma levels of leucine, phenylalanine, and valine markedly increase. Urinary excretion of alanine, valine, serine, threonine, glycine, and glutamic acid have also been found to increase upon cold exposure.[15,16]

Effects of moderate cold exposure on two enzymes directly involved in protein metabolism have also been reported. Schayer et al.[17] found a marked increase of histidine decarboxylase in mice exposed to 2°C for 6 hr. By allowing cold-exposed rats to eat only as much protein as their warm mates, Klain and Vaughan[18] showed that the activities of tryptophan peroxidase and tyrosine-α-ketoglutaric acid transaminase were increased directly by the cold stress and not by increased food consumption. In contrast, the increased arginase activity was a direct result of a higher protein intake.

Excretion of nitrogenous compounds other than amino acids also increased in the cold when food intake was equalized[19,20] or when rats were allowed to feed ad libitum.[21-23] Greater excretion has also been reported for urea, allantoin, creatine,[15,16,24] creatinine,[25,26] and uric acid.[25]

In spite of all these alterations in protein metabolism during cold exposure, protein has never been found to be the most efficient source of energy for the extra heat required in cold climates. Animal experimentation,[27,28] as well as studies on humans,[29,30] yielded negative results when a comparison was made between a normally adequate protein intake and a high dietary level of that nutrient. Increasing the amount of protein in the diet may not improve cold tolerance, but supplementing a diet with an individual amino acid may be a different question. Animals subjected to cold and given 10% glycine in the diet exceed their controls in ability to maintain liver glycogen during fasting.[31] Upon sudden severe cold exposure, maintenance of liver glycogen might be a definite advantage. Incorporation of 1% glutamic acid to the diet, however, failed to prolong survival of rats exposed to cold.[32]

Stevenson[11] found that during complete starvation at 2 to 5°C, rats previously fed high-protein, high-carbohydrate, or high-fat diets survived essentially the same length of time.

In comparison with fats and sugars, Keeton and co-workers[29] found that proteins exert a depressing effect on tolerance to cold in man. According to Mitchell and Edman,[30] the specific dynamic action of proteins cannot contribute significantly to total heat production in nonresting subjects exposed to cold.

Finally, when animals are restricted to a single nutrient, protein is hardly better in the cold than complete starvation.[33]

However, the fact remains that under moderately cold conditions, rats can consume an imbalanced diet and grow as well as controls, whereas in warm environment a similar diet causes a considerable decrease in food intake and a severe retardation[18] in growth. The imbalance was caused by adding to the basic diet either 5% L-leucine or an amino mixture lacking histidine, or by incorporating 0.4% DL-methionine and 0.6% DL-phenylalanine to a 6% fibrin diet or by omitting isoleucine or isoleucine and valine. The observations by Pastro et al.[34,35] that body temperature is increased and thyroid activity is diminished when chicks are fed a lysine-deficient diet have raised the possibility that the improved utilization of diets imbalanced or deficient in amino acids may occur because cold stress facilitates the dissipation of excess heat. The capacity of rats to gain weight with an imbalanced low protein diet in moderately cold environments gives no indication as to their degree of cold tolerance upon exposure to severely cold temperature.

Lipids

Through animal experimentation, much evidence has been obtained indicating that lipid metabolism is greatly increased in chronic cold exposure:

1. The turnover and oxidation rates of fatty acids are greater[36]
2. The rate of synthesis from glucose is increased[37]
3. Synthesis of fatty acids in adipose tissue as measured in vitro is much greater[38]
4. Serum levels of triglycerides and VLD lipoproteins are depressed[39] and activity of lipoprotein lipase is greater,[40] indicating greater uptake of triglycerides in peripheral tissues[41,42]
5. Noradrenaline induces an increase in triglyceride hydrolysis in brown fat tissue, resulting in the release of fatty acids from their storage form[43]

As early as 1937, Kayser claimed that lipids were preferentially used for cold thermogenesis,[44] or, in other words, that a greater proportion of lipids and consequently a smaller proportion of carbohydrates were utilized for heat production in cold environments than at warm temperatures. In 1960, however, Depocas and Masironi[45] showed by measuring various parameters of glucose metabolism using C^{14} glucose that lipids cannot be considered as preferentially used for cold thermogenesis under steady state conditions, since carbohydrates were involved in the same proportion at 6°C as under basal warm conditions.

Lipids may not be preferentially used in the cold, but the fact remains that during depletion of energy reserves the major portion of the extra heat produced by cold-exposed animals is obtained from noncarbohydrate reserves, most likely from lipids.[45] From this large utilization of lipids, the possibility arises that perhaps for maximum cold resistance it would be preferable to supply the organism with more dietary lipids than with carbohydrates to be transformed by the body into lipids for extra heat production.

There is evidence in the literature that supports this possibility. In 1945, Dugal and his collaborators[46] studied the ability of warm-acclimated rats to resist cold temperatures (-2 or -4°C) when fed equal amounts of vitamins and isocaloric diets in which only the proportions of proteins, carbohydrates, and fats varied. Rats on high-fat diet (51% of calories coming from lipids) showed a survival rate of 80% after 20 days at -2°C, as compared to 40% for the high-carbohydrate group (79% of calories provided by dextrose). Later on, Pagé and Babineau[28] showed that in a cold environment, rats on a high-fat diet had larger gains in body weight without being significantly fatter. In 1957, Leblanc[47] observed a much greater cold resistance in rats fed a high-fat semisynthetic diet containing 17% oil or lard than in rats fed a laboratory chow containing 3.5% fat. It is impossible to attribute the increased cold resistance to the amount or type of fat in the diets because there were many other differences between laboratory chow and the semisynthetic diets. That the type of fat can influence cold resistance in rats was clearly demonstrated in Beare's experiment. Rats fed a semipurified diet containing 20% corn oil gained weight at 4°C, whereas rats fed the same diet containing 20% rapeseed oil instead of corn oil lost weight and died in 4 to 38 days, with a mean survival time of 15 days.[48]

It is generally believed that in a cold environment men prefer foods of higher caloric density (rich in fat).[49] Milan, Elsner, and Rodahl[13] have reported an increased avidity for fat in personnel at an Antarctic base. In 1947, on the other hand, Johnson and Kark[9] had reported "no evidence of the appetite for fat supposed to develop during a sojourn in the Arctic." This was corroborated by Swain et al.[10] 2 years later.

Mitchell et al.[50] have shown that high-fat rations are better than high-carbohydrate ones in cold environments. Criteria of efficiency included body temperature, psychomotor tests, and visual efficiency.

Eskimos may have a diet rich in fat and protein by necessity because of a lack of available carbohydrates, but this cannot be taken as an indication that high fat diets are better in cold environments. In fact, since metabolic measurements done on Eskimos[51] revealed no marked physiological differences between Eskimos and Caucasians, it was concluded that the principal adaptation of the Eskimo was to increase his insulation technologically with clothing and shelter.

Since high-fat diets containing 2% cholesterol have been shown by Sellers and Baker[52] to increase the incidence or severity of coronary atherosclerosis in rats chronically exposed to cold, the possible advantage gained by a high-fat diet in terms of cold resistance will have to be weighed against permanent damage it could cause to arterial vessels.

Carbohydrates

High-carbohydrate, low-protein meals are more potent than high-protein, low carbohydrate meals in combatting the effect of cold by slowing the rate of deep tissue and surface cooling. On the other hand, high fat diets fed for long periods of time are better than high carbohydrate ones.[30] These experiments were carried out in a small experimental chamber (14 X 10.5 X 8.5 ft) which restricted activity; provisions made for exercise were rarely used. Moreover, clothing was purposely planned not to protect the subjects completely from cold since it was essential to the purpose of the experiments that thermal equilibrium not be maintained.

Under more natural conditions in the field, where human beings may have to carry on heavy work for many hours in severely cold weather without access to food, prefeeding of a high-carbohydrate diet for a few days may produce definite advantages. It is known that during prolonged heavy exercise (80% of maximal oxygen consumption [VO_2]) glycogen content in muscle drops to zero or very close to zero within 80 min, at which time the subject is exhausted.[53] Whenever the glycogen depot is depleted, it is no longer possible for the subject to perform at this high work level. On the other hand, it is also known that the higher the initial glycogen store, the longer a heavy work load can be maintained.[54,55] Moreover, after 72 hr of feeding on a high-carbohydrate diet (2300 kcal carbohydrates and 500 kcal protein), the glycogen store is twice as high as after 3 days of a mixed diet. As pointed out by the author of these studies,[53-55] the results showed clearly the importance of available carbohydrate stores for the subject's capacity to perform prolonged heavy exercise. In cold exposure, available carbohydrates may be an important limiting factor for prolonged work performance.

Vitamins

The need for a greater dietary concentration of certain specific nutrients such as vitamins and minerals in cold environments is at this time only vaguely suspected. As mentioned by Pagé,[56] "It is clear that increased requirements of certain vitamins in cold environment may not be due specifically to cold per se but may result from the greater wear and tear of enzymes entailed by a higher metabolic rate. Other vitamins may achieve a greater importance than at ordinary environmental temperature because of the coming into preeminence of some particular biochemical process."

Many have suspected that the daily requirements for vitamins may be much higher than the recommended allowances under stressful conditions such as disease, reproduction, cold environments, climatic changes, etc. In 1956, Krehl[57] even spoke of an optimum nutrition which he described as "that which provides all dietary nutrients in respect to kind and amount, and in proper state of combination or balance so that the organism may always meet the varied exogenous and endogenous stresses of life, whether in health or disease, with a minimal demand or strain on the body's natural homeostatic mechanisms." According to Mitchell,[58] "Among the foreseeable stresses for which vitamin defenses may be set up in time are seasonal or climatic stresses."

Multivitamin Supplements

Assuming that massive doses of vitamins would with time increase cellular reserves and provide cells with a greater intrinsic capacity to respond to stressful conditions, numerous studies have been conducted on human beings to verify if vitamin supplementation would increase health, physical fitness, endurance, work performance, or resistance to fatigue, cold, or infections.

When elementary-school children in England[59] were provided with vitamin supplements containing vitamins A, D, C, and three of the B complex, thiamine, riboflavin, and nicotinamide, in minimal concentrations recommended by the Committee on Nutrition of the British Medical Association, no beneficial effects were found on growth, muscular strength, or absence from school on account of illness. On the other hand, when aircraft workers in California[60] were provided with the same vitamins but in concentrations five to ten times higher than the recommended allowances, a definite improvement was observed which resulted in a savings of 10.5 working days per man per year.

When soldiers were provided with vitamins C and B (no A or D) in concentrations that were from 2 to 6 times greater than the recommended allowances, no improvement in cold endurance was observed,[61] but when soldiers were provided with the same vitamins (no A or D) in concentrations 20 to 30 times higher than the recommended allowances, a significant improvement in cold resistance was found.[62]

From these studies, it can be concluded that the beneficial effect of vitamin supplementation on resistance to stress will be ascertained only (1) when different concentrations are tested for different lengths of time, and (2) when the initial assumption is verified, that is, whether high vitamin intake can increase vitamin reserves in tissues and whether resistance to stress is correlated with this vitamin build up.

Individual Vitamin Supplements
Ascorbic Acid

About 20 years ago, Dugal[63] showed very convincingly that high doses of ascorbic acid increased cold resistance in rats, guinea pigs, and monkeys. These studies are perhaps the only ones showing that (1) the feeding of massive doses of a vitamin results in the accumulation of that vitamin in tissues, and (2) the facility to adapt to cold is proportional to the level of ascorbic acid in tissues, especially in adrenals. These observations tend to substantiate the assumption mentioned above that massive doses would with time increase cellular reserves and provide cells with a greater intrinsic capacity to respond to stress. In fact, Dugal and his colleagues found that the typical enlargement of the adrenals under the influence of cold was completely prevented in rats and guinea pigs if they received large doses of ascorbic acid. Those which had the smaller adrenals were more resistant to cold.

Resistance to $-20°C$ in preadapted monkeys was substantially increased with doses of 325 mg/day of ascorbic acid as opposed to 25 mg/day. On a 0.74 body-weight basis, an effective dose in human beings would have been 2135 mg/day, but when experiments on men were conducted, only 200 mg,[61] 500 mg,[64] or 1200 mg[62] were used, resulting in negative results except with the highest dose, where a slight but significant increase in cold tolerance was found. However, since in this latter study other vitamins were also given, it cannot be said conclusively that the improvement was due to ascorbic acid.

In 1974, Canadian investigators[62a] showed that a daily 1000-mg supplement of vitamin C reduced significantly the incidence and severity of colds in troops undergoing operational training in the Arctic. Wilson et al.[62b] reached essentially the same conclusion: 500 mg/day of ascorbic acid for 9 months had definite beneficial effects in schoolgirls reducing the severity and intensity of colds. On the other hand, Walker et al.[62c] reported that after 3 days of a treatment of 3 g of ascorbic acid daily, volunteers receiving intranasal drops of influenza virus developed colds with the same incidence and severity as controls treated with placebo tablets. These divergent results suggest that the length of time high doses of vitamin C are given may be more important than the dose itself.

Dietary intake of 300 mg/day of ascorbic acid has been found to increase performance in situations where higher energy production was required. Scheunert,[65] for example, reported a reduced rate of absenteeism due to illness in workers of a factory in Leipzig receiving a vitamin C supplement for 242 days. Work performance on an ergometer was found to increase by 21% with a daily supplemental dose of 300 mg.[66] In both cases, the beneficial effect might have been due to an insufficient initial intake.

When large doses of vitamins, well above the minimum dose required to prevent deficiencies, are recommended, the danger of hypervitaminosis with undesirable consequences and even permanent damage is raised immediately. In 1968, Raskin wrote a review article on hypervitaminosis in man[66a] in which he refers to different Russian studies presenting scientific evidence that large doses of vitamin C lead to hypervitaminosis and cause pathological damage. It had been shown that high concentrations of vitamin C (1 to 1.5 g) caused glycosuria.[66b] Urine sugar level remained elevated for 30 days after the vitamin C treatment was stopped, even though vitamin C levels in serum and urine had returned to normal. This latter observation led Raskin to conclude in his review that glycosuria was the result of toxic damage to the epithelium of the renal tubules, even though no histological examination of the kidneys had been done and no other functional tests had been performed to evaluate the integrity of the kidneys. Since the old and unspecific method of Szomogyi-Nelson[66c] was used to determine glucose in urine, it is difficult to attach great importance to these results. However, they are sufficient to raise some doubts and to justify a new study with more modern and more specific methods.

In another study, Gordonoff[66d] showed that guinea pigs who received very large doses of vitamin C (500 mg s.c./day) previous to a scurvy diet fell prey to and died of scurvy earlier than those having previously received physiological amounts of vitamin C.

Large doses of ascorbic acid may also have undesirable effects on the course of pregnancy; with 6 g of vitamin C for 3 days, pregnancy in guinea pigs was interrupted.[66a]

The possibility that large doses of vitamin C given to healthy unstressed subjects may have deleterious effects cannot be ruled out, and more research is definitely required to provide a clear-cut answer to this problem. The fact still remains, however, that under stressful conditions such as severe cold exposure the vitamin C requirement may increase. It is possible that under such circumstances a rapid utilization could preclude any damage, which still remains hypothetical. It must be noted here that in 1972, Körner et al.,[66e] following an extensive and critical review of the literature, could find no evidence of prejudicial effect on health caused by vitamin C, even if administered in high doses.

Pantothenic Acid

The second vitamin that has been shown to increase cold resistance both in animals and human subjects is pantothenic acid.[67] After 6 weeks of 10 g of calcium pantothenate per day, a higher body temperature was maintained by men immersed in water at 9°C for 8 min than before vitamin supplementation. The increased level of blood ascorbic acid and the decreased fall in eosinophil count upon cold stress following the pantothenate treatment was interpreted by the investigator as indicating a reduced output of adrenal cortical hormones, owing to a greater intrinsic capacity of cells to response to stress.

Claim for increased requirement of other vitamins has not been based on direct measurement of cold resistance but on parameters such as weight gain or urinary loss of the vitamins.

Pyridoxine

György[68] observed that acrodynia, a symptom of pyridoxine deficiency, appears in rats earlier at 40°F than at comfortable temperatures. György called attention to the striking similarity between acrodynia in the rat and the well-known syndrome of chilblains in man, and suggested that susceptibility to chilblains may be a function of pyridoxine reserves in the body, and that pyridoxine medication may be of value in the prevention of chilblains.

Thiamine

On the basis of body weight gain, Hegsted and McPhee[69] estimated the daily requirement of thiamine in rats to be 62 μg/kg body weight at 55°F and 42 μg at 78°F.

Riboflavin

In an unpublished experiment on pigs, it was found in the Division of Animal

Nutrition at the University of Illinois that at 40°F the urinary loss of riboflavin was less than the loss at 85°F, which was interpreted as indicating a greater requirement for riboflavin in a cold environment.

Vitamin A

In 1952, Ershoff showed a daily oral requirement of 0.9 μg of vitamin A for rats at room temperature and 1.7 μg for rats maintained in the cold.[70] More recently, Sundaresan and co-workers[71] demonstrated that when rats were fed a vitamin A-deficient diet at least a daily injection of 100 μg of retinoic acid was necessary for survival and growth at 5°C, whereas approximately 5 μg was sufficient at 25°C. On the basis of a lowered blood carotene and vitamin A level during cold weather, Keener et al.[72] also concluded that the vitamin A requirement of calves increases in cold weather.

Not only does the vitamin A requirement appear to be greater in cold than in warm environments, cold resistance is severely reduced when animals are fed a diet deficient in vitamin A, without any vitamin A supplementation.[70,71]

The storage of vitamin A in liver was found to be directly related to the intake of that vitamin. Judging from appearance, survival, and body weight, Rapport[73] found that, with vitamin A intake close to the minimum requirement of rats living at ordinary temperature, i.e., 40 IU per week, cold-acclimated rats do not seem to be unfavorably affected, except for a reduced liver storage. After 4 months, rats kept at 25°C and consuming 40 IU of vitamin A per week had a total of 103 ± 10.4 μg of vitamin A in their liver, while rats at 0 to 2°C with the same intake had only 57 ± 7.8 μg in their liver. When rats were fed an excess of vitamin A (with Master Lab Chow, a rat would consume 3314 IU per week at 25°C and approximately 5565 IU at 0 to 2°C), the vitamin A content of the liver of rats kept at 25°C for 4 to 7 months was 12,850 μg, while the vitamin A liver content of rats kept at 0 to 2°C was 22,100 μg. Rapport also found that the longer the animal stayed in the cold, the more vitamin A it accumulated.

Apparently, an animal in the cold supplied with a large amount of vitamin A in its diet, can store it and live successfully for months. However, no one knows what, if any, is the long-term effect of such a large storage.

A low vitamin A intake resulting in a low vitamin A storage in the liver may not interfere with adaptation to moderately cold temperatures in rats[71] or in humans,[4-6] but it has not yet been demonstrated how successful these rats or men would be in resisting severely cold conditions.

The experimental evidence that cold tolerance in animals is greatly affected by a vitamin A deficiency in their diets, that the vitamin A requirement is greater in cold temperatures than in warm, and the recent demonstration that one quarter of the Canadian population show a low vitamin A reserve in liver raises an important question: How would such a low reserve affect cold resistance, health, and performance of workers transferred to the Arctic?

Other Vitamins

The requirements in cold environments for any of the other vitamins, i.e., vitamins D, E, K, B_{12}, niacin, pyridoxine, folic acid, and biotin, have not been studied. A greater requirement for the B vitamins in the cold could be surmised from their function as coenzymes involved in chemical reactions taking place in energy production. When metabolic energy is increased by dessicated thyroid administration, the thiamine requirement is also increased;[74] muscular exercise has the same effect.[75]

Minerals

As far as the author knows, no one has verified whether a high mineral intake could improve cold resistance, as measured by maintenance of homeothermy upon exposure to severely cold temperature.

Despite numerous observations showing that low environmental temperature affects electrolyte metabolism, dietary requirements of potassium, sodium, phosphorus, calcium, and chlorine have never been studied.

Magnesium

The requirement for magnesium in the rat as influenced by environmental temperature was evaluated only on the basis of weight gain. Hegsted and co-workers[76] found that twice as much magnesium was needed at 55°F than at 78°F. McAleese and Forbes,[77] on the other hand, could not see any effect of environmental temperature on the Mg^{++} requirement for maximum weight gain. Upon acute exposure to cold, an increase in the serum Mg^{++} values was reported in rats.[78] It is most probable that the initial increase in magnesium is due to secretion of adrenaline,[80] which is known to result from sudden cold exposure. Its physiological significance, however, is unknown. Whereas Hannon et al.[81] found the Mg^{++} level in serum to remain elevated after 30 days of cold exposure, Neubeiser et al.[78] found that this electrolyte returned to its initial level after the same length of time in the cold.

After 7 to 11 weeks of chronic cold exposure, the urinary excretion of Mg^{++} in rats was found to be more than twice as high as at normal temperatures.[82] The validity of these excretion rates is doubtful, however, because they were obtained after a 24-hr fasting period, which may have a very different effect on animals kept at 5°C and maintaining a high metabolic rate than in rats at 25°C which have a much lower metabolic rate.

Subarctic exposure (3 winter months) of men at Fort Churchill, Manitoba, resulted in a significant drop in Mg^{++} serum level.[83] Without any measurements of heat loss or cold resistance, the hypothesis was advanced that the lowered serum magnesium level induced a decrease in the sensitivity of the heat loss center of the hypothalamus, potentiating the action of the heat conservation center during cold acclimatization.

All these contradictory results regarding the effect of low environmental temperatures on magnesium metabolism indicate clearly that the role of magnesium in cold acclimation and its dietary requirement will be known only when studies are performed under conditions of controlled Mg^{++} intake, and when resistance is correlated with Mg^{++} intake, serum Mg^{++} level, and urinary Mg^{++} loss.

Magnesium being a cofactor for all enzymes involved in the production of energy, it would not be surprising to find that cold resistance can be improved by high magnesium intake, as long as all the other necessary nutrients are present in optimum quantities. In an unpublished study conducted in our laboratory, it was found that a chronic suboptimal intake of magnesium was much more detrimental in rats living at 6°C than in rats living at 28°C. In comparing two groups of rats fed a semisynthetic diet, which satisfied the recommended daily allowances for rats and which contained 52 mg of magnesium/100 g of diet for the control group and only 12.5 mg of magnesium for the experimental group, it was observed that at 6°C the low Mg^{++} group displayed retarded growth, had twice as much calcium in the heart, had more severe and more numerous cardiomyopathies, and had a much shorter lifespan than the control group. At 28°C the feeding of a suboptimal amount of magnesium also resulted in reduced growth, but it did not result in an accumulation of Ca^{++} in the heart, greater incidence of cardiomyopathies, or reduced lifespan. In the absence of any overt sign of magnesium deficiency, a prolonged suboptimal intake of magnesium at 28°C led with age to a gradual reduction in cold resistance, a reduction that did not take place in control rats.

Potassium

As found for magnesium, plasma potassium concentration increases during sudden cold exposure in rats[84-86] as well as in men.[66,70] It also increases during exercise[87] and after injection of isoproterenol[88] or after the release of epinephrine during the crisis of an illness.[89]

The initial increase in potassium plasma level observed during acute cold exposure may be due to the high release of epinephrine or to the increased metabolic activity in muscle, but it may also result from kidney retention of potassium. While a positive balance has been found in the first few days of cold exposure,[84] upon prolonged cold exposure urinary and fecal loss of potassium increases significantly in rats.[78,82,90] The intake, however, is sufficiently large to compensate and to result in a positive balance. According to Baker and Sellers,[84] the plasma level of potassium gradually returns to normal in chronic cold exposure.

Sodium

Initial responses to cold in man include sodium retention,[25,79,84,91] increased plasma sodium level,[84] diuresis,[92,91] reduced water content,[93] and hemoconcentration.[49,94,95] Upon prolonged exposure, even though blood volume, plasma volume, and total body water become greater,[79,86,96,97] sodium concentration in the plasma remains high.[84] Blood volume is also higher in Eskimos than in whites during the winter.[98,99]

In relation to cold resistance and especially resistance to cold injury, changes in peripheral tissue electrolyte composition may be much more important than systemic changes throughout the body. In rats exposed to cold for 7 weeks, the total water content of the skin was increased[100] due to an increase in the chloride "space" and intracellular sodium was decreased. As mentioned by Baker,[101] "Reader[102] found the thermal conductivity of tissues dependent on the water content. A generalized dehydration of peripheral tissues would thus tend to conserve body heat. Conversely, the slowed heat transfer would make the peripheral tissues more prone to cold injury. An increase in extracellular fluid accompanied by a decrease in intracellular fluid might provide for an optimum tolerance to cold." Although only a subjective impression, an observation by Frazier,[103] who was the medical officer of the U.S. Antarctic Service Expedition and who spent a year in Little America III, is of interest. He found that men who had spent considerable time outside had a greater resistance to frostbite than those whose occupations kept them inside. He commented on the apparent dryness of the skin of the outdoor group and considered that dehydration was partially responsible for their resistance to cold injury.

It appears that the early water loss, hemoconcentration, and increase in plasma magnesium, potassium, and sodium are transient and gradually disappear or even become reversed as a result of cold acclimation.

DIETARY INFLUENCE ON STRESS TOLERANCE

Even though both laboratory chow and semisynthetic diets are usually prepared to meet daily nutrient requirements, it is apparent from a review of the literature that they do not provide the same degree of tolerance to stress.

Commercial laboratory chows are usually prepared with distillers dried molasses solubles, dried whey, brewers dried yeast, dehydrated alfalfa meal, fish meal, meat meal, soybean oil meal, cooked corn, cooked wheat, shorts, molasses, apple pomace, and added salts and vitamins. Protein, carbohydrate, and fat sources are then of a mixed nature. The apple pomace, vegetable fibers, and relative undigestibility of the complex protein of animal origin brings down the overall digestibility of the diet to a low level of 67%.

Semisynthetic diets are usually prepared with casein as a source of protein, corn oil, cottonseed oil, or soybean oil as a fat source, cornstarch, or sucrose, for carbohydrates and vitamin and salt mixtures. The absence of fiber and pomace as well as the high degree of digestibility of casein results in an overall digestibility over 97%.

Detailed analysis of typical chow and casein diets (which were used in our experiments) is given in Table 3.

These diets are usually formulated to provide intensive reproduction, lactation, and rapid growth of young in animals kept at room temperature (22 to 23°C). Capacity to tolerate stress is never used as a parameter in the formulation of these diets, yet greater tolerance with synthetic diets than with laboratory chow has been observed under at least six different stressful conditions.

Cold

In warm-acclimated rats as well as in cold-acclimated ones, a semisynthetic, low-iodine, bulk-free diet (T_4F), supplemented with potassium iodide in drinking water, was found to provide the animals with a much greater degree of cold resistance when exposed to $-20°C$ than when fed laboratory chow (MLC).[104,105] One of the main features of this semisynthetic diet ($T_4 F$) is to permit cold adaptation without increased thyroid activity. Since a lower energy balance was found to be maintained with this diet than with MLC,

Table 3
COMPOSITION OF MASTER LABORATORY CHOW (MLC) AND A
SEMISYNTHETIC CASEIN DIET ($T_4 F$)

	MLC(%)	$T_4 F$(%)		MLC(%)	$T_4 F$(%)
Moisture	10.5	11.1	Carbohydrate	49.3	49.8
Protein	22.9	24.0	Fiber	3.5	0.0
Fat	4.7	12.4	Ash	9.6	2.7

Amino Acids (Grams of Amino Acid Residue per 100 g of Wet Diet)

Lysine	1.159	2.720	Serine	0.424	0.090
Histidine	0.453	0.818	Glutamic acid	2.349	3.938
Threonine	0.481	0.518	Proline	1.305	3.423
Valine	0.435	1.163	Hydroxyproline	a	0.050
Methionine	0.093	0.348	Tryptophane	0.240	0.290
Leucine	0.988	1.889	Glycine	1.160	0.092
Isoleucine	0.495	1.066	Alanine	0.468	0.337
Phenylalanine	0.641	0.756	Tyrosine	0.483	0.847
Arginine	1.242	1.007	Cystine	0.300	0.216
Aspartic acid	1.231	1.070			

Fatty Acids (mol %)

Myristic	0.9	0.7	Oleic	23.8	21.2
Palmitic	19.1	20.5	Linoleic	44.6	55.0
Stearic	5.1	2.6	Linolenic	6.0	0.0

Vitamins[b]

A (units/%)	1894	1982	Ca-pantothenate (mg/%)	1.586	6.61
D (units/%)	308	220	Inositol (mg/%)	—	11.01
B_1 (mg/%)	0.749	2.20	E (mg/%)	7.27	11.01
B_2 (mg/%)	1.320	2.20	K (mg/%)	0.11	4.96
B_6 (mg/%)	0.132	2.20	B_{12} (μg/%)	1.76	2.97
C (mg/%)	$-^c$	99.1	H (μg/%)	15.4	44.05
Choline (mg/%)	132	165.2	Folic acid (μg/%)	300	198
Niacin (mg/%)	7.05	9.91			
p-Aminobenzoic acid (mg/%)	—	11.01			

Table 3 (continued)
COMPOSITION OF MASTER LABORATORY CHOW (MLC) AND A
SEMISYNTHETIC CASEIN DIET (T_4F)

	MLC(%)	T_4F(%)		MLC(%)	T_4F(%)
			Minerals (mg/%)		
Calcium	1570	780	Zinc	15	1.4
Magnesium	250	31	Lead	0.8	0.4
Sodium	380	120	Copper	1.1	1.1
Potassium	760	360	Nickel	0.3	0.1
Iron	21	8.3	Cobalt	0.4	0.08
Manganese	14	1.2	Iodine	0.1	—
Phosphorus	720	130			
			Hormones (μg/%)		
Thyroxine	52.0	0			

[a] Undetectable.
[b] Vitamin values are those reported by the manufacturer.
[c] Not given by the manufacturer.

its slightly higher caloric content (4.9 cal/g vs. 4.3 cal/g for MLC) does not appear to be the responsible factor for providing greater cold resistance.

The fact that metabolic sensitivity to norepinephrine (NE) was the same in both groups[106] suggests that some factor other than catecholamine secretion was responsible for the increased cold resistance of rats fed the T_4F diet. A low caloric uptake, accompanied by faster growth and maintenance of a higher body temperature in T_4F-fed rats than in MLC-fed rats,[107] indicates strongly that the T_4F diet permits a lower heat loss. Since MLC and T_4F diets are different in many respects,[105] it is impossible to attribute the superiority of T_4F to any particular dietary factor. A systematic screening is required.

In 1945, Dugal and his collaborators[46] compared the ability of rats to resist extreme temperatures (−2 or −4°C) when fed equal amounts of vitamins and isocaloric diets in which only the proportions of proteins, carbohydrates, and fats varied. Rats on the high-fat diet (51% of calories coming from lipids) preadapted to their diet (2 weeks) showed a survival of 80% after 20 days at −2°C, as compared to 40% for the high-carbohydrate group (79% of caolories provided by dextrose).

In our studies mentioned above,[104] non-cold-acclimated rats fed the semisynthetic diet could withstand much more extreme temperature (−20°C) than the rats in Dugal's experiment (−2 or −4°C)[46] for at least 5 hr without becoming hypothermic. Rats fed the usual commercial chow performed comparably only if they were preadapted to cold (+6°C).

Leblanc[47] also observed a much greater cold resistance in rats fed a high-fat semisynthetic diet containing 17% oil or lard than in rats fed a laboratory chow containing 3.5% fat.

Dugal's, Leblanc's, and our own studies demonstrate clearly that cold resistance is a diet-dependent phenomenon.

Hypophysectomy

Between 60 and 70% of rats fed casein diets ad libitum after surgical removal of the hypophysis survived for experimental periods of at least 88 and 112 days. Only 10% of comparable rats offered laboratory chow survived beyond 45 days, and none survived more than 63 days.[107]

DDT

In 1966, Ortega[108] reported that rats fed a semipurified diet were able to survive a dose (1000 ppm) of DDT which proved in an earlier study to be quickly toxic to similar rats fed lab chow.

Hemorrhage

The development of extraintestinal lesions (heart, kidney, and lungs) in dogs submitted to severe hemorrhagic shock was found to be correlated with the appearance of a necrotic degeneration of the intestinal mucosa.[109] These pathological sequelae could be prevented from occurring if a pure chemical diet was used in place of the regular kennel chow.

Radiation

Thirty days after irradiation with 900 R (X-rays), 85% of the mice on lab chow were dead, but only 55% of those on a semisynthetic diet succumbed.[110]

Antimetabolite

In patients eating a normal hospital diet, treatment of advanced metastatic carcinoma with 5-fluorouracil (5FU) is associated with significant weight loss and specific lesions of the rectal mucosa. A comparable group of patients eating a hydrolysed elemental diet (Mead Johnson 3200 AS) prepared with a casein hydrolysate 4 days before and throughout the 6 to 9 days of 5 FU treatment had no rectal lesions and maintained their pretreatment body weight.[111]

In this case as well as in those above, it may be noted that the source of protein in the synthetic diets was either casein, a casein hydrolysate, or a mixture of pure amino acids in proportions found in casein. Not only do casein diets provide rats with a greater degree of stress tolerance than does lab chow, it also increases their longevity. Average lifespan of rats kept at 23°C and fed Purina lab chow was found to be 729 days, while life spans of rats fed different casein diets varying only in their proportion of casein and cane sugar ranged between 840 and 925 days.[112] However, the numerous differences between lab chows and the different semisynthetic diets preclude any attempt at attributing the greater stress tolerance provided by the synthetic diet to any given nutrient.

CONCLUSIONS

As far as calories and sources of calories are concerned, the preceding review of the literature reveals quite clearly that:

1. Calorie requirement is increased in cold environments.
2. The most efficient source of energy for extra heat in cold climates is not protein.
3. In chronic cold exposure, high-fat diets appear preferable to high-protein or high-carbohydrate diets, but more clear-cut evidence is required.

It remains to be seen whether prefeeding of a high-carbohydrate diet in order to build up glycogen stores would be beneficial in practical situations where a man has to work hard in severely cold weather for several hours without eating. The possibility that cold tolerance may be influenced by different quality of protein, carbohydrate, or fat remains to be fully explored.

As for vitamin needs in cold environments, there is sufficient experimental evidence to conclude with reasonable certitude that:

1. In specific avitaminosis, the animal body is more susceptible to climatic stress than in a condition of adequate nutrition.

2. On the basis of survival or maintenance of body temperature, animals chronically exposed to cold have greater requirements for ascorbic acid, pantothenic acid, or vitamin A than those in warm environments. Thiamin and riboflavin have also been claimed to be required in greater amounts in the cold, not on a cold resistance basis (as measured by maintenance of body temperature) but on a weight basis or urinary loss basis. The need for any of the other vitamins in cold environments is unknown.

3. The accumulation of vitamin C in tissues, especially in the adrenals, and of vitamin A in liver when large dietary supplements are given, as well as the correlation between the degree of cold resistance and the degree of vitamin C accumulation, strongly supports the concept that large supplements of vitamins can increase vitamin stores and result in greater cold tolerance.

The limited success obtained with humans in attempts to raise cold tolerance with vitamin supplementation may have been due to supplementation of too-low concentrations of vitamins for too short a period of time, or too-short preexposures to cold which prevented a significant accumulation of vitamins in tissues.

Whether a high mineral content in the diet can have an effect on the initial electrolyte changes taking place during cold exposure and whether this would be beneficial in terms of cold resistance remains to be seen.

Finally, sufficient experimental evidence exists to demonstrate that different diets may in all appearances satisfy the minimum requirements, promote reasonable growth, and yet provide animals with a very different degree of stress resistance.

In previous cold-environment nutritional studies, emphasis was always placed on caloric expenditure, caloric requirements, and optimal proportion of main nutrients (protein, fat, carbohydrates, and quantity of certain vitamins). In the future, more attention will have to be paid to minerals, vitamins, and quality of the main nutrients.

REFERENCES

1. *Recommended Dietary Allowances,* 8th rev. ed., National Academy of Sciences, Washington, D.C., 1974.
2. **Johnson, R. F.,** Caloric requirements under adverse environmental conditions, *Fed. Proc.,* 22(6), 1439–1446, 1963.
3. **Erschoff, B. J.,** Comparative effects of pantothenic acid deficiency and inanition on resistance to cold stress in the rat, *J. Nutr.,* 49, 373–385, 1953.
4. **Hoppner, K., Phillips, W. E. J., Murray, T. K., and Campbell, J. S.,** Survey of liver vitamin A stores of Canadians, *Can. Med. Assoc. J.,* 99, 983–985, 983, 1968.
5. **Hoppner, K., Phillips, W. E. J., Erdody, P., Murray, T. K., Perrin, D. E.,** Vitamin A reserves of Canadians, *Can. Med. Assoc. J.,* 101(12), 84–90, 1969.
6. **Murray, K.,** *Proc. Western Hemisphere Nutr. Conf.,* in press.
7. Committee of Animal Nutrition, *Nutrient Requirements of Laboratory Animals,* Publ. 990, National Academy of Sciences, Washington, D.C., 1962.
8. **Héroux, O.,** unpublished.
9. **Johnson, R. E. and Kark, R. M.,** Environment and food intake in man, *Science,* 105, 378–379, 1947.
10. **Swain, H. L., Toth, F. M., Consolazio, F. C., Fitzpatrick, W. H., Allen, D. I., and Koehn, C. J.,** Food consumption of soldiers in a subarctic climate (Fort Churchill, Manitoba, Canada, 1947–1948), *J. Nutr.,* 38, 63, 1949.
11. **Stevenson, J. A. F.,** *Conf. on Cold Injury, Trans. 3rd Conf. Josiah Macy, Jr. Foundation,* New York, 165–188, 1955.

12. **Hart, J. S.,** Physiological responses to cold in nonhibernating homeotherms, *Temperature − Its Measurement and Control in Science and Industry,* Vol. 3, Part 3, Reinhold, New York, 373–406, 1963.

13. **Milan, F. A., Elsner, R. W., and Rodahl, K.,** The effect of a year in the Antarctic on human thermal and metabolic responses to an acute standardized cold stress, USAF, *Arct. Aeromed. Lab. U.S. Tech. Rep.,* 60(9), 1–21, 1961.

14. **Williams, J. N., Jr., Schurr, P. E., and Elvehjem, C. A.,** Influence of chilling and exercise on free amino acid concentrations in rat, *J. Biol. Chem.,* 182, 55–59, 1950.

15. **Hale, H. B. and Mefferd, R. B., Jr.,** Factorial study of environmentally-induced metabolic changes in rats, *Am. J. Physiol.,* 194, 469–475, 1958.

16. **Mefferd, R. B., Jr., Hall, H. B., and Martens, H. H.,** Nitrogen and electrolyte excretion of rats chronically exposed to adverse environments, *Am. J. Physiol.,* 192, 209–218, 1958.

17. **Schayer, R. M., Houlihan, P., Sestokas, E., and Chapin, L.,** Relation of induced histidine decarboxylase activity and histidine synthesis to shock from stress and from endotoxin, *Am. J. Physiol.,* 198, 1187–1192, 1960.

18. **Klain, G. J. and Vaughan, D. A.,** Alterations of protein metabolism during cold-acclimation, *Fed. Proc.,* 22(3), 862–867, 1963.

19. **Ingle, D. J., Meeks, R. C., and Humphrey, L. M.,** Effects of exposure to cold upon urinary nonprotein nitrogen and electrolytes in adrenalectomized and nonadrenalectomized rats, *Am. J. Physiol.,* 173, 387–389, 1953.

20. **Lathe, G. H. and Peters, R. A.,** Some observations on the comparative effects of cold and burns on protein metabolism in rats, *Q. J. Exp. Physiol.,* 35, 55–64, 1949.

21. **Hannon, J. P. and Young, D. W.,** Effect of prolonged cold exposure on the gross blood composition of the rat, *Am. J. Physiol.,* 197, 1008–1012, 1959.

22. **Treichler, R. and Mitchell, H. H.,** Influence of the plane of nutrition and of environmental temperature on the relationship between basal metabolism and endogenous nitrogen metabolism subsequently determined, *J. Nutr.,* 22, 333–343, 1941.

23. **You, S. S., You, R. W., and Sellers, E. A.,** Effect of thyroidectomy, adrenalectomy and burning on the urinary nitrogen excretion of the rat maintained in a cold environment, *Endocrinology,* 47, 156–161, 1950.

24. **Young, D. R. and Cook, S. F.,** Effect of environmental temperature and dietary protein on urinary and nitrogen excretion of rats, *Proc. Soc. Exp. Biol. Med.,* 89, 482–484, 1955.

25. **Chinn, H. J., Oberst, F. W., Nyman, B., and Fenton, K.,** The Biochemical Changes During Exposure to Cold, USAF School of Aviation Medicine, Proj. Rep. No. 21-23-027, Randolph AFB, Tex., 1950.

26. **Selye, H. J.,** The general adaptation syndrome and the diseases of adaptation, *J. Clin. Endocrinol. Metab.,* 6, 117–230, 1946.

27. **Leblond, C. P., Dugal, L. P., and Thérien, M.,** Les aliments choisis par le rat blanc au froid et à la chaleur, *Rev. Can. Biol.,* 3, 127–129, 1944.

28. **Pagé, E. and Babineau, L. M.,** The effects of diet and cold on body composition and fat distribution in the white rat, *Can. J. Med. Sci.,* 31, 22–40, 1953.

29. **Keeton, R. W., Lambert, E. H., Glickman, N., Mitchell, H. H., Last, J. H., and Fahnestock, M. K.,** The tolerance of man to cold as affected by dietary modifications: proteins versus carbohydrates, and the effect of variable protective clothing, *Am. J. Physiol.,* 146, 66–83, 1946.

30. **Mitchell, H. H. and Edman, M.,** *Nutrition and Resistance to Climatic Stress with Particular Reference to Man,* Charles C Thomas, Springfield, Ill., 1951.

31. **Todd, W. R.,** Maintenance of carbohydrate stores during stress of cold and fatigue in rats prefed diets containing added glycine, *Arct. Aeromed. Lab. U.S. Tech. Rep.,* 60(13), 1, 1961.

32. **Dugal, L. P. and Thérien, M.,** Effets de l'acide glutamique et d'extraits de foie sur la résistance du rat blanc à un froid intense, *Rev. Can. Biol.,* 11, 180–184, 1952.

33. **Giaja, I. and Gelineo, M. S.,** Physiologie − alimentation et résistance au froid, *C.R. Soc. Biol.,* 198, 2277–2278, 1934.

34. **Pastro, K. R., March, B. E., and Biely, J.,** Body temperature of chicks in response to lysine deficiency, *Can. J. Physiol. Pharmacol.,* 47, 339–342, 1969.

35. **Pastro, K. R., March, B. E., and Biely, J.,** Diminished thyroidal activity in chicks in response to lysine deficiency, *Can. J. Physiol. Pharmacol.,* 47, 645–647, 1969.

36. **Masironi, R. and Depocas, F.,** Effect of cold exposure on respiratory $C^{12}O_2$ production during infusion of albumin-bound palmitate-1-C^{14} in white rats, *Can. J. Biochem. Physiol.,* 39, 219–224, 1961.

37. **de Freitas, A. S. W.,** The effects of cold on glyceride, glycerol and fatty-acid synthesis in *Proc. 9th Cold Physiol. Conf.,* Edmonton University of Alberta, Edmonton, Canada, 1–3, 1967.

38. **Patkin, J. K. and Masoro, E. J.,** The effect of cold acclimation on lipid metabolism in adipose tissue, *Arct. Aeromed. Lab. U.S. Tech.Rep.,* 60(41), 1, 1961.

39. **Radomski, M. W.,** Effect of cold exposure on serum lipids and lipoproteins in the rat, *Can. J. Physiol. Pharmacol.,* 44, 711–719, 1966.

40. **Grafnetter, J., Grossi, E., and Morganti, P.,** Effect of catecholamines and cold exposure on lipolytic activity of rat heart, *Med. Pharmacol. Exp.,* 12, 266–273, 1965.

41. **Ballard, F. B., Danforth, W. H., Naegle, S., and Bing, R. J.,** Myocardial metabolism of fatty acids, *J. Clin. Invest.,* 39, 717–723, 1957.

42. **Gousios, A., Felts, J. M., and Havel, R. J.,** The metabolism of serum triglycerides and free fatty acids by the myocardium, *Metabolism,* 12, 75–80, 1963.

43. **Beyer, R. E.,** in *Biochemical Responses to Environmental Stress,* Bernstein, I. A., Ed., Plenum, New York, 1971.

44. **Kayser, C.,** Variations du quotient respiratoire en fonction de la température du milieu chez le rat, le pigeon et la cobaye, *C.R. Soc. Biol.,* 126, 1219–1222, 1937.

45. **Depocas, F. and Masironi, R.,** Body glucose as fuel for thermogenesis in the white rat exposed to cold, *Am. J. Physiol.,* 199, 1051–1055, 1960.

46. **Dugal, L. P., Leblond, C. P., and Thérien, M.,** Resistance to extreme temperatures in connection with different diets, *Can. J. Res.,* 23, 244–258, 1945.

47. **Leblanc, J.,** Prefeeding of high fat diet and resistance of rats to intense cold, *Can. J. Biochem. Physiol.,* 35, 25–30, 1957.

48. **Beare, J. L., Murray, T. K., McLaughlan, J. M., and Campbell, J. A.,** Relative effects of rapeseed oil and corn oil on rats subjected to adrenalectomy, cold, and pyridoxine deprivation, *J. Nutr.,* 80(2), 157–161, 1963.

49. **Burton, A. C., Scott, J. C., McGlone, B., and Bazett, H. C.,** Slow adaptations in the heat exchanges of man to changed climatic conditions, *Am. J. Physiol.,* 129, 84–101, 1940.

50. **Mitchell, H. H., Glickman, N., Lambert, E. H., Keeton, R. W., and Fahnestock, M. K.,** The tolerance of man to cold as affected by dietary modification: carbohydrate versus fat and the effect of frequency of meals, *Am. J. Physiol.,* 146, 84–96, 1946.

51. **Hart, J. S., Sabean, H. B., Hildes, J. A., Depocas, F., Hammel, H. T., Andersen, K. L., Irving, L., and Foy, G.,** Thermal and metabolic responses of coastal Eskimos during a cold night, *J. Appl. Physiol.,* 17(6), 953–960, 1962.

52. **Sellers, E. A. and Baker, D. G.,** Coronary atherosclerosis in rats exposed to cold, *Can. Med. Assoc. J.,* 83, 6–13, 1960.

53. **Saltin, B. and Hermansen, L.,** Glycogen stores and prolonged severe exercise, in *Symp. of the Swedish Nutr. Foundation,* Blixt, G., Ed., Almquist and Wiksell, Uppsala, Sweden, 32–46, 1967.

54. **Hermansen, L., Haltman, E., and Saltin, B.,** Muscle glycogen during prolonged severe exercise, *Acta Physiol. Scand.,* 71, 129–139, 1967.

55. **Bergstrom, J., Hermansen, L., Haltman, E., and Saltin, B.,** Diet muscle glycogen and physical performance, *Acta Physiol. Scand.,* 71, 140–150, 1967.

56. **Pagé, E.,** Low temperature considerations, in *Nutrition Under Climatic Stress. A Symposium,* National Academy of Sciences, Washington, D.C., 183–191, 1954.

57. **Krehl, W. A.,** A concept of optimal nutrition, *Am. J. Clin. Nutr.,* 4, 634–641, 1956.

58. **Mitchell, H. H.,** Vitamin requirements in terms of dietary equivalents, in *Comparative Nutrition of Man and Domestic Animals,* Vol. 2, Academic Press, New York, 1964.

59. **Bransby, E. R., Hunter, J. W., Magee, H. E., Milligan, E. H. M., and Rodgers, T. S.,** The influence of supplements of vitamins A, B, B$_2$, C, and D on growth, health, and physical fitness, *Br. Med. J.,* 1, 77–78, 1944.

60. **Borsook, H., Alpert, E., and Keighley, G. L.,** Nutritional status of aircraft workers in southern California. II. Clinical and laboratory findings, *Milbank Mem. Fund Q.,* 21, 115–157, 1943.

61. **Glickman, N., Keeton, R. W., Mitchell, H. H., and Fahnestock, M. K.,** The tolerance of man to cold as affected by dietary modifications: high versus low intake of certain water-soluble vitamins, *Am. J. Physiol.,* 146, 538–558, 1946.

62. **Ryer, R., III, Grossman, M. I., Friedemann, T. E., Best, W. R., Consolazio, C. F., Kuhl, W. J., Insull, W., Jr., Hatch, F. T.,** and the Staff of the U.S. Army Nutrition Laboratory, Vitamin supplementation of soldiers residing in a cold environment. Part I. Physical performance and response to cold exposure, *J. Clin. Nutr.,* 2, 97–132, 1954.

62a. **Sabiston, B. H. and Radowski, M. W.,** DCIEM Rep. No. 74-R-1012, Defense and Civil Institute of Environmental Medicine, Donsview, Ont., 1, 1974.

62b. **Wilson, C. W. M., Loh, H. S., and Foster, F. G.,** *Eur. J. Clin. Pharmacol.,* 6, 26, 1973.

62c. **Walker, G. H., Bynoe, M. L., and Tyrrell, D. A. J.,** *Br. Med. J.,* 1, 603, 1967.

63. **Dugal, L. P.,** Acclimatization to cold environment, in *Nutrition Under Climatic Stress,* National Academy of Sciences, 70–81, 1954.

64. **Leblanc, J., Stewart, M., Marier, G., and Whillans, M. G.,** Acclimatization and the affect of ascorbic acid in men exposed to cold, *Can. J. Biochem. Physiol.,* 32, 407–427, 1954.

65. **Scheunert, A.,** Daily requirement of the adult for vitamin C, *Int. Z. Vitaminforsch.,* 20, 374–386, 1949.

66. **Hoitink, A. W. J. H.,** Vitamin C and work. Inquiries into the influence of work and of the administration of vitamin C on the human organism, *Verh. Inst. Praevent. Geneesk,* No. 4, 1, 1946.

66a. **Raskin, I. M.,** Hypervitaminosis in man, *Hyg. Sanit.,* 33, 235, 1968.

66b. **Hruba, F. and Mašek, J.,** Einige Aspekte der Wirkung hoher Dosen von L-Ascorbinsäure auf den gesunden Menschen, *Nahrung,* 6, 507–517, 1962.

66c. **Nelson, N.,** A photometric adaptation of the Szomogyi method for the determination of glucose, *J. Biol. Chem.,* 153, 380–395, 1944.

66d. **Gordonoff, Van T.,** Darf man wasser lösliche Vitamine überdosieren, *Schweig. Med. Wochenschr.,* 90(27), 726–729, 1960.

66e. **Körner, W. F. and Weber, F.,** *Int. Z. Vitam. Ern. Forsch.,* 42, 528, 1972.

67. **Ralli, E. P.,** The effect of certain vitamins on the response of normal subjects to cold water stress, in *Nutrition Under Climatic Stress,* National Academy of Sciences, Washington, D.C., 81–90, 1954.

68. **György, P.,** Environmental temperature and 'rat acrodynia', *J. Nutr.,* 16, 69–77, 1938.

69. **Hegsted, M. D. and McPhee, G. S.,** The thiamine requirement of the adult rat and the influence on it of a low environmental temperature, *J. Nutr.,* 41, 127–136, 1950.

70. **Ershoff, B. H.,** Effects of vitamin A malnutrition on resistance to stress, *Proc. Soc. Exp. Biol. Med.,* 79, 580–584, 1952.

71. **Sundaresan, P. R., Winters, V. G., and Therriault, D. G.,** Effect of low environmental temperature on the metabolism of vitamin A (retinol) in the rat, *J. Nutr.,* 92, 474–478, 1967.

72. **Keener, H. A., Bechdel, S. I., Guerrant, N. B., and Thorp, W. T. S.,** Carotene in calf nutrition, *J. Dairy Sci.,* 25, 571, 1942.

73. **Rapport, D.,** Metabolism of fatty acids and related substances in animals exposed to cold, *Arct. Aeromed. Lab. U.S. Tech. Note,* 1–12, 1961.

74. **Cowgill, G. R. and Palmieri, M. L.,** Physiology of vitamins. XXII. The effect of experimentally induced hyperthyroidism on the vitamin B requirement of pigeons, *Am. J. Physiol.,* 105, 146–150, 1933.

75. **Cowgill, G. R., Rosenberg, H. A., and Rogoff, J.,** The physiology of vitamins. XVI. The effect of exercise on the time required for the development of the anorexia characteristic of lack of undifferentiated vitamin B, *Am. J. Physiol.,* 98, 589–594, 1931.

76. **Hegsted, D. M., Vitale, J. J., and McGrath, H.,** The effect of low temperature and dietary calcium upon magnesium requirement, *J. Nutr.,* 58, 175–188, 1956.

77. **McAleese, D. M. and Forbes, R. M.,** Requirement and tissue distribution of Mg in the rat as influenced by environmental temperature and dietary Ca, *J. Nutr.,* 73, 94–106, 1961.

78. **Neubeiser, R. E., Platner, W. S., and Shields, J. L.,** Magnesium in blood and tissues during cold acclimation, *J. Appl. Physiol.,* 16, 247–249, 1961.

79. **Quinn, M., Bass, D. E., and Kleeman, C. R.,** Effect of acute cold exposure on serum potassium and magnesium and the electrocardiogram in man, *Proc. Soc. Exp. Biol. Med.,* 83, 660–661, 1953.

80. **Larvor, P.,** Effect of adrenaline and noradrenaline on magnesemia and glycemia. Influence of dihydroergotamine and insulin, *Ann. Biol. Anim. Biochim. Biophys.,* 8, 461–464, 1968.

81. **Hannon, J. P., Larson, A. M., and Young, D. W.,** Effect of cold acclimatization on plasma electrolyte levels, *J. Appl. Physiol.,* 13, 239–240, 1958.

82. **Mefferd, R. B., Hale, H. B., and Martens, H. H.,** Nitrogen and Electrolyte Excretion of Rats Ohronically Exposed to Adverse Environments, *USAF School of Aviation Medicine Rep. 57-66,* Randolph AFT, Tex., 1957, 1.

83. **Daniels, F., Jr., Quinn, M., Kleeman, C. R., and Marino, J.,** Plasma magnesium changes during cold acclimatization in man, *Fed. Proc.,* 12, 31, 1953.

84. **Baker, D. G. and Sellers, E. A.,** Electrolyte metabolism in the rat exposed to a low environmental temperature, *Can. J. Biochem. Physiol.,* 35, 631–636, 1957.

85. **Booker, W. M., Hayes, R. L., DaCosta, F. D., Jones, W., Hill, R., and Titus, P.,** Analysis of the electrolyte changes in rats during cold stress, *Fed. Proc.,* 11, 15–16, 1952.

86. **Schales, O. and Schales, S. S.,** A simple and accurate method for the determination of chloride in biological fluids, *J. Biol. Chem.,* 140, 879–884, 1941.

87. **Kilburn, K. H.,** Muscular origin of elevated plasma potassium during exercise, *J. Appl. Physiol.,* 21, 675–678, 1966.
88. **Lehr, D., Krukowski, M., and Colon, R.,** Correlation of myocardial and renal necrosis with tissue electrolyte changes, *JAMA,* 197, 105–112, 1966.
89. **D'Silva, J. L.,** Action of adrenaline on serum potassium, *J. Physiol.,* 90, 303–309, 1937.
90. **Fregly, M. J.,** Water and electrolyte exchange in rats exposed to cold, *Can. J. Physiol. Pharmacol.,* 46, 873–881, 1968.
91. **Gibson, A. G.,** On the diuresis of chill, *Q. J. Med.,* 3, 52–60, 1909.
92. **Bader, R. A., Eliot, J. W., and Bass, D. E.,** Hormonal and renal mechanisms of cold diuresis, *J. Appl. Physiol.,* 4, 649–658, 1952.
93. **Eliot, J. W., Bader, R. A., and Bass, D. E.,** Blood changes associated with cold diuresis, *Fed. Proc.,* 8, 41, 1949.
94. **Scott, J. C., Bazett, H. C., and Mackie, G. C.,** Climatic effects on cardiac output and the circulation in man, *Am. J. Physiol.,* 129, 102–122, 1940.
95. **Adolph, E. F. and Molner, G. W.,** Exchange of heat and tolerances to cold in men exposed to outdoor weather, *Am. J. Physiol.,* 146, 507–537, 1946.
96. **Deb, G. and Hart, J. S.,** Hematological and body fluid adjustments during acclimation to a cold environment, *Can. J. Biochem. Physiol.,* 34, 959–966, 1956.
97. **Everett, N. B. and Matson, L.,** The red cell and plasma volumes of the rat and of its individual tissues and organs during acclimatization to cold, *Arct. Aeromed. Lab. U.S. Tech. Rep.,* 60(35), 1, 1961.
98. **Meehan, J. P.,** Racial and individual differences in the peripheral vascular response to a cold stimulus, *Am. J. Physiol.,* 179, 657, 1954.
99. **Brown, G. M., Bird, G. S., Boag, T. J., Boag, L. M., Delahaye, J. D., Green, J. E., Hatcher, J. D., and Page, J.,** The circulation in cold acclimatization, *Circulation,* 9, 813–822, 1954.
100. **Baker, D. G.,** Electrolyte metabolism in the rat exposed to a low environmental temperature, *Can. J. Biochem. Physiol.,* 38, 205–211, 1960.
101. **Baker, D. G.,** Influence of cold exposure on electrolyte metabolism (in man and rat), *Fed. Proc.,* 19, Suppl. 5, 125–130, 1959.
102. **Reader, S. R.,** The effective thermal conductivity of normal and rheumatic tissues in response to cooling, *Clin. Sci.,* 11, 1–12, 1952.
103. **Frazier, G.,** Acclimatization and the effects of cold on the human body as observed at Little America III, on the United States Antarctic Service Expedition 1939-1941, *Proc. Am. Philos. Soc.,* 89, 249–255, 1945.
104. **Deslauriers, R., Zoami, J., McCullough, R. S., and Héroux, O.,** Caloric uptake and cold resistance in cold-acclimated rats fed commercial chow or semipurified diet, *Can. J. Physiol. Pharmacol.,* 49(7), 707–712, 1971.
105. **Héroux, O., Russel, D. S., Wong, T. K., and Campbell, J. S.,** Diet-induced cold resistance and focal myocytolysis of heart in warm-acclimated rats exposed to −18°C, *Rep. Proc. Int. Symp. Environ. Physiol. (Bioenergetics),* FASEB, Washington, D. C., 185–189, 1972.
106. **Héroux, O.,** Thyroid parameters and metabolic adaptation to cold in rats fed a low-bulk thyroxide-free diet, *Can. J. Physiol. Pharmacol.,* 46(6), 843–846, 1968.
107. **Shaw, J. H. and Greep, R. O.,** Relation of diet to the duration of survival, body, weight and composition of hypophysectomized rats, *Endocrinology,* 45, 520, 1949.
108. **Ortega, P.,** Light and electron microscopy of dichlorodiphenyltrichloroethane (DDT) poisoning in the rat liver, *Lab. Invest.,* 15(4), 657–679, 1966.
109. **Bounous, G., Cronin, R. F. P., and Gurd, F. N.,** Dietary prevention of experimental shock lesions, *Arch. Surg.,* 94, 46–60, 1967.
110. **Hugon, J. S. and Bounous, G.,** unpublished, *Can. J. Surg.,* 15, 1, 1972.
111. **Bounous, G., Gentile, J. M., and Hugon, J.,** Elemental diet in the management of the intestinal lesion produced by 5-fluorouracil in man, *Can. J. Surg.,* 14, 312–323, 1971.
112. **Ross, M. H.,** Protein, calories and life expectancy, *Fed. Proc.,* 18, 1190–1207, 1959.

NUTRITIONAL FACTORS IN ACCLIMATIZATION TO HEAT

Robert E. Johnson

DEFINITION OF ACCLIMATIZATION

Acclimatization to heat has been studied most extensively in man among homoiotherms and in fish among poikilotherms. We shall deal only with man.

Acclimatization is defined as an increase in tolerance to heat stress upon repetition of exposure. Upon initial exposure, a given heat stress will cause some measurable physiological response. After several subsequent exposures, the same stress will cause a different response, and a lesser strain. If we express this concept in terms of Hooke's law, for an acclimatized man

$$Thermal\ stress/Strain = K$$

but with deacclimatization, or dysacclimatization, the constant K becomes smaller.

If we take a change in the rectal temperature as a strain, and working at a fixed pace in a hot, dry environment as a stress, then with repetition on a daily basis, the change in rectal temperature decreases, and the constant K increases. At the same time, the man who develops heat exhaustion in an hour or two on Day 1 may become tolerably comfortable after repetition of the stress and be able to continue for hours on Day 7, limited only by his need for water, food, and energy. The sedentary man or woman does not acclimatize to heat stress that is associated with physical work.

The measurable effects of acclimatization are found in cardiovascular function, thermal regulation, and several metabolic correlates of these. For a given submaximal stress of combined work and heat, acclimatization is characterized by a lower pulse rate, a decrease in peripheral vasodilatation, lower rectal and skin temperatures. a decrease in the rate of sweating, and production of a more dilute sweat. If the acclimatized subject is now stressed maximally, all these measurements return to or above preacclimatization levels, and he is able to sweat more profusely. Autonomic and adrenocortical functions are profoundly affected by repetitive heat stress.

PATHOPHYSIOLOGY OF STRESS IN DRY HEAT

Lee[1] has summarized the various syndromes that appear in dry heat as a result of failure in adaptation. These may occur singly or simultaneously in the same patient. Disturbances of the central nervous control system for thermoregulation may result in reversible fever (pyrexia) or in irreversible heat stroke (hyperpyrexia). Cardiovascular syncope may occur as a result of lack of acclimatization or of its loss (dysacclimatization). Sometimes it is a result of hypohydration even in a fully acclimatized healthy person. A negative balance of sodium chloride may lead to heat cramps. Primary hypohydration leads to a reduced blood volume and ultimately to reduce kidney function, uremia, and death. The skin may suffer in sunny dry heat and develop a variety of lesions; photochemical lesions include sunburn, urticaria solare of Blum, and phototoxic reactions following external applications of sensitizing agents. Cancer of the skin is most common where exposure to solar radiation is the greatest. Diminution of sweating (hidromeiosis) and total cessation of sweating (anhidrosis) often precede heat stroke. Miliaria occurs in dry heat, but is not common.

PATHOPHYSIOLOGY OF STRESS IN MOIST HEAT

Ladell[2] has summarized the ills which may befall persons in the tropics. Disturbances of central nervous control systems lead to fever or heat stroke (hyperpyrexia). Cardiovascular problems may manifest themselves in the syncope of heat exhaustion, which may come about from excessive heat stress, lack of or loss of acclimatization, and hypohydration. Skin problems are common, especially miliaria, and with it come defects in the ability to sweat and superimposed infections of the skin. Primary hypohydration can lead to hypovolemia, renal dysfunction, uremia, and death. Undue loss of salt may lead to heat cramps. Water and salt are the two main nutritional problems in all types of heat stress.

NUTRITIONAL REQUIREMENTS FOR TEMPERATE CONDITIONS AND THEIR MODIFICATION BY HEAT STRESS

If we accept the recommendations of the U.S. Food and Nutrition Board[3] for temperate conditions, then we should consider water, energy, the macronutrients (proteins, fats, and carbohydrates), the major minerals, the trace minerals, the fat-soluble vitamins, the water-soluble vitamins, and miscellaneous nutrients not conveniently classified above such as additives, spices, and herbs.

In the clinical nutrition of deficiency disorders (i.e., a negative balance), there may be a primary deficiency (insufficient intake, ingestion of foodstuffs that are not digested or not absorbed) or a secondary deficiency (conditioned deficiency due to increased metabolic demand, failure of digestion, failure of absorbed nutrients to reach tissue, failure of diffusion of nutrients into the cells, failure of metabolism in the cell, or presence of antimetabolites or enzyme poisons). There are also disorders caused by plethora (i.e., a positive balance) due to primary overconsumption, secondary interference with normal metabolism or excretion, or decreased metabolic demand.[4]

Energy

The basic equation for heat balance[5-7] is

$$
\begin{aligned}
\text{Stored heat} \;=\; & + \text{metabolic heat} \\
& - \text{evaporative heat} \\
& \pm \text{physical work performed} \\
& \pm \text{radiation} \\
& \pm \text{conduction} \\
& \pm \text{convection}
\end{aligned}
$$

Metabolic heat may be regarded as of two portions: maintenance (or resting) and heat due to activity. If resting metabolism is expressed in terms of units of body size (weight, surface area), heat has little if any effect. The metabolic heat of activity is related to the effective temperature. It may be diminished in the comfort zone by moderate heat that does not tax the mechanisms for dissipation of heat. However, under heat stress there is an increase in the work of the sweat glands and an increase in heat production per unit of external work. Thus, the energy cost of a given specific task may be increased by heat stress.

Water

This is the most urgent of nutrient requirements in heat stress. Even total deprivation of food energy (starvation) may take a day or two (depending on the work rate) to cause serious trouble. Lack of minerals or water-soluble vitamins have a time schedule of days or weeks; lack of fat-soluble vitamins may not cause difficulties for weeks or months. By contrast to all of the other nutrients, lack of water can cause heat exhaustion in a matter of hours if heat stress is accompanied by physical exertion.

Proteins

There is little evidence that either heat stress or exercise change the requirements for essential amino acids. A diet high in protein does not affect performance in the heat, despite its specific dynamic action (heat increment due to feeding). However, the concentrations of urea and ammonia in sweat are of the same order of magnitude as in blood plasma. Therefore, a copious loss of sweat probably does raise the requirements for nonessential nitrogen in the diet.

Carbohydrates

In the typical U.S. diet, about 50% of the energy is derived from carbohydrates, mostly sucrose and starch. This proportion is not changed by residence in the desert or the tropics. Whether it is "good" or "bad" is a matter for debate.

Fats

There has been little research on the effects of environment on the requirements for fats and essential fatty acids. The proportion of energy from fat is about 35% in a typical U.S. diet, and this is not changed by residence in the desert or the tropics. Sargent and colleagues[8] showed that a warm environment decreased the severity of post-exercise ketosis as contrasted with a cool environment. This observation has interesting implications for the relationship between intermediary metabolism and the ambient environment.

Minerals

In osmotic concentration, sweat is generally hypotonic to blood plasma, rarely isotonic, and almost never hypertonic except in patients with cystic fibrosis. Nevertheless, it does contain sodium, chloride, potassium, and calcium in concentrations sufficient to cause significant depletions when the daily loss of sweat is large. Unless balanced by an adequate intake, loss of minerals in the sweat can lead to hyponatremia and its effects on renal function, hypokalemia with its circulatory effect, and hypocalcemia with its effect upon neuromuscular function.

Trace Minerals

It has been argued that losses of iron and zinc in the sweat may become significant in continued heat stress. This view is not universally accepted, owing to the difficulty of collecting "pure" sweat, uncontaminated with dermal debris. However, there is a continuous loss of hair, epithelial cells, and sebum even in temperature conditions, and this loss is accelerated by heat stress.

Water-soluble Vitamins

Some of the classical nutritional diseases have been endemic in warm or tropical regions. Examples are pellagra, dry beriberi, wet beriberi, and tropical sprue. It can be argued that foods peculiar to warm regions, such as maize and polished rice, just happen to be lacking in niacin, tryptophan, or thiamine. By this argument there is no specific effect of living in the tropics or the desert. Acute heat stress has never been demonstrated to increase the requirement for any water-soluble vitamin. They are present in sweat, but the amounts are too small to be contributory to any disease.

Fat-soluble Vitamins

Among the diseases caused by lack of one or another of the fat-soluble vitamins, only rickets has classically been related to temperate or cold climates, where sunshine does not reach the human species nearly as much as it does in warm places. Keratomalacia and nyctalopia are due to deficiency of vitamin A, and are more common in the tropics than elsewhere. These are also regions typical of diets low in fat. There is no convincing evidence that acute or chronic heat stress relates in any way to a need for increased amounts of fat-soluble vitamins or essential fatty acids.

Miscellaneous

Traditionally, the diets in many warm countries are highly spiced as with curry, or hot with cayenne pepper, or both. There is no concrete evidence that any herb or spice is essential in human nutrition. All modern cultures have beverages that contain caffeine or related substances, including coffee, tea, cocoa, and mattè, and all modern cultures have fermented or distilled alcoholic beverages, or both, with the possible exception of orthodox Moslems. There is no evidence that either caffeine or ethyl alcohol is essential for human nutrition, although they are considered to add pleasure to life.

ACCLIMATIZATION TO HEAT AND ITS NUTRITIONAL IMPLICATIONS

We have taken the position that heat stress in working men may increase the requirements (for a given regimen or task) for water, sodium, chloride, potassium, calcium, nonessential nitrogen, and, in severe stress, energy. These increases are related to strain on the mechanisms for heat dissipation (mainly sweating), increased cardiovascular strain, and changes in body composition in the direction of hypovolemia. The autonomic nervous system and the endocrine system are both involved in physiological responses to heat stress.[9]

Paradoxically, acclimatization may be responsible for increasing a nutrient requirement under one set of circumstances and for decreasing it under another. The reason is that, for a given heat stress, an acclimatized person can go on for a longer time before exhaustion than he can when unacclimatized or when he has lost acclimatization (dysacclimatization). At the same time, when pushed by maximal heat stress, the acclimatized person can sustain a higher rectal temperature and sweats more profusely than he did when unacclimatized.

The nutritional implications of acclimatization must, therefore, take into account the nature and severity of the heat stress and the time of exposure. By far the most pressing problem is water. For a given moderate heat stress, the rate of sweating may be decreased by acclimatization because the skin is kept cooler and evaporation is more efficient. However, the acclimatized person can work longer than the unacclimatized person, and so will lose more sweat and also more water vapor from the lungs. Under maximal heat stress the acclimatized person can sweat faster and longer than can the unacclimatized; both factors increase the requirement for water.

As a rule of thumb in planning for water under heat stress, a base supply of 3ℓ of fluid daily is the minimum. For each hour of moderate work add 500 mℓ and for each hour of hard work 1000 mℓ.

Sweat is the only body fluid in which the concentration of sodium equals that of chloride. Usually, as in plasma, the sodium is higher. The concentrations of sodium and chloride are regulated. At least five factors have been identified as affecting these concentrations: dietary intake, the skin temperature, adrenocortical function, the rate of sweating, and acclimatization. At a given moderate heat stress, the acclimatized person has a lower sweat rate, a cooler skin, and a lower sodium concentration in the sweat than does the unacclimatized. Therefore, the sodium and chloride loss per hour is less, but a longer work day before exhaustion may cause a greater total loss. By contrast, in severe heat stress acclimatization can permit higher rectal and skin temperatures and a higher sweat rate with quite concentrated sweat. Hence, the loss of sodium and chloride per hour will be greater for the acclimatized than for the unacclimatized, and the duration can be longer.

In planning diets for heat stress, the sedentary person under moderate stress needs a minimum of 5 g of NaCl per day. For each hour of work, an extra gram of salt may be added. Under severe stress, an extra 2g may be needed. For all practical purposes, salt added at mealtime from the shaker will suffice. Only in the hottest, hardest-working occupations it is necessary to add salt to the beverages ingested. Unfortunately, man's appetite for salt is not an accurate guide to its need. Current dietetic thinking leans toward a diminished, not a raised, salt intake for man in a temperate environment. Carried to extremes, this could be dangerous for men working in the heat.

So far as concerns protein, fats, carbohydrates, minerals (other than sodium, potassium, and calcium), trace elements, fat-soluble vitamins, water-soluble vitamins, and miscellaneous other nutritional factors, there is no evidence that acclimatization to heat has nutritional implications.

REFERENCES

1. Lee, D. H. K., Terrestrial animals in dry heat: man in the desert, in *Adaptation to the Environment,* Dill, D. B., Ed., American Physiological Society, Bethesda, Md., 1964, 551—582.
2. Ladell, W. S. S., Terrestrial animals in humid heat, in *Adaptation to the Environment,* Dill, D. B., Ed., American Physiological Society, Bethesda, Md., 1964, 625—661.
3. U.S. National Academy of Science, National Research Council, Food and Nutrition Board, *Recommended Dietary Allowances,* National Research Council, Washington, D.C., 1979.
4. Carlson, L. D. and Hatch, A. C. L., *Control of Energy Exchange,* Macmillan, New York, 1970.
5. Edholm, O. G. and Lewis, H. S., Terrestrial animals in cold: man in polar regions, in *Adaptation to the Environment,* Dill, D. B., Ed., American Physiological Society, Bethesda, Md., 1964, 435—446.
6. Hardy, J. D., Gagge, A. P., and Stolwijk, J. A., *Physiological and Behavioral Temperature Regulation,* Charles C Thomas, Springfield, Ill., 1970.
7. Judy, W. V., Body temperature regulation, in *Physiology,* 4th ed., Selkurt, E., Ed., Little, Brown, Boston, 1976, 696—699.
8. Sargent, F., Johnson, R.E., Robbins, E., and Sawyer, L., Effects of environment and other factors on nutritional ketosis, *Q.J. Exp. Physiol.,* 43, 345—351, 1958.
9. Sargent, F., Johnson, R. E., Effects of diet on renal function in healthy men, *Am. J. Clin. Nutr.,* 4, 466—481, 1956.

NUTRITION AND ALTITUDE ACCLIMATIZATION

J. T. Maher

The land surface of our planet covers approximately 148 million square kilometers, of which some 7 million are above 3000 m. This amounts to nearly 5% of the total land mass with a permanent human population of no more than a few percent.[1] Although men have climbed without supplemental oxygen to 8500 m,[2] the limiting altitude to which human acclimatization is possible appears to be approximately 5500 m, i.e., where the ambient barometric pressure is about one half of a standard atmosphere. Since acclimatization is not achieved above this altitude, it is axiomatic that prolonged residence will result in progressive deterioration. The members of one Himalayan expedition spent 5 months at 5800 m, at the end of which time they found themselves in considerably worse condition than their newly arrived cohorts.[3] The extent to which dietary and nutritional factors may have contributed is unknown. More telling, perhaps, is the fact that no mining camps have been established above 5300 m in South America or elsewhere.

While many of us are often prone to equate the stress of altitude with *hypoxic hypoxia,* i.e., the low partial pressure of oxygen, numerous other stressful factors are commonly operative. At high elevations, the average temperatures are lower and severe cold is not unusual. The decrease in temperature with altitude approximates 2°C for every 300 m. The alteration in caloric requirement imposed by cold exposure is addressed elsewhere in this handbook. Other stress factors at altitude include increased solar radiation, high winds, aridity, and rough terrain. A frequent scarcity of natural resources of food, water, and shelter imposes added difficulties, as do sterilization and food preparation because of the reduced boiling point of water. It has been suggested that the factor limiting population growth and expansion at altitude is the limited nutritional base, rather than hypoxia.[4] One of the few redeeming features of high terrestrial altitude, from the standpoint of nutrition, is that food preservation may be facilitated if freezing temperatures prevail.

Abrupt exposure of the unacclimatized person to terrestrial or simulated altitudes above 3000 m commonly results in the development of acute mountain sickness. Gastrointestinal symptoms, including anorexia, nausea, and vomiting, are among the more prominent manifestations of the disorder. Studies carried out at 4300 m have shown food intakes to be decreased by 25 to 50% during acute exposures,[5-7] with minimal values observed, by and large, during the first 3 days of exposure. The degree of anorexia may be markedly influenced by the palatability of the diet. Although similar in magnitude, the anoretic response is a more transient phenomenon in women than in men (J.P. Hannon, personal communication). A caloric deficit secondary to appetite suppression inevitably results in weight loss. Losses ranging from 3.5%[7] to 5%[8] of preexposure body weight have been recorded at 4300 m after 8 and 12 days, respectively. The loss in body weight has been densitometrically partitioned into losses of body fat, water, and dry protein.[8] A diminution of appetite, caloric consumption, and growth rate characterizes the early response of experimental animals to altitude as well.[9,10] The incidence and severity of this nutritional problem increase with increasing elevation and rapidity of ascent.

The problem of inadequate energy intake is compounded by increased rates of energy expenditure which have been recorded in man under basal,[11] resting,[12] and exercise[13] conditions. Animals acclimatizing to altitude also invoke an increased metabolic response.[14] The consequent energy deficit results in the catabolism of body tissues with a diminution of body fat[7,8] and protein.[5,8] This observation has stimulated inquiries regarding the adequacy at altitude of the National Research Council's daily allowances of

0.8 g of protein per kilogram of body weight.[15] Negative nitrogen balances with intakes of 0.9 g of protein per kilogram of body weight have been reported, and the results of serum albumin turnover studies have suggested an impairment in protein biosynthesis during the first week of altitude exposure.[16] Other metabolic disturbances and biochemical alterations that occur during this acute phase of acclimatization include negative water balances,[5,17] abnormal electrolyte shifts,[6,18] and decreased fasting glucose levels and disappearance curves.[19] Because these abnormalities mimic those observed during caloric restriction and acute starvation, the question arose as to whether the altitude-induced metabolic alterations are attributable to the anorexia and resultant caloric deprivation or to hypoxia *per se.*

This problem has been addressed in recent years and apparently resolved — at least in man. With minimization of symptomatology by a progressive staging of ascent or in other ways,[20,21] the daily caloric (~3500 kcal/day) and protein consumption in human subjects can be maintained after exposure to high altitude. Under such conditions, body weight losses can be greatly reduced, positive nitrogen balances can be achieved, blood electrolyte levels are normal, mineral balances are positive, and fasting glucose levels and glucose tolerance curves are normal.[21] Digestion and absorption are also normal by sea-level standards. Contrary to popular belief, the digestibility, absorption, and utilization of dietary fats are not disturbed in men at elevations up to 4700 m.[22] This finding argues for the adequacy of secretion of gastric and pancreatic lipases as well as bile salts. Thus, it would appear that many of the metabolic and biochemical changes that attend abrupt altitude exposures are directly related to anorexia and voluntary caloric deficit rather than to a direct effect of hypoxia. Furthermore, the growth rate depression in young animals at high altitude also seems to be entirely attributable to reduced food consumption.[10]

The weight losses not due to caloric restriction are probably the result of hypohydration[17,23] which occurs during the first days at altitude. The daily water flux of members of the 1960-1961 Everest Expedition was approximately 30% higher at 5800 m than at sea level.[3] The hyperventilation caused by the low ambient oxygen pressure coupled with the dry atmosphere and reduced surface tension of water bring about a three- to four-fold increase in water loss via the lungs. The hypohydration may also be associated in part with a transient fall in plasma and urinary aldosterone levels.[24] Furthermore, the cold altitude environment usually evokes a diuresis. Unfortunately, thirst does not appear to be an accurate guide to the need for water at altitude, at least during the early stages of the sojourn, so dehydration poses a serious threat. In light of these considerations, it is not unreasonable to recommend that a liter of water be imbibed every 4 hr by active adults at high elevations. That hypohydration is a transient and adaptive response to acute altitude exposure is suggested by the report that total body water content is the same in Andean native populations as in sea-level residents.[25]

With the subsidence of acute symptoms and progressive acclimatization, the loss of weight generally abates. However, if anorexia continues throughout altitude exposure, essential nutrient reserves may be depleted, resulting in deficiency states.

Factors other than anorexia appear to be responsible for the inability of certain mammalian species to acclimatize with prolonged exposure. Whereas sheep are commonly grazed without ill effect well above the timberline in high mountain areas, this is not the case with cattle. Cattle are distinguished from many other species by a failure to show a satisfactory weight gain during chronic exposure to moderately high altitudes — even when rations are heavier than provided at lower elevations.[26] In contrast to the carcasses of sheep which showed excellent nutrition after a prolonged sojourn at 3870 m,[27] the carcasses of steers after a comparable exposure were strikingly depleted of fat and were given the low commercial grading of "canners and cutters."[26] It is unlikely that these observations are explicable on the basis of altered gastrointestinal function. It has been shown that the motility, secretion, and absorption of the gastrointestinal tract are relatively resistant to hypoxia.[28] Moreover, both species exhibit marked similarities in oxygen transport. The bovine species, however, is remarkable for the severe pulmonary hypertension which develops during chronic hypoxia. Whether the steers' failure to thrive is related to this circulatory disorder is not clear.

The effects of altitude on human nutritional requirements have been reviewed previously.[29] On the basis of available information, the authors concluded that "the interaction of many of the indirect effects of hypoxia usually served to stabilize caloric intake at levels comparable to those found at sea level for the man performing like amounts of work." However, more recent data suggest that alterations, albeit minor, in certain nutrient requirements as well as utilization[31] attend exposure to moderate and high altitudes. Increases in energy expenditure ranging from 6.9%[13] to 25%[30] have been reported in soldiers performing heavy work at altitude. An increase in energy intake commensurate with the altitude-induced increase in energy expenditure is obviously essential if balance is to be achieved. In this connection, the advantages of high-carbohydrate feedings in mountain climbers were recognized early in this century.[32] The superiority of carbohydrate as a metabolic fuel at altitude becomes apparent when one considers that pulmonary uptake of one liter of oxygen yields approximately 5.05 kcal in the combustion of carbohydrate, but only 4.69 in the combustion of fat.[33] Other advantages of a high-carbohydrate diet (~68% of the kcal) include an increase in pulmonary ventilation and diffusion capacity with elevated alveolar and arterial oxygen pressures, a reduction in clinical symptomatology, and an improvement in physical work capacity and mental efficiency.[34-37] In contrast, the metabolism of ethyl alcohol (theoretical RQ of 0.67) materially lowers respiratory gas exchange and arterial oxygenation.[38] On the basis of controlled studies designed to assess the efficacy of various nutrients at altitude, daily minimal carbohydrate requirements of 320 g have been established for moderately active young adults.[39] Whether fortuitous or otherwise, a marked preference, indeed craving, for sugar and other sweets characterizes the newcomer's response to altitude. It is interesting to note that the diet of the Andean natives contains 79 to 89% of their calories as carbohydrate.[40] These highlanders exhibit no discomfort from their environment and little limitation in their physical activity.

Cardinal among the numerous physiologic adjustments that occur during exposure to altitude is an augmentation of erythrocyte production in response to increased levels of erythopoietin. This observation prompts inquiry into the adequacy of iron available from normal body stores and usual dietary intake in relation to the polycythemic response. While normal stores plus daily dietary (10 to 15 mg) iron have been found adequate to meet the needs of increased hemoglobin synthesis in men at high altitude,[41] there are data suggestive of an additional iron requirement in women.[42]

Repression of ascorbic acid synthesis with the development of scurvy has been reported in the rabbit under hypoxic conditions.[43] An increased thiamine requirement has also been postulated on the basis of extensive dephosphorylation of tissues in animals subjected to hypoxia.[44] However, it has not been clearly established that the requirement of man for ascorbic acid, thiamine, or other vitamins is greater at altitude.

REFERENCES

1. Clegg, E. J., Harrison, G. A., and Baker, P., *Hum. Biol.*, 42, 486–518, 1970.
2. Wilson, R., *Ann. Intern. Med.*, 78, 421–428, 1973.
3. Nevison, T. O., Roberts, J. E., and Lackey, W. W., in *Proc. Symp. on Arct. Biol. and Med., V. Nutritional Requirements for Survival in the Cold and at Altitude*, Vaughan, L., Ed., Arctic Aeromedical Laboratory, Fort Wainwright, Alaska, 1965, 343.
4. Mazess, R. B., in *Physiological Anthropology*, Damon, A., Ed., Oxford University Press, New York, 1975, 167–209.
5. Consolazio, C. F., Matoush, L. O., Johnson, H. L., and Daws, T. A., *Am. J. Clin. Nutr.*, 21, 154–161, 1968.
6. Janoski, A. H., Whitten, B. K., Shields, J. L., and Hannon, J. P., *Fed. Proc.*, 28, 1185–1189, 1969.
7. Surks, M. I., Chinn, K. S. K., and Matoush, L. O., *J. Appl. Physiol.*, 21, 1741–1746, 1966.
8. Krzywicki, H. J., Consolazio, C. F., Matoush, L. O., Johnson, H. L., and Barnhart, R. A., *Fed. Proc.*, 28, 1190–1194, 1969.
9. Hannon, J. P., Krabill, L. F., Woolridge, T. A., and Schnakenberg, D. D., *J. Nutr.*, 105, 278–287, 1975.
10. Schnakenberg, D. D., Krabill, L. F., and Weiser, P. C., *J. Nutr.*, 101, 787–796, 1971.
11. Hannon, J. P. and Sudman, D. M., *J. Appl. Physiol.*, 34, 471–477, 1973.
12. Billings, C. E., Brashear, R. E., Mathews, D. K., and Bason, R., *Arch. Environ. Health*, 18, 978–995, 1969.
13. Johnson, H. L., Consolazio, C. F., Daws, T. A., and Krzywicki, H. J., *Nutr. Rep. Int.*, 4, 77–82, 1971.
14. Phillips, R. W., Knox, K. L., House, W. A., and Jordan, H. N., *Fed. Proc.*, 28, 974–977, 1969.
15. Reco
15. *Recommended Dietary Allowances*, 8th ed., Food and Nutrition Board, National Research Council, Washington, D.C., 1974, 37–48.
16. Surks, M. I., *J. Clin. Invest.*, 45, 1442–1451, 1966.
17. Krzywicki, H. J., Consolazio, C. F., Johnson, H. L., Nielsen, W. C., Jr., and Barnhart, R. A., *J. Appl. Physiol.*, 30, 806–809, 1971.
18. Johnson, H. L., Consolazio, C. F., Matoush, L. O., and Krzywicki, H. J., *Fed. Proc.*, 28, 1195–1198, 1969.
19. Janoski, A. H., Johnson, H. L., and Sanbar, S. S., *Fed. Proc. Abstr.*, 28, 593, 1969.
20. Maher, J. T., Cymerman, A., Reeves, J. T., Cruz, J. C., Denniston, J. C., and Grover, R. F., *Aviat. Space Environ. Med.*, 46, 826–829, 1975.
21. Consolazio, C. F., Johnson, H. L., and Krzywicki, H. J., in *Physiological Adaptations, Desert and Mountain*, Yousef, M. K., Horvath, S. M., and Bullard, R. W., Eds., Academic Press, New York, 1972, 227–241.
22. Rai, R. M., Malhotra, M. S., Dimri, G. P., and Sampathkumar, T., *Am. J. Clin. Nutr.*, 28, 242–245, 1975.
23. Johnson, H. L., Consolazio, C. F., Burk, R. F., and Daws, T. A., *Aerosp. Med.*, 45, 849–854, 1974.
24. Maher, J. T., Jones, L. G., Hartley, L. H., Williams, G. H., and Rose, L. I., *J. Appl. Physiol.*, 39, 18–22, 1975.
25. Siri, W. E., Reynafarje, C., Berlin, N. I., and Lawrence, J. H., *J. Appl. Physiol.*, 7, 333–334, 1954.
26. Grover, R. F., Reeves, J. T., Will, D. H., and Blount, S. G., Jr., *J. Appl. Physiol.*, 18, 567–574, 1963.
27. Reeves, J. T., Grover, E. B., and Grover, R. F., *J. Appl. Physiol.*, 18, 560–566, 1963.
28. Van Liere, E. J. and Stickney, J. C., *Hypoxia*, University of Chicago Press, Chicago, 1963, 274.
29. Buskirk, E. R. and Mendez, J., *Fed. Proc.*, 26, 1760–1767, 1967.
30. Malhotra, M. S., Ramaswamy, S. S., and Sen Gupta, J., in *Proc. Symp. on Human Adaptability to Environments and Physical Fitness*, Malhotra, M. S., Ed., Defence Institute of Physiology and Allied Sciences, Madras-3, India, 1966, 180–194.
31. Chinn, K. S. K. and Hannon, J. P., *Fed. Proc.*, 28, 944–947, 1969.
32. Boycott, A. E. and Haldane, J. S., *J. Physiol. London*, 37, 354–377, 1908.
33. Durnin, J. V. G. A. and Passmore, R., *Energy, Work and Leisure*, Heinemann, London, 1967, 16.
34. Consolazio, C. F., Matoush, L. O., Johnson, H. L., Krzywicki, H. J., Daws, T. A., and Isaac, G. J., *Fed. Proc.*, 28, 937–943, 1969.

35. **Dramise, J. G., Inouye, C. M., Christensen, B. M., Fults, R. D., Canham, J. E., and Consolazio, C. F.,** *Aviat. Space Environ. Med.,* 46, 365–368, 1975.
36. **Hansen, J. E., Hartley, L. H., and Hogan, R. P.,** *J. Appl. Physiol.,* 33, 441–445, 1972.
37. **Mitchell, H. H. and Edman, M.,** *Nutrition and Climatic Stress,* Charles C Thomas, Springfield, Ill., 1951, 136–143.
38. **Hansen, J. E. and Claybaugh, J. R.,** *Aviat. Space Environ. Med.,* 46, 1123–1127, 1975.
39. **Consolazio, C. F., Johnson, H. L., Krzywicki, H. J., and Daws, T. A.,** *J. Physiol. Paris,* 62, 232–235, 1971.
40. **Mazess, R. B. and Baker, P. J.,** *Am. J. Clin. Nutr.,* 15, 341–351, 1964.
41. **Hornbein, T. F.,** *J. Appl. Physiol.,* 17, 243–245, 1962.
42. **Hannon, J. P., Shields, J. L., and Harris, C. W.,** in *The Effects of Altitude on Physical Performance,* Goddard, R. F., Ed., The Athletic Institute, Chicago, 1966, 37–44.
43. **Borsuk, V. N.,** *Chem. Abstr.,* 43, 4740, 1949.
44. **Govier, W. M.,** *JAMA,* 126, 749–750, 1944.

NUTRITION AND RESISTANCE*

W. P. Faulk and R. K. Chandra

INTRODUCTION

Epidemiological data and experience indicate that malnourished persons have a greater mortality and morbidity from infectious diseases than do well-nourished subjects.[1] Since the major host defense mechanism against infections is immunological,[2,3] this suggests that the immune response in malnutrition is inadequate. Research into the effects of malnutrition on the immune responses supports the concept that the immunological system in malnourished persons is damaged.[4-6]

Another aspect of the malnutrition-infection problem is that infections can often cause malnutrition, particularly in a marginally nourished child.[7] This is a difficult problem to study because it is influenced by environmental and social factors such as weather and crowding, and by customs and traditions such as feeding habits and diet. Nevertheless, it is broadly accepted that many infections cause children to be irritable and not eat, and such infections often cause diarrhea and vomiting with subsequent loss of fluid, electrolytes, and nutrients.[8] Those children who do eat sometimes do not have adequate absorption from the gut, depending on the infection, and the net effect of all these factors is negative nitrogen balance and malnutrition.[9] Whatever the initiating event might be, it is obvious that infection and malnutrition can perpetuate themselves in a vicious cycle (Figure 1).[5,6,10]

The problem is of major public health importance because it affects a great number of people in both developing and developed countries. The problem is also interesting because it attracts both clinical and research efforts, and is a point of intersection for immunologists, nutritionists, infectious diseases experts, and persons involved in many aspects of public health. Because of this, the problem has attracted the attention of a great number of scientists. In addition, the World Health Organization has coordinated an international collaborative study of the effects of malnutrition on the immune response with particular emphasis on public health aspects of the nutrition-infection cycle.[11] Considerable data have accumulated as a result of these studies, and a profile of the immunological capabilities of malnourished children is beginning to emerge.[5,6,12-16] The pathogenesis of this profile is not presently clear, but it is likely to be better defined through continuing studies in this area.

THE IMMUNOLOGICAL SYSTEM

Modern immunology has established that the lymphoid system is composed of at least two components, both apparently arising from the same stem cell series (Figure 2): one in the thymus and the other in the bone marrow.[17] Lymphocytes of thymus origin are called T-cells, and are responsible for many cell-mediated immune (CMI) reactions such as graft rejection, delayed hypersensitivity, and cytotoxicity. Lymphocytes of bone marrow origin are called B-cells, and are responsible for immunoglobulin (Ig) and antibody production.[17] T- and B-cells and their products, along with macrophages, complement, and certain nonspecific factors of resistance, constitute the bulwarks of host defense against infections (Table 1).[18,19] It is thus important to learn the effects of malnutrition on these components of host resistance. The T- and B-cells work together in healthy

*This is Publication No. 53 from the Department of Basic and Clinical Immunology and Microbiology, Medical University of South Carolina. Research supported in part by USPHS Grant HD-09938 and in part by the World Health Organization.

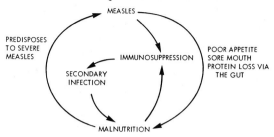

FIGURE 1.   Interactions of infection and malnutrition. Measles has been chosen as an example because it is a common problem. Many other infections follow this general scheme.

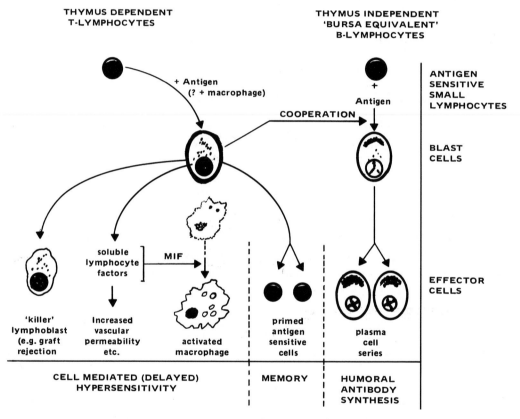

FIGURE 2.   Role of T-lymphocytes and B-lymphocytes in immunological responses. Many of the events involve active cell proliferation, but for simplicity this has been indicated at two stages. Different subsets mediate the various T-cell functions. (From Roitt, I. M., Greaves, M. F., Torrigiani, G., Brostoff, J., and Playfair, J. H. L., *Lancet,* ii, 367–371, 1969. With permission.)

persons to produce an adequate immune response to most infections, but some infections such as pneumococcal pneumonia are relatively more dependent on adequate B-cell function while other infections such as tuberculosis are relatively more dependent on T-cell function.[18] This division of labor within the immune system has been revealed largely as a result of extensive studies on patients suffering from primary immunodeficiency diseases such as defects of humoral and cellular immune responses and leukocyte bactericidal function (Table 2).

T-cells can be quantified according to their ability to form rosettes with sheep red blood cells, and one aspect of their function can be measured by their proliferative

Table 1
SOME COMPONENTS OF HOST RESISTANCE

General category	Specific items
Immunoglobulins	IgG, IgM, IgA, secretory IgA, IgD, IgE
Nonimmunoglobulin serum factors	Complement C-reactive protein Transferrins
Nonimmunoglobulin nonserum factors	Lysozyme Interferon Lactoferrin

Cells	Phagocytes: macrophages, neutrophils, etc.
	Lymphocytes: T-cells,
	  B-cells, K-cells
	Cells of reticuloendothelial system: Kupffer
	  cells, fibroblasts, etc.

Table 2
PATHOGENS THAT CAUSE INFECTIONS IN PATIENTS WITH IMMUNODEFICIENCIES

Type of immunodeficiency	Type of pathogens generally responsible for infections in each immunodeficiency group	
Humoral immune responses	*Pneumococcus* *Haemophilus influenzae* *Streptococcus* sp. *Meningococcus* sp.	*Pseudomonas aeruginosa* Hepatitis virus *Pneumocystis carinii*
Cellular immune responses	Rubeola Varicella Vaccinia Cytomegalic-inclusion-body virus	*Mycobacterium tuberculosis* *Candida albicans* Histoplasmosis
Disorders of phagocytosis	*Staphylococcus* *Klebsiella* sp. *Aerobacter aerogenes* *Serratia marcescens*	*C. albicans* *Aspergillus* *Nocardia*

Note: Data have been assembled from patients suffering from immunodeficiency diseases and leukocyte bactericidal functional defects.[18] Complement deficiencies have not been included, but it should be recalled that these patients show an increased susceptibility to bacterial infections.

response to phyto-hemagglutinin, a plant glycoprotein that has a nonspecific mitogenic effect on T-cells. B-cells can be quantified according to their ability to form rosettes with either antibody- or antibody-and-complement-coated sheep red blood cells. They can also be measured by membrane immunofluorescence because they bear Ig on their cell membranes, and the type of Ig can be determined by using fluoresceinated class-specific antisera.[20] Since B-cells produce antibodies and all antibodies are Ig, one of the most commonly used measurements of B-cell function simply estimates serum Ig levels or measures the production of antibody subsequent to antigenic stimulation.

HISTOPATHOLOGICAL CONSIDERATIONS

T- and B-lymphocytes are produced in the central lymphoid organs of the immunological system, the thymus and bone marrow, and are seeded to peripheral lymphoid organs such as lymph nodes, spleen, tonsils, Peyer's patches, and other lymphoid aggregates in the gastrointestinal tract. Both the central and peripheral organs of the immunological system demonstrate morphological and histopathological evidence of damage during malnutrition.[21-23] Lymphocytopenia sometimes occurs, and low lymphocyte counts have been reported in marasmic and kwashiorkor children,[24,25] as well as in nutritionally deprived mice and guinea pigs.[26,27] Plasmacytoid cells have also been observed by electron microscopy in the peripheral blood of malnourished children.[16]

Thymus glands from healthy 4-month-old children weigh about 25 g, but thymuses from malnourished children of comparable age weigh less than 10 g, frequently about 1 g, or even less. In addition, thymuses from healthy neonates during the first several days of life weigh about 20 g, but those from neonates who sustain intrauterine malnutrition also reveal morphological alterations and reduction in weight.

Histological examination of the thymus of a normal child reveals lobules that are well demarcated by thin connective-vascular fascia, and each lobule is differentiated into medullary and cortical regions. The medullary region contains large lymphocytes and structures of unestablished function called Hassall bodies. T-lymphocytes arise from the cortex. The histology of thymuses from children with malnutrition varies according to the degree of undernutrition.[21] A progressive loss of corticomedullary differentiation and lymphocytic depletion is seen in the initial or intermediate stages of malnutrition, and this can ultimately lead to the complete loss of normal thymus architecture with lymphocyte depletion, interstitial fiborsis, and degenerative changes of Hassall bodies in severe cases (Figure 3).

The peripheral lymphoid organs of the immune system show gross and microscopic evidence of damage in malnutrition. Lymph nodes and spleen are small, and they contain fewer and smaller germinal centers. Cells from these organs taken from malnourished rats and mice incorporate much less tritiated thymidine than do comparable cells from well-nourished animals.[29] This is consistent with the observation that dividing cells are rarely seen in lymph nodes or splenic tissues from malnourished humans. Lymphoid aggregates such as Peyer's patches and palatine tonsils are extremely hypoplastic in patients suffering from malnutrition. However, it is not clear whether these morphological changes in the thymus and peripheral lymphoid tissues are primarily the result of malnutrition or the secondary effects of infection or stress.[30,31] Histopathological findings in thymuses from intrauterine malnourished neonates might suggest that the changes are primarily due to malnutrition, but the possibility of transplacental transport of maternal stress hormones, endotoxins, or viruses as possible augumenting factors has not been excluded. Whatever the cause, it is clear that both the central and peripheral components of the immune system undergo drastic changes during malnutrition, and these histopathological alterations are clinically associated with a compromised ability of the host to deal effectively with infections.

CELL-MEDIATED IMMUNITY

Cell-mediated immunity (CMI) in malnourished humans seems to be considerably depressed. The numbers of circulating T-cells in peripheral blood are often depressed, as measured by spontaneous rosette formation with sheep red blood cells.[32-34] Also, several investigators have observed depressed responses of peripheral blood lymphocytes to phytohemagglutinin,[22,24,35-37] although it is possible that this depression is due to

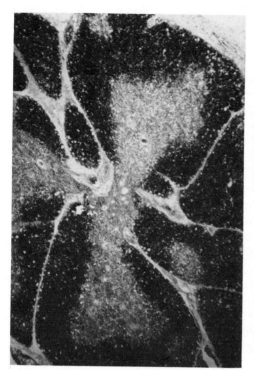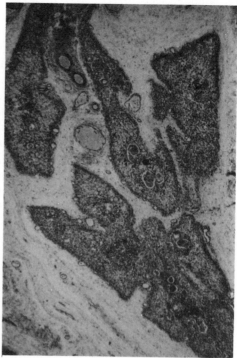

FIGURE 3.   Thymus gland from nourished and malnourished children. A: Note clear demarcation into medullary and cortical regions. This is a normal thymus (× 35). B: Thymus from a severely malnourished child of same age as in A. Note loss of corticomedullary demarcation and general depletion of cells and increase of connective tissue (× 35). (Photographs taken by Dr. R. Pinto-Paes, from Faulk, W. P., Pinto-Paes, R., and Marigo, C., *Br. J. Nutr.,* in press, 1976. With permission.)

circulating inhibitors.[38,39] Suppressor cells may play a part in reducing CMI in malnutrition.[40] Very little is presently known about the role of CMI mediators such as lymphokines in malnutrition. The most reproducible measure of decreased T-cell function in malnutrition is the skin test response to antigens, such as PPD following BCG immunization, that are characterized by delayed hypersensitivity reactions. Many different antigens have been used in PCM, and they uniformly fail to elicit normal delayed hypersensitivity reactions.[24,35,39-43] One assumes that the skin test for delayed hypersensitivity is an accurate measure of CMI, but nonimmune factors such as hormones or biochemical alterations in the skin[44] can presumably depress the skin test. Many virus infections can also depress delayed hypersensitivity reactions in the skin,[45] and the role of either superimposed virus infections or the activation of latent viruses in PCM has not been adequately explored. Finally, it is interesting that some immediate skin test reactions are also depressed in PCM.[46]

PHAGOCYTOSIS

One of the primary methods of resistance is that of phagocytosis and intracellular digestion. This mechanism is found in animals who lack a well-organized immunological system, and in mammals it is more specialized and integrated with a protease-containing system of lysosomes.[47] Organisms are recognized and bound by phagocytic cells either by virtue of membrane receptors or by the presence of cytophilic antibodies. The organism is then endocytozed into a phagosome, and the phagosome fuses with lysosomes to form phagolysosomes. Acid proteases are released from the lysosome into the phagolysosome, and the phagocytozed organism is degraded and killed.[48] Successful killing of microorganisms thus requires (a) recognition and binding, (b) endocytosis, (c) phagolysosome formation, and (d) enzymatic degradation. Defects can occur in each of these steps, and several diseases in man such as chronic granulomatous disease and Chediak-Higashi syndrome are associated with increased infections due to faulty phagocytosis and killing.[49]

Studies done on phagocytic cells, mostly neutrophils, from malnourished children have shown that recognition and endocytosis of bacteria are normal, but that these cells have a delayed chemotactic response, particularly in the presence of infection.[50,51] There is no characteristic abnormality in the enzymes from leukocytes of malnourished individuals, but they do demonstrate increased resting activity of the hexose-monophosphate shunt, and they do not release acid phosphatase from lysosomes during phagocytosis, unlike those from controls.[52] Experimentally, they also manifest a decreased extent of iodination as measured by radiolabeled incorporation into trichloracetic-acid-precipitable proteins by phagocytozing neutrophils, suggesting an impairment in intracellular myeloperoxidase-H_2O_2-iodide-mediated killing.[53] However, myeloperoxidase activity is reported to be normal in neutrophils from malnourished children.[54] The role of dietary iron in maintaining efficient myeloperoxidase activity is not clear, but it is anticipated to be of importance. Iron deficiency is associated with a reversible reduction of myeloperoxidase[55] and reduced intraleukocytic bacterial killing.[56-58]

The most direct association of phagocytes with an increased incidence of infections in malnutrition is that of defective or delayed killing of phagocytozed organisms.[59-61] This has been known with several organisms including *Candida*[51] a common pathogen in malnourished children. The defective in vitro candidacidal activity of neutrophils from malnourished patients may contribute to the increased susceptibility of these children to *Candida* infections. However, *Candida* infections also frequently occur in patients with impaired cell-mediated immunity,[52] which is also known to be depressed in kwashiorkor, suggesting that multiple immunological factors may be involved.

IMMUNOGLOBULINS AND ANTIBODIES

Nutritional deprivation is usually not associated with a significant change in the proportion or absolute number of B-lymphocytes.[63] Indeed, in occasional patients with prolonged infection, these cells may be slightly increased.[40] The serum concentrations of all immunoglobulin classes are often elevated in malnutrition,[22,24,35,63] and are likely to be the result of frequent and prolonged infections. In some subjects, IgA is increased more than other immunoglobulins, perhaps as a consequence of gastrointestinal and respiratory infections. Serum IgE is also often elevated, particularly in patients with certain parasitic infestations.[64] In addition, concomitant depression of cell-mediated immunity may contribute to the elevated IgE levels, since T-lymphocytes seem to have an inhibitory effect on IgE synthesis.[65] In a few undernourished infants, low levels of IgG and sometimes of IgA and IgM are seen,[24] but many such children have low birth weights and are small for their gestational ages.

There is a paucity of data on the metabolism of immunoglobulins in malnutrition. Preliminary observations suggest that the plasma half-life of IgG is prolonged in individuals with low IgG levels and shortened in those with high IgG levels.[5,6,64] Elevated IgG levels are a common finding in association with infection, and this is also true in malnutrition. For instance, in malnourished individuals without significant infection, the distribution and turnover of γ-globulin are relatively unaffected. However, synthesis is increased and catabolism is slightly diminished when infection supervenes.[66]

Specific serum antibody responses in human malnutrition are variable,[13,64] and may relate to the difficulty of controlling many critical variables such as the extent and type of nutritional deficiency, associated infections, liver function, administration of nutritional supplements, etc. The dose and nature (i.e., live vs. killed) of the antigen and the presence and type of adjuvants are also important. Studies in laboratory animals can be planned to control some of these complicating factors, but the experimental design must ensure that the animal chosen for study does have an obligatory requirement for the nutrient being studied. A reduction in antibody response has been demonstrated in a variety of nutritional deficiencies, including those of protein, calories, thiamine, pyridoxine, cobalamine, pantothenic acid, folate, biotin, ascorbic acid, and vitamins A and D.[1] However, it must be stressed that impaired antibody production is not necessarily synonymous with reduced resistance to infection.

Deprivation of even a single nutrient can reduce an animal's appetite and dietary intake and thereby lead to multiple deficiencies. Antibody response to thymus-dependent antigens such as heterologous red blood cells is markedly reduced by general starvation as well as by the specific lack of individual dietary substances such as pyridoxine, pantothenic acid, lipotropic factors, etc. Maternal nutritional deprivation can also reduce antibody responses in both the first and second generation offspring.[67,68] Data on antibody formation in response to various antigens are summarized in Table 3.

The recognition that mucosal immune responses are largely independent of systemic immunity has led to the concept of locally produced immunoglobulins. IgA present in secretions is a dimer composed of two 7S IgA monomers connected by a joining, or J-,chain and linked to another molecule called secretory-piece (mol. wt. 58,000) that is produced by epithelial cells.[116] In malnourished children the concentration of IgA in nasopharyngeal secretions is significantly depressed relative to the mild decrease in levels of total proteins and albumin.[109,117] Consequently, IgA-antibody response to viral antigens on musocal surfaces is impaired (Figure 4). Indeed, in many malnourished children no secretory-IgA antibody activity can be detected in upper respiratory washings.[109] This reduction in mucosal immune response may contribute to an increased frequency and severity of infections associated with nutritional deficiency. Systemic spread (septicemia) may also occur more easily because of the impaired ability of mucosa to prevent pathogenic organisms from penetrating gastrointestinal and respiratory epithelia. Other antigens seem to also take advantage of this impairment; for instance, protein antigens in the diet get across the gut wall and stimulate the formation of food antibodies.[118] It remains to be established if the incidence of other immunopathologic diseases known to be associated with defective mucosal immunity such as atopy, autoimmunity, and neoplasia are increased in malnourished populations.

The biologic significance of impaired antibody response to some antigens in malnutrition remains unclear. In any event, the variable data on humoral antibody production are not in themselves a sufficient reason to deny or unnecessarily delay a much-needed immunization. This is important because immunization-induced active immunity is one of the principal mechanisms of resistance to infectious diseases (Table 4).

THE COMPLEMENT SYSTEM

The complement system is a complex set of interacting proteins present in the serum in an inactive form which can be activated by a variety of agents such as antibodies, microbial products, and enzymes.[121] There are two major pathways of complement activation: (a) the classical pathway in which C1 serves as the recognition unit, C4, C2, and C3 the activation system, and C5, C6, C7, C8, and C9 the membrane attack unit, and (b) the alternate pathway which bypasses C1, C4, and C2 and is activated by

Table 3
SERUM ANTIBODY RESPONSE IN NUTRITIONAL DEFICIENCY

Antigen	Group[a]	Antibody production[b] Normal	Antibody production[b] Reduced
Bacterial			
Tetanus toxoid	H	24	90,91
Friedlander's bacillus	A		98
Diphtheria toxoid	H		106
	A	87	69,70,71,78
Pneumococcus	H	35	
	A		95
Escherichia coli	A		94
Brucella	H		94
Salmonella	H	90	24,91,104,105,107,112
	A	72,89	73,75,84,94,95,102
Cornybacterium kutscheri	A	82,83	82,83
Pasteurella	H		93
	A		97
Klebsiella	A		102
Viruses			
Poliomyelitis	H	92,109,110	109
Measles	H	109	109
Yellow fever	H		111
Tobacco mosaic	H		103
Influenza	H	86	115
	A	88	79
Hepatitis	H	145	
Western equine encephalomyelitis	A		110
Miscellaneous			
Heterologous red blood cells	H		103
	A	77	67,68,72,74—77,94
Keyhole limpet hemocyanin	H	35	
Tumor antigens	H		
	A		113,114
Rickettsia	A	87	80,101
Ascaris	A		85
Heterologous proteins	A		99

[a] H = human, A = Experimental animals.
[b] Numbers refer to source articles. In some instances, the same reference is given for normal and reduced, since antibody production was affected by deficiency of some nutrients but not by others.

From Chandra, R. K., Chakraburty, S., and Chandra, S., *Indian J. Pediatr.,* Vol. 42, 1976. With permission.

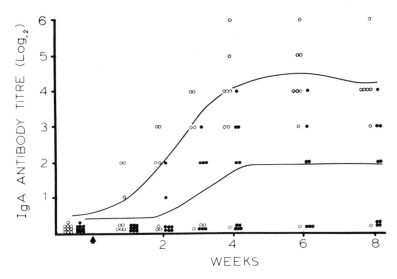

FIGURE 4. Preimmunization and postimmunization measles IgA antibody titers. o: healthy children; o: malnourished children. (From Chandra, R. K., *Br. Med. J.*, 2, 583–585, 1975. With permission.)

Table 4
MECHANISMS OF RESISTANCE TO INFECTIONS

Type	Examples
A. Nonspecific immunity	Phagocytosis, lysozyme, interferon
B. Specifically acquired immunity	

Passive { Natural	Maternally derived IgG in baby
Passive { Induced	Protection by homologous or heterologous antibody or gamma globulin

Active { Natural	Exposure to infection
Active { Induced	Immunization with toxoid, or with killed or attenuated organisms

immunoglobulin aggregates and polysaccharides; this consists of the initiating factors, properdin, C3 proactivator, and C3 proactivator convertase. The two pathways merge with each other at the C3 stage, sharing the membrane attack unit. The end result of the activated complement system may be membrane damage, leading to cell death by lysis. In addition, several molecules involved in the reaction have contributing roles in chemotaxis, blood clotting, anaphylaxis, and other systems that amplify the immune response.

Complement System in Malnutrition

Total hemolytic complement activity and levels of almost all complement components except C4 are reduced in malnourished patients.[122-124] The reduction is more pronounced in those with infection, which contrasts with the raised levels seen in infected well-nourished subjects (Table 5). In many samples, electrophoretically altered complement fractions are detectable, suggesting activation in vivo. There is an inverse correlation between serum C3 concentrations and immunoconglutinin titers (i.e., antibodies to activated C3 and C4), as is also reported in other conditions where complement fixation has been demonstrated.[125] In a significant proportion of malnourished children the

Table 5
HEMOLYTIC COMPLEMENT, C3, AND IMMUNOCONGLUTININ (IK) IN HEALTHY AND MALNOURISHED CHILDREN WITH OR WITHOUT INFECTION

	Well nourished		Undernourished	
	No infection	With infection	No infection	With infection
Number	20	10	23	12
CH_{50} (units/ml)	58 ± 13	105 ± 21	39 ± 15	28 ± 11
C3 (mg/100 ml)	132 ± 18	245 ± 57	89 ± 23	57 ± 19
Altered C3 on IEP[a] (number positive)	0	6	9	5
IK ($-\log_2$) (range)	1	5	3	4
		2—8	1—5	1—8

Note: Mean ± standard deviation are given.

[a] Immunoelectrophoresis.

From Chandra, R. K., *Arch. Dis. Child.*, 50, 225—229, 1975. With permission.

direct antiglobulin (Coombs') test is positive[22] due to the presence of C4 (and occasionally other complement components) and immunoglobulins on the surface of red cells. Nutritional recovery is associated with a return of complement levels and function to normal.

Impaired complement activity in nutritional deficiency is likely to be the consequence of reduced protein synthesis. Some complement proteins are produced by liver and gut cells as well as by lymphocytes, and in malnutrition atrophic changes of the liver, gut, and lymphoid systems are common. In addition, loss of complement proteins may occur through associated protein-losing gastroenteropathy. Another likely factor in the diminution of blood complement levels in PCM is its activation and subsequent consumption by antigen-antibody reactions. Complement activation in vivo is evidenced by the presence of fractions with altered mobility on immunoelectrophoresis, and by raised immunoconglutinin titers. Infection is probably an initiating factor in these reactions. Also, endotoxemia is frequently detected in malnourished children, and endotoxin can activate certain aspects of the complement systems, thus allowing another mechanism for in vivo complement activation.

NONSPECIFIC FACTORS OF RESISTANCE

Humoral immunity includes strictly Ig, antibodies, complement, and specialized cells, but there are other humoral factors that influence immunity and resistance. These are generally classified as nonspecific factors of resistance, and include many substances such as C-reactive protein, lysozyme, beta-lysins, and hormones.[125] Many of these factors are affected by alterations in the status of particular nutrients (Table 6). There is very little information about nonspecific factors in malnutrition, but some attention has focused on the transferrins, iron-binding proteins that reportedly bear a bad prognosis if depressed.[127] It is not altogether clear why depressed serum transferrin values should herald a poor prognosis, but it is thought to be related to their iron-binding capacity.[128-130] Iron is important in the killing of endocytozed bacteria by phagocytes,[56-58,131] and certain bacteria require iron to manifest their pathogenecity.[132] Studies of the general role of iron and transferrins in host resistance are needed, and it would seem to be particularly

Table 6
NONSPECIFIC FACTORS OF RESISTANCE THAT ARE AFFECTED BY ALTERATIONS IN THE STATUS OF PARTICULAR NUTRIENTS

Nonspecific factors	Relevant nutrient	Nutrient status[a]
Anatomic barriers		
Mucosa, connective tissue	Protein	Deficiency
Skin, secretions, etc.	Vitamin A	Deficiency
	Vitamins B_1, B_2, B_6, niacin	Deficiency
	Vitamin C	Deficiency[b]
	Zinc	Deficiency[b]
Achlorhydria	B_{12}	Deficiency
Ventilatory capacity	Vitamin D	Deficiency
	Calories, fat	Excess
Intestinal flora alterations	Protein-calorie	Deficiency
	Vitamin A	Deficiency
	Iron	Excess
Fever (endogenous pyrogens)	Protein-calorie	Deficiency – presumptive
Hormonal response		
Cortisone (stress)[c]	Protein-calorie	Deficiency
Cortisone[c]		
Thyroxin	Iodine	Deficiency
Interferon	Protein	Deficiency – presumptive
	Vitamin A	Deficiency
Lysozyme	Protein	Deficiency – presumptive
	Vitamin A	Deficiency – presumptive
Properdin	Protein	Deficiency – presumptive
	Pantothenic acid	Deficiency
Metal-binding proteins		
Transferrin and lactoferrin	Protein	Deficiency
Albumin	Protein	Deficiency
Ceruloplasm (in infection)	Protein	Deficiency – presumptive
α-2-Macroglobulin	Protein	Deficiency – presumptive

[a] Precedes infection and not as a result of the infection.
[b] Relative deficiency; wound healing improves when normal levels are supplemented.
[c] In kwashiorkor, infection, and marasmus, total levels may be reduced but free cortisol is elevated.

Compiled by Dr. Charlotte Neumann, Department of Pediatrics, UCLA School of Medicine.

useful to know more about transferrins in malnutrition. Indeed, the transferrin-iron relationship may even be important in protecting the human fetus *in utero* because transferrin has been reported in trophoblasts as early as the 6th week of development. This persists throughout gestation and is observed in trophoblasts of term placentae.[133]

The diets of many malnourished persons also lack adequate vitamins, and several vitamins have been shown to be important in mounting an adequate immune response. This topic has been comprehensively reviewed in a W.H.O. monograph.[1] Data on the effect of vitamin deficiency on antibody production were summarized in the earlier section on Immunoglobulins and Antibodies. Pyridoxine deficiency is associated with defective cell-mediated immunity.[134] Regarding nonspecific resistance, chickens fed diets deficient in vitamin A demonstrated a replacement of their normal mucociliated epithelium by keratinized squamous cells,[135] and the multiplication of both Newcastle disease and influenza viruses was much higher in these birds.[136] Iron deficiency may alter epithelial structure, which permits fungal infection to take hold. The consequent antigenic load may contribute to a depression of CMI.[137-139] Selective vitamin deficiencies are less common than multiple deficiencies in malnutrition, but these studies are important in terms of understanding the role of vitamins in basic concepts of the immune response. In this regard, it is interesting that vitamin A can serve an adjuvant-like effect, and its administration in nontoxic doses to well-nourished animals results in an augmentation of humoral immunity as well as a reduction in rejection times of skin grafts.[140]

For many years it has been speculated that breast milk contains nonspecific factors of resistance because breast-fed infants seem to thrive better than bottle-fed babies. For instance, significant levels of resistance to enteric infection is observed among breast-fed babies, even if they are living under very deficient environmental sanitation.[141] Mechanisms for this resistance are poorly understood, though one appears to be rendered by certain indigenous microflora which form a protective barrier against pathogenic organisms. Breast-fed infants develop a predominant flora of Gram-positive anaerobic bacilli (*Bifidobacterium*), probably as a result of the combined action of bifidus factor(s), lysozyme, secretory IgA, other antibodies, and macrophages and lymphocytes present in human milk.[142] Bifidobacteria synthetize considerable amounts of acetic and lactic acids. Lysozyme and immunoglobulins are thought to exert a suppressing and/or lytic effect on Gram-negative facultative bacilli (enterobacteriaceae). These actions result in a milieu unfavorable for *Shigella* and other enteropathogenic agents.[143] As a consequence, incidence of infection among small infants in highly contaminated environments is low if infants are breast-fed. The progressive weaning and concomitant decrease in natural resistance may account for increasing rates of infection and infectious disease as weaning progresses.

FETAL MALNUTRITION

Infants with low birth weight (LBW) who are small for gestational age (SGA) represent the fetal form of malnutrition (FM). Several factors are known to contribute to intrauterine growth retardation, including maternal variables such as short stature, hypertension, metabolic illnesses, parity greater than four, age over 35 years, previous induced abortions, uterine anomalies, toxemia, infections, chronic illness, and "stress."[144] Fetal factors such as malformations, multiple pregnancy, and infections, and placental factors such as the "insufficiency" syndromes are also important. In addition, the health-socioeconomic background of the mother, including factors such as low social class, inadequate prenatal care, ethnic group, high altitude, drug abuse, and smoking, plays a significant role.

Intrauterine infections significantly affect the morbidity and mortality of low-birth-weight infants. The etiologic agent in these instances may be of low virulence, and systemic spread with poor localization is common. Several aspects of immunocompetence are impaired in such infants,[145,146] and diminished host defenses may be severe and long lasting.[5,6,39,147] Cell-mediated immunity as measured either by delayed hypersensitivity reactions in the skin or by lymphocyte responses to in vitro stimulation are usually depressed. In addition, quantitative measurements of T-lymphocytes in the blood reveal that they are reduced in number.[5,6,34,39,147] Hypoimmunoglobulinemia, especially involving IgG, is frequent and pronounced (Figure 5). The maternofetal transfer of IgG is reduced, IgG$_1$ transport being affected to a greater extent than that of IgG$_2$.[148] The blood concentration of the third component of complement is low, the opsonic function of plasma is reduced, and the bacterial killing by polymorphonuclear leucocytes is slightly impaired.[145] It is suspected that these functional defects in the host resistance of LBW-SGA infants can persist in extrauterine life for several months.[5,6,39,147] These children often sustain repeated infections, and clinically they tend to resemble children with immunodeficiency diseases.

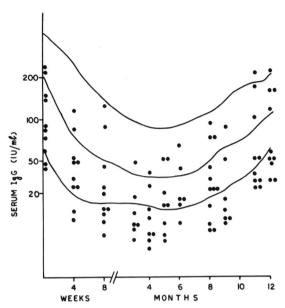

FIGURE 5. Longitudinal follow-up of serum IgG levels in ten infants with fetal growth retardation, plotted on mean and range of values for healthy children. (From Chandra, R. K., *Am. J. Dis. Child.*, 129, 450–455, 1975. Copyright 1975, American Medical Association.)

CLOSING COMMENTS

This review of resistance to infection in undernutrition has attempted to bring together several of the known mechanisms of host defense, and has obviously been biased towards immunological considerations. One reason for this emphasis is that the immune system has been clearly established as one of the principal bulwarks of host defense,[18] not only to infection but also to cancer, transplants, and other special circumstances such as blood transfusions, pregnancy, and aging. However, this is not to be interpreted as being either the only or the most important aspect of lowered resistance in malnutrition, for the roles of hormones,[31] trace elements,[149] and nonspecific factors[126] might be equally as important. Studies of malnourished populations are greatly complicated by uncontrollable variables such as concommitant infections, regional diets and customs, weather, altitude, and lack of appropriate genetic data. Some of these aspects can be controlled in studies of animal models, and this approach continues to add valuable information about basic immunological aspects that are altered by nutritional manipulations.[113,114]

One encouraging observation made in studies of human populations is that some of the immune defects seem to rapidly return to normal following dietary therapy,[33,150,151] suggesting that the immune lesions may not be irreversible. This also has implications for mass vaccine administrations and other public health programs that deal with infectious diseases among malnourished populations. However, these observations must be tempered with other reports of prolonged suppression of immunoglobulin production in man[152] and of T-lymphocytes in low-birth-weight infants,[5,6,39,147] and with animal studies that show immunological depressions in the progeny of malnourished parents.[67,68] Long-term follow-up studies of immunological responses are badly needed in nutritionally supplemented human populations that have sustained various degrees of malnutrition, as well as in children who have been diagnosed as having intrauterine malnutrition.

The clinical and biochemical profiles of malnourished children are extraordinarily complex, and it is unwise to make generalities about their capacities to resist infections. However, several years ago children with immunodeficiency diseases were an equally heterogeneous and baffling lot. Research on these diseases has developed a systematic approach to diagnosis and treatment based on the pathophysiology of each deficiency, and this has led to improved prognoses in many immunodeficiency diseases.[153] As research broadens current understanding of the immune response in malnutrition, it seems to be increasingly possible to think of the immune defects in undernutrition as being analogous to those in immunodeficiency diseases, and it has been suggested that malnourished children might be considered as having a type of secondary or acquired immunodeficiency disease.[5,6,154,155] This approach is useful in establishing a more intelligent understanding of patterns of host resistance in malnourished children as well as in helping to build new concepts in the treatment and prevention of infections in malnourished populations.[156] Immunology has a great deal to offer the science of nutrition, and it would seem that the combined approaches of nutrition, public health, and immunology may have something of value to offer the malnourished child.

REFERENCES

1. Scrimshaw, N. S., Taylor, C. E., and Gordon, J. E., *WHO Monogr. Ser.*, No. 57, 1968.
2. Faulk, W. P., in *Medicine*, 2nd Ser., Infectious Diseases, Vol. 1, Smith, H. and Ronald, P. D., Eds., Medical Education International, London, 1976.
3. Chandra, R. K., in *Manual of Pediatrics*, Prasad, L. S. N. and Robinson, P., Eds., Orient Longmans, Bombay, 1976.
4. Awdeh, Z., Bengoa, J., Demaeyer, E., Dixon, H., Edsall, G., Faulk, W. P., Goodman, H. C., Hopwood, B. E. C., Jose, D., Keller, W., Kumate, J., Mata, J., McGregor, I., Miescher, P., Rowe, D., Taylor, C., and Torrigiani, G., *Bull. WHO*, 26, 537–546, 1972.
5. Chandra, R. K., *World Rev. Nutr. Diet.*, 25, 166–188, 1976.
6. Chandra, R. K., in *Food and Immunology*, Hambreaus, L., Ed., Almquist and Wiksell International, Stockholm, 1976.
7. Faulk, W. P., DeMaeyer, E., and Davies, A. J. S., *Am. J. Clin. Nutr.*, 27, 638–646, 1974.
8. McGregor, I. A., Rahman, A. K., and Thomson, A. M., *Trans. R. Soc. Trop. Med. Hyg.*, 64, 48–77, 1970.
9. Beisel, W. R., *Am. J. Clin. Nutr.*, 25, 1254–1259, 1972.
10. Faulk, W. P. and Greenwood, B. M., in *Medical Immunology*, Holborow, E. J. and Reeves, G., Eds., Academic Press, New York, 1976.
11. Faulk, W. P., in *Immunodeficiency in Man and Animals*, Bergsma, D., Ed., Sinauer Associates, Sunderland, Mass., 1975.
12. Faulk, W. P., Mata, L. J., and Edsall, G., *Trop. Dis. Bull.*, 72, 89–102, 1975.
13. Chandra, R. K., in *Progress in Immunology II*, Vol. 4, Brent, L. and Holborow, J., Eds., North Holland/American Elsevier, Amsterdam, 1974, 355–358.
14. Chandra, R. K., in *Proc. X Int. Congr. Nutr.*, Kyoto, in press, 1976.
15. Suskind, R. M., Ed., *Malnutrition and the Immune Response*, Raven Press, New York, 1976.
16. Douglas, S. D. and Schopfer, K., *Clin. Immunol. Immunopathol.*, in press.
17. Roitt, I. M., Greaves, M. F., Torrigiani, G., Brostoff, J., and Playfair, J. H. L., *Lancet*, ii, 367–371, 1969.
18. Good, R. A., Finstad, J., and Gatti, R. A., in *Infectious Agents and Host Resistance*, Mudd, S., Ed., W. B. Saunders, Philadelphia, 1970, 76–114.
19. Chandra, R. K., in *Text Book of Pediatrics*, Udani, P. M., Ed., Orient Longmans, Bombay, 1976.
20. Faulk, W. P. and Hijmans, W., *Prog. Allergy*, 16, 9–36, 1972.
21. Watts, T., *J. Trop. Pediatr.*, 15, 155–158, 1969.
22. Smythe, P. M., Brereton-Stiles, G. G., Grace, H. G., Mafoyane, A., Schonland, M., Coovadia, H. M., Loening, W. E. K., Parent, M. A., and Vos, G. H., *Lancet*, ii, 939–943, 1971.

23. Schonland, M., *J. Trop. Pediatr.*, 18, 217–224, 1972.
24. Chandra, R. K., *J. Pediatr.*, 81, 1194–1200, 1972.
25. Rosen, E. V., Geefhuysen, J., Anderson, R. K., Joffe, J., and Rabson, A. R., *Arch. Dis. Child.*, 50, 220–225, 1975.
26. Chandra, R. K., Sharma, S., and Bhujwala, R. A., *Indian J. Med. Res.*, 61, 93–97, 1973.
27. Bhuyan, U. N. and Ramalingaswami, V., *Am. J. Pathol.*, 75, 315–326, 1974.
28. Faulk, W. P., Pinto-Paes, R., and Marigo, C., *Br. J. Nutr.*, in press, 1976.
29. Krishnan, S., Ghuyan, U. N., Talwar, G. P., and Ramalingaswami, V., *Immunology*, 27, 383–392, 1974.
30. Rao, K. S. S., Srikantia, S. G., and Gopalan, C., *Arch. Dis. Child.*, 43, 365–367, 1968.
31. Gardner, L. I. and Amacher, P., Eds., *Endocrine Aspects of Malnutrition*, Kroc Foundation, Santa Ynez, Calif., 1973.
32. Bang, F. B. and Bang, D. G., *J. Nepal Med. Assoc.*, 11, 43–49, 1973.
33. Chandra, R. K., *Br. Med. J.*, 3, 608–609, 1974.
34. Ferguson, A. C., Lawlor, G. C., Jr., Neumann, C. G., Oh, W., and Stiehm, E. R., *J. Pediatr.*, 85, 717–723, 1974.
35. Neumann, C. G., Lawlor, G. C., Stiehm, E. R., Swedseid, M. E., Newton, C., Herbert, J., Ammann, A. J., and Jacob, M., *Am. J. Clin. Nutr.*, 28, 89–99, 1975.
36. Grace, H. J., Armstrong, D., and Smythe, P. M., *S. Afr. Med. J.*, 46, 402–403, 1972.
37. Sellmeyer, E., Bhettay, E., Truswell, A. S., Meyers, O. L., and Hansen, J. D. L., *Arch. Dis. Child.*, 47, 429–435, 1972.
38. Moore, D. L., Heyworth, B., and Brown, J., *Clin. Exp. Immunol.*, 17, 647–656, 1974.
39. Chandra, R. K., in *Malnutrition and the Immune Response*, Suskind, R. M., Ed., Raven Press, New York, in press, 1976.
40. Chandra, R. K., in preparation.
41. Harland, P. S. E. G., *Lancet*, ii, 719–721, 1965.
42. Edelman, R., Suskind, R., Olson, R. E., and Sirisinha, S., *Lancet*, i, 506–509, 1973.
43. Bistrian, B. R., Blackburn, G. L., Scrimshaw, N. S., and Flatt, J. P., *Am. J. Clin. Nutr.*, 28, 1148–1155, 1975.
44. Vasantha, L., Srikantia, S. G., and Gopalan, C., *Am. J. Clin. Nutr.*, 23, 78–82, 1970.
45. Mims, C. A., in *Microbial Pathogenecity in Man and Animals*, Smith, H. and Pearce, J. H., Eds., Cambridge University Press, Cambridge, 1972, 333–358.
46. Abbassy, A. S., Badr El-din, M. K., and Hassan, A. I., *J. Trop. Med. Hyg.*, 77, 18–21, 1974.
47. Douglas, S. D., *Blood*, 35, 851–866, 1970.
48. Stossel, T., *New Engl. J. Med.*, 290, 717–723, 1974.
49. Douglas, S. D., *Br. J. Haematol.*, 21, 493–496, 1971.
50. Chandra, R. K., Chandra, S., and Ghai, O. P., *J. Clin. Pathol.*, 29, 224–227, 1976.
51. Schopfer, K. and Douglas, S. D., in preparation, 1976.
52. Selvaraj, R. J. and Bhat, K. S., *Biochem. J.*, 127, 255–259, 1972.
53. Klebanoff, S. J. and Green, W. L., *J. Clin. Invest.*, 52, 60–72, 1973.
54. Avila, J. L., Valazquez-Avila, G., Correa, C., Castillo, C., and Convit, J., *Clin. Chim. Acta*, 19, 5–10, 1973.
55. Higashi, O., Sato, Y., Takamatsu, H., and Oyama, M., *Tohoku J. Exp. Med.*, 93, 105–109, 1967.
56. Chandra, R. K., *Arch. Dis. Child.*, 48, 864–866, 1973.
57. Chandra, R. K., *J. Pediatr.*, 86, 899–902, 1975.
58. MacDougall, L. G., Anderson, R., McNab, G. M., and Katz, J., *J. Pediatr.*, 86, 833–843, 1975.
59. Seth, V. and Chandra, R. K., *Arch. Dis. Child.*, 47, 282–284, 1972.
60. Selvaraj, R. J. and Bhat, K. S., *Am. J. Clin. Nutr.*, 25, 166–174, 1972.
61. Douglas, S. D. and Schopfer, K., *Clin. Exp. Immunol.*, 17, 121–128, 1974.
62. Kirkpatrick, C. H., Rich, R. R., and Bennett, J. E., *Ann. Intern. Med.*, 74, 955–978, 1971.
63. Mata, L. J. and Faulk, W. P., *Arch. Latinoam. Nutr.*, 23, 345–362, 1973.
64. Chandra, R. K., in *Malnutrition and the Immune Response*, Suskind, R. M., Ed., Raven Press, New York, in press, 1976.
65. Kikkawa, V., Kamimura, K., Hamajima, T., Sekiguchi, T., Kawai, T., Takenaka, M., and Tada, T., *Pediatrics*, 51, 690–694, 1973.
66. Chen, S. and Hansen, J. D. L., *Clin. Sci.*, 23, 351–359, 1962.
67. Gebhardt, D. M. and Newberne, P. M., *Immunology*, 26, 489–495, 1974.
68. Chandra, R. K., *Science*, 190, 289–290, 1975.
69. Arkwright, J. A. and Zilva, S. S., *J. Pathol. Bacteriol.*, 27, 346–351, 1924.
70. Bieling, R., *Z. Hyg. Infektionskr.*, 104, 518–521, 1925.
71. King, C. G. and Menten, M. L., *J. Nutr.*, 10, 129–137, 1935.

72. Greene, M. R., *Am. J. Hyg.,* 17, 60–64, 1933.
73. Blackberg, S. N., *Proc. Soc. Exp. Biol. N.Y.,* 25, 770–772, 1928.
74. Stoerk, H. C., Eisen, H. N., and John, H. M., *J. Exp. Med.,* 85, 365–371, 1947.
75. Agnew, L. R. C. and Cook, R., *Br. J. Nutr.,* 2, 321–326, 1954.
76. Axelrod, A. E., Carter, B. B., McCoy, R. H., and Geisinger, R., *Proc. Soc. Exp. Biol. N.Y.,* 66, 137–139, 1947.
77. Axelrod, A. E., *Am. J. Clin. Nutr.,* 6, 119–124, 1958.
78. Axelrod, A. E. and Pruzansky, J., *Ann. N.Y. Acad. Sci.,* 63, 202–207, 1955.
79. Axelrod, A. E. and Hopper, S., *J. Nutr.,* 72, 325–330, 1960.
80. Wertman, K. and Sarandria, J. L., *Proc. Soc. Exp. Biol. N.Y.,* 76, 388–391, 1951.
81. Zucker, T. F. and Zucker, L. M., *Proc. Soc. Exp. Biol. N.Y.,* 85, 517–520, 1954.
82. Zucker, T. F., Zucker, L. M., and Seronde, J., Jr., *J. Nutr.,* 59, 299–303, 1956.
83. Seronde, J., Jr., Zucker, T. F., and Zucker, L. M., *J. Nutr.,* 59, 287–291, 1956.
84. Panda, B. and Combs, G. F., *Proc. Soc. Exp. Biol. N.Y.,* 113, 530–536, 1963.
85. Leutskaja, Z. K., *Dokl. Akad. Nauk SSSR,* 159, 938–942, 1964.
86. Feller, A. E., Roberts, L. B., Ralli, E. P., and Francis, T., Jr., *J. Clin. Invest.,* 21, 121–128, 1942.
87. Klimentova, A. A. and Frajazinova, I. B., *Z. Mikrobiol. Moskow,* 42, 96–103, 1965.
88. Underdahl, N. R. and Young, G. A., *Virology,* 2, 415–421, 1956.
89. Harmon, B. G., Miller, E. R., Hoefer, J. A., Ullrey, D. E., and Luecke, R. W., *J. Nutr.,* 79, 263–268, 1963.
90. Hodges, R. E., Bean, W. B., Ohlson, M. A., and Bleiler, R. E., *Am. J. Clin. Nutr.,* 11, 85–91, 1962.
91. Hodges, R. E., Bean, W. B., Ohlson, M. A., and Bleiler, R. E., *Am. J. Clin. Nutr.,* 11, 180–186, 1962.
92. Hodges, R. E., Bean, W. B., Ohlson, M. A., and Bleiler, R. E., *Am. J. Clin. Nutr.,* 11, 180–186, 1962.
93. Morey, G. R. and Spies, T. D., *Proc. Soc. Exp. Biol. N.Y.,* 49, 519–523, 1942.
94. Orr, J. B., MacLeod, J. J. R., and Mackie, T. J., *Lancet,* i, 1177–1179, 1931.
95. Cannon, P. R., Chase, W. E., and Wissler, R. W., *J. Immunol.,* 47, 133–36, 1943.
96. Wissler, R. W., Woolridge, R. L., and Steffe, C. H. J., *J. Immunol.,* 52, 267–270, 1946.
97. Berry, L. J., Davis, J., and Spies, T. D., *J. Lab. Clin. Med.,* 30, 684–688, 1945.
98. Benditt, E. P., Wissler, R. W., Woolridge, R. L., Rowley, D. A., and Steffee, C. H., *Proc. Soc. Exp. Biol. N.Y.,* 70, 240–243, 1949.
99. Gemeroy, D. G. and Koffler, A. H., *J. Nutr.,* 39, 299–303, 1949.
100. Ruckman, I., *J. Immunol.,* 53, 51–56, 1946.
101. Klimentova, A. A. and Frjazinova, I. B., in *Voprosy Infekcionnoj Patologii i Immunologii,* Zdrodovskij, P. F., Ed., Soviet Academy of Medical Sciences, Moscow, 1963.
102. Wissler, R. W., Fitch, F. W., LaVia, M. F., and Gunderson, C. H., *J. Cell Comp. Physiol.,* 50, 265–269, 1957.
103. Gell, P. G. H., *Proc. R. Soc. Med.,* 41, 323–325, 1948.
104. Wohl, M. G., Reinhold, J. G., and Rose, S. B., *Arch. Intern. Med.,* 83, 402–405, 1949.
105. Budiansky, E. and da Silva, N. N., *Hospital (Rio de Janeiro),* 52, 251–256, 1957.
106. Olarte, J., Cravioto, J., and Campos, B., *Biol. Med. Hosp. Infant. Mex.,* 13, 467–471, 1956.
107. Reddy, V. and Srikantia, S. G., *Indian J. Med. Res.,* 52, 1154–1158, 1964.
108. Chandra, R. K., *Am. J. Dis. Child.,* 129, 450–455, 1975.
109. Chandra, R. K., *Br. Med. J.,* 2, 583–585, 1975.
110. Brown, R. E. and Katz, M., *Trop. Geogr. Med.,* 18, 125–128, 1966.
111. Brown, R. E. and Katz, M., *Trop. Geogr. Med.,* 18, 129–133, 1966.
112. Hodges, R. E., Bean, W. B., Ohlson, M. A., and Bleiler, R. E., *Am. J. Clin. Nutr.,* 10, 500–505, 1962.
113. Jose, D. G. and Good, R. A., *Cancer Res.,* 33, 807–809, 1973.
114. Jose, D. G. and Good, R. A., *J. Exp. Med.,* 137, 1–11, 1973.
115. Jose, D. G., Welch, J. S., and Doherty, R. L., *Aust. Paediatr. J.,* 6, 192–203, 1970.
116. Hanson, L. A. and Brandtzaeg, P., in *Immunologic Disorders in Infants and Children,* Stiehm, E. R. and Fulginiti, V. A., Eds., W. B. Saunders, Philadelphia, 107–126.
117. Sirisinha, S., Suskind, S., Edelman, R., Asuapaka, C., and Olson, R. E., *Pediatrics,* 55, 116–170, 1975.
118. Chandra, R. K., *Arch. Dis. Child.,* 50, 532, 1975.
119. Bergsma, D., Ed., *Immunologic Deficiency Diseases in Man,* National Foundation, New York, 1968.
120. Chandra, R. K., Kaveramma, B., and Soothill, J. F., *Lancet,* I, 687–689, 1969.

121. Muller-Eberhard, H. J., in *Progress in Immunology II,* Vol. 1, Brent, L. and Holborow, J., Eds., North Holland/American Elsevier, Amsterdam, 1974, 173–182.
122. Sirisinha, S., Suskind, R., Edelman, R., Charupatana, C., and Olson, R. E., *Lancet,* i, 1016–1019, 1973.
123. Chandra, R. K., *Arch. Dis. Child.,* 50, 225, 1975.
124. Chandra, R. K., in *Malnutrition and the Immune Response,* Suskind, R. M., Ed., Raven Press, New York, in press, 1976.
125. Ngu, J. and Soothill, J. F., *Clin. Exp. Immunol.,* 5, 557–563, 1969.
126. Braun, W. and Ungar, J., Eds., *Nonspecific Factors Influencing Host Resistance,* Karger, Basel, 1973.
127. Antia, A. U., McFarlane, H., and Soothill, J. F., *Arch. Dis. Child.,* 43, 459–462, 1968.
128. Weinberg, E. D., *JAMA,* 231, 39–41, 1975.
129. Bullen, J. J., Rogers, H., and Leigh, L., *Br. Med. J.,* 1, 69–72, 1972.
130. Elin, R. J. and Wolff, S. M., *J. Immunol.,* 112, 737–742, 1974.
131. Arbeter, A., Echeverri, L., Franco, D., Munson, D., Velez, H., and Vitale, J. J., *Fed. Proc.,* 30, 1421–1428, 1971.
132. Editorial, *Iron and Resistance to Infection,* Lancet, i, 325–326, 1974.
133. Faulk, W. P. and Johnson, P. M., to be published.
134. Axelrod, A. E., *Am. J. Clin. Nutr.,* 24, 265–276, 1971.
135. Bang, F. B. and Bang, D. G., *Proc. Soc. Exp. Biol. N.Y.,* 132, 50, 1969.
136. Bang, F. B. and Foard, M. A., *Johns Hopkins Med. J.,* 129, 100–108, 1971.
137. Higgs, J. M. and Wells, R. S., *Br. J. Dermatol.,* 86, 88–94, 1972.
138. Fletcher, J., Mather, J., Lewis. M. J., and Whiting, G., *J. Infect. Dis.,* 131, 44–50, 1975.
139. Chandra, R. K., *Nutr. Rev.,* 34, 129–132, 1976.
140. Jorin, M. and Tannock, I. F., *Immunology,* 23, 283–287, 1972.
141. Mata, L. J. and Wyatt, R. G., *Am. J. Clin. Nutr.,* 24, 976–986, 1971.
142. Goldman, A. S. and Smith, C. W., *J. Pediatr.,* 82, 1082–1090, 1973.
143. Mata, L. J. and Urrutia, J. J., *Ann. N. Y. Acad. Sci.,* 176, 93–109, 1971.
144. Sinclair, J. C. in *Pediatrics,* Barnett, H. L. and Einhorn, A. H., Eds., Appleton-Century-Crofts, New York, 1972, 88–116.
145. Chandra, R. K., unpublished data.
146. Chandra, R. K., *Lancet,* ii, 1393–1394, 1974.
147. Chandra, R. K., Ali, S. K., Chandra, S., and Kutty, K. M., *Biol. Neonat.,* in press, 1976.
148. Chandra, R. K., in *Maternofoetal Transmission of Immunoglobulins,* Hemmings, W. A., Ed., Cambridge University Press, New York, 1975, 77–90.
149. Smith, J. C., Jr., McDaniel, E. G., Fan, F. F., and Halsted, J. A., *Science,* 181, 954–955, 1973.
150. Mathews, J. D., Whittingham, S., Mackay, I. R., and Malcolm, L., *Lancet,* ii, 675–678, 1972.
151. Ziegler, H. D. and Ziegler, P. B., *Johns Hopkins Med. J.,* 137, 59–64, 1975.
152. Aref, G. H., Badr El-Din, M. K., Hassau, A. I., and Braby, I. I., *J. Trop. Med. Hyg.,* 73, 186–189, 1970.
153. Cooper, M. D., Faulk, W. P., Fudenberg, H. H., Good, R. A., Hitzig, W., Kunkel, H. G., Rosen, F. S., Seligann, M., Soothill, J., and Wedgewood, R. J., *Clin. Immunol. Immunopathol.,* 2, 416–445, 1974.
154. Faulk, W. P., *Nature,* 250, 283–284, 1974.
155. Good, R. A. and Jose, D., in *Immunodeficiency in man and animals,* Bergsma, D., Ed., *Birth Defects Orig. Artic. Ser.,* 10 (1), 219–222, 1975.
156. Douglas, S. D. and Faulk, W. P., *Advances in Clinical Immunology,* Churchill Livingston, London, Vol. 1, in press, 1976.

INDEX

general, effects on populations, I: 113
gonadotropin content affected by, I: 409
height/intelligence correlation in effects, I: 344
immune reactions in, II: 555
lymphoid organs affected by, II: 558
postnatal, effects of, I: 340
prenatal, effects of, I: 323, 339
protein energy, endocrine secretion changes
    resulting from, II: 163—166
reproduction, effects on, 397
Mammary cancer, see also Carcinogenesis
diet relationships, I: 155—157
Mammary glands
metabolism, I: 446
structure, I: 439, 444
Manganese
actions on differentiation, I: 65
behavioral disturbances associated with
    elevated intake, II: 505
cadmium metabolism affected by, II: 342
cadmium-produced anemia reduced by, II: 329
cancer relationship, I: 160
deficiency
    behavioral effects, II: 505
    effect on bone formation, I: 240
    prenatal effects, I: 130, 335
    reproduction affected by, I: 419
egg production requirements, I: 505
role in fertility, I: 429
role in fetal development, I: 420
role in synthesis of glycosaminoglycans, I: 241
Marasmus
bone abnormalities in, I: 219
conditions associated with, I: 345
endocrine changes associated with, II: 163—166
incidence associated with decline of breast
    feeding, I: 498
motor nerve effects in, I: 338
overhydration in, II: 165
protein energy malnutrition causing, II: 163
Marrow
leukocyte production, II: 19, 558
protein malnutrition, effect of, I: 108
starvation affecting, II: 29
Maternal nutrition, effect on fetal development,
    see Fetal development
Mental retardation
amino acid excess associated with, I: 333
congenital galactosemia associated with, I: 117
folic acid deficiency associated with, I: 332
low birth weight associated wit, I: 339
maternal phenylketonuria associated with, I:
    116
Mercury
effect on cadmium in tissue, II: 329
toxicity and metabolism, II: 337, 344, 373
Metabolism
maintenance, I: 386
of drugs, see Drugs
work effects, II: 399
Metals, see also particular metals
interaction with dietary components, II: 325

Metamorphosis
amino acids affecting, I: 20, 22, 23, 25, 26, 83
amphibian, nutrition affecting, I: 81
arsenic affecting, I: 52
carbohydrates affecting, I: 81
copper affecting, I: 63, 64
fatty acids affecting, I: 35, 82
food intake affecting, I: 7, 11, 12, 14
iodine affecting, I: 53
lipids affecting, I: 81
proteins affecting, I: 83
vitamins affecting, I: 29, 30, 33, 50, 84—87
Methionine, role in wound healing, I: 259
Microcephaly
maternal phenylketonuria associated with, I:
    116
maternal vitamin A deficiency associated with,
    I: 119
Milk
composition, I: 439, 443, 497
consumption, relationship to colon cancer, I:
    152
fat, absorption and retention, II: 150, 151
human
    composition and volume, I: 496
    disease resistance associated with feeding, II:
    566
    nutritional requirements, I: 495
lactose content, I: 497
milk-fat composition, dietary fat affecting, I:
    442, 467—483
milk-fat content, changes in on change of diet,
    I: 441, 453—459
milk-lactose content, variations in, I: 442, 461
milk-protein content, changes in on change of
    diet, I: 442, 460—466
mineral content, I: 497
nitrogen absorption by infants, II: 135, 136
protein, digestion, postnatal changes in, II: 156
secretion, diet affecting, I: 440
sow's milk, nutrition affecting, I: 443,
    484—491
synthesis, I: 439
yield
    carbohydrate feed change affecting, I: 440,
    446—452
    dietary fat affecting, I: 442, 467—483
    protein deficiency affecting, I: 442, 462—466
Mineralization, see Bone formation
Miscarriage, incidence during food shortage, I:
    113
Mitochondria
DNA synthesis, food deprivation affecting, I:
    99
effect on associated with myopathic muscle, I:
    277, 278
of adrenal cortex, thiamin deficiency affecting,
    I: 37
of liver, degeneration in vitamin E deficiency,
    I: 33
Molybdenum
deficiency, hematopoiesis affected by, II: 13

W

Z